Cartilage Repair and Joint Preservation of the Knee

Second Edition

Edited by

Tom Minas, MD, MS

Professor Emeritus
Harvard Medical School
Cambridge, Massachusetts
Director, Cartilage Repair Center
Paley Orthopedic & Spine Institute
West Palm Beach, Florida

ELSEVIER

Elsevier
1600 John F. Kennedy Blvd.
Ste 1800
Philadelphia, PA 19103-2899

CARTILAGE REPAIR AND JOINT PRESERVATION OF THE KNEE,
SECOND EDITION ISBN: 978-0-323-69808-5

Library of Congress Cataloging-in-Publication: 2021946510

Senior Content Strategist: Belinda Kuhn
Senior Content Development Specialists: Laura Klein/Denise Roslonski
Content Development Manager: Laurie Gower
Publishing Services Manager: Shereen Jameel
Senior Project Manager: Umarani Natarajan
Designer: Brian Salisbury

Printed in the United States of America

Last digit is the print number: 9 8 7 6 5 4 3 2 1

Contributors

Luca Andriolo, MD
Clinica Ortopedica e Traumatologica 2
Applied and Translational Research (ATR) Center
IRCCS Istituto Ortopedico
Rizzoli Orthopaedic Institute
Bologna, Italy

Angelo Boffa, MD
Clinica Ortopedica e Traumatologica 2
IRCCS Istituto Ortopedico
Rizzoli Orthopaedic Institute
Bologna, Italy

Alessandro DiMartino, MD
Clinica Ortopedica e Traumatologica 2
Applied and Translational Research (ATR) Center
IRCCS Istituto Ortopedico
Rizzoli Orthopaedic Institute
Bologna, Italy

Giuseppe Filardo, MD, Ph
Applied and Translational Research (ATR) Center
Rizzoli Orthopaedic Institute
Bologna, Italy
Orthopaedic and Traumatology Unit, Ospedale Regionale di Lugano, EOC
USI-Università della Svizzera Italiana, Facoltà di Scienze Biomediche
Lugano, Switzerland

Lisa A. Fortier, DVM, PhD
James Law Professor of Large Animal Surgery
Clinical Sciences
Cornell University College of Veterinary Medicine
Ithaca, New York

Andreas H. Gomoll, MD
Associate Professor of Orthopedic Surgery
Hospital for Special Surgery
New York, New York

John G. Kennedy, MD, FRCS
Department of Orthopedic Surgery
New York University Langone
New York, New York

Brendan Maloney, BS
Research Assistant, Clinical Sciences
Cornell University
Ithaca, New York

Tom Minas, MD, MS
Professor Emeritus, Orthopedics
Harvard Medical School
Cambridge, Massachusetts
Director, Cartilage Repair Center
Paley Orthopedic & Spine Institute
West Palm Beach, Florida

Bridgette Nixon, BS
Research Assistant, Clinical Sciences
Cornell University
Ithaca, New York

Takahiro Ogura, MD
Sports Medicine and Joint Center
Funabashi Orthopaedic Hospital
Chiba, Japan

Dedication

I would like to dedicate the second edition of this book to Lars Peterson, MD, PhD, Gothenburg, Sweden. The reality of joint preservation in young adults with articular cartilage injuries has only become possible because of his vision and courage to persevere with the premise that cultured articular chondrocytes may affect repair. He translated a hypothesis to a preclinical rabbit model in 1982 and then to clinical application in 1987. Thirty-four years later, the majority of his patients continue to do well.

He is a pioneer in the field of orthopedics. I thank him and his co-workers, Anders Lindahl, MD, PhD, and Matts Brittberg, MD, PhD, for allowing me to be a part of their team. Lars has been a mentor and a great friend over the years as we have tried to promote the field of cartilage repair around the world together. Working with him and knowing him has been a true honor and privilege for me.

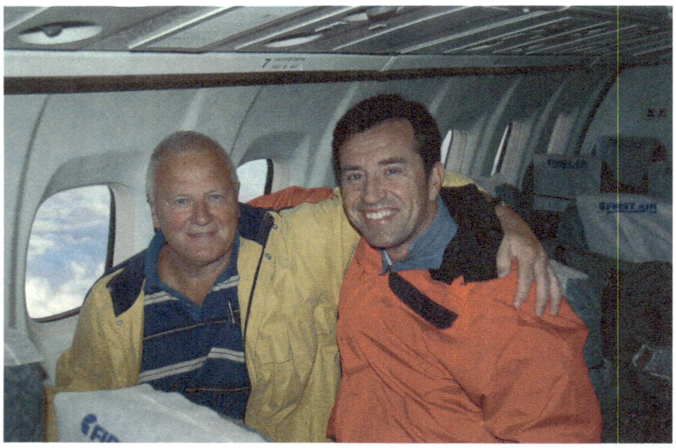

Lars Peterson, MD, PhD, and author Tom Minas, MD, MS, on their way to Great Slave Lake, Northwest Territories, Canada, 2005.

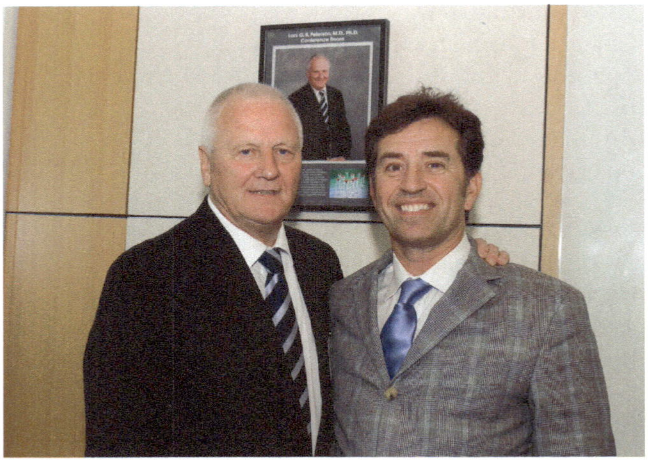

Lars Peterson, MD, PhD, and author Tom Minas, MD, MS, at the dedication of the Lars Peterson Library in Cambridge, Massachusetts in 2009.

Special Thanks

I would like to thank all the readers of my first edition who encouraged me to update my book with the field of cartilage repair and techniques that I have modified to write a second edition.

Certainly, my children Krista and Lucas remember well when I wrote my first edition taking time away from them when they were children every Saturday for 3 years. They have always been very encouraging and clearly the light of my life. They are now in college, and just laughed, but remained very encouraging when I told them I would do a second edition. Thank you both!

Finally, I would like to thank my parents, Mary and Angelo Minas for their unconditional love and support throughout my life. They have been role models for me with their dedication to both career and family.

Introduction

While I was at the Brigham and Women's Hospital, Harvard Medical School (1988–2018), my residents and fellows asked me to write a syllabus for them on the newly developing field of cartilage repair in the 1990s and 2000s. The first edition of this book was the result. It has since been useful for residents, fellows, and experienced surgeons. That continues to be my intent, and I hope that you enjoy the book.

I performed the first periosteal autologous chondrocyte implant (ACI) procedure in the United States 26 years ago. Early on I worked with Lars Peterson to develop specialized techniques combining previous principles of internal fixation, osteotomy, ligamentous and meniscal surgical repairs and transplants in combination with ACI to obtain excellent joint-preserving clinical outcomes by managing what we collectively called "Background Factors" (predisposing factors) when doing cartilage repair.

Since then, a careful prospectively gathered database has proven through peer-reviewed articles that this was the right approach. The clinical outcomes are excellent and durable. This second edition reviews the progression from periosteal ACI (p-ACI) to collagen ACI (c-ACI) and then matrix ACI (MACI). In addition, two new chapters have been added to review the usefulness of biologics such as platelet-rich plasma (PRP), bone marrow aspirate concentrate (BMAC), stem cells and others in treating cartilage injuries and early osteoarthritis. We have also added several videos that demonstrate the surgical techniques visually which includes my commentary.

Acknowledgments

My career has been influenced by many people. James Waddell, MD, and Robin Sullivan, MD (deceased), who inspired me to be an orthopedist. Martin Tile, MD, a great mentor and friend who guided me in critical thinking in the principles of internal fixation. Robert Salter, MD (deceased), my Orthopedics Professor at the University of Toronto, who continued to inspire and encourage me into my clinical path of joint preservation and cartilage repair. Clement Sledge, MD, who introduced me to the basic science of cartilage repair in Boston.

Thomas Thornhill, MD, my former chairman, mentor, and lifelong friend who helped me set up the first Cartilage Repair Center (CRC) in the United States at the Brigham and Women's Hospital in 1999. Richard Scott, MD, who has taught me so much about knee surgery and gave me the idea to write this book. Julie Glowacki, PhD, and Shuichi Mizuno, PhD, who guided and helped me understand the basic science of cartilage cell biology. The teamwork that resulted at the CRC in excellent clinical care of my patients and through subsequent follow-up research has advanced the field of cartilage repair. My collaboration with Carl Winalski, MD, Department of Radiology, first started at the CRC when evaluating cartilage repair by noninvasive MRI methods has been invaluable. Tim Bryant, RN, BSN, was involved in my practice from 1993 until 2018. It is because of his professionalism, persistence, and kindness that my patient follow-up program under his guidance has given us such thorough and comprehensive clinical outcome results. Andreas Gomoll, MD, contributed tremendously to the clinical research papers that came out in the late 2000s. Takahiro Ogura, MD (Tokyo, Japan), who was my clinical research fellow for 3 years (2015-2018), arrived with tremendous enthusiasm and work ethic, and has been my most prolific co-author. Thank you, Taka!

For the second edition, I would like to thank Lisa Fortier DVM, PhD, for her expertise and adding a chapter to the basic science of biologics, as well as Giuseppe Filiberto, MD, PhD, who reviewed the worldwide literature on clinical outcomes of biologics for the care of patients with cartilage injuries and early osteoarthritis.

After working at the Brigham and Women's Hospital, Harvard Medical School for the last 30 years, I now find myself in West Palm Beach, Florida, working at the Paley Institute. I continue my career in Cartilage Repair, Joint Preservation, and Joint Replacement. I continue to do clinical research with my research assistant, Liana Leja, MS, who works tirelessly and is invaluable. Finally, I would like to thank my medical illustrator, Dan Nichols, MS, for his superb work in both my first and second editions. Working with Dan was both easy to do and a pleasure. After making a sketch and sending it to him, a brief description of what I intended to do was beautifully portrayed in his illustrations. This has added greatly to the quality of my book. Thank you, Dan! I apologize in advance if I have omitted anyone.

Such a wonderful career only occurs by being offered and seizing opportunities and working with excellent team members and co-workers. This is my blessing.

Contents

1 Chondral Injury and Osteoarthritis: The Impact of Articular Cartilage Lesions

TOM MINAS, MD, MS

CHAPTER OUTLINE

Introduction

Damage to the articular cartilage comprises a spectrum of disease entities ranging from single, focal chondral defects to more advanced degenerative disease and end stage osteoarthritis (OA). Long implicated in the subsequent development of osteoarthritis, focal chondral defects result from various causative factors and those factors that may genetically predispose to early breakdown and wear.

Genetics may predispose to early cartilage wear and OA in addition to metabolic, inflammatory, and developmental diseases, which may lead to articular cartilage damage. These may include Gaucher disease, hemophilia, hemochromatosis, ochronosis, Ehlers-Danlos syndrome, Paget disease, acromegaly, avascular necrosis, neuropathic arthropathy, and joint dysplasia.

Patients are approximately evenly split in reporting a traumatic versus an insidious onset of symptoms; athletic activities are the most common inciting event associated with the diagnosis of a chondral lesion.[1] Traumatic events and developmental causative agents such as OCD predominate in younger age groups. Several large studies have found high-grade chondral lesions (Outerbridge grades III and IV) in 5% to 11% of younger patients (<40 years) and up to 60% of older patients.[1–3] The most common locations for these defects are the medial femoral condyle (up to 32%) and the patella,[2,3] and most are detected incidentally during meniscectomy or anterior cruciate ligament reconstruction.[1,4] Notably, despite this relatively high incidence, many of these defects are incidental in nature and asymptomatic. It is agreed that articular cartilage lesions have no spontaneous repair potential and a propensity to worsen with time. Even though the natural history is still not completely understood, those involved in cartilage repair agree that one must look for background factors that predispose to the formation of these defects—malalignment and compartment overload of the tibiofemoral or patellofemoral compartments, joint laxity, contracture, meniscal insufficiency, and of course, genetic predisposition to OA—for which we are just beginning to scratch the surface through advancements in genetic, genomic, and epigenetic research.

Effect of Running and Other Sports on Osteoarthritis

Long distance running and its relationship to the development of OA is an issue of great interest. Several studies have suggested that recreational long distance running is not associated with the progression of knee OA.[5–8] However, the presence of risk factors such as obesity, muscle weakness, or previous joint injury can make the knee more susceptible to the demands associated with participation in sports or athletics.[9] In contrast to recreational involvement, participation in several athletic and sporting activities at the elite level has been associated with an increased risk of lower extremity OA.[10–12] These activities include those involving torsion and impact such as soccer, weightlifters, and sprinters.[11,13] Ignoring a known cartilage injury and continuing to participate in torsional impact sports such as soccer has been shown to cause progression of articular cartilage injuries with large areas of delamination developing.[14] Other studies have demonstrated that known articular injury greater than 1 cm^2 have progressed to OA with greater than 14 years follow-up in greater than half the patients observed when allowed to participate in sports.[15] Even when known cartilage injuries are treated with articular cartilage repair by the use of microfracture or autologous chondrocyte implantation (ACI), OA may develop in as much as one-third of the patients[16] as early as 5 years later. This may be a result of missed axial alignment versus the severity of the instigating initial injury to produce the articular cartilage injury because this has not been found with ACI alone when alignment has been carefully assessed and treated.[17,18]

Anterior Cruciate Ligament Injury

Another consideration that often directly relates to athletic participation is injury to the anterior cruciate ligament (ACL) and subsequent development of knee OA. For patients with an ACL injury, OA susceptibility is reported to be as high as 60% to 90%.[19]

This severe trauma is generally associated with bone bruising at the time of the subluxation of the tibiofemoral joint with tear of the ACL.[20,21] In fact, biopsies of the overlying articular cartilage[22] to the bone bruise have demonstrated that the superficial and middle zones of articular cartilage have greater than 50% cartilage apoptosis in addition to loss of proteoglycans, indicating severe injury to the overlying cartilage surface with a propensity for late articular cartilage loss and delamination and the possibility of progression to OA. Bone bruises in the study have been shown to occur in greater than 80% of ACL injured knees.[22]

The untreated chronic ACL deficient knee, however, has an increased risk of articular cartilage injury especially as the time from initial injury increases.[23,24]

Long-term follow-up of ACL injured patients has consistently demonstrated an association with ACL injury and the development of knee OA. It has been postulated that disruption of the normal mechanics of the knee and continued instability with resultant shear forces to the articular surfaces also predispose to injury to the meniscus as the secondary stabilizer of the knee. The role of the loss of the meniscus as a shock absorber plays a significant contributor to subsequent OA development.

Surgical repair of the ACL aims to restore normal biomechanics to the knee. However, ACL repair has not been shown to reduce the incidence of knee OA when compared with nonoperative management.[25] This may support the theory that the initial trauma and bone bruising with overlying cartilage injury eventually fail, leading to OA, which is the author's belief. Additionally, surgery cannot fully restore normal joint biomechanics. Gait analysis studies revealed altered kinematics of the ACL-reconstructed knee compared with the uninjured contralateral knee. Titchenal et al. identified greater medial compartment motion in 26 ACL-reconstructed knees.[26] Is it speculated that the altered joint loading patterns may still contribute to progression of knee OA despite surgery.

Neuman et al.[27] reported that the primary risk factor for development of knee OA after ACL injury was whether a meniscectomy had been performed. This would seem to support the view that maintenance of knee loading and chondroprotection from the meniscus is an important consideration in this issue.

In general, several causative factors are thought to be involved in the progression of OA in this ACL-injured population, including biological, structural, mechanical, and neuromuscular factors.[28] Further investigation is needed to determine the precise mechanism responsible for early OA development in this population.

Posterior Cruciate Ligament Injury

The posterior cruciate ligament (PCL) is rarely injured compared with the anterior cruciate ligament. Occasionally patients are asymptomatic with PCL injured knees; when they are symptomatic, they generally exhibit pain and disability rather than functional instability as seen in the ACL-deficient knee. The medial femoral condyle is injured more frequently than the lateral femoral condyle.[29,30] Varus alignment of the limb predisposes to medially based pain in this situation. To prevent further progression of a medial articular injury, PCL reconstruction is recommended. However, valgus tibial osteotomy combined with increased flexion in the sagittal plane decreases posterior translation of the tibia and in itself may unload and add enough stability. A careful assessment of instability, alignment, and cartilage injury is required to make an appropriate treatment pathway.

Meniscal Injury

The role of the meniscus in load distribution and shock absorption has long been understood. The absence of a meniscus has been shown predictably to result in OA of the affected compartment with the characteristic radiographic changes being noted such as flattening of the femoral condyles with peripheral osteophyte formation and sclerosis of the tibial surface.[31–33]

It has been noted that the medial compartment of the knee develops these changes within 10 to 15 years after total meniscectomy; however, the lateral compartment may degenerate within 2 to 5 years after total meniscectomy.

This leads me to consider that the compartments are quite different in their susceptibility to loss of the meniscus. The medial compartment comprises 60% of the weight-bearing surfaces compared with 40% in the lateral compartment. The medial compartment is congruent in that the femoral articular surface is convex and the tibial articular surface is concave. The broad medial collateral ligament in addition to the meniscus stabilizes the medial compartment such that there is a rolling motion of the femur on the tibia without translation and shear. Hence the term "medial pivot" with the medial side of the knee being relatively stable and the lateral side exposed to more shear. The medial meniscus does not capture the entire medial femoral condyle because the anterior horn attachment varies and often rolls off the anterior aspect of the tibia, providing less surface to the femoral articular condyle. It is therefore less crucial to the medial compartment than the posterior horn of the medial meniscus, which is loaded continuously during flexion of the knee. The articular surfaces in addition to being congruous have firmer and harder surfaces than the lateral compartment. This increased stability, congruence, and hardness is more protective and in the presence of normal alignment wear is slow to progress. However, varus alignment on the medial compartment usually results in a more rapidly degenerating medial compartment in OA. For this reason, I consider the medial compartment of the knee very alignment-dependent.

The lateral compartment, however, is very different. The lateral tibial plateau surface is convex, the articular surface softer than the medial compartment. The lateral collateral ligament is thin and posteriorly based and provides little stability to the lateral compartment itself. The meniscus, however, is almost circular and makes up for the lack of congruence of the tibial articulation to the femoral articulation. Loss of the lateral meniscus therefore allows incongruence of the lateral compartment and increased translation and shear with point loading of the femoral condyle on the softer lateral tibial plateau articulation and therefore predisposing to rapid articular wear as seen clinically. For this reason, I consider the lateral compartment very meniscal-dependent as opposed to the medial compartment, which is more alignment-dependent.

Alignment: Tibiofemoral and Patellofemoral

The role of alignment cannot be underestimated in the progression of an articular cartilage injury and OA. Sharma[34] noted that if there was malalignment of the tibiofemoral joint, the risk of progression of arthritis in the knee was four times greater in the medial compartment in cases of varus of just 2 degrees and five times in the lateral compartment when only 2 degrees of valgus was present over a period of 18 months. Other studies[35,36] have shown that malalignment plays a role in articular cartilage degeneration by placing abnormal stresses on the articular cartilage. Corrective osteotomy to normalize the forces of the tibiofemoral joint will arrest progression of disease and in the event of cartilage repair will improve the environment for optimal reconstitution of the articular surface.

Patellar lateral maltracking, patella baja, and arthrofibrosis of the infrapatellar fat pad all result in abnormal forces across the articulation of the patellofemoral joint. Isolated lateral patellar facet arthritic change may develop with isolated lateral maltracking and pan-patellar articular loss is more common with patella baja and patellar contracture. Addressing the underlying causes, through possible soft tissue releases, tibial tubercle osteotomy, vastus medialis oblique (VMO) quadriceps advancement, and trochleoplasty, is necessary to halt the progression of disease or to allow cartilage repair without overload and failure.

Chondral Defect Size

The initiation of an articular cartilage defect as noted is frequently traumatic in over half of the cases that are detected and the remainder arise insidiously.[1]

The progression of an articular cartilage lesion to a bipolar articular injury and then to OA is multifactorial as previously discussed. When considering cartilage repair for such a defect, the size of the defect factors into the choice of repair. The natural history of disease for a known size cartilage defect is unknown. However, it is known that even a small defect such as 1 cm^2 may progress if activity is unrestricted.[15] All other factors being equal after background factors have been corrected, the size of the chondral defect in the treatment is critical. If the defect is well shouldered when weight-bearing forces are placed across it (Fig. 1.1), the shoulders take up the load protecting the subchondral bone of the defect from stimulation and hence pain. If the defect is asymptomatic and can be observed over time to determine disease progression, treatment might be unnecessary or it might be adequate to give a treatment that would provide a fibrocartilage repair that protects and stabilizes the existing shoulders dispersing the forces throughout the defect. However, if the defect is large, there may not be shoulders that are participating in the loadbearing, and the subchondral bone of the defect then becomes abrasive to the opposite articular surface producing bipolar degenerative changes. A repair tissue for this situation would need to bear all of the forces and require durability and viscoelastic mechanical properties that would be durable and nonabrasive such as hyaline articular cartilage. This will determine treatment options for the patient and will be discussed in the later chapters on treatment options.

Effect of BMI on Osteoarthritis

Obesity is a well-documented risk factor for the development of OA of the knee and it has been demonstrated that weight reduction lowers the risk of developing OA.[37,38] Body mass index (BMI) is often used as a measure of obesity. However, these measures do not accurately capture the components of body composition such as muscle and fat, only giving a measure of total weight or the ratio of weight to height. Wang et al.[39] examined the relationship between fat mass (FM), fat-free mass (FFM) and their effect on tibial cartilage volume. Their analysis showed a positive correlation between increased FFM and tibial cartilage volume. Additionally, increased FM was correlated with an increased risk for tibial articular cartilage defects. These defects have previously been shown to be predictive of cartilage loss.[40,41]

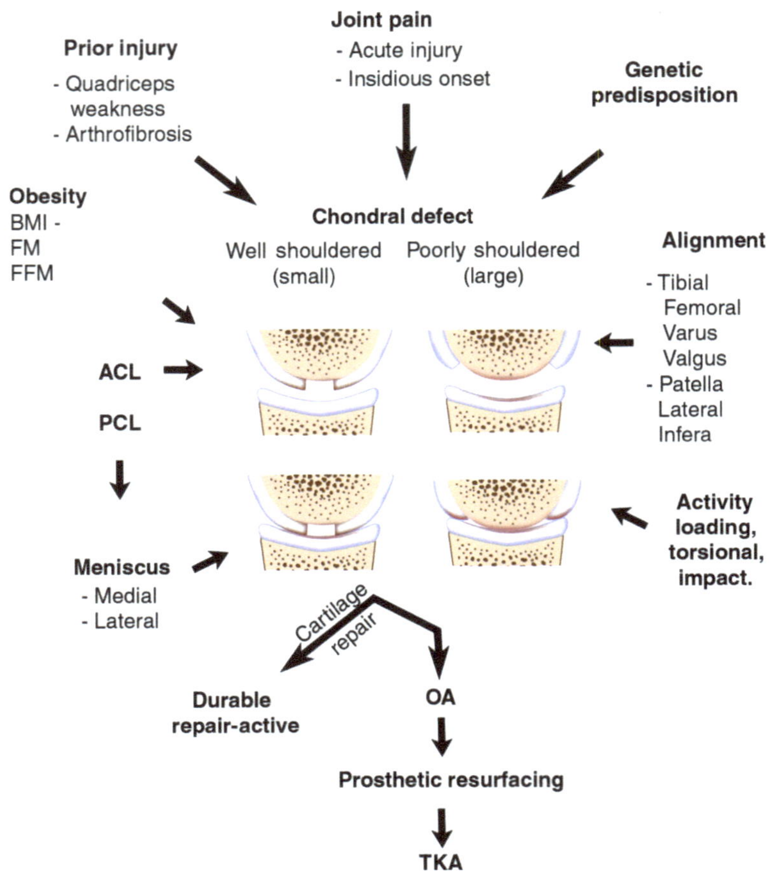

• **Fig. 1.1** Multiple factors influence the progression of cartilage damage to OA. Cartilage repair may be successful in halting the progression of disease if these factors are managed. These factors are frequently referred to as "background factors" when assessing and managing chondral defects with cartilage repair. *ACL*, anterior cruciate ligament; *FFM*, fat-free mass; *FM*, fat mass; *OA*, osteoarthritis; *PCL*, posterior cruciate ligament; *TKA*, total knee arthroplasty.

In addition to biomechanical factors, recent literature suggests that alterations of cartilage composition may also contribute to obesity-related OA and disease progression. The presence of OA in non-weight bearing joints (i.e., wrist and hand) of obese individuals supports this notion.[42,43] When investigating cartilage strain in response to treadmill walking using T1rho imaging, Collins et al. found lower proteoglycan content of the tibiofemoral cartilage in subjects with higher BMI.[44] A previous study presented similar findings. Using delayed gadolinium-enhanced magnetic resonance imaging of cartilage (dGEMRIC) to estimate proteoglycan content, Anandacoomarasamy et al. found improved levels and reduced cartilage thickness losses in subjects after undergoing a weight loss program.[45] Additional studies show that metabolic factors occurring with obesity enhance the activity of inflammatory cytokines associated with OA.[46,47] It is well known that increased inflammatory cytokine activity can lead to chondrocyte catabolism and thus degenerative changes of articular cartilage. Although the exact mechanism remains unclear, adipose-related inflammation in combination with mechanical loading probably plays a role in obesity-related OA. Future studies are needed to validate this relationship.

Prevalence of Osteoarthritis

OA of the knee is a disease that has a profound presence and impact upon our society. However, because of the varied diagnostic criteria available, it is difficult to estimate the incidence and prevalence of this disease accurately. Estimates of prevalence can vary widely based on whether a radiological, symptomatic, or combination diagnosis is used. Although radiological methods are more accurately reproducible for longitudinal studies, patient reports of pain and disability give a better picture of the impact on both society and the health care system.

Perhaps the most well-known study of the prevalence of OA is the Framingham Osteoarthritis Study.[48] This study utilized a combination of patient responses to a standardized questionnaire, radiographic evidence, and physician assessment. The study demonstrates a clear linear relationship between increasing age and prevalence of OA, with radiographic evidence of disease in 11.5% of patients >70 years of age and 19.4% of patients ≥ 80 years of age. However, by no means did all patients with radiographic diagnosis report pain. The proportion of patients reporting symptoms rose from 7.6% of patients with no radiographic evidence of disease to 40% of patients with grade 3 or 4 disease. It is interesting to observe that even in the most severe radiographic categories of disease, less than 50% of patients report symptoms of OA. Each year, approximately 25% of adults over 55 years of age experience knee pain lasting for at least 1 month. Of this group, about half of the patients show radiographic evidence of OA. By using stricter criteria for diagnosis including both symptoms and radiographic evidence, the prevalence is often estimated at <15%.[49] This figure is widely regarded to be a significant underestimate.[48]

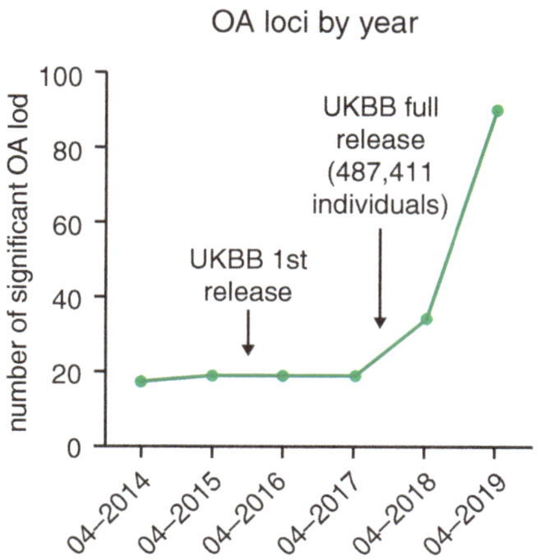

• **Fig. 1.2** Number of OA-associated loci from 2014 to 2019. (From Reynard LN, Barter MJ. Osteoarthritis year in review 2019: genetics, genomics and epigenetics. *Osteoarthr Cartil*. 2020;28(3):275–284.)

More recent published findings from the National Health Interview Survey estimated that nearly 14 million people in the United States (6.9% of the total US population ≥ 25 years of age) have both radiographic OA and symptomatic OA of the knee. Of this population, notably over 3 million individuals are among racial/ethnic minorities.[50]

Genetics of Osteoarthritis

Advancements in DNA sequencing and epigenetic studies have enhanced our understanding of the pathophysiological mechanism underlying OA. The number of identified OA loci leaped from 19 to 90 with the publication of the UK biobank (UKBB) genotype data (Fig. 1.2). Recently published findings of several large genome-wide association studies using the UKBB data identified robustly replicated genetic

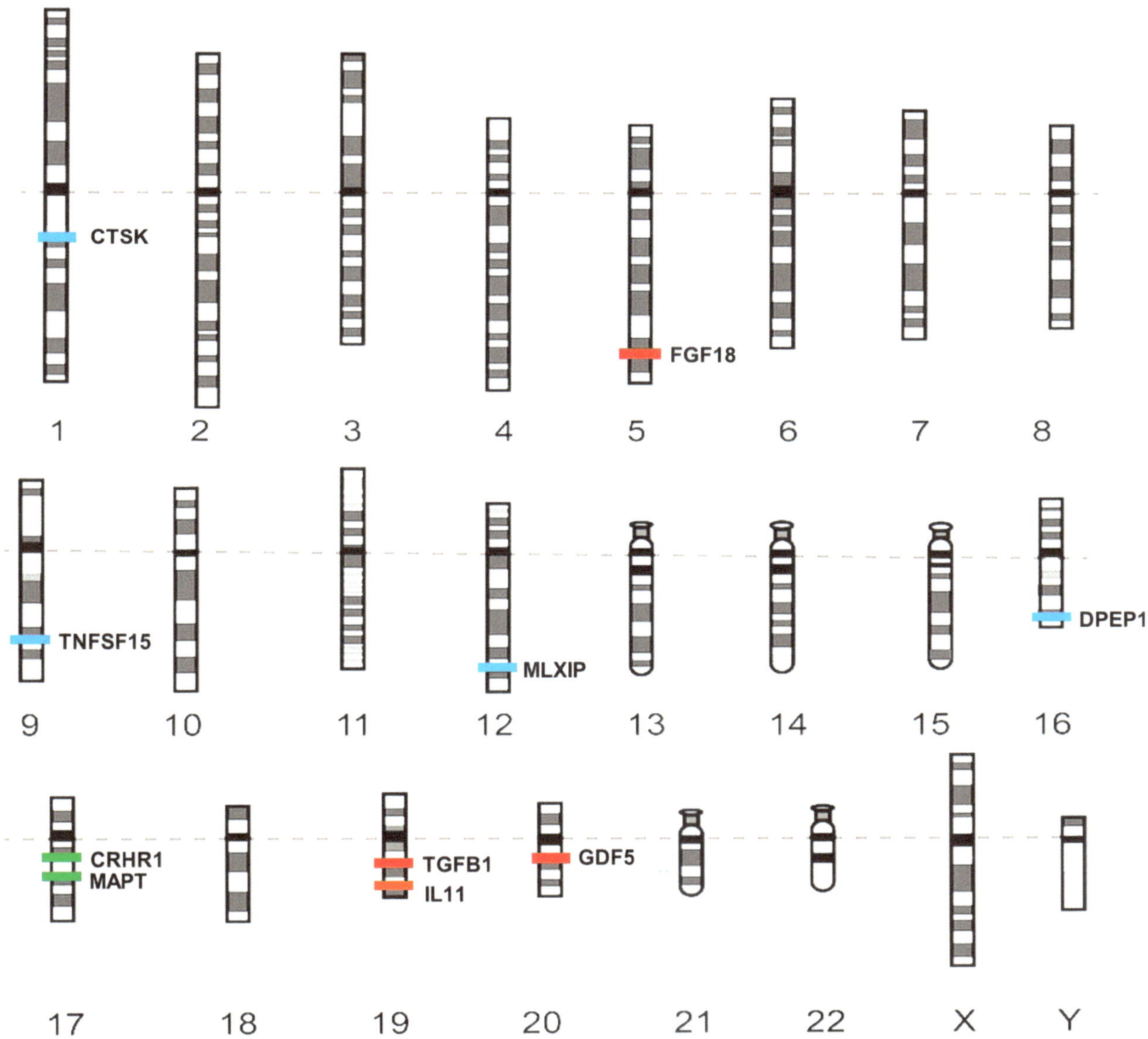

• **Fig. 1.3** Current OA-associated genes targeted in therapeutic treatment. Colors indicate suspected mechanism of action: red: agonist/upregulator; blue: inhibitor; green: unknown; orange: ↑ IL11 signaling. (Adapted from Tachmazidou I, Hatzikotoulas K, Southam L, et al. Identification of new therapeutic targets for osteoarthritis through genome-wide analyses of UK Biobank data. *Nat Genet*. 2019;51(2):230–236.)

TABLE 1.1 Current OA-Associated Genes Targeted in Therapeutic Treatment

Mapped gene	OA chromosome: variant-risk allele	Reported OA phenotype	Targeting drug: developmental phase
TGFB1	19: rs75621460-A	Knee OA Hip OA OA	INVOSSA: Registered
FGF18	5: rs3884606-G	Knee OA Hip OA	NAS-902330: Clinical development
GDF5	20: rs143384-A	Knee OA	HMR-4052: Clinical development
CTSK	1: rs10888395-C	Hip OA OA	CTSK Inhibitor: Clinical development
IL11	19: rs4252548-T	Hip OA	Oprelvekin: Approved
MLXIP	12: rs11059094-T	Hip OA	LCL-161: Clinical development
DPEP1	16: rs1126464-G	OA	Cilastatin: Approved
CRHR1	17: rs62063281-?	Hip OA	NBI-74788: Clinical development
MAPT	17: rs62063281- G	Hip OA	Flortaucipir F18, leuco-methylthioninium: Clinical development
TNFSF15	9: rs919642-T, rs1330349-C	Knee OA Hip OA OA	PF-06480605: Clinical development

variants associated with OA susceptibility. To date, the largest OA genetic study assessing the genomes of over 450,000 individuals in the UK identified 52 novel genetic variants of OA, including 24 signals for OA at any site, 15 for hip OA, 7 for knee OA, and 6 signals for OA of the hip and/or knee.[51]

Further analysis revealed several genes causally linked to OA etiology. These particular genes were found either to encode structural bone and/or cartilage proteins or to play a vital role in bone/cartilage development.[51] Additionally, this study highlighted 10 genes currently targeted for OA therapeutic treatment (Fig. 1.3 and Table 1.1). Notably, only one of the 10 genes (GDF5) was found to be genetically associated with OA susceptibility.[51]

There has also been an increased interest in epigenetic modifications associated with OA, evidenced by recent publications assessing genome-wide methylation,[52–54] posttranslational histone modifications in OA,[55] and OA noncoding RNA.[56,57]

With over 60 biological processes associated with OA from bone, cartilage, and chondrocyte morphology to collagen and extracellular matrix organization, there is more to learn. Further work is needed to characterize the genetic contributors of OA and to identify novel pathways for therapeutic targets.

Present Versus Future Total Knee Arthroplasty Numbers

As our population ages, the number of both primary and revision total knee arthroplasty procedures performed is predicted to rise by over 600%.[58] Between 2005 and 2030, primary total knee arthroplasty demand has been projected to rise by 673%, from 450,000 procedures annually in 2005 to 3,481,000 annually in 2030.[58] The total number of revision knee arthroplasty procedures is projected to rise from 38,300 in 2005 to 268,200 in 2030, an increase of 601%. These numbers have even more impact when compared with the corresponding figures for hip arthroplasty. The numbers of primary and revision total hip arthroplasties are projected to rise by 174% and 137%, respectively. It has been predicted that the current supply of orthopedic surgeons will be unable to accommodate such a vast increase in surgical volume.[59]

Economic Burden

In 2013, OA was deemed the second most costly health condition in the United States.[60] The cost of arthritis-attributable conditions was estimated to be 1% of gross domestic product, accounting for $16.5 billion (4.3%) of total hospitalization costs.[60] This number is quite significant, especially considering that knee and hip OA have a disproportionate impact on patient disability and health care costs as compared with OA in other joints.[61] It is important to consider not only the direct costs associated with OA, but also the indirect costs. The CDC reported $164 billion in lost wages in 2013 primarily attributed to substantially fewer adults with OA working compared with adults without OA.[60] Also accounted for were the lost wages of the informal caregivers, such as relatives. Studies have reported substantial personal costs to OA patients.[62,63]

Conclusion

Symptomatic chondral defects represent a difficult clinical treatment pathway. When managing knee injury, an injured articular surface is truly the "Holy Grail." Despite excellent reconstructive measures of associated injuries to the athlete, a career-ending injury is frequently an articular cartilage injury. When managing such an injury, the associated background factors must be assessed and treated either prior to or at the time of the articular cartilage injury.

Former athletes frequently develop degenerative arthritis of their joints. They wish to maintain healthy and active lifestyles as our society of baby boomers now become retirees. In order to do so we must continue to strive to preserve the joint yet maintain the option for total knee arthroplasty if necessary. OA of the knee represents a tremendous social and economic burden to our society. Maintaining an enjoyable quality of life through joint preservation has become a reality because of biologic advances in technology and imaging. This book will focus on this possibility through addressing background factors, cartilage repair, and truly regenerative medicine.

References

1. Aroen A, Loken S, Heir S, et al. Articular cartilage lesions in 993 consecutive knee arthroscopies. *Am J Sports Med.* 2004;32(1):211–215.
2. Curl WW, Krome J, Gordon ES, et al. Cartilage injuries: a review of 31,516 knee arthroscopies. *Arthroscopy.* 1997;13(4):456–460.
3. Hjelle K, Solheim E, Strand T, et al. Articular cartilage defects in 1,000 knee arthroscopies. *Arthroscopy.* 2002;18:730–734.
4. Piasecki DP, Spindler KP, Warren TA, Andrish JT, Parker RD. Intraarticular injuries associated with anterior cruciate ligament tear: findings at ligament reconstruction in high school and recreational athletes. An analysis of sex-based differences. *Am J Sports Med.* 2003;31(4):601–605.
5. Chakravarty EF, Hubert HB, Lingala VB, Zatarain E, Fries JF. Long distance running and knee osteoarthritis. A prospective study. *Am J Prev Med.* 2008;35(2):133–138.
6. Cheng Y, Macera CA, Davis DR, et al. Physical activity and self-reported, physician-diagnosed osteoarthritis: is physical activity a risk factor? *J Clin Epidemiol.* 2000;53(3):315–322.
7. Hannan MT, Felson DT, Anderson JJ, Naimark A. Habitual physical activity is not associated with knee osteoarthritis: the Framingham Study. *J Rheumatol.* 1993;20(4):704–709.
8. Panush RS, Schmidt C, Caldwell JR, et al. Is running associated with degenerative joint disease? *Jama.* 1986;255(9):1152–1154.
9. Felson DT. An update on the pathogenesis and epidemiology of osteoarthritis. *Radiol Clin North Am.* 2004;42(1):1–9. v.
10. Kujala UM, Kaprio J, Sarna S. Osteoarthritis of weight bearing joints of lower limbs in former elite male athletes. *Br Med J.* 1994;308(6923):231–234.
11. Kujala UM, Kettunen J, Paananen H, et al. Knee osteoarthritis in former runners, soccer players, weight lifters, and shooters. *Arthritis Rheum.* 1995;38(4):539–546.
12. Teitz CC, Kilcoyne RF. Premature osteoarthrosis in professional dancers. *Clin J Sport Med.* 1998;8(4):255–259.
13. Lindberg H, Roos H, Gardsell I. Prevalence of coxarthrosis in former soccer players. *Acta Orthop Scand.* 1993;64:165–167.
14. Levy AS, Lohnes J, Sculley S, et al. Chondral delamination of the knee in soccer players. *Am J Sports Med.* 1996;24:634–639.
15. Messner K, Maletius W. The long-term prognosis for severe damage to weight-bearing cartilage in the knee: a 14-year clinical and radiographic follow-up in 28 young athletes. *Acta Orthop Scand.* 1996;67(2):165–168.
16. Knutsen G, Engebretsen L, Ludvigsen TC, et al. A randomized trial comparing autologous chondrocyte implantation with microfracture. Findings at 5 years. *J Bone Joint Surg Am.* 2007;89:2105–2112.
17. Peterson L, Brittberg M, Kiviranta I, et al. Autologous chondrocyte transplantation. Biomechanics and long-term durability. *Am J Sports Med.* 2002;30(1):2–12.
18. Minas T. Autologous chondrocyte implantation for focal chondral defects of the knee. *Clin Orthop Relat Res.* 2001;391 Suppl:S349–S361.
19. Meunier A, Odensten M, Good L. Long-term results after primary repair or non-surgical treatment of anterior cruciate ligament rupture: a randomized study with a 15-year follow-up. *Scand J Med Sci Sports.* 2007;17(3):230–237.
20. Rosen M, Jackson D, Berger P. Occult osseous lesions documented by MRI associated with anterior cruciate ligament rupture. *Arthroscopy.* 1991;7:45–51.
21. Spindler K, Schils JP, Bergfield J, et al. Prospective study of osseous articular, and meniscal lesions in recent anterior cruciate ligame tears by magnetic resonance imaging and arthroscopy. *Am J Sports Med.* 1993;21:551–557.
22. Johnson D, Urban W, Carbon D, et al. Articular cartilage changes seen with magnetic resonance imaging: Detected bone bruises associated with acute anterior cruciate ligament rupture. *Am J Sports Med.* 1998;26:409–414.
23. Gillquist J, Messner K. Anterior cruciate ligament reconstruction and the long-term incidence of gonarthrosis. *Sports Med Arthrosc.* 1999;27:143–156.
24. Roos H, Adalberth T, Dahlberg L, Lohmander LS. Osteoarthritis of the knee after injury to the anterior cruciate ligament or meniscus: the influence of time and age. *Osteoarthritis Cartilage.* 1995;3:261–267.
25. Kessler MA, Behrend H, Henz S, Stutz G, Rukavina A, Kuster MS. Function, osteoarthritis and activity after ACL-rupture: 11 years follow-up results of conservative versus reconstructive treatment. *Knee Surg Sports Traumatol Arthrosc.* 2008;16(5):442–448.
26. Titchenal MR, Chu CR, Erhart-Hledik JC, Andriacchi TP. Early changes in knee center of rotation during walking after anterior cruciate ligament reconstruction correlate with later changes in patient-reported outcomes. *Am J Sports Med.* 2017;45(4):915–921.
27. Neuman P, Englund M, Kostogiannis I, Friden T, Roos H, Dahlberg LE. Prevalence of tibiofemoral osteoarthritis 15 years after nonoperative treatment of anterior cruciate ligament injury: a prospective cohort study. *Am J Sports Med.* 2008;36(9):1717–1725.
28. Wang LJ, Zeng N, Yan ZP, Li JT, Ni GX. Post-traumatic osteoarthritis following ACL injury. *Arthritis Res Ther.* 2020;22(1):57.
29. Geissler V, Whipple T. Intraarticular abnormalities in association with posterior cruciate ligament injuries. *Am J Sports Med.* 1993;21:846–849.
30. Torg J, Barton T, Pavlov H. Natural history of the posterior cruciate ligament-deficient knee. *Clin Orthop Relat Res.* 1989;246:208–216.

31. Fairbank T. Knee joint changes after meniscectomy. *J Bone Joint Surg Br.* 1948;30:664–670.
32. Tapper E, Hoover N. Late results after meniscectomy. *J Bone Joint Surg Am.* 1969;51:517–526.
33. Johnson R, Kettelkamp D, Clark W, et al. Factors affecting late results after meniscectomy. *J Bone Joint Surg Am.* 1974;56:719–729.
34. Sharma L, Song J, Felson DT, Cahue S, Shamiyeh E, Dunlop DD, et al. The role of knee alignment in disease progression and functional decline in knee osteoarthritis. *JAMA.* 2001;286(2):188–195.
35. Tetsworth K, Paley D. Malalignment and degenerative arthropathy. *Orthop Clin North Am.* 1994;25:367–377.
36. Wu D, Burr D, Boyd R, et al. Bone and cartilage changes following experimental varus or valgus tibial angulation. *J Orthop Res.* 1990;8:572–585.
37. Felson DT, Anderson JJ, Naimark A, Walker AM, Meenan RF. Obesity and knee osteoarthritis. The Framingham Study. *Ann Intern Med.* 1988;109(1):18–24.
38. Felson DT, Zhang Y, Anthony JM, Naimark A, Anderson JJ. Weight loss reduces the risk for symptomatic knee osteoarthritis in women. The Framingham Study. *Ann Intern Med.* 1992;116(7):535–539.
39. Wang Y, Wluka AE, English DR, et al. Body composition and knee cartilage properties in healthy, community-based adults. *Ann Rheum Dis.* 2007;66(9):1244–1248.
40. Cicuttini F, Ding C, Wluka A, Davis S, Ebeling PR, Jones G. Association of cartilage defects with loss of knee cartilage in healthy, middle-age adults: a prospective study. *Arthritis Rheum.* 2005;52(7):2033–2039.
41. Ding C, Cicuttini F, Scott F, Boon C, Jones G. Association of prevalent and incident knee cartilage defects with loss of tibial and patellar cartilage: a longitudinal study. *Arthritis Rheum.* 2005;52(12):3918–3927.
42. Grotle M, Hagen KB, Natvig B, Dahl FA, Kvien TK. Obesity and osteoarthritis in knee, hip and/or hand: an epidemiological study in the general population with 10 years follow-up. *BMC Musculoskelet Disord.* 2008;9:132.
43. Oliveria SA, Felson DT, Cirillo PA, Reed JI, Walker AM. Body weight, body mass index, and incident symptomatic osteoarthritis of the hand, hip, and knee. *Epidemiology.* 1999;10(2):161–166.
44. Collins AT, Kulvaranon ML, Cutcliffe HC, et al. Obesity alters the in vivo mechanical response and biochemical properties of cartilage as measured by MRI. *Arthritis Res Ther.* 2018;20(1):232.
45. Anandacoomarasamy A, Leibman S, Smith G, et al. Weight loss in obese people has structure-modifying effects on medial but not on lateral knee articular cartilage. *Ann Rheum Dis.* 2012;71(1):26–32.
46. Aygun AD, Gungor S, Ustundag B, Gurgoze MK, Sen Y. Proinflammatory cytokines and leptin are increased in serum of prepubertal obese children. *Mediators Inflamm.* 2005;2005(3):180–183.
47. Wellen KE, Hotamisligil GS. Inflammation, stress, and diabetes. *J Clin Invest.* 2005;115(5):1111–1119.
48. Felson DT, Naimark A, Anderson J, Kazis L, Castelli W, Meenan RF. The prevalence of knee osteoarthritis in the elderly. The Framingham Osteoarthritis Study. *Arthritis Rheum.* 1987;30(8):914–918.
49. D'Ambrosia RD. Epidemiology of osteoarthritis. *Orthopedics.* 2005;28(2 Suppl):s201–s205.
50. Vina ER, Kwoh CK. Epidemiology of osteoarthritis: literature update. *Curr Opin Rheumatol.* 2018;30(2):160–167.
51. Tachmazidou I, Hatzikotoulas K, Southam L, et al. Identification of new therapeutic targets for osteoarthritis through genome-wide analyses of UK Biobank data. *Nat Genet.* 2019;51(2):230–236.
52. Zhao L, Wang Q, Zhang C, Huang C. Genome-wide DNA methylation analysis of articular chondrocytes identifies TRAF1, CTGF, and CX3CL1 genes as hypomethylated in osteoarthritis. *Clin Rheumatol.* 2017;36(10):2335–2342.
53. Wang X, Tang D, Shen P, et al. Analysis of DNA methylation in chondrocytes in rats with knee osteoarthritis. *BMC Musculoskelet Disord.* 2017;18(1):377.
54. Wang W, Yu Y, Hao J, et al. Genome-wide DNA methylation profiling of articular cartilage reveals significant epigenetic alterations in Kashin-Beck disease and osteoarthritis. *Osteoarthritis Cartilage.* 2017;25(12):2127–2133.
55. Monteagudo S, Cornelis FMF, Aznar-Lopez C, et al. DOT1L safeguards cartilage homeostasis and protects against osteoarthritis. *Nat Commun.* 2017;8:15889.
56. Kung LHW, Ravi V, Rowley L, Bell KM, Little CM, Bateman JF. Comprehensive expression analysis of microRNAs and mRNAs in synovial tissue from a mouse model of early post-traumatic osteoarthritis. *Sci Rep.* 2017;7(1):17701.
57. Si HB, Zeng Y, Liu SY, et al. Intra-articular injection of microRNA-140 (miRNA-140) alleviates osteoarthritis (OA) progression by modulating extracellular matrix (ECM) homeostasis in rats. *Osteoarthritis Cartilage.* 2017;25(10):1698–1707.
58. Kurtz S, Ong K, Lau E, Mowat F, Halpern M, et al. Projections of primary and revision hip and knee arthroplasty in the United States from 2005 to 2030. *J Bone Joint Surg Am.* 2007;89(4):780–785.
59. Iorio R, Robb WJ, Healy WL, et al. Orthopaedic surgeon workforce and volume assessment for total hip and knee replacement in the United States: preparing for an epidemic. *J Bone Joint Surg Am.* 2008;90(7):1598–1605.
60. *Arthritis Cost Statistics.* 2020 February 27, 2020 [cited 2020 September 21, 2020]; Available from: https://www.cdc.gov/arthritis/data_statistics/cost.htm.
61. Surgeons AAoO, ed. *Burden of Musculoskeletal Diseases in the United States: Prevalence, Societal and Economic Cost.* 1st Ed. American Academy of Orthopaedic Surgeons; 2008.
62. Gabriel SE, Crowson CS, Campion ME, O'Fallon WM. Direct medical costs unique to people with arthritis. *J Rheumatol.* 1997;24(4):719–725.
63. Lapsley HM, March LM, Tribe KL, Cross MJ, Brooks PM. Living with osteoarthritis: patient expenditures, health status, and social impact. *Arthritis Rheum.* 2001;45(3):301–306.

2

Cartilage Repair and Regeneration

TOM MINAS, MD, MS, AND TAKAHIRO OGURA, MD

CHAPTER OUTLINE

Cartilage Structure and Function

The Chondrocyte as an Anabolic/Catabolic Cell

Chondrocytes are highly specialized cells that differentiate from clusters of mesenchymal cells during skeletal embryogenesis. The chondrocyte synthesizes and secretes the components of the extracellular matrix, primarily proteoglycans and type II collagen. Most of the immature cartilage is temporary and is replaced by bone during epiphyseal development, whereas the regions nearest the synovial cavity remain as the permanent articular cartilage of the adult. During growth and development, immature cartilage undergoes cellular replication in both the superficial and deep zones. However, as skeletal maturity approaches, replication occurs only in the deep zone. Cell replication after skeletal maturity is rare. The cell content of articular cartilage is low, occupying no more than 10% of the tissue volume in humans. Cell density has been estimated as 10^5 cells per cubic millimeter in newborns and 1/10 of that in adult cartilage. Values are higher in the superficial zone than in the deeper zone. Experimental animals have far greater cellularity. For example, adult rabbits have nearly 10-fold greater cell density than human cartilage and mice have 25-fold greater cell density.[1] The general cellular morphology ranges from flattened and discoidal in the most superficial zones to ovoid in the deeper regions. The ovoid cells display enlarged Golgi bodies, a characteristic of cells actively secreting proteins, and cellular processes that extend into the adjacent pericellular matrix.

Chondrocytes are normally long-lived cells. They are not replaced by new cells as occurs in the turnover of other tissues. However, the capacity for cell division is manifest when the integrity of the matrix is compromised, as in osteoarthritis. Cartilage fibrillation is associated with necrosis in the superficial zone and with clusters of cells in deep zones. Metabolic studies show increased sulfate incorporation by the cells in the clusters surrounded by proteoglycan-poor matrix. If viewed as an attempt to repair, the cells in clusters are active in matrix synthesis but are not capable of matrix replacement at distances from the clusters. Thus, the overall content of proteoglycan is low in fibrillated cartilage.

Chondrocytes are embedded in an avascular matrix in which nutrients and waste products must diffuse. Oxygen tension is approximately 1/3 that measured between capillaries in soft tissues. On a per-cell basis, oxygen uptake is 1/50 that of kidney, but the rates of glycolysis between chondrocytes and kidney are comparable. Thus, chondrocytes engage in relatively anaerobic metabolism.

Chondrocytes are dynamic cells with anabolic and catabolic activity; they mediate both synthesis and degradation of the matrix. Proteoglycan metabolism has been studied extensively. As is typical for other cells, the protein components are synthesized in the cytoplasmic rough endoplasmic reticulum and sulfation of the polysaccharides occurs in the Golgi bodies. Ex vivo studies with radioactive tracer isotope of ^{35}S-sulfate show incorporation into glycosaminoglycans by intermediate and deep cells and subsequent movement into the matrix. Type II collagen is synthesized and secreted as separate procollagen chains with extensions on its ends, converted to tropocollagen, and organized into fibrils with small amounts of type IX and type XI collagen. In contrast to the dense, thick, highly oriented collagen fibers of bone, cartilage fibrils are thin and cross-linked into an open meshwork. The fibrils contain variable amounts of noncollagenous macromolecules, notably decorin. The half-life of type II collagen is more than 200 years in humans. Thus, the major component of the native fibrils does not appear to be renewed or reparable in the normal setting. The collagen fibrillar network is under tension and serves to contain the glycosaminoglycans in a compressed state. It is difficult to imagine how that network could be turned over without compromising the mechanical integrity of the tissue or how denatured foci could be mended. Evidence shows damage to the fibrillar network in osteoarthritis. Osteoarthritis drastically affects the mechanical properties of cartilage. Excessive swelling of osteoarthritic samples in dilute salt solution is taken as evidence of the loss of resistance afforded by the fibrillar net to absorption of water by the polysaccharides. Although there appears to be little turnover of the fibrillar network, the entrapped proteoglycans undergo turnover that can be accelerated by local cytokines. Chondrocytes are responsible for maintaining the matrix environment in which they are encased and hence ensure the tissue's mechanical charactericss.[2] They are protected from osmotic and mechanical damage by the rigid pericellular matrix, called the *chondron*. Maintenance of the matrix involves degradation by proteinases and free radicals generated by the chondrocyte. Matrix metalloproteinases and aggrecanase catalyze the turnover of cartilage matrix in normal as well as in diseased cartilage. Because many of the matrix components in cartilage are specific to that tissue, there is great interest in developing and validating assays for their degradation products in plasma or synovial fluid as markers for turnover.[3]

In the modern view, osteoarthritis is considered to result from an imbalance between dynamic anabolic and catabolic activities that are normally well balanced. The chondrocyte functions as the agent of these two processes. This is in contrast to bone tissue, for example, in which anabolic activities are ascribed to the osteoblast and catabolic or osteolytic activities to the osteoclast. Although normally interaction between the two cell types maintains skeletal mass constant within the remodeling process, imbalance occurs with aging, osteoporosis, and infection. The situation in cartilage is distinct. Evidence suggests that the earliest stages of osteoarthritis are balanced by an upregulation of the biosynthetic processes. Synovial fluid collects a byproduct of procollagen II processing, called *chondrocalcin* or *C-propeptide*, whose levels are elevated in traumatic and primary osteoarthritis.

Previously, cartilage was regarded to be immunologically privileged because of either the absence of transplantation antigens or the protective effect of the matrix. These states were invoked to explain the endurance of allografts in heterotopic sites. It is now appreciated that chondrocytes do display major transplantation antigens and that components of the matrix are weakly antigenic. In healthy intact cartilage, these determinants are probably shielded from antibodies because of steric hindrance caused by the proteoglycans in the matrix. Preservation of matrix integrity appears to be essential to prevent exposure of the cells and rejection of the tissue.

The heterogeneous group of inflammatory joint diseases involve underlying disturbances in immune regulation. In rheumatoid arthritis, the synovial lining is the initial target of inflammatory pathology. Proliferation of synovial lining cells and infiltration by lymphocytes and activated macrophages produce a tissue mass called the *pannus*. The pannus can invade and destroy the integrity of articular cartilage. Products of the pannus act as cytokine mediators of both chondrolysis and osteolysis. The major agents are interleukin-1 (IL-1) and tumor necrosis factor-α. These agents signal the cascade of release of IL-6, IL-8, IL-17, cyclooxygenase-2, and nitric oxide, all of which are actual or potential targets of pharmacologic management. In vitro models have been useful to describe the mechanisms by which these immunomodulatory cytokines change gene expression in chondrocytes, thus promoting chondrolysis.

Mechanical Properties of Articular Cartilage

Articular cartilage is a hypocellular, viscoelastic tissue that lines synovial joints, providing them with a nearby frictionless environment. Synovial cartilage articulations provide a coefficient of friction for joint motion that is less than 1/5 that of ice on ice.[4] The mechanical properties of articular cartilage depend upon its composition and its architecture. Normally, the hydrophilic proteoglycans and collagen constitute 30% of the tissue mass; the remainder is water. Cartilage matrix can be viewed as a biphasic material in which the fluid phase flows upon mechanical deformation of its solid phase. Although the water is constrained by the proteoglycan molecules, the fluid phase can also be called the *porosity* of the cartilage. The high water content of the tissue also generates its high viscoelasticity. Its elastic module is low at slow rates of loading but is two orders greater at physiologic rates.

The surface cartilage layer or "skin" is resistant to compressive loads or penetration. The vertically arranged collagen fibers of the radial and calcified zones are resistant to shear. Upon application of pressure to articular cartilage through weight bearing, the water contained within the cartilage exudes upon pressure. With diminished pressure, water is drawn back to the aggrecan. The surface protein dermatan sulfate also acts as an antiadhesion substance. The fine filaments of the superficial zone combine with water so that articulation with the opposite joint surface also occurs with combined water and superficial zone filaments.[2] Therefore, the lubricating barrier between joint surfaces is mostly water. Water is released during weight-bearing pressure from hyperhydrated negatively charged proteoglycans in articular cartilage. With damage or degeneration, loss of proteoglycans and water results in impaired mechanical properties and joint function.

Incidence of Cartilage Lesions

The true incidence of cartilage lesions and their natural history are unknown. It has been proposed that between 5% and 10% of acute knee hemarthroses after a work-related or sports injury is associated with an acute chondral injury.[5] In a retrospective review of 31,516 knee arthroscopies, the prevalence of chondral lesions was 63%. However, isolated unipolar chondral defects in patients younger than 40 years were rare, occurring in only 5% of this patient population.[6] Both clinical and experimental evidence showed that with time focal cartilage injuries will enlarge and progress to osteoarthritis.[7]

Mechanical injury to articular cartilage during sporting injuries may occur with shearing forces secondary to disruption of the anterior cruciate ligament. Shearing osteochondral fractures occurring at the time of ligament disruption have been noted. Blunt injury to the joint surfaces may cause injury to and death of articular chondrocytes. If the articular chondrocyte cannot continue to synthesize and remodel its matrix macromolecules, the pericellular matrix will eventually degenerate. This may account for the high incidence of osteoarthritis encountered with anterior cruciate ligament injuries. Acutely the incidence of chondral injuries is approximately 2% but may approach 20% in the long run.[8]

In a study performed by Repo and Finlay,[9] blunt force to articular chondrocytes in excess of 25 MPa reproducibly resulted in death of articular chondrocytes. Hence there appears to be a threshold to which articular chondrocytes can withstand blunt trauma. This may be an important factor in understanding articular cartilage degeneration after injury and may be an important technical factor during new repair techniques, such as osteochondral graft transfers. Large impaction forces needed to introduce osteochondral grafts to recipient sites may result in injury and cell death to the cartilage cap of the osteochondral grafts, leading to failed long-term results.

Magnetic resonance imaging scans demonstrated bone bruises after blunt injuries sustained during work-related and sporting activities. Arthroscopic biopsy studies of cartilage overlying bone bruises demonstrated superficial chondrocyte death and matrix dehydration.[10] Cartilage cell death is proposed to arise directly from the blunt trauma exceeding this threshold.

The natural history of osteoarthritis itself is unknown. A Swedish longitudinal study notes radiographic progression of osteoarthritis in the knee occurs over a 20-year time course when greater than 50% joint space narrowing is present at initial evaluation (Ahlbäck stages 2–4).[11] However, only 60% of patients with Ahlbäck stage 0 (peripheral osteophytes and a normal joint space) or Ahlbäck stage 1 (<50% joint space narrowing) at initial presentation will progress radiographically. Not all radiographic osteoarthritis will progress.

In the United States, more than 450,000 total knee replacements are performed annually. The disability and economic hardship encountered by osteoarthritis are substantial. This is especially true if a cartilage injury occurs at a young age when socioeconomic productivity and recreational activities are especially affected. The problem arises from the unique structure, function, and repair mechanisms of articular cartilage.

Cartilage Injuries and Repair

Articular cartilage is devoid of a nerve supply. Cartilage covers and protects the richly innervated subchondral bone plate from stimulation. Once articular cartilage is damaged, pain can result from contact of the subchondral bone plate. If a healing response does not develop, load will be borne by the shoulders of the chondral defects in addition to the exposed subchondral bone. This situation will result in overload and breakdown of the shoulders of the defect, with progressive enlargement of the defect. The opposing articulation would be exposed to a bare bone surface with resultant erosive degradation of its cartilage surface. The resultant bone-on-bone articulation is by definition osteoarthritis. Symptoms from direct stimulation of the subchondral bone plate or from indirect stimulation to the bone via an attached cartilage flap may occur. Breakdown products from the cartilage along with liberated enzymes may cause effusions in the joint, capsular distention, or synovitis as other mechanisms of pain. As the subchondral bone plate hardens, secondary vascular venous congestion in the medullary cavity results and may cause deep aching pain.

Cartilage repair would be beneficial in the short term to alleviate symptoms and in the long term to prevent progressive breakdown of the articulations of the joint and the development of osteoarthritis. Thus, the goal of cartilage repair is to produce a tissue that will fill the defect, integrate with the adjacent articular cartilage and subchondral bone plate, have the same viscoelastic mechanical properties, and maintain its matrix over time without breakdown. That is, the goal is to restore the osteochondral functional unit with a repair tissue that approaches regeneration.

Clinical and experimental evidence shows that damage involving the articular cartilage surface and confined to the cartilage undergoes little restoration. Cartilage has little intrinsic ability to heal. Chondrocytes in mature articular cartilage rarely divide and their density declines with age. In contrast, lesions that extend to the subchondral marrow may heal clinically.[12] Therefore, a cell source for cartilage regeneration or repair must arise from the underlying subchondral bone marrow, the adjacent synovial tissue, or an exogenous source.

Absence of blood supply and endogenous source of new cells contribute to cartilage's incapacity for repair. The typical wound healing response of hemorrhage, fibrin clot formation, and mobilization of cells and growth factors is absent. The only spontaneous repair reaction may occur at the edge of superficial articular cartilage lesions. Articular cartilage is isolated from the subchondral bone marrow cells by the dense subchondral bone and cartilage matrix.

Cartilage repair is dependent on the mobilization of cells derived from the subchondral bone marrow, which include multipotential cells, osteoblasts, chondroblasts, fibroblasts, and hematoprogenitor cells.[13] Therefore, the repair tissue that results may be variable based on the predominant cell line that proliferates and its modulation by local growth factors, cytokines, and the local mechanical environment.

Clinical Repair for Full-Thickness Cartilage Defects

The spectrum of repair tissue is clinically variable, depending on the clinical technique used as well as intrinsic and local factors. Repair tissue may be fibrous tissue, transitional tissue, fibrocartilage, hyaline cartilage, articular cartilage, bone, or a mixture of these tissues.[14] Fibrous tissue consists of fibrocytes and a type I collagen fibrous matrix. Transitional tissue consists of ovoid cells that may produce proteoglycans as well as a fibrous matrix. The matrix may stain positively with safranin O for proteoglycan production. Fibrocartilage consists of round chondrocyte-appearing cells with a type I collagen fibrous matrix. Hyaline cartilage consists of chondrocytes in a matrix of type II collagen and proteoglycans, with a hyaline, ground-glass appearance by light microscopy. The cellular and matrix organization may be different than normal articular cartilage. Articular cartilage resembles normal articular cartilage. Articular cartilage is essentially a regenerating tissue with articular chondrocytes, arranged in the usual palisading columns found in normal articular cartilage, with markers of normal articular cartilage matrix including type II collagen, proteoglycans, etc. A mixture of all these components may be present at a single repair site. The predominant repair tissue type will determine the long-term outcome of the patient. If the majority of the repair tissue is hyaline or articular cartilage, the viscoelastic properties found with a type II collagen framework and proteoglycans will give a durable repair and usually a superior clinical result. Fibrocartilage and fibrous repairs consist of type I collagen, which is usually not as strong as type II collagen and often contains short-chain proteoglycans. Fibrocartilage and fibrous repairs do not maintain a high negative charge density, are soft, and break down (Fig. 2.1).

Factors that may influence the quality of repair tissue noted clinically include acuteness of injury, age, size of defect, ligament stability, axial alignment, and presence or absence of the meniscus.[12,15] In a study conducted by Nehrer and associates[14] (Table 2.1), failed repair tissues were analyzed after three techniques of marrow stimulation: drilling, abrasion, and microfracture. The repair tissues retrieved were composed predominantly of fibrous and fibrocartilaginous tissues. The tissues were soft and degenerating. They had poor mechanical viscoelastic properties even though they filled the defects. The repair tissues clinically failed by 2.5 years after treatment, with an average defect size greater than 3 cm^2. Cartilage defects that were treated by perichondrial grafting had an excellent clinical result early postoperatively. By 4 to 5 years postoperatively, however, the repair tissue had undergone enchondral ossification. The perichondrial chondrocytes had features of hypertrophic chondrocytes, notably type X collagen, a precursor to mineralization (Fig. 2.2). Although those grafts had a high percentage of hyaline cartilage, they also contained bone.

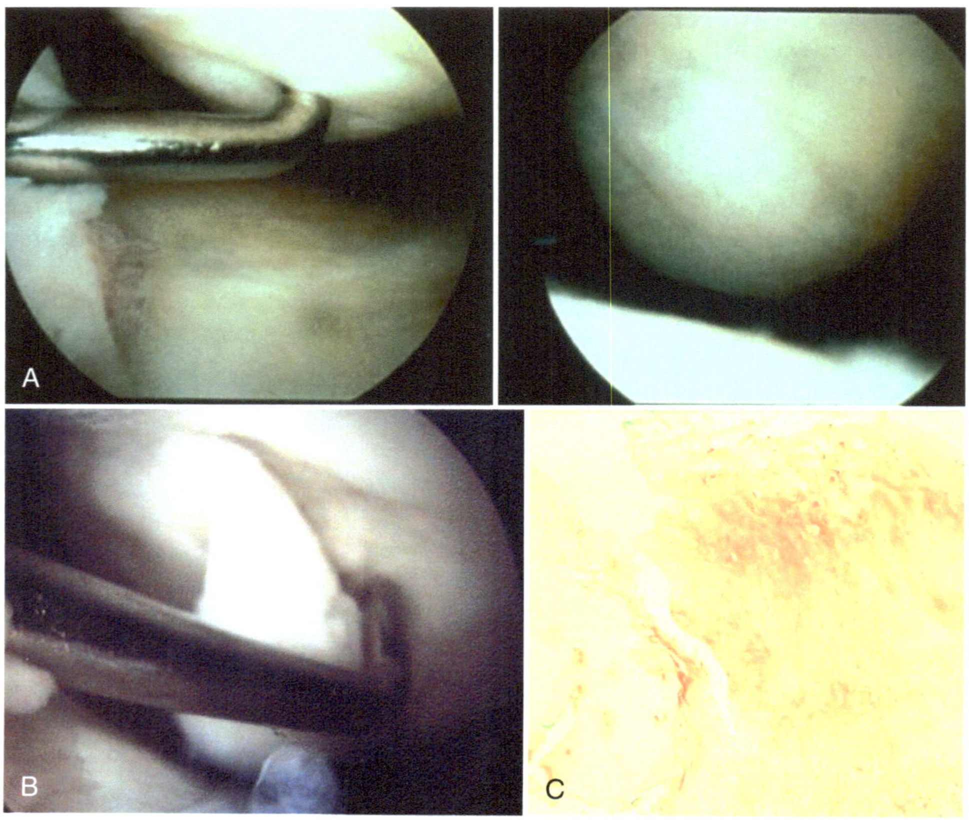

• **Fig. 2.1** (A) Arthroscopic appearance of a symptomatic fibrocartilage repair after drilling. Repair tissue is evident from native articular cartilage. Complete fill of defect with white repair tissue is evident. However, its mechanical properties are insufficient and soft, with resultant symptoms. (B) Arthroscopic appearance of a symptomatic fibrocartilage flap after drilling. Poor integration and mechanically soft tissue have resulted in a poor clinical result. (C) Low-power photomicrograph of retrieved fibrocartilage repair stained for proteoglycans with safranin O. Alternating layers of fibrous and fibrocartilage repair tissue have a porous appearance and a degenerating surface. This human retrieval resulted from a failed arthroscopic abrasion arthroplasty with resultant filled defect and soft repair tissue as shown in (A).

TABLE 2.1 Evaluation of Tissue Retrieved After Failed Articular Cartilage Repair Procedures: Histologic and Immunohistochemical Comparative Analysis

--	Treatment			P value
--	Arthroscopic abrasion arthroplasty ($n = 12$)	Perichondrial rib grafting ($n = 4$)	Autologous chondrocyte implantation ($n = 6$)	$P < .05$ (ANOVA)
Follow-up (months)	21 ± 4	31 ± 8	3 ± 1	--
Tissue Type (%)				
Articular cartilage	2 ± 1	3 ± 2	0	NS
Hyaline cartilage	30 ± 10	47 ± 7	2 ± 1	Sig.
Fibrocartilage	28 ± 7	15 ± 4	6 ± 2	NS
Transition tissue	18 ± 2	12 ± 3	31 ± 7	NS
Fibrous tissue	22 ± 9	4 ± 2	61 ± 9	Sig.
Bone	0	19 ± 6	0	Sig.

Quantities of tissue types for failed cartilage repair procedures (arthroscopic abrasion arthroplasty, perichondrial rib grafting, and autologous chondrocyte implantation) in a human series at various time intervals after treatment are listed. *NS*, Not significant.
From Nehrer S, Spector M, Minas T. Histologic analysis of failed cartilage repair procedures. *Clin Orthop Relat Res*. 1999;365:149-162.

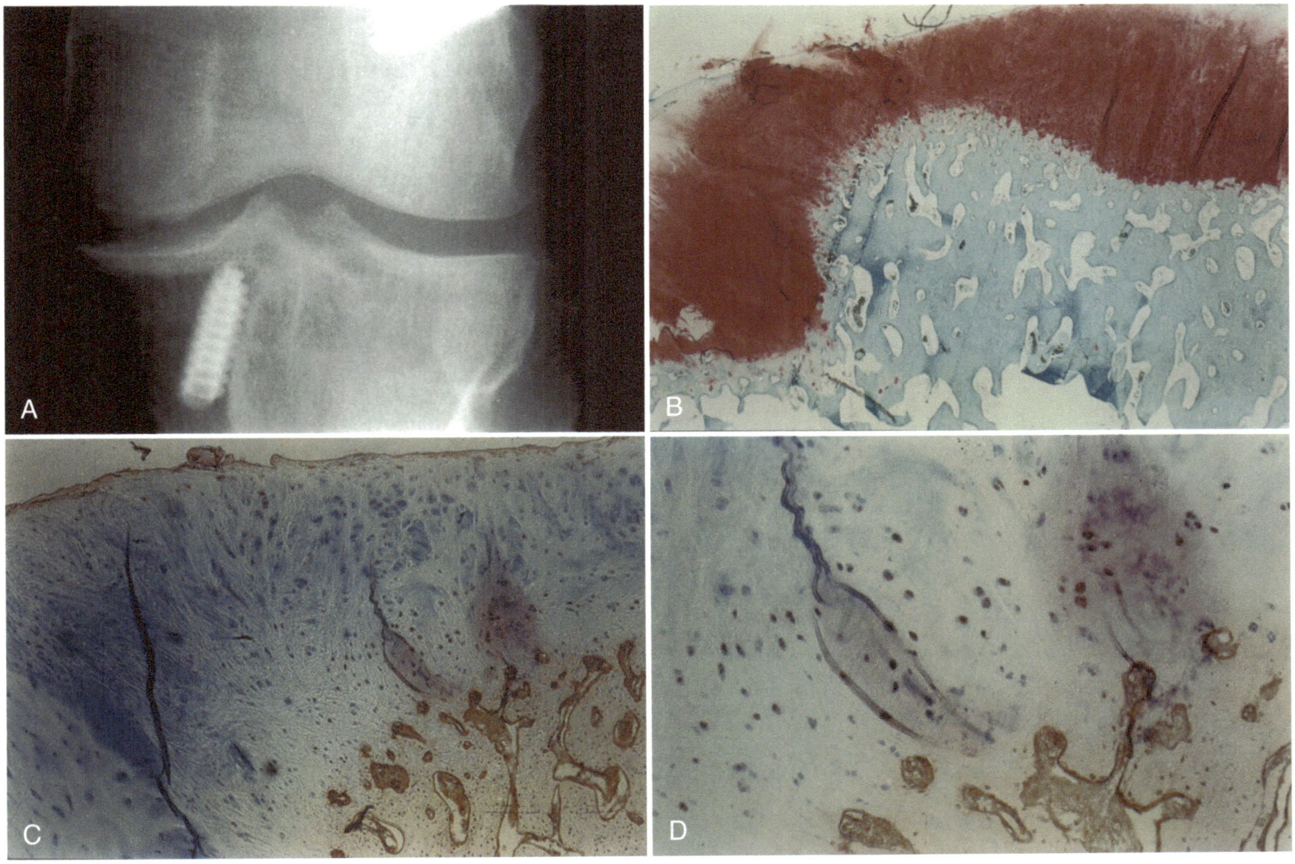

• **Fig. 2.2** (A) X-ray appearance of medial femoral condyle autologous perichondrial graft undergoing ossification. Ossification developed 3 years after cartilage repair, with initial excellent clinical result. Revision cartilage repair with autologous chondrocyte implantation graft resulted in successful clinical outcome. Retrieval of failed perichondrial graft specimen allowed histologic analysis. (B) Low-power photomicrograph of retrieved perichondrial autograft undergoing enchondral ossification stained with safranin O. Notice excellent proteoglycan production as demonstrated by *red staining*. However, an advancing front of bone formation *(blue stain)* will eventually ossify the entire cartilage graft without stabilization with a tidemark. (C) Low-power photomicrograph of antibody staining *(brown)* to type X collagen demonstrating intracellular production of type X collagen as expressed by hypertrophic chondrocytes undergoing enchondral ossification. (D) High-power photomicrograph demonstrating intracellular antibody staining to type X collagen of hypertrophic chondrocytes. This is a common mechanism of failure of perichondrial autografts seen clinically.

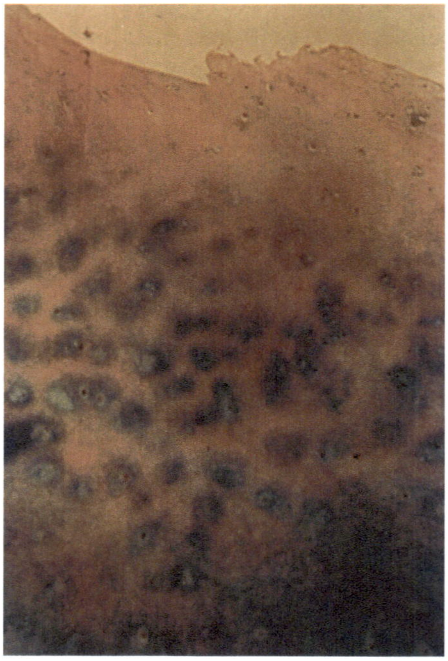

• **Fig. 2.3** High-power photomicrograph of biopsy stained with safranin O of autologous chondrocyte implantation in a human. Note homogeneous ground-glass appearance of matrix and abundant chondrocyte formation.

The autologous chondrocyte implantation grafts that failed did so early (<6 months after implantation) as a result of trauma as the grafts were growing. At this early stage of repair, a high percentage of the repair tissue was fibrous or transitional in nature. Mature autologous chondrocyte implant grafts (>2 years after implantation) may have excellent clinical outcomes, with hyaline cartilage repair having firm viscoelastic properties (Fig. 2.3).

Intrinsic repair in the acute situation is possible by marrow stimulation repair if chondral injury involves the underlying subchondral bone. However, appropriate rehabilitation after injury is critical (Table 2.2). The factors previously described delineating the possibility of a successful repair are important. Rehabilitation after such an injury is also important. However, there may be a critical size of subchondral bone involvement that will result in cystic degeneration rather than repair. This occurs specifically in osteochondritis dissecans or when lesions are deep. A study with experimental osteochondral defects greater than 8 mm in diameter and deep in adult goats demonstrated cystic enlargement of the defects rather than repair.[16] Therefore, repair of osteochondral defects is more complex. A staged reconstruction using autogenous tissues is required. Other options include allogeneic osteochondral reconstruction or autologous-derived tissue engineering solutions (Fig. 2.4).

TABLE 2.2 Clinical Recommendations for Careful Rehabilitation After Autologous Chondrocyte Implantation

	Time		
--	**0–6 Weeks**	**7–12 Weeks**	**>13 Weeks–3 years**
Stage	Proliferation	Transition	Remodeling and maturation
Histology	Rapid proliferation of spindle-shaped cells with defect fill. Mostly type I collagen with early formation of colonies of chondrocytes forming type II collagen.	Matrix formation, mostly chondrocytes producing type II collagen and proteoglycans Poor integration to underlying bone and cartilage	Ongoing remodeling of matrix with reorganization and quantity of type II collagen, and integration to bone (arcades of Benninghoff) and adjacent host cartilage Large-chain aggregates of proteoglycans, with increased water content of cartilage
Viscoelastic arthroscopic appearance	Filled, soft, white tissue	Jelly-like firmness, with "wavelike" motion when probed, not yet firm and integrated to underlying bone	Firm "indentable" but not "wave-like" when probed 4–6 months after autologous chondrocyte transplantation Graft whiter than host cartilage and may demonstrate periosteal hypertrophy (20%) Equal firmness to host cartilage 9–18 months after autologous chondrocyte transplantation
Activity level	• CPM starts 6 hours after surgery for 6–8 hours/day for 6 weeks • Touch WB • Isometric muscle exercises and ROM	• Discontinue CPM • Active ROM • Partial graduated WB to full WB by 12 weeks • Functional muscle usage, stationary bicycle, treadmill	• Discontinue assistive devices 4–5 months postoperatively if free of pain, catching, swelling • Distance walking, resistance walking • Nonpivoting running at 9–12 months • Pivoting allowed at 14–18 months

From Minas T, Peterson LL. Autologous chondrocyte transplantation. *Oper Tech Sports Med*. 2000;8:144-157.
Clinical recommendations made for careful rehabilitation after autologous chondrocyte implantation based on correlative observations on the basic science repair process learned from a canine model and arthroscopic evaluations in humans (with biopsies) at various stages of repair to determine viscoelastic mechanical maturation over time and prevent premature overloading of healing grafts. *CPM*, Continuous passive motion; *ROM*, range of motion; *WB*, weight bearing.

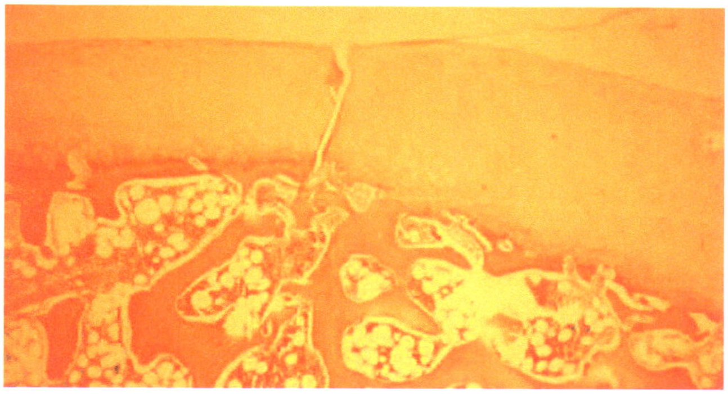

• **Fig. 2.4** Low-power photomicrograph of canine biopsy specimen at the junction of the osteochondral graft transfer and native cartilage margin. Note the persistent cleft without integration at the cartilage junctures and the various thicknesses of articular cartilage with the different tidemark junctures. Excellent bony remodeling is noted in the subchondral bone marrow. (Courtesy Laszlo Hangody, MD, Budapest, Hungary.)

Experimental Models and Usefulness

Selection of an appropriate animal model to assess the mechanisms and outcomes of procedures for cartilage repair has been problematic. The ideal is a skeletally mature animal with anatomic and morphologic similarities to the human clinical situation. Inclusion of multiple control groups is essential to assess the hypothesis that a certain treatment is superior. In this way the relative value of a therapy can be assessed but with limited translation to humans. However, this is not always feasible because bilateral simultaneous treatments may not be ethically or physiologically sound for the repair model. The duration of the experiment needed to confirm endurance of cartilage repair and prevention of osteoarthritis usually is cost prohibitive.

Use of periosteum to treat full-thickness chondral defects under the influence of continuous passive motion has been investigated in a rabbit model.[17] An elegant experiment demonstrated that periosteum was capable of undergoing neochondrogenesis and that, under the influence of continuous passive motion, the quality of the repair tissue was similar to hyaline cartilage.

The translation of this model to demonstrate proof of principle in humans has not been fully realized.[18,19] Whether the rabbit is capable of an unusually robust healing response and whether technical differences in the experimental methodology account for unpredictable results in patients are not known.

The technique of autologous chondrocyte implantation has been controversial.[20–23] Much of the controversy apparently has been due to the conflicting results with two different animal models. The Swedish model was based on a pilot study performed in patellar chondral defects in rabbits.[24] The rabbit model showed that the implanted in vitro–labeled chondrocytes were largely responsible for the repair tissue that developed to fill chondral defects. The repair tissue was superior to that of periosteum alone.

The quality and quantity of repair tissues remained consistently higher in the rabbit model when compared to empty defects, periosteum, periosteum plus autologous

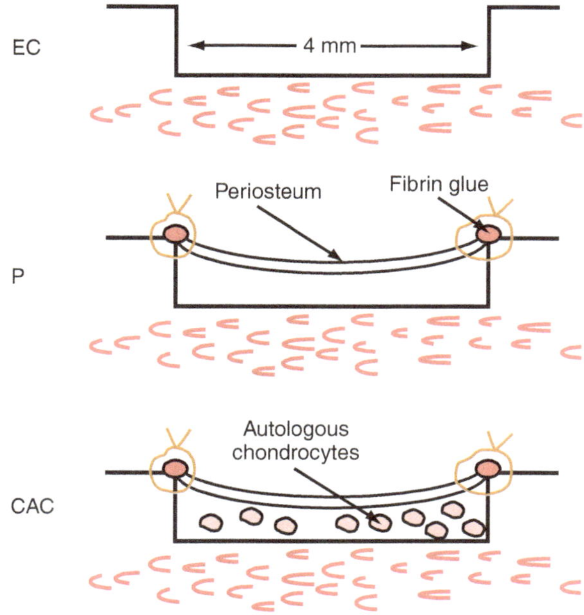

• **Fig. 2.5** Schematic representation of canine experiment evaluating the effect of autologous chondrocyte implantation using cultured articular chondrocytes (CAC), versus periosteal resurfacing alone (P), versus empty control (EC), 4-mm defect. The periosteum was microsutured using absorbable suture to the native articular margins with the cambium layer of periosteum facing the bony surface. The margins were then sealed with autologous fibrin glue. The animal was protected with an external fixation device for 10 days and then allowed to bear weight as tolerated. Two chondral defects were made per knee in the femoral sulcus or the trochlea (see Fig. 2.6).

chondrocytes, and carbon fiber pads plus autologous chondrocytes.[25] A similar study was performed in a rabbit model with bilateral patellar chondral defects, unlike the human situation in which defects are most commonly found on the femoral condyles.

When the experiment was completed in a canine model using the femoral sulcus, the results comparing empty defects, periosteum, and periosteum plus autologous chondrocytes were similar in the early postoperative period (<6 months) but were uniformly osteoarthritic in the long term (12–18 months).[13,26] No treatment difference could be detected. A clear species difference between rabbit and dog was seen at 12 months (Figs. 2.5–2.12).

Translational Research

It may be that there is no perfect animal model with repair characteristics similar to the human species. However, new technologies and treatment options may be evaluated in an animal model with control groups. In this way, the efficacy of repair may be assessed. In general, proof of principle involves the progression of scientific methodology from in vitro methods to small animal experimentation to larger animal validation prior to human clinical trials and is the desired scientific method. The hypotheses for the scientific methods are derived from clinical problems or failures

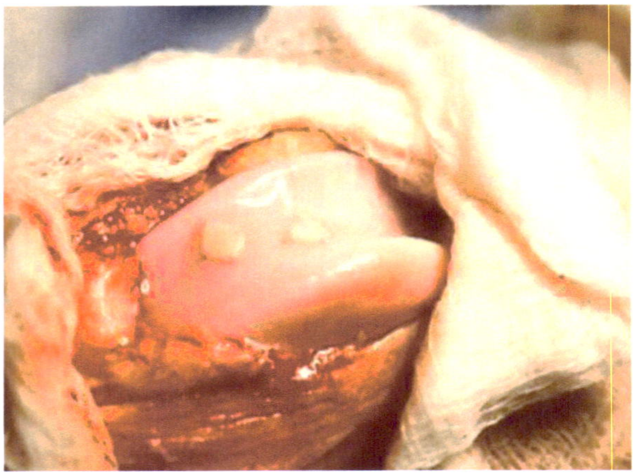

• **Fig. 2.6** Gross appearance of periosteal patches sutured to chondral defects undergoing autologous chondrocyte implantation on the femoral sulcus in a canine model. The chondral defects measured 4 mm in diameter.

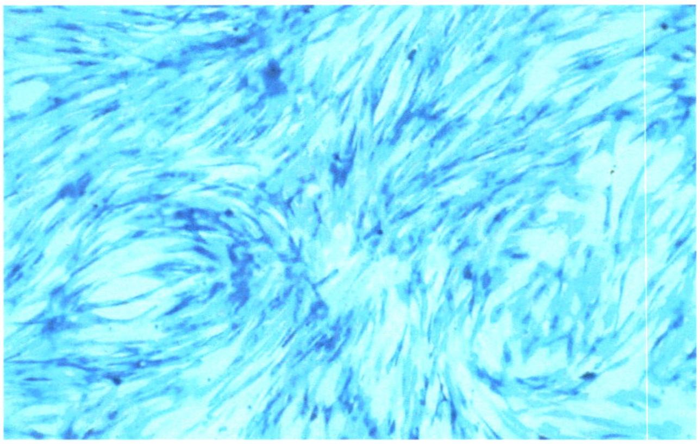

• **Fig. 2.7** High-power photomicrograph of beta-galactosidase–labeled reporter gene *(blue)* in chondrocyte culture in monolayer approaching confluence. The reporter gene allows tracking of implanted chondrocytes over time. The label was no longer effective after 3 months in vivo.

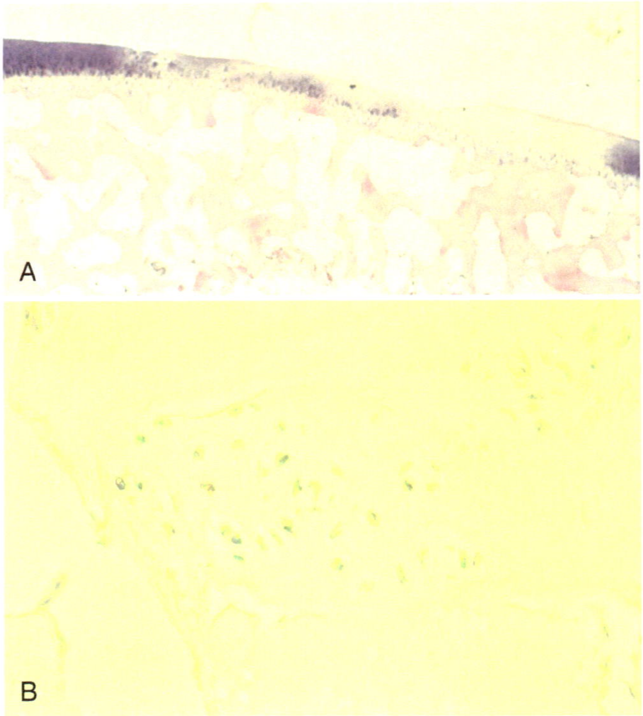

• **Fig. 2.8** (A) Low-power histologic section with hematoxylin and eosin staining of canine defect treated by autologous chondrocyte implantation at 3 months. The defect appears filled but has poor staining characteristics, although the repair tissue appears to consist predominantly of cellular chondrocytes. (B) High-power photomicrograph of area that is poorly staining in (A), demonstrating the persistence of beta-galactosidase reporter gene labeling of implanted chondrocytes 3 months after implantation. This image demonstrates that the implanted chondrocytes are responsible for the repair tissue and not local cellular repair.

of existing techniques. The methodology of pursuing a hypothesis rendered from a clinical situation taken to the basic science laboratory is the basis of translational research. The topic of cartilage repair is an especially difficult clinical problem and field. The concept of translational research is especially suited in the field of cartilage repair.

State of the Art

Tissue Engineering

Because cartilage is a relatively simple tissue because of its cellular homogeneity and avascularity, it has been a model for research of in vitro engineered tissues.[27] Progress has been slow and obstructed on several levels. The adult chondrocyte has limited capacity for proliferation and has both catabolic and anabolic functions. These metabolic features must be optimized and controlled for engineered tissue to endure. The motivation for tissue engineering is to promote biologic repair or regeneration. Conceptual approaches include implantation of inert substitutes for discontinuities or missing parts, drug or matrix treatments to stimulate tissue regeneration, autogenous cell or tissue transfer, and in vitro production of tissues or tissue equivalents for implantation. Three considerations when designing a construct for engineered tissue are (1) the source of cells, if any; (2) the nature of the carrier or scaffold; and (3) the use, if any, of genes, biochemical and biomechanical factors, or adjuvants.

Interestingly, cultured chondrocytes under the influence of constant hydrostatic pressure perfusion versus intermittent perfusion demonstrate improved cartilage matrix production (Fig. 2.13). Experimental work was performed at our laboratory (Skeletal Biology Laboratory, Orthopedic Research, Cartilage Repair Center, Brigham and Women's Hospital, and Harvard Medical School, Boston, MA) to assess this effect in an in vivo evaluation of cartilage repair in an animal model (Minas et al., Autologous Cartilage Repair in Rabbits with Chondrocytes in 3D Collagen Sponges Precultured with Hydrostatic Pressure, unpublished data).

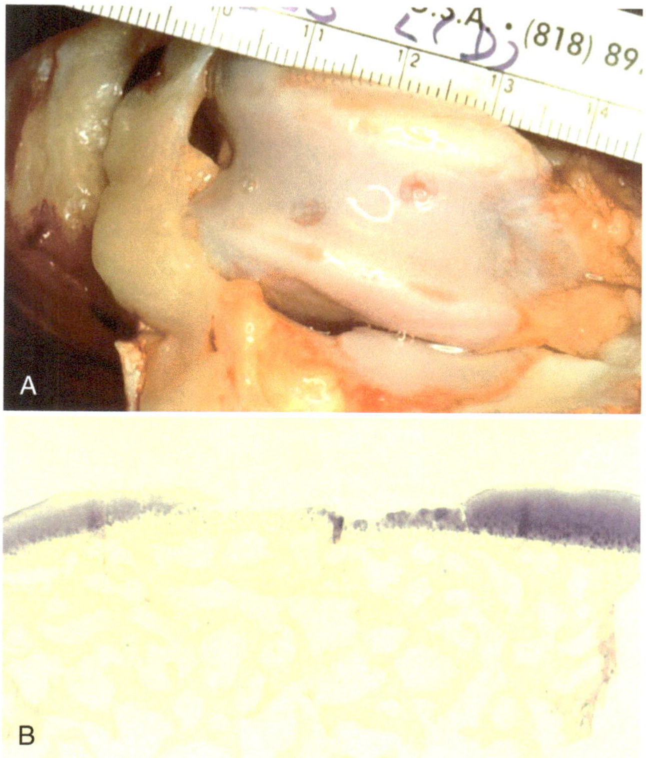

• **Fig. 2.9** (A) Gross appearance of empty canine defects 6 months after treatment. Minimal repair tissue is seen around the margins. (B) Low-power histologic section with hematoxylin and eosin staining of canine defect as control defect at 6 months. Note lack of repair tissue fill except around the margins.

The goal of our study was to assess a collagen sponge seeded with autologous cultured chondrocytes under the influence of hydrostatic pressure as a tissue-engineered construct, versus the gold standard of autologous cultured chondrocyte implantation under a periosteal flap, versus control groups of empty defect, empty sponge, periosteum without cells. Information on the treatment groups is given in Table 2.3.

Seven-month-old New Zealand white male rabbits were used in the study. After a medial parapatellar incision was made, the patella was dislocated laterally, and a 3-mm-diameter defect was created in the center of the patella using a circular stainless-steel punch. Cartilage tissue was harvested using a beaver blade and a sharp edge of host cartilage was created using a curette. The defects were cylindrical in shape and extended over the tide mark. The knee was closed.

Chondrocyte Isolation. The cartilage slices were harvested and digested. The isolated chondrocytes were seeded to T-25 culture flasks and incubated for 6 days. The chondrocytes were harvested using trypsin and 300,000 cells in 25 μL of medium were injected into collagen sponges. The sponges were incubated using a pressure/perfusion culture system at 0.7 MPa, 0.015 Hz, and 0.3 mL/min for 7 days (Fig. 2.13A).

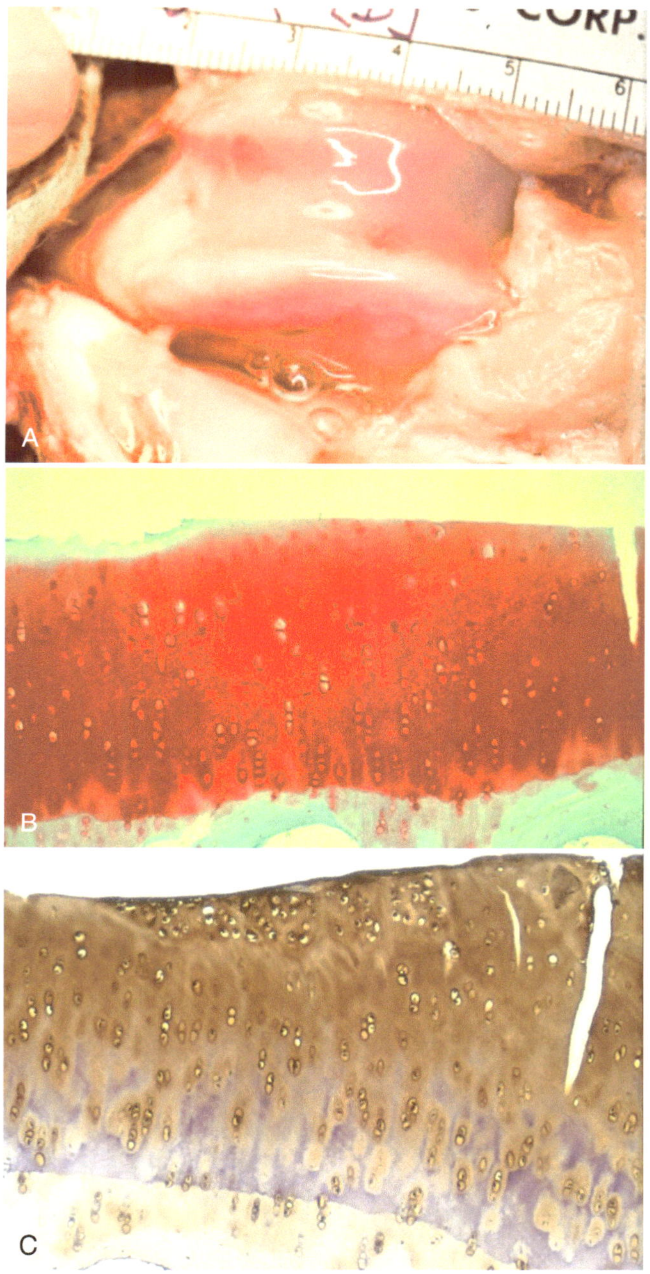

• **Fig. 2.10** (A) Gross appearance of defects in a canine model 6 months after treatment with autologous chondrocytes. Note the complete fill and smoothness of the surface. (B) High-power photomicrograph with safranin O staining of retrieved tissue shown in (A). Hyaline cartilage repair tissue with deep proteoglycan staining, palisading chondrocyte arrangement, and excellent subchondral bone integration with tidemark formation are seen. However, note the cleft to the far right of the cartilage integration. This is a common finding early after treatment with autologous chondrocyte implantation grafting. (C) Same specimen stained with antibody to type II collagen *(brown)*. Note uniform density of staining.

Engineered Cartilage Implantation

The second operation was performed after 2 weeks of in vitro monolayer culture and pressure/perfusion culture. A full-thickness defect (3-mm diameter and over the

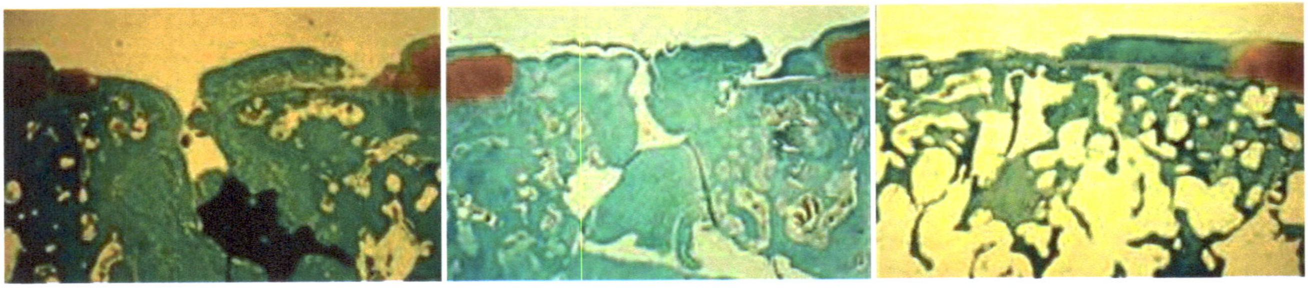

• **Fig. 2.11** Low-power photomicrographs of empty defect *(left)*, periosteum alone *(center)*, and autologous chondrocyte implantation *(right)* in canine experiment 12 months postimplantation. The worst-case scenario demonstrates collapse of the subchondral bone plate with fibrous tissue formation in an empty defect in both the empty control and periosteum alone groups. The autologous chondrocyte implantation treatment group similarly has a poor repair tissue that is delaminating, but the subchondral bone is intact. Difference between the three treatments could not be graded by independent observation by a histologist.

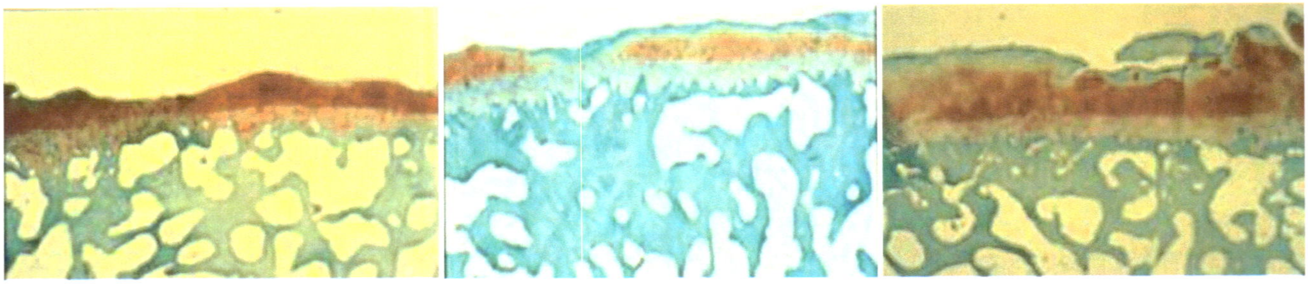

• **Fig. 2.12** Low-power photomicrographs of the same treatments as shown in Fig. 2.11. In the best-case scenario, repair tissue in all three treatment arms could not be graded as different. No difference in treatment effect was apparent. The canine model for cartilage repair for periods of time greater than 12 months demonstrated spontaneous repair or degeneration to a similar treatment end point. However, autologous chondrocyte implantation for less than 6 months demonstrated a superior repair.

TABLE 2.3 Treatment Groups

Group	Left knee	Right knee
1	Periosteum + autologous cultured chondrocytes	Periosteum
2	Periosteum + autologous cultured chondrocytes	Empty defect
3	Engineered cartilage	Periosteum + autologous cultured chondrocytes
4	Engineered cartilage	Collagen sponge control
5	Allo-engineered cartilage	Periosteum + allo-autologous cultured chondrocytes

tidemark) through the articular cartilage was created in the femoral weight-bearing condyle using a circular stainless steel punch. The lesion produced was a deep defect that extended through all chondral layers into the calcified zone. It was termed a *full-thickness lesion* to distinguish it from an osteochondral bone plate.

Under aseptic conditions, the autologous cartilage was trimmed using a 4-mm punch and directly sutured into the defect. The knee was closed in separate layers.

Rabbits from each treatment group (see Table 2.3) were euthanized at time points of 4 weeks and 12 weeks. The tissue around the defect was harvested for histologic analysis.

Histologic Evaluation. The sections were graded as poor, fair, good, or excellent by three blinded individuals.

Results. Sponges with chondrocytes that were cultured for 5 days with hydrostatic pressure accumulated more metachromatic matrix than did those cultured without hydrostatic pressure.

Clinically, some of the control empty defects and those with cell-free collagen sponges were partially filled, but the collagen sponge + cells scored consistently higher than the other treatment groups.

Histologically, most of the empty controls showed poor repair (Fig. 2.14). Collagen sponge + cells showed better

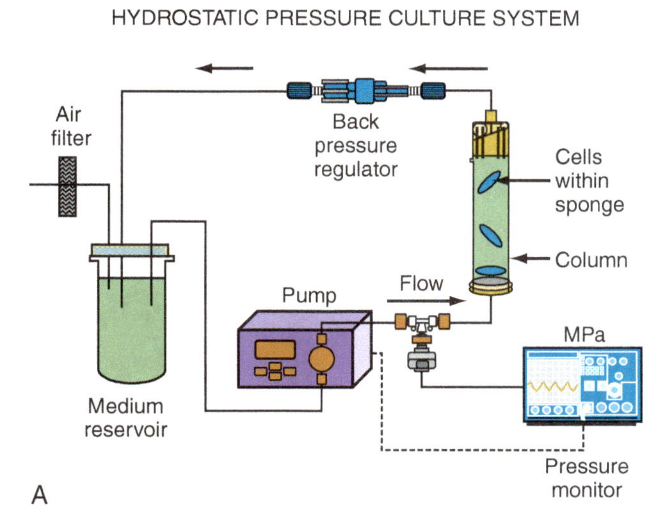

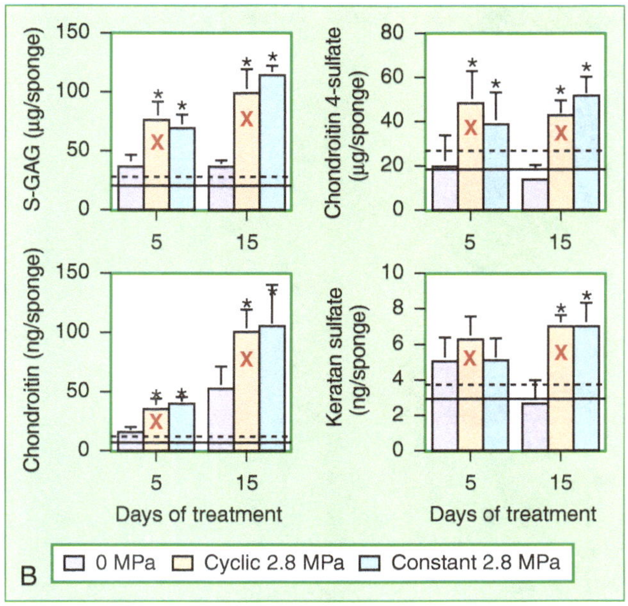

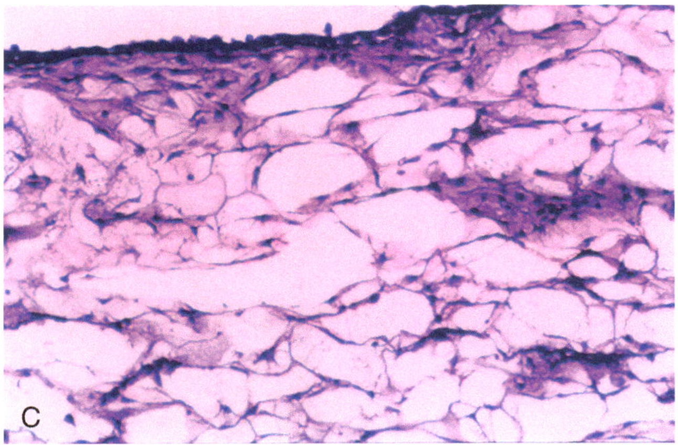

• **Fig. 2.13** (A) Illustration of hydrostatic pressure culture system used for the experimentation described in text to produce a tissue-engineered cartilage implant evaluated in the New Zealand rabbit model. (B) Graphs which demonstrate the production of proteoglycan macromolecules found in articular cartilage increase with time under pressure perfusion which is improved with constant perfusion versus intermittent perfusion or no pressure. (C) Photomicrograph of type I collagen sponge seated with autologous rabbit chondrocytes under the influence of 0.7-MPa constant pressure perfusion (magnification ×50). Note distribution of cells throughout the sponge producing early matrix 7 days after onset of perfusion. (A from Mizuno S, Ushida T, Tateishi T, Glowacki J. Effects of physical stimulation on chondrogenesis in vitro. *Mat Sci Eng C.* 1998;6:301-306. B from Mizuno S, Tateishi T, Ushida T, Glowacki J. Hydrostatic fluid pressure enhances matrix synthesis and accumulation by bovine chondrocytes in three-dimensional culture. *J Cell Physiol.* 2002;193:319-327.)

repair than collagen sponge alone. Collagen sponge + cells were similar to the autologous chondrocyte implantation group.

We concluded that tissue-engineered cartilage demonstrated histologic repair superior or similar to that of autologous chondrocyte implantation and was better than the controls of empty defect, periosteum alone, or empty sponge. However, some of the empty sponge defects did demonstrate a reasonable repair tissue migration into the sponge and partial repair.

From an experimental translational research model, this work was continued and was the basis for the formation of a clinically relevant human cartilage repair trial (see the NeoCart system in Chapter 16).

Effect of Mechanical Stress on hACs

Recently, various cell culture technologies using mechanical stimuli have been developed to engineer chondrocyte constructs for improving clinical outcomes. Using an engineering strategy, the application of cyclic pure hydrostatic pressure (HP) was shown to be effective on anabolic turnover by chondrocytes. Previous studies demonstrated that intermittent HP-loading (1-10 MPa, 0.5-1 Hz, 4 hours per day for 4 days) increased Col-2 and Agg expressions by monolayer cultures of bACs or hACs compared with a single HP-loading.[28–31] reference 33 For further optimization of extracellular matrix synthesis and accumulation, a repetitive hydrostatic pressure–atmospheric pressure (HP-AP) regimen was investigated using our well-validated culture system.[31–33] We focused on the effects of HP-AP (HP-loading followed by AP regimen, Fig. 2.15) on anabolic (Aggrecan, Col-2), catabolic (MMP-13), and chondroprotective (TIMP-2) activities by hACs seeded within a 3D collagen gel/sponge scaffold to improve accumulation of ECM within chondrocyte constructs. Our data indicated that the HP-AP upregulated anabolic function, whereas it downregulated catabolic function with hACs by day 14 (Fig. 2.16). Additionally, intense accumulation of Col-2 in HP-AP and Rep HP-AP (Fig. 2.17) and significantly greater accumulation of sulfated glycosaminoglycan (S-GAG) in HP-AP were observed (Fig. 2.18). These characteristics suggested that HP-AP may be beneficial to engineer a mature chondrocyte construct in vitro prior to implantation.[34]

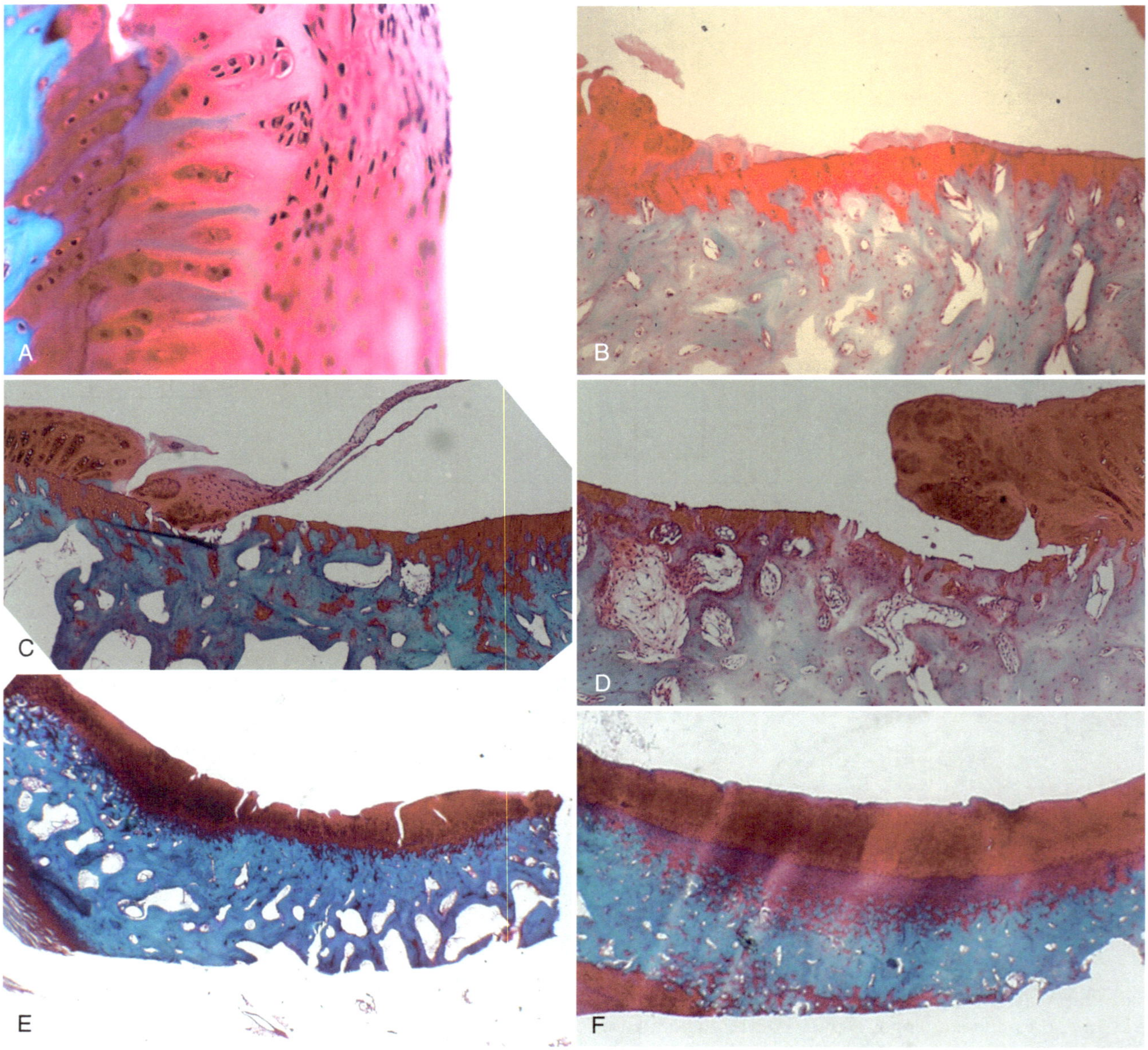

• **Fig. 2.14** (A) One-month patellar defect of tissue-engineered implant in a New Zealand rabbit (safranin O staining, magnification ×100). Note excellent integration, fill, and cellular proliferation within the defect. (B) Three-month patellar empty defect (magnification ×25). Note complete absence of repair tissue in the defect except for the margins. (C) Three-month patellar defect repaired with an empty sponge. Poor filling and only marginal repair are seen. (D) Three-month patellar defect repaired with periosteum alone without cells. No tissue repair is seen except for the margins of the defect. (E) Three-month patellar defect repaired with autologous chondrocyte implantation under a periosteal patch. Excellent cellular response in the defect with fill and subchondral bone integration are seen. Some minor fissuring at the edges of the defect has occurred. (F) Tissue-engineered cartilage implant produced under the influence of constant hydrostatic pressure perfusion of a collagen sponge implanted into a 4-mm diameter chondral defect. Excellent fill, integration, and proteoglycan staining with cellular proliferation and organization are seen.

Additionally, as any kind of engineered chondrocytes construct is exposed to compressive stress caused by weight bearing and joint loading after implantation, the effects of compressive stresses that included HP and deviatoric stress (DS) were evaluated. These are theoretically independent but practically coexist in articular cartilage. Results showed that changes in HP alone, DS alone, and combined HP and DS followed by offloading altered the cell proliferation capacity and metabolism of ESM of hACs within an agarose hydrogel (Fig. 2.19). HP will be useful to stimulate production of cartilage ECMs within a cell construct, whereas DS may have a catabolic role on the ECM.[35] Understanding the mechanisms underlying HP and DS in chondrocyte metabolism and proliferation will broaden treatment strategies including stem cell therapy for osteoarthritis (Fig. 2.20).

Cell Based

One of the main components of cartilage tissue engineering is cells. In general, chondrocytes, stem cells, genetically modified cells, and fibroblasts have been tested in cartilage tissue engineering. However, chondrocytes and stem cells are the main chondrogenic cells in cartilage regeneration and engineering.

Autologous chondrocyte implantation has been shown to be a promising treatment over a long-term follow-up. Mesenchymal stem cells (MSCs) are multipotent cells that can be differentiated into various cells, including osteoblasts, adipocytes, chondrocytes, as well as neuronal and myogenic cells. MSCs are isolated from adipose tissue, bone marrow, synovial membrane, muscle, and periosteum.

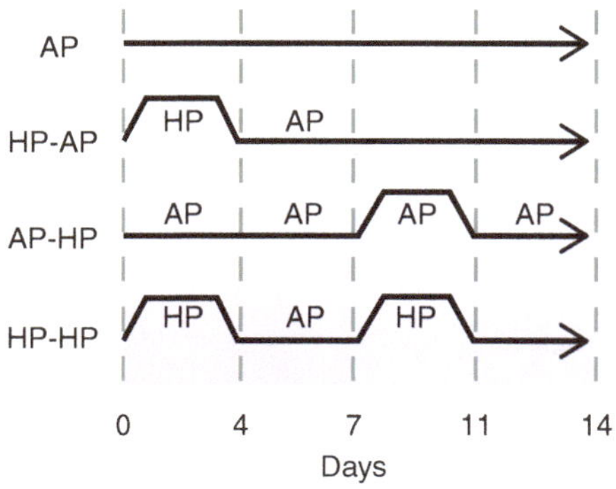

• **Fig. 2.15** The loading regimen of application of HP and AP. *AP*, atmospheric pressure *HP*; hydrostatic pressure.

Recently, the use of human induced pluripotent stem cells (hiPSCs) has been reported. hiPSCs are obtained from somatic cells by reprogramming transcription factors (SCX2, Oct4, Myc and Klf4). The other type of cells includes embryonic stem cells (ESCs). Despite their usefulness in cartilage tissue engineering, the extraction of these cells is subject to ethical and political issues. Additionally, undifferentiated ESCs can cause tumors and increase the risk of developing teratomas in the body, which is another limitation of the use of these potent cells.

Gene Therapy

Bioactive proteins are challenging to apply effectively; however, gene transfer approaches are being developed to provide their sustained synthesis at transferred sites. Advances in gene transfer technology have been translated to clinical applications. Proof of principle has been demonstrated for in vivo and ex vivo transfection of genes into articular chondrocytes. Efficient transfection requires vectors, materials, or methods to promote uptake and expression of the gene of interest. In principle, different methods may result in transient or more enduring expression of the gene product. For chondrocytes, some of the useful genes include insulin-like growth factor-I, transforming growth factor-α, and IL-1 receptor antagonist. Although promising preclinical data are

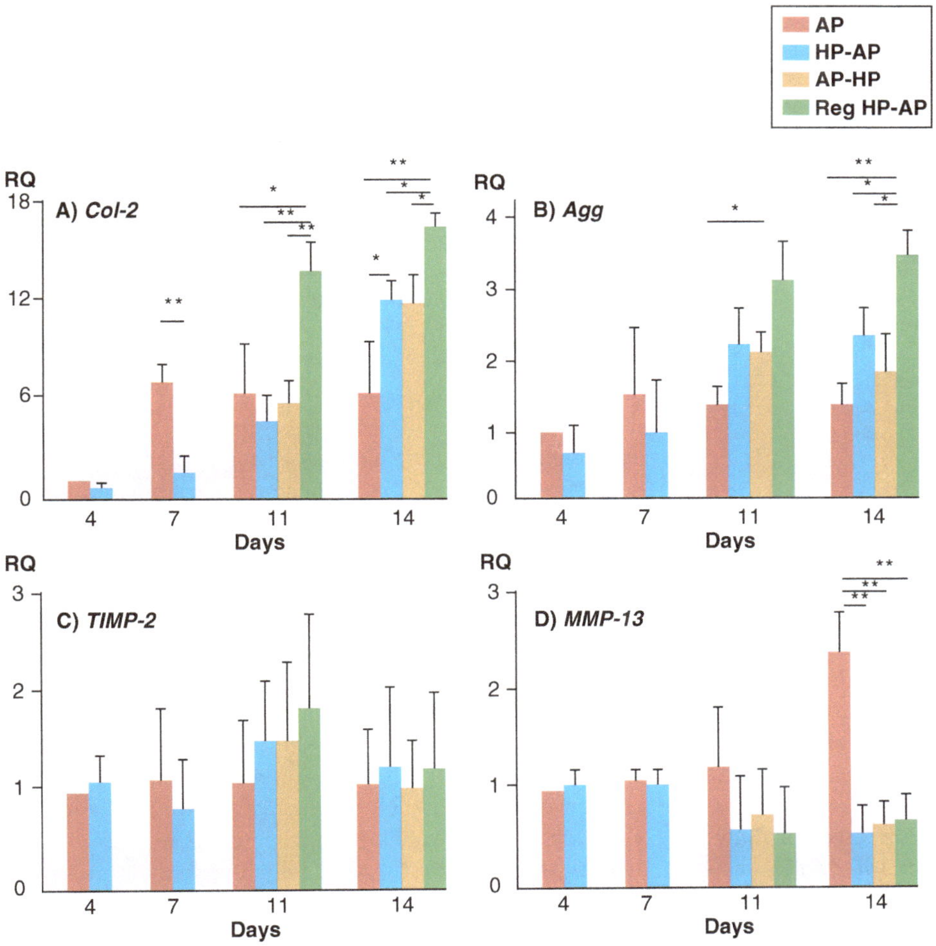

• **Fig. 2.16** Relative quantity (RQ) of chondrocyte phenotype, chondroprotective, and degenerative markers. (A) Col-2, (B) Agg, (C) TIMP-2, and (D) MMP-13 expression compared with each gene expression under atmospheric pressure (AP) at each time point (AP at day 4 as a control of value 1.0). Asterisks indicate significant difference among groups (*P <.05, **P <.01). Error bar indicates SD.

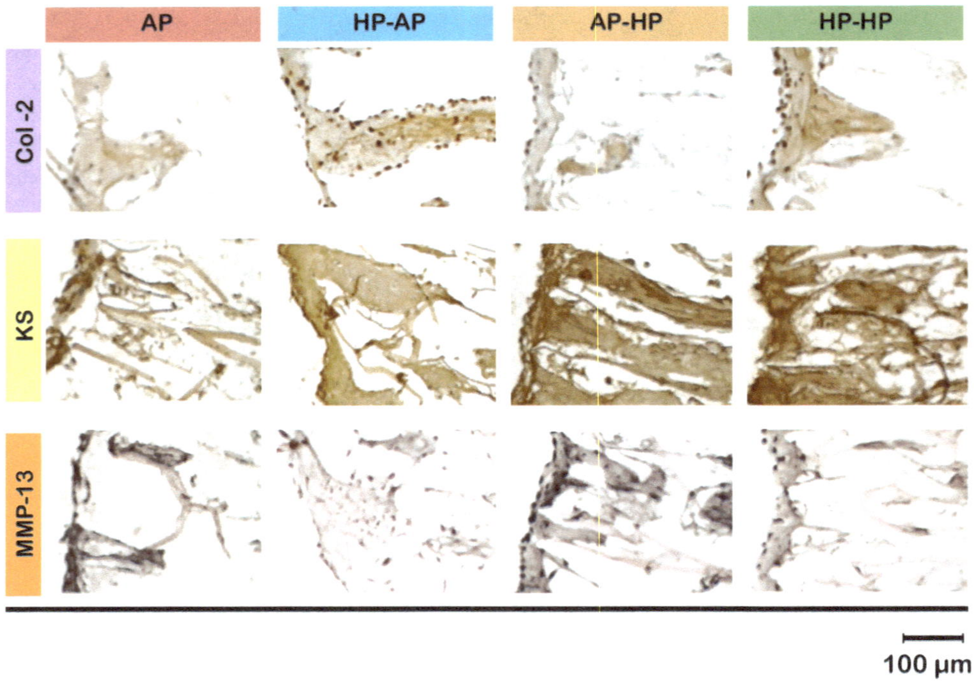

• **Fig. 2.17** Immunohistology of human articular chondrocytes (hACs) within a collagen sponge at day 14. Intense accumulation of Col-2 was seen in the construct in HP-AP and Rep HP-AP compared with AP-HP and AP. *AP*, Atmospheric pressure; *Col-2*, collagen type II; HP, hydrostatic pressure; *KS*, keratan sulfate; MMP-13, matrixmetalloproteinase-13.

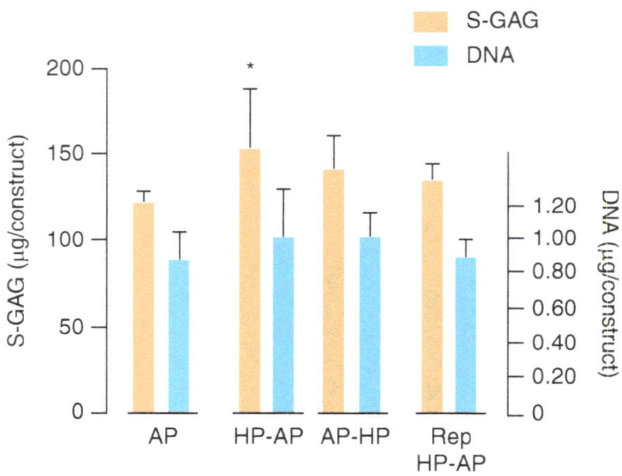

• **Fig. 2.18** Accumulation of sulfated glycosaminoglycan (S-GAG) and DNA at day 14. **P* <.05. Error bar indicates SD. *AP*, Atmospheric pressure (no HP); *HP*, hydrostatic pressure (0.5 MPa, 0.5 Hz).

arising, the concept of genetic approach needs to be proven by the future clinical researches.

Materials

Delivery of simple cell suspensions is of limited value in musculoskeletal applications because of the requirement for cells to be retained at the desired site. Isolated chondrocytes lack adherence to lesion sites and suspensions may produce fibrocartilage or small foci of cartilage. Fluid carriers or three-dimensional scaffolds can be used for delivery and retention of cells. Popular natural hydrogels such as alginates, fibrin, denatured collagen gels, hyaluronan, and admixtures are useful for containing or immobilizing cell suspensions. In addition to their important function as a carrier of cells, three-dimensional scaffolds are useful for defining the space for new tissue and potentially for enhancing the maturation and function of regenerated tissue. Candidate scaffolds include natural polymeric materials such as collagen lattices, synthetic polymers, biodegradable polymers, and polymers with adsorbed proteins or immobilized functional groups.

The key requirements of bioresorbable materials are that (1) their rates of degradation must be compatible with the intended use and (2) the products of their degradation must be nontoxic. Of the synthetic materials, polyglycolic acid, polylactic acid, and their copolymers are most widely studied.

Future Directions

Although novel technologies are being developed, treatment of cartilage lesions is still challenging. Combination of different approaches, including efficiently differentiated chondrocytes, advanced scaffolds, and gene transfer might greatly improve the regeneration of articular cartilage. The ultimate goal of cartilage repair is to delay progression of OA and to avoid arthroplasty. In addition to treating focal chondral defect, biologic environment of the knee joint needs to be considered. To reach this ultimate goal, joint homeostasis is the important key to successful cartilage repair as well as delay progression of OA. As an augmentation, therefore, the concomitant use of PRP, bone marrow aspirates, and stem cells with surgical cartilage repair procedures are presently investigated in clinical studies, which possibly improves the biological environment of the knee and leads to satisfactory outcomes. Future well-designed, randomized, double-blind,

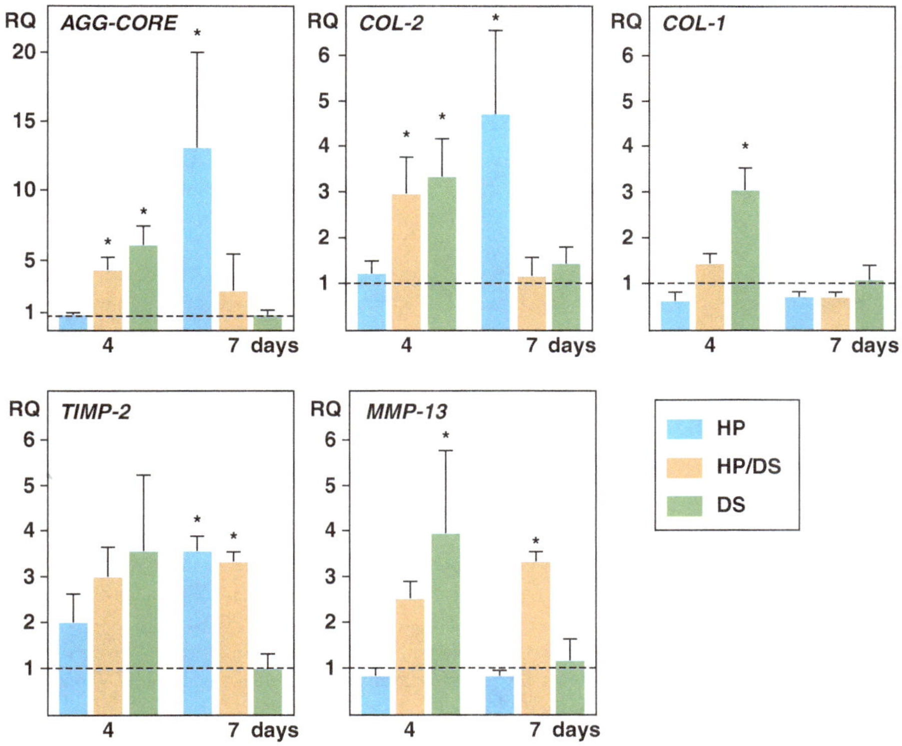

• **Fig. 2.19** Gene expression profiles by human articular chondrocytes in response to hydrostatic pressure (HP) alone, combined HP and deviatoric stress (DS), and DS alone. Relative quantity (RQ) of aggrecan core protein (AGG-CORE), collagen type II (COL-2), collagen type I (COL-1), tissue inhibitor for metalloproteinase-II (TIMP-2), and matrix metalloproteinase-13 (MMP-13) expression compared with no-stress control normalized as value 1.0 at each time point. Asterisks indicate $P < .05$ versus no stress. Means ± SD ($n = 3$).

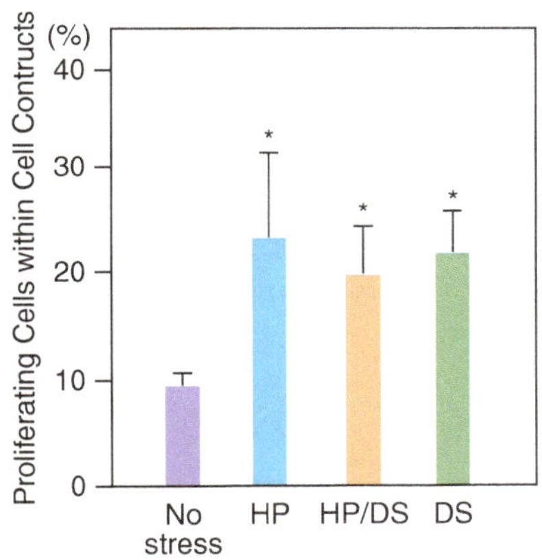

• **Fig. 2.20** Proliferating cells within the cell construct stained with antibody against proliferating cell nuclear antigen (PCNA) at Day 7, incubated with HP, HP/DS, and DS, expressed as percentage (*$P < .05$). *HP*, Hydrostatic pressure; *DS*, deviatoric stress.

long-term studies are necessary to confirm the best treatment in this field.

References

1. Stockwell RA, Meachim G. The chondrocytes. In: Freeman MAR, ed. *Adult Articular Cartilage*. Kent: Pitman Medical; 1979; 69–144.
2. Mankin HJ, Mos VW, Buckwalter JA, Iannotti JP, Ratcliffe A. Articular cartilage structure, composition and function. In: Buckwalter JA, Einhorn TA, Simon SR, eds. *Orthopaedic Basic Science*. Rosemont, IL: American Academy of Orthopaedic Surgeons; 2000.
3. Seibel MJ, Robbins SP, Bilezikian JP, eds. *Dynamics of Bone and Cartilage Metabolism*. San Diego: Academic Press; 1999.
4. Mow VC, Ratcliffe A. Structure and function of articular cartilage and meniscus. In: Mow VC, Hayes WC, eds. *Basic Orthopaedic Biomechanics*. Philadelphia: Lippincott-Raven Publishers; 1997.
5. Noyes FR, Bassett RW, et al. Arthroscopy in acute traumatic hemarthrosis of the knee: incidence of anterior cruciate tears and other injuries. *J Bone Joint Surg Am*. 1980;62:687–695.
6. Curl W, Krome J, et al. Cartilage injuries: a review of 31,516 knee arthroscopies. *Arthroscopy*. 1997;13:456–460.
7. Messner K, Maletius W. The long-term prognosis for severe damage to weight-bearing cartilage in the knee. A 14-year clinical and radiographic follow-up in 28 young athletes. *Acta Orthop Scand*. 1996;67:165–168.
8. Minas T, Nehrer S. Current concepts in the treatment of cartilage defects. *Orthopedics*. 1997;20:525–538.
9. Repo RU, Finlay J. Survival of articular cartilage after controlled impact. *J Bone Joint Surg Am*. 1977;59:1068–1076.
10. Johnson DL, Urban WP, Caborn NNM, Carlson C, Van Arthros W. February 25, 1996. *Articular cartilage pathology associated with MRI detected "bone bruises" after ACL rupture*. American Academy of Orthopaedic Surgeons Society for Sports Medicine Specialty Day: Atlanta, February 25, 1996.
11. Sahlström A, Johnell O, Redlund-Johnell I. The natural course of arthrosis of the knee. *Clin Orthop Relat Res*. 1997;40:152–157.
12. Dzioba RB. The classification and treatment of acute articular cartilage lesions. *Arthroscopy*. 1988;4:72–80.
13. Breinan H, Minas T, Hsu HP, et al. Effect of cultured articular chondrocytes on repair of chondral defects in a canine model. *J Bone Joint Surg Am*. 1997;79:1439–1451.

14. Nehrer S, Spector M, Minas T. Histologic analysis of failed cartilage repair procedures. *Clin Orthop Relat Res.* 1999;365:149–162.
15. Friedman MJ, Berasi CC, Fox JM, et al. Preliminary results with abrasion arthroplasty in the osteoarthritic knee. *Clin Orthop Relat Res.* 1984;182:200–205.
16. Jackson DW, Lalor PA, Aberman HM, Simon TM. Spontaneous repair of full-thickness defects of articular cartilage in a goat model: a preliminary study. *J Bone Joint Surg Am.* 2001;83:53–64.
17. O'Driscoll SW, Salter R. The induction of neochondrogenesis in free intra-articular periosteal autografts under the influence of continuous passive motion. *J Bone Joint Surg Am.* 1984;66:1248–1257.
18. Angermann P, Riegels-Nielsen P, Pedersen H. Osteochondritis dissecans of the femoral condyle treated with periosteal transplantation. *Poor outcome in 14 patients followed for 6–9 years. Acta Orthop Scand.* 1998;69:595–597.
19. Madsen BL, Noer HH, Carstensen JP, Normark F. Longterm results of periosteal transplantation in osteochondritis dissecans of the knee. *Orthopedics.* 2000;23:223–226.
20. Brittberg M, Lindahl A, Nilsson A, Ohlsson C, et al. Treatment of full-thickness cartilage defects in the human knee with cultured autologous chondrocytes. *N Engl J Med.* 1984;331:889–895.
21. Messner K, Gillquist J. Cartilage repair: a critical review. *Acta Orthop Scand.* 1996;67:523–529.
22. Brittberg M. A critical analysis of cartilage repair. *Acta Orthop Scand.* 1999;88:186–191.
23. Jackson DW, Simon T. Current concepts. Chondrocyte transplantation. *Arthroscopy.* 1996;12:732–738.
24. Grande DA, Pitman ML, et al. The repair of experimentally produced defects in the rabbit articular cartilage by autologous chondrocyte transplantation. *J Orthop Res.* 1989;7:208–218.
25. Brittberg M, Nilsson A, Lindahl A, et al. Rabbit articular cartilage defects treated with autologous cultured chondrocyte. *Clin Orthop Relat Res.* 1995;326:270–283.
26. Breinan H, Minas T, Barone L, et al. Histological evaluation of the course of healing of canine articular cartilage defects treated with cultured chondrocytes. *Tissue Eng.* 1998;4:101–114..
27. Glowacki J. In vitro engineering of cartilage. *J Rehabil Res Dev.* 2000;37:171–177.
28. Li Y, Zhou J, Yang X, Jiang Y, Gui J. Intermittent hydrostatic pressure maintains and enhances the chondrogenic differentiation of cartilage progenitor cells cultivated in alginate beads. *Dev Growth Differ.* 2016;58:180–193.
29. Zhu G, Mayer-Wagner S, Schroder C, Woiczinski M, Blum H, Lavagi I, et al. Comparing effects of perfusion and hydrostatic pressure on gene profiles of human chondrocyte. *J Biotechnol.* 2015;210:59–65.
30. Ikenoue T, Trindade MC, Lee MS, Lin EY, Schurman DJ, Goodman SB, et al. Mechanoregulation of human articular chondrocyteaggrecan and type II collagen expression by intermittent hydrostatic pressure in vitro. *J Orthop Res.* 2003;21:110–116.
31. Smith RL, Lin J, Trindade MC, Shida J, Kajiyama G, Vu T, et al. Time-dependent effects of intermittent hydrostatic pressure on articular chondrocyte type II collagen and aggrecan mRNA expression. *J Rehabil Res Dev.* 2000;37:153–161.
32. Mizuno S. Novel cell culture model using pure hydrostatic pressure and a semipermeable membrane pouch. *Cell Transplant.* 2011;20:767–774.
33. Watanabe S, Inagaki S, Kinouchi I, Takai H, Masuda Y, Mizuno S. Hydrostatic pressure/perfusion culture system designed and validated for engineering tissue. *J Biosci Bioeng.* 2005;100:105–111.
34. Ogura T, Tsuchiya A, Minas T, Mizuno S. Optimization of extracellular matrix synthesis and accumulation by human articular chondrocytes in 3-dimensional construct with repetitive hydrostatic pressure. *Cartilage.* 2018;9:192–201.
35. Ogura T, Minas T, Tsuchiya A, Mizuno S. Effects of hydrostatic pressure and deviatoric stress on human articular chondrocytes for designing neo-cartilage construct. *J Tissue Eng Regen Med.* 2019;13:1143–1152.

3

Imaging: The Basis for a Sound Decision in Joint Preservation

TOM MINAS, MD, MS

CHAPTER OUTLINE

Introduction

Radiological assessment of the knee may provide a tremendous amount of information when proper radiographs are performed and a knowledge of patterns of wear are recognized. A standard series of digital radiographs that we perform at our center include a 54-inch anteroposterior (AP) axial alignment x-ray image (with radiographic markers for magnification), standing bilateral AP, 45-degree bent standing posteroanterior (PA) (Rosenberg views[1]), and a tangential patellar skyline view at 45 degrees supine. However, *supine AP radiographs of the knee should not be performed* because they are not useful in determining the cartilage joint space and hence the potential for joint-preserving surgery.

Patients sent to us with articular cartilage injuries have frequently had high-resolution MRI scans and arthroscopy photographs; however, they have never had standing x-rays to demonstrate that they have preexisting bone-on-bone osteoarthritis. Simple radiographs would give us the answers that these patients are not suitable for cartilage repair, based on their bone-on-bone changes; however, they may still be suitable for osteotomy or the possibility of unicompartmental replacement.

Radiological Patterns of Osteoarthritis

Advanced tricompartmental osteoarthritis (OA) is exceedingly rare unless there is advanced unicompartmental disease with tibiofemoral subluxation. Ahlbäck[2] reviewed a Swedish population in the region of Stockholm and published his report in 1968. He reviewed approximately 1200 patients, 1800 knees reviewing weight-bearing radiographs from these patients. In reviewing a series for arthrosis, 281 patients were reviewed comprising 370 knees with joint space narrowing. Standing AP projections were taken but not PA projections, loading 20 degrees bent axial patellofemoral views, and supine lateral views. The following Venn diagrams were constructed depicting the wear patterns noted (Fig. 3.1).

The predominance of arthritic wear patterns was in the medial and patellofemoral articulations in 80% of patients. However, because the lateral compartment usually wears posteriorly[1] these numbers may have changed slightly if the standing PA views had been included. In any case, the Venn diagrams demonstrate that unicompartmental and bicompartmental wear is more common than tricompartmental wear. Total knee arthroplasty may therefore be an overly aggressive solution to osteoarthritis in a younger patient population. Cartilage repair, possibly combined with osteotomy or when bone-on-bone changes are present, unicompartmental or bicompartmental resurfacing arthroplasty may be more suitable in an attempt to preserve the joint for as long as possible.

Medial Osteoarthritis

Standing AP x-rays will generally demonstrate early joint space narrowing for the medial wear pattern of osteoarthritis (Fig. 3.2). With medial OA, a standing PA may demonstrate increased posterior joint space unless anterior cruciate

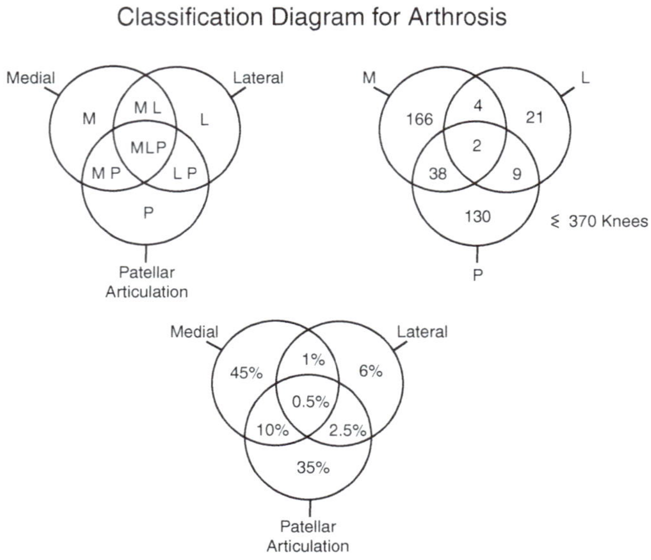

• **Fig. 3.1** The Venn diagrams demonstrate the predominance of osteoarthritic joint space narrowing in the medial and patellar articulations of the knee. This classic study, which was the basis for the classification proposed by Ahlbäck,[2] notes that tricompartmental arthritis is exceedingly rare in this Swedish cohort of 370 knees performed in the 1960s in the Stockholm region.

ligament (ACL) deficiency is present, whereby tibial translation anteriorly permits a posterior wear pattern on the medial side (see Fig. 3.3).[3]

Lateral Tibiofemoral Osteoarthritis

Lateral osteoarthritic changes usually occur in the central to posterior aspect of the lateral tibial plateau. This is irrespective of whether this is caused by valgus malalignment, post-meniscectomy, or ACL deficiency. Early joint space narrowing with peripheral osteophyte formation may be noted in a standing AP x-ray examination. However, the standing 45-degree Rosenberg PA[1] x-ray image usually demonstrates loss of articular space and should always be included (Fig. 3.4).

Patellofemoral Dysplasia and Degenerative Osteoarthritis of the Patellofemoral Joint

Just as there is dysplasia of the hip joint resulting in early osteoarthritis secondary to abnormal contact forces in patients in their early 40s and 50s, a similar condition exists in the patellofemoral joint. Dysplasia of the trochlea has been discussed in Europe, especially France, since the 1970s. However, it is just starting to become recognized in the United States in the last decade. Dejour[4] has done much work to demonstrate the radiographic abnormalities that are present in patients with dysplasia of the trochlea (Fig. 3.5). Dysplasia may present as a poorly formed or flattened sulcus or a convex trochlea and is discussed further in Chapter 12. The lateral x-ray demonstrates a lack of a "crossing sign," which is characteristic of someone with dysplasia in that a poorly formed sulcus does not demonstrate a double dip on the lateral x-ray. These patients frequently present with an adolescent dislocation of the patella or anterior knee pain or both. The pain may persist through young adulthood and by the fourth or fifth decades presents with end-stage patellofemoral isolated osteoarthritis.

Magnetic Resonance Imaging of Articular Cartilage

The clinical suspicion of an articular cartilage defect may be confirmed by magnetic resonance (MR) imaging or at arthroscopic surgery. Although arthroscopy is the gold standard for evaluation of articular surface lesions, MR imaging

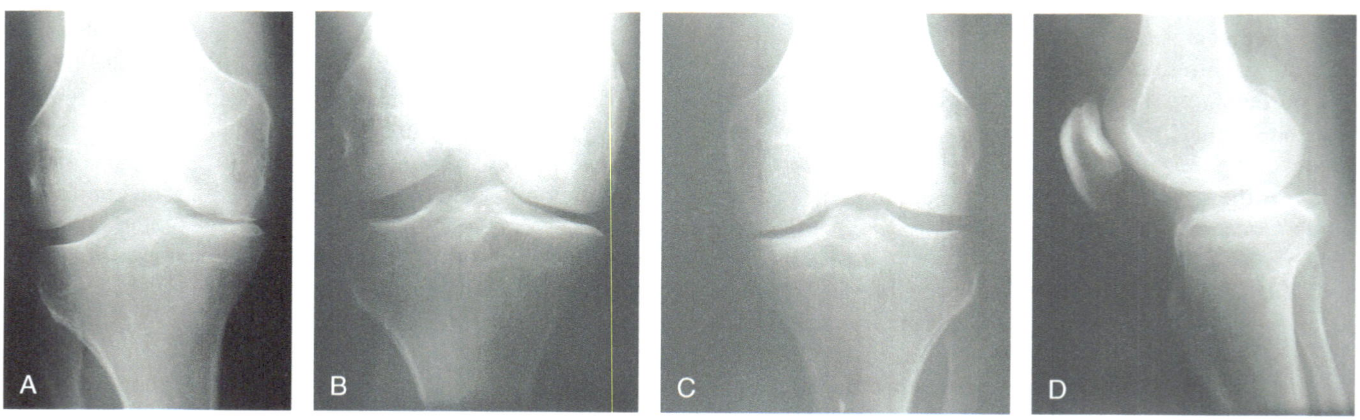

• **Fig. 3.2** 40-year-old male with bilateral varus knees. He demonstrates a classic anterior medial wear pattern of osteoarthritis. (A) Standing AP demonstrating loss of joint space in full extension. (B) Standing 45 degrees bent PA demonstrating a preserved posterior medial joint space. He had childhood medial femoral condyle osteochondritis dissecans. (C) The left knee in the same patient again demonstrating loss of joint space in extension on the AP x-ray to the left and (D) an anterior wear pattern noted on the lateral x-ray on the right.

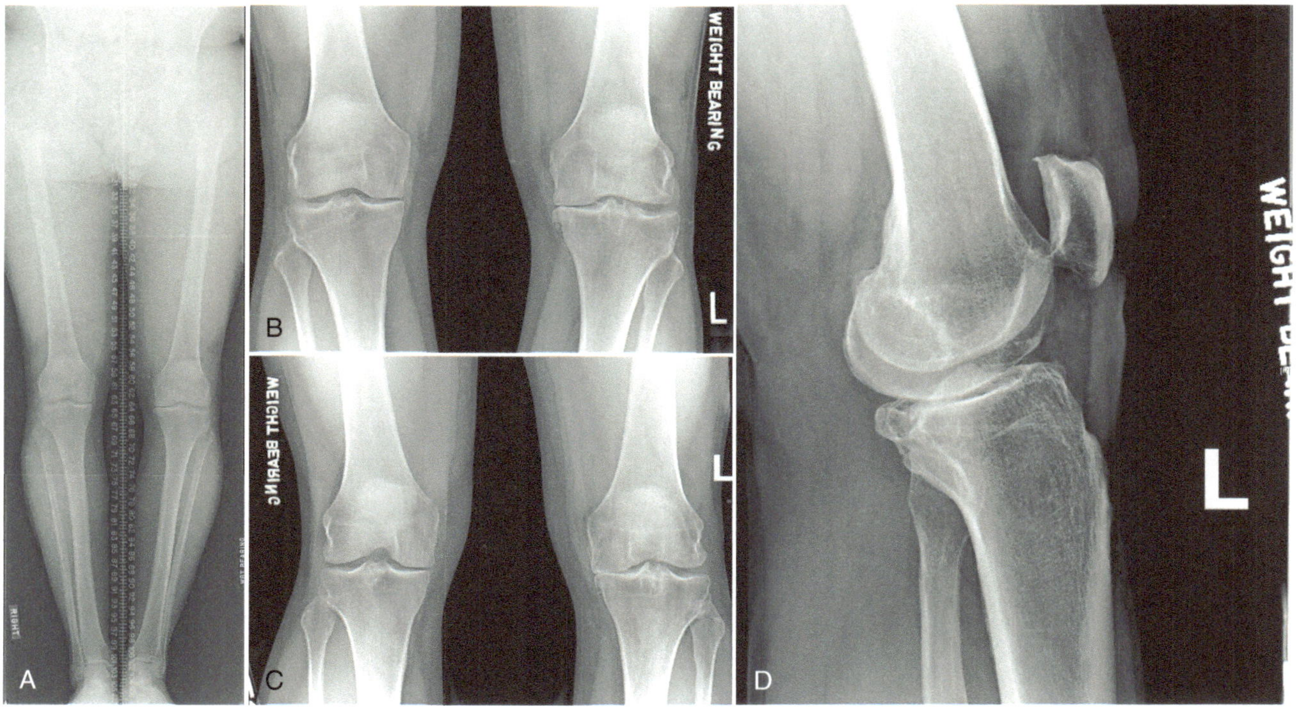

• **Fig. 3.3** Effect of anterior cruciate ligament deficiency in a 40-year-old male with long-standing alignment issues. X-ray images (A) demonstrate varus alignment of the lower extremities. (B) Standing AP x-ray image demonstrates medial joint space loss with peripheral osteophyte formation with residual joint space remaining. However, (C) standing PA x-ray image demonstrates complete obliteration of the posterior medial joint space. This is typical of a chronic anterior cruciate ligament (ACL)-deficient knee with the tibial wear translating further posterior as the tibia subluxes anterior secondary to the ACL deficiency. (D) Lateral x-ray image demonstrates atypical "cupola" or cupped appearance of the tibia.

is currently considered the best noninvasive means of diagnosis.[5] We have found that sequences used with a standard 1.5 Tesla magnet with thinner slice thicknesses and longer acquisition times have provided excellent imaging of the articular surfaces.[6] Our standard series have been published and are outlined in Tables 3.1 and 3.2.

Setting up slice sequences that are orthogonal to the articular surfaces to be imaged is important to obtain accurate full thickness assessments of the articular cartilage (Fig. 3.6). Tangential cartilage volume defect artifact may otherwise occur.

The literature reports that MR is 50% to 96% sensitive in detecting articular cartilage lesions.[7] Fat-suppressed T1-weighted gradient echo (e.g., spoiled gradient recalled echo) and intermediate-weighted fast spin echo (FSE) have become among the most commonly used sequences for cartilage imaging. Improved sensitivity to edema-like signal in the subchondral bone marrow may be achieved through the addition of fat suppression to FSE sequences, either with a fat selective pre-saturation pulse or a short tau inversion recovery (STIR) sequence.[5,8–10] The presence of focal edema-like signal in the subchondral marrow may indicate the presence of an overlying cartilage defect and may, in fact, be easier to detect than the cartilage defect itself.[11] (Fig. 3.7).

MR arthrography (MRA) with enhancement of the joint fluid by a contrast agent, performed with either the direct injection of a dilute gadolinium-based contrast agent (direct MRA) or an intravenous (IV) injection of contrast followed by joint motion (IV or indirect MRA) (Fig. 3.8), may be used to provide additional image contrast for the evaluation of cartilage defects.[12,13]

Direct MRA has proven useful in the evaluation of the stability of osteochondral lesions.[14] More recent work has shown the ability to determine the relative proteoglycan concentration of articular cartilage in vivo using an IV MRA technique called delayed gadolinium-enhanced MR imaging of cartilage (dGEMRIC) (Fig. 3.9).[15] This particular technique holds great promise not only for following the progression or regression of a cartilage lesion, but also to evaluate cartilage success of a cartilage repair noninvasively by assessing the progression of glycosaminoglycan synthesis (Fig. 3.10).[16]

Although MR imaging has proved very sensitive for the detection of defects, there are limitations with regard to accurately defining the depth (grade) and size of articular cartilage lesions. The accuracy of MR for detecting, grading, and sizing defects is very sensitive to the acquisition parameters used. Because most of the diagnostic difficulties arise from partial volume artifacts caused by the combination of

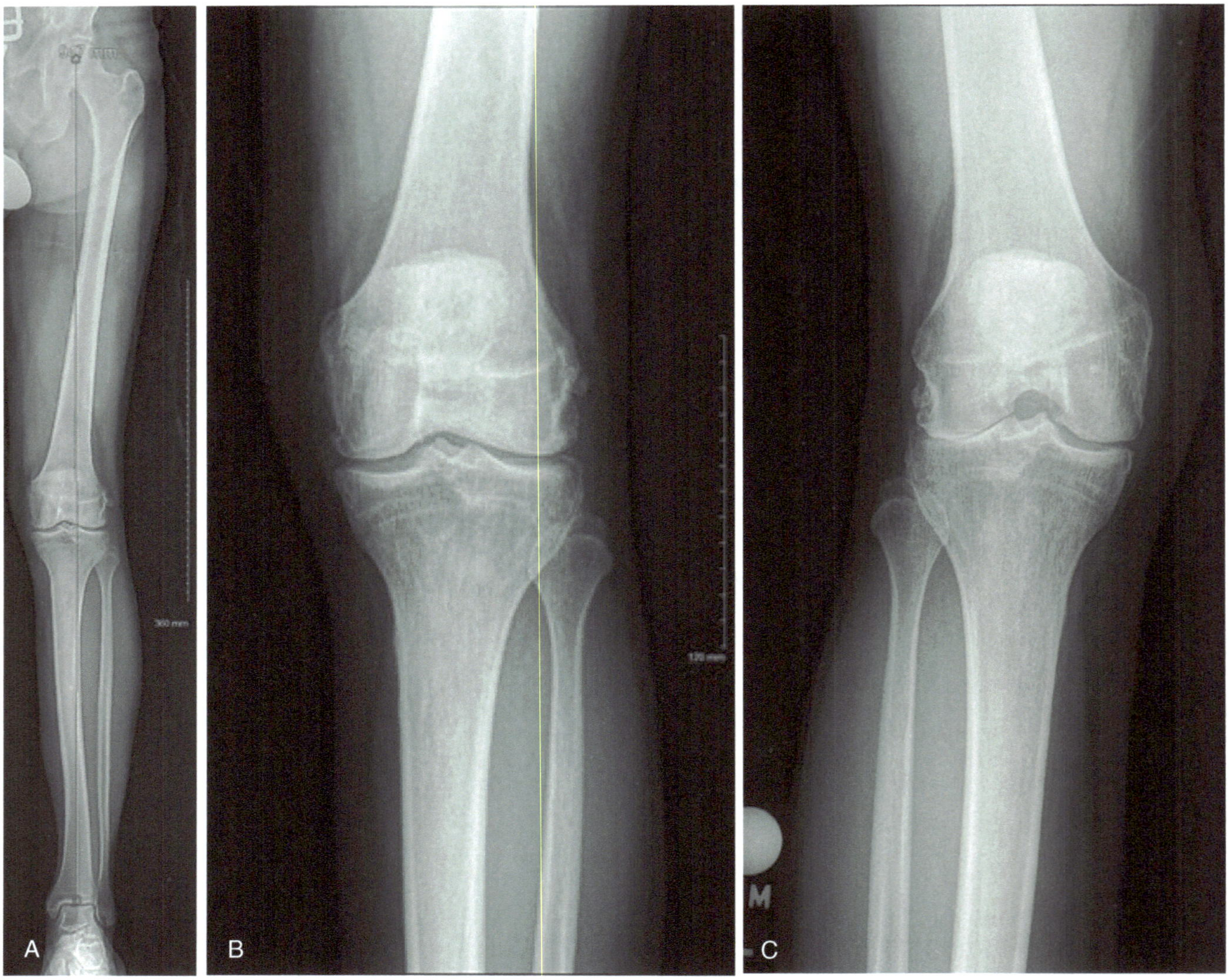

• **Fig. 3.4** A 67-year-old patient with mild valgus alignment of the lower limb on long alignment (A) AP x-ray and lateral joint pain. (B) Standing AP x-ray notes the joint space to be intact. (C) Rosenberg view demonstrates the bone-on-bone changes that would be otherwise missed on a standard AP x-ray examination.

the curved surfaces of the joint surfaces and relatively large voxel dimensions of MR images, close attention should be paid to obtaining the highest resolution images possible. In our experience,[17] we have found that MR images tend to underestimate the size and depth of cartilage lesions, that significant lesions may exhibit very subtle findings on MR images, and that lesions may be visualized accurately on only one slice plane (Fig. 3.11).

Despite these limitations, the sensitivity of MR imaging for articular cartilage defects is valuable not only for the diagnosis of a cartilage lesions, but may also be useful in planning treatment, particularly for the knee. For example, when considering a valgus producing high tibial osteotomy or unicompartmental arthroplasty for a knee with varus alignment resulting from severe medial compartment cartilage loss, it is important to assess the status of the articular cartilage in the joint compartments. If there are significant cartilage lesions in the other lateral and patellofemoral joint compartments, the osteotomy or unicompartmental arthroplasty may fail to relieve symptoms because of the increased load on this diseased cartilage produced by the change in the mechanical axis. Prior to surgery, the overall assessment of the cartilage is traditionally done arthroscopically. This arthroscopy is not required for the performance of the surgery and adds potential morbidity and expense. However, a preoperative MR that can accurately assess the status of the articular cartilage in all compartments can alert the surgeon to the presence of cartilage abnormalities in the other portions of the joint and help determine the feasibility of reconstructive procedures that address only specific compartments of the knee. Furthermore, such an assessment can help the physicians better prepare

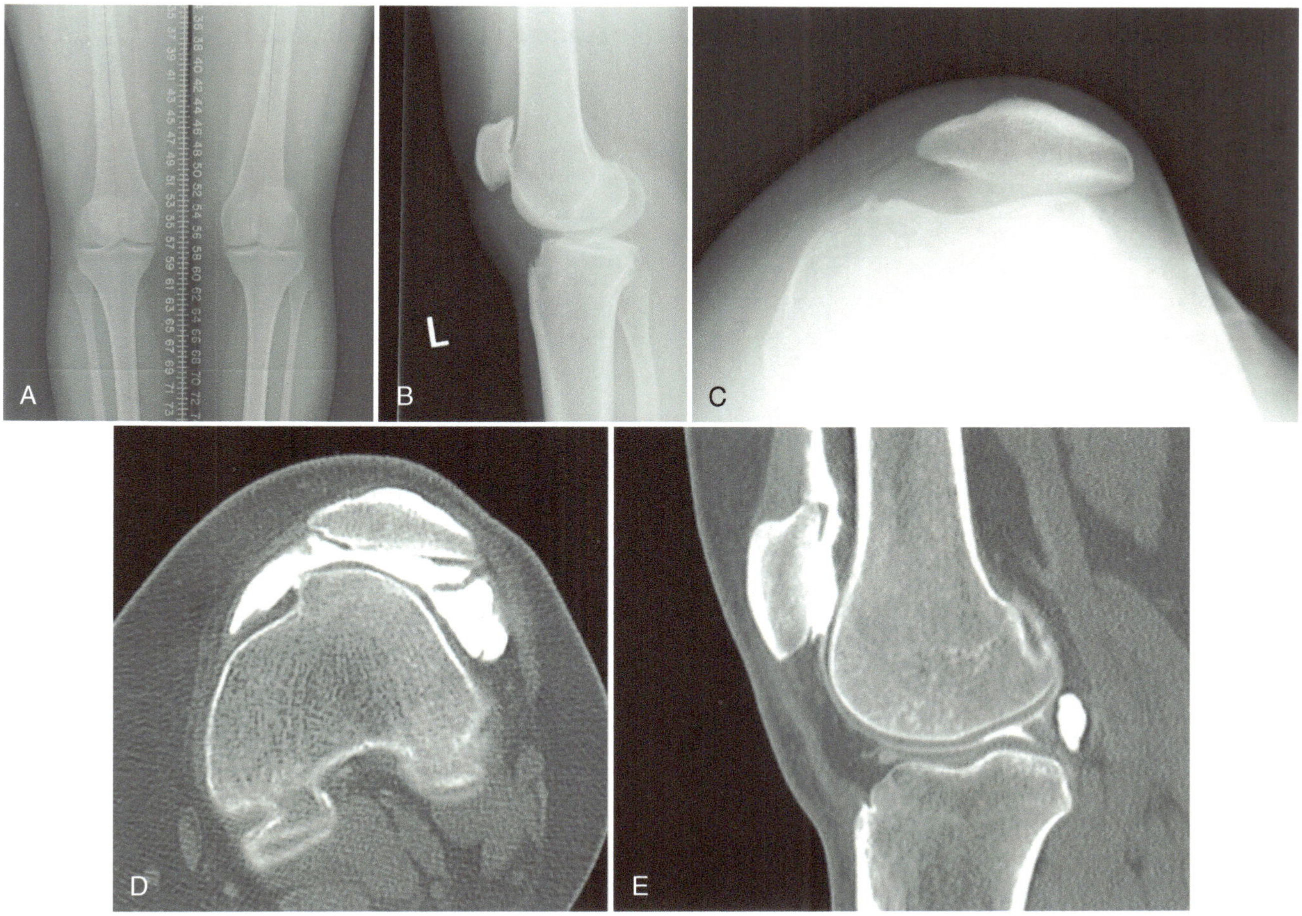

• **Fig. 3.5** (A) Cropped image of long alignment x-ray images in a 19-year-old young woman with severe anterior knee pain and recurrent dislocations. The left knee is most symptomatic. The axial alignment is neutral to slight varus. (B) The lateral x-ray image demonstrates lack of a "crossing sign" of Dejour[4] of the proximal trochlea as the patella engages the sulcus. The trochlea is either barrel-shaped or convex at its entry site. (C) The skyline x-ray image demonstrates both tilt and subluxation of the patella; however, the dysplasia of the trochlea and the loss of articular cartilage on the patella were demonstrated clearly only when a CT arthrogram was performed. CT arthrogram is my preferred study for assessment of patellofemoral dysplasia as well as for damage to the articular surfaces. (D) The axial image of the CT arthrogram demonstrates clearly the dysplastic nature of the trochlea with a very prominent and convex proximal lateral facet with cartilage loss to the central and lateral facet of the patella. (E) The sagittal image of the CT arthrogram demonstrates that the articular surface of the trochlea remains intact; however, at the inferior two-thirds of the articular surface, cartilage on the patella is completely lost (centrally). Notice the excellent visualization of the tibiofemoral cartilage and the meniscus with this spiral CT arthrogram. However, a CT arthrogram does not demonstrate the subtle nature of subchondral changes such as bone marrow edema (BME) or cartilage fluid update, which may indicate softening and early degeneration and is better visualized with an MRI scan. Hence both studies are occasionally required to get the complete picture of the situation.

their patients for the most likely treatment than with the standard combination of diagnostic arthroscopy followed by either a unicompartmental treatment approach or total arthroplasty. We currently use the global assessment of knee cartilage by MR to exclude patients from unicompartmental therapy when cartilage lesions are found in other compartments.[17]

A similar approach has been suggested for preoperative assessment of the knee prior to meniscal allograft surgery.[18]

MR imaging is also valuable in assessing the status of articular cartilage repair tissue after reconstructive efforts.[19,20] It can assess repair site surface congruity and incorporation following many repair techniques, as well as identify many of the complications that may occur following cartilage repair. At the moment, the application of carefully performed MR imaging studies may preclude the need for invasive arthroscopic evaluation of articular cartilage lesions and reconstructions.

MRI for Predicting the Success of ACI Bone Marrow Edema

Bone marrow edema (BME) on fat-suppressed MRI images represents an abnormality in the osteochondral unit from mild inflammation to osseous cyst formation and collapse. The intensity can be classified[21] as I-IV, Grade I absent, Grade II mild, Grade III moderate, with Grade IV being severe (see Fig. 3.12).

TABLE 3.1 Standard Knee Protocol for ACI Imaging Without Intravenous Contrast Enhancement

Plane	Sequence	TR (ms)	TE (ms)	TI (ms)	ETL	Slice (thickness/ gap in mm)	Matrix	Fat saturation
Coronal	T1W	500–800	20	–	–	3.5/0.5	512 × 256	No
Coronal	IRFSE	2000–3000	8	160	8	4/1	256 × 192	No
Sagittal	FSE	3000–4000	25	–	8	3.5/0.5	512 × 256	Yes
Sagittal	FSE	3000–4000	38	–	8	3.5/0.5	512 × 256	No
Axial	FSE	3000–4000	25 and 130	–	12	4/1	256 × 256	No
Oblique[a]	FSE	3000–4000	25	–	8	3.5/0.5	512 × 256	Yes

[a]Oblique scan is oriented orthogonal to the ACI site (e.g., for ACI in the inferior part of the trochlea, an oblique coronal plane parallel to the roof of the intercondylar notch is chosen).

Note: All scans are performed with a field of view between 14 and 16 cm. Field of view and matrix size are adjusted to patient size and signal-to-noise ratio of the magnetic resonance imaging system. *ACI*, Autologous chondrocyte implantation; *ETL*, echo train length; *FSE*, fast spin echo; *IRFSE*, inversion recovery fast spin echo; *T1W*, T1 weighted.

From Alparslan L, Minas T, Winalski CS. Magnetic resonance imaging of autologous chondrocyte implantation. *Semin Ultrasound CT MR*. 2001;22(4):341-351.

TABLE 3.2 IV (Indirect) Arthrography Knee Protocol for ACI Imaging

Plane	Sequence	TR (ms)	TE (ms)	TI (ms)	ETL	Slice (thickness/ gap in mm)	Matrix	Fat saturation
Coronal	T1W	500–800	20	–	–	3.5/0.5	512 × 256	No
Coronal	IRFSE	2000–3000	8	160	8	4/1	256 × 192	No
Sagittal	FSE	3000–4000	25	–	8	3.5/0.5	512 × 256	Yes
Sagittal	FSE	3000–4000	38	–	8	3.5/0.5	512 × 256	No
Axial	FSE	3000–4000	25 and 130	–	12	4/1	256 × 256	No
Sagittal	T1W	500–800	14	–	–	3.5/0.5	512 × 256	Yes
Oblique[a]	T1W	500–800	14	–	–	3.5/0.5	512 × 256	Yes

[a]Oblique scan is oriented orthogonal to the ACI site (e.g., for ACI in the inferior part of the trochlea, an oblique coronal plane parallel to the roof of the intercondylar notch, or for a patellar ACI, a true axial image plane is chosen).

Note: All scans are performed with a field of view between 14 and 16 cm. Field of view and matrix size are adjusted to patient size and signal-to-noise ratio of the magnetic resonance imaging (MRI) system. Before imaging, 0.1 mmol/kg of intravenous (IV) gadolinium-DTPA is administered. The patient is then asked to perform 15 minutes of motion exercise within the limits of their rehabilitation protocol, usually walking, to promote uniform joint fluid enhancement. MRI can begin any time after the exercise period. Because joint fluid enhancement persists for over 1 hour, the start of imaging can be delayed for up to 45 minutes without severe loss of joint fluid enhancement. *ACI*, Autologous chondrocyte implantation; *ETL*, echo train length; *FSE*, fast spin echo; *IRFSE*, inversion recovery fast spin echo; *T1W*, T1 weighted.

From Alparslan L, Minas T, Winalski CS. Magnetic resonance imaging of autologous chondrocyte implantation. *Semin Ultrasound CT MR* 2001;22(4):341-351.

In a matched case control study[22] assessing preoperative BME when articular defects were treated by autologous chondrocyte implantation (ACI), Grade IV BME had little influence on the outcome or failure rate of ACI (control group Fig. 3.13) except if prior microfracture had been performed. After microfracture, if done when Grade IV BME was present, the failure rate was dramatically worse: 83.7% at 5 years versus 21.4% at 5 years in the control group (Fig. 3.14). Hence MR imaging is valuable in predicting ACI graft failure after microfracture if Grade IV BME is present preoperatively. This would imply failure of the osteochondral unit, which should be replaced in its entirety by a combined ACI sandwich technique with autologous bone graft or an osteochondral allograft.

In summary, a knowledge of existing radiographic patterns of wear for medial and lateral tibiofemoral disease, patellofemoral dysplasia, and ACL deficiency assists in subtle diagnoses that are critical for an understanding of a patient's

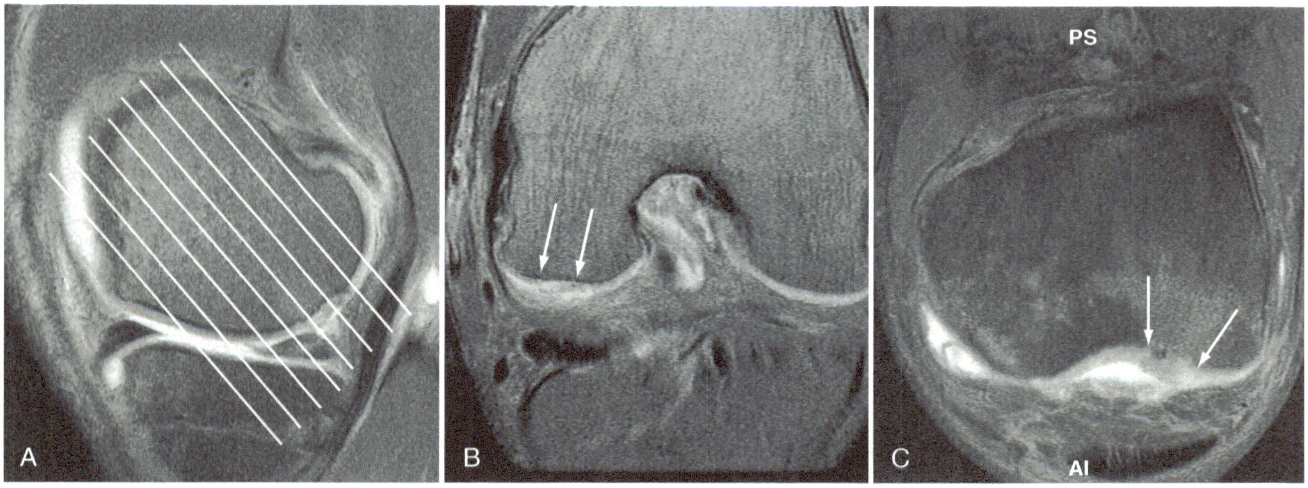

• **Fig. 3.6** Example of an oblique scan being taken to demonstrate (*arrows*) a posterior medial femoral condyle ACI graft (B) and a lateral trochlea facet ACI graft (C). The scan must be positioned orthogonal to the graft sites (A) to ensure an appropriate image acquisition. This underlines the importance of a good relationship between the orthopedist and the musculoskeletal radiologist who is performing the images to maximize the information gained from the evaluation. (Images courtesy Dr. Carl Winalski.)

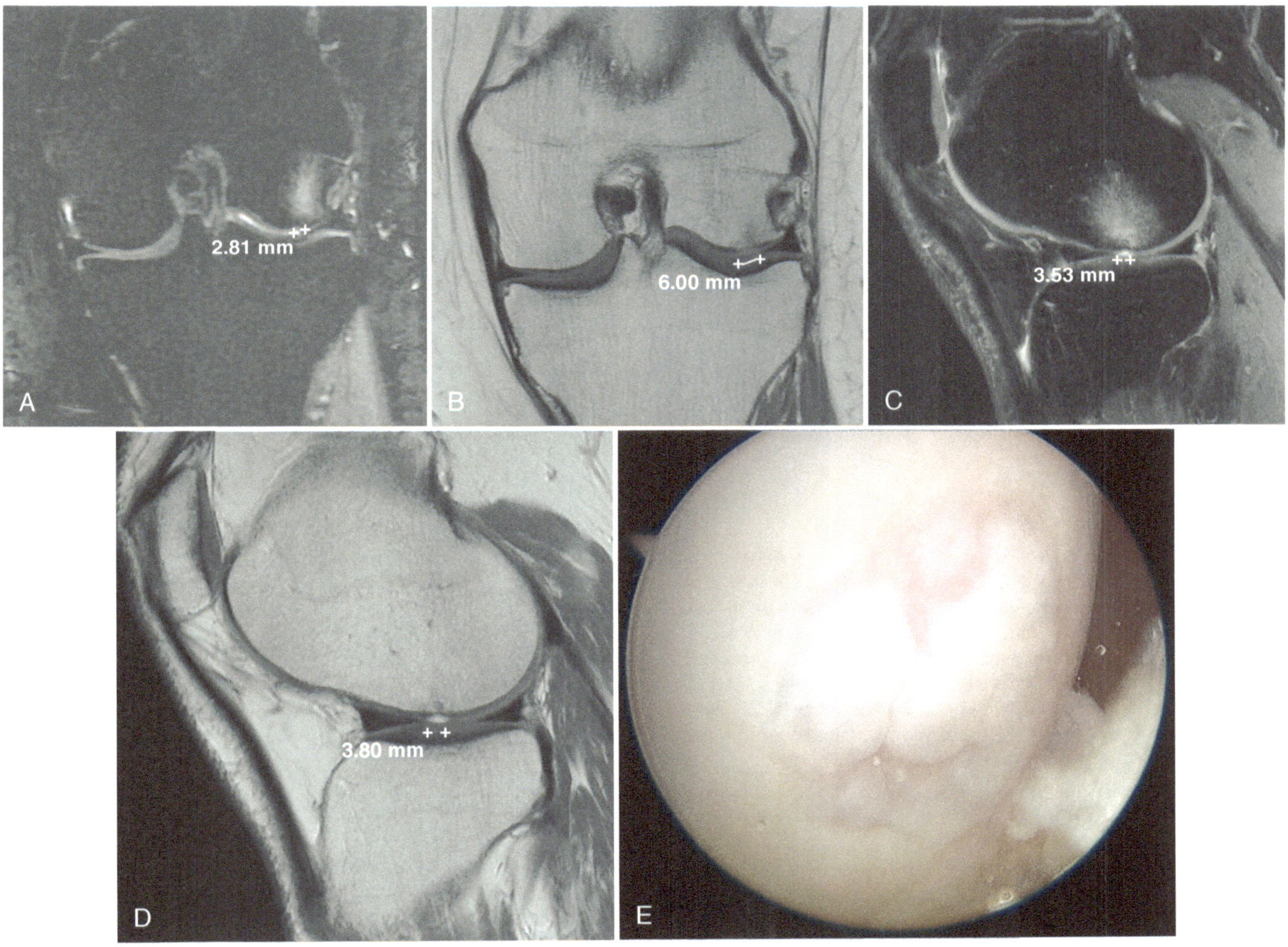

• **Fig. 3.7** Coronal MRI images (A) with and (B) without fat suppression. The bone marrow edema on the fat suppression image brings attention to an overlying articular cartilage injury that occurred 2 years after microfracture to the lateral femoral condyle. The defect might have otherwise been missed on the (B) proton density image alone. Sagittal MRI images with (C) fat-suppressed and (D) non-fat suppressed images of same patient demonstrating bone marrow edema that brings attention to the small overlying articular cartilage defect. E, Arthroscopic appearance of cartilage defect shown by MRI 2 years following microfracture. This patient had a bony repair tissue with large intralesional osteophyte formation with a thin fibrous film covering it.

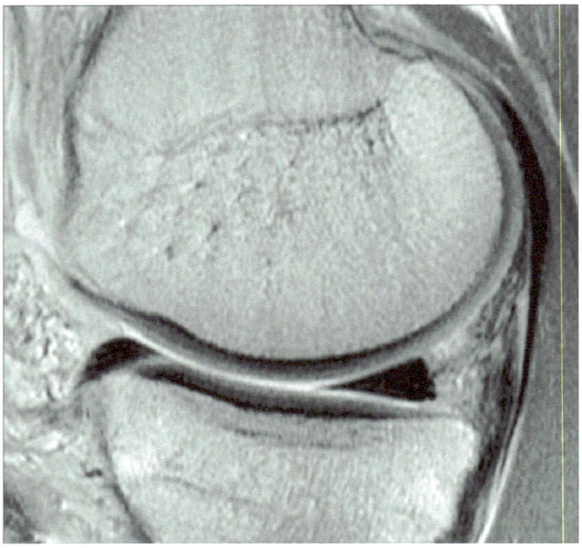

• **Fig. 3.8** Enhancement of the articular surface with intravenous MR arthrography demonstrates an excellent interface between cartilage and joint space on the sagittal image of the medial femoral condyle. (Image courtesy Dr. Carl Winalski).

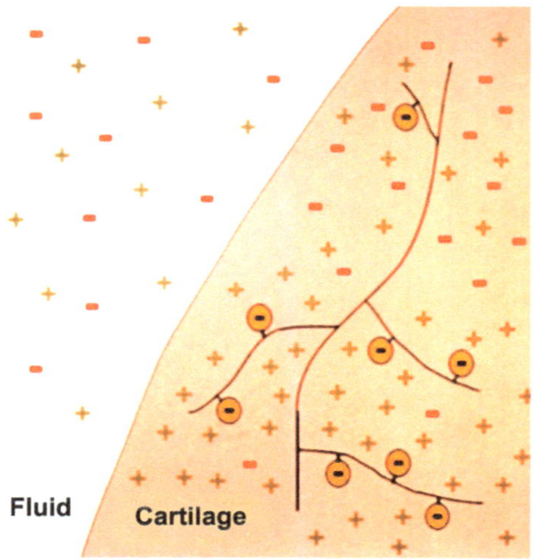

• **Fig. 3.9** Schematic delayed gadolinium-enhanced magnetic resonance imaging of cartilage (dGEMRIC) works on the premise that proteoglycans found in articular cartilage are negatively charged molecules. Using gadolinium-DTPA^{2-}, intra-articular contrast agent and allowing this to set and equilibrate over time, the gadolinium DTPA distribution in the articular cartilage will be inversely proportional to the proteoglycan content of the articular cartilage. Abnormal areas will therefore have a lower T1 signal and therefore T1 maps will quantify abnormal areas in the articular cartilage. A clinical example is given in Fig. 3.10.

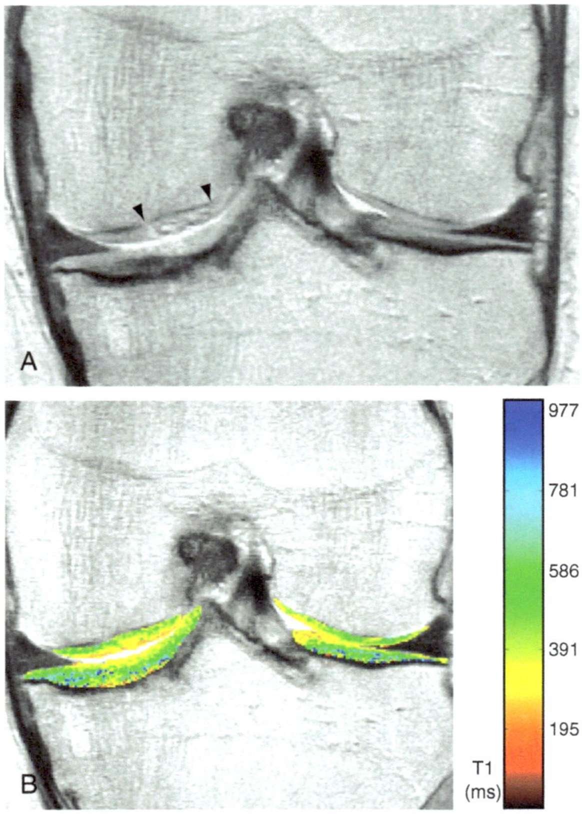

• **Fig. 3.10** (A) A non-dGEMRIC (delayed gadolinium-enhanced magnetic resonance imaging of cartilage) image with *arrows* denoting an ACI on the MFC (medial femoral condyle). The patient is doing well and is clinically symptom-free. (B) The highest numbers on the dGEMRIC scale represent high proteoglycan content and are *blue-green*. The lowest numbers (*yellow-red*) represent lessened proteoglycan content. The highest proteoglycan content is generally in the deep and middle layers of the articular cartilage as is seen in this image. The *yellow* represents the fibrous surface of the periosteum on the MFC of this ACI repair or the fibrous lamina splendens of the native articular cartilage. (Images courtesy Dr. Carl Winalski).

disease pattern. In addition to a careful history and physical examination along with high-quality digital x-ray images and long alignment x-ray images, the surgeon should have a good idea of the diagnosis towards the patient's clinical disability. High resolution MRI scan with a standard 1.5 Tesla magnet, and now 3.0 Tesla magnet, set with the appropriate sequences, slice orientation and image acquisition time with the possibility of image contrast will give excellent quality assessment of the articular cartilage surfaces of the knee joint. CT scan with image contrast may complement and supplement the images obtained with MRI scan specifically to help address bony deficiencies with osteoarticular fragments, maltracking of the patella and trochlea dysplasia, as well as articular, meniscal, or ligamentous injury associated with unicompartmental knee replacements due to the high-quality software that is available to limit artifact from a prosthesis.

I have found that it is rare to require an arthroscopy for a diagnosis of articular cartilage injury and treatment plan based on the excellent quality of available MRI and CT present-day imaging. The key to high-quality imaging, however, is a team approach with a dedicated musculoskeletal radiologist who understands the needs of the orthopedist and will set the parameters for the images needed.

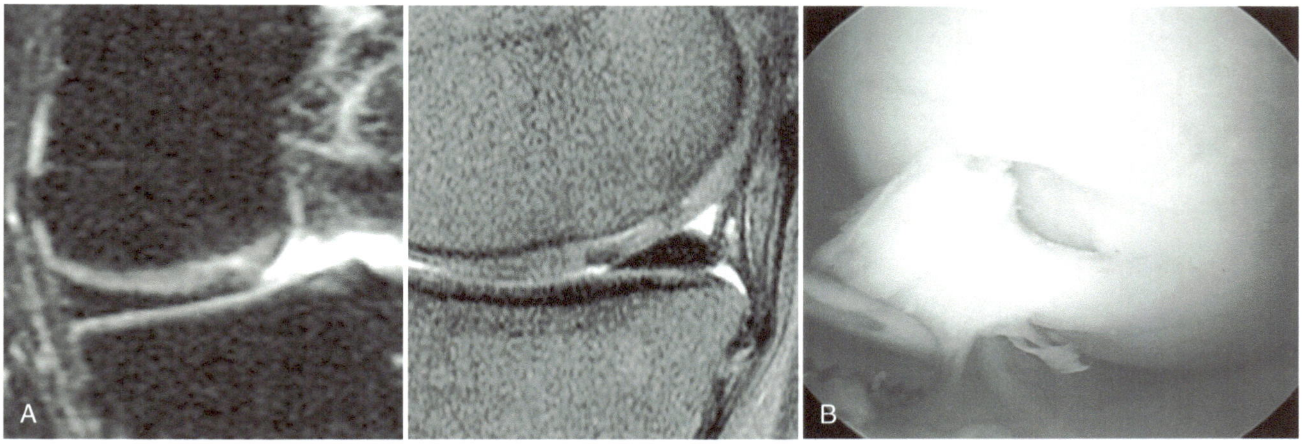

• **Fig. 3.11** (A) MRI images of fast spin echo with fat-suppressed and non-fat-suppressed sequences demonstrating subtle fluid signal under articular cartilage. This chondral flap is confirmed at the time of arthroscopy. (B) Undermined articular cartilage at the time of arthroscopy which was noted by MRI scan. (A, courtesy Dr. Carl Winalski).

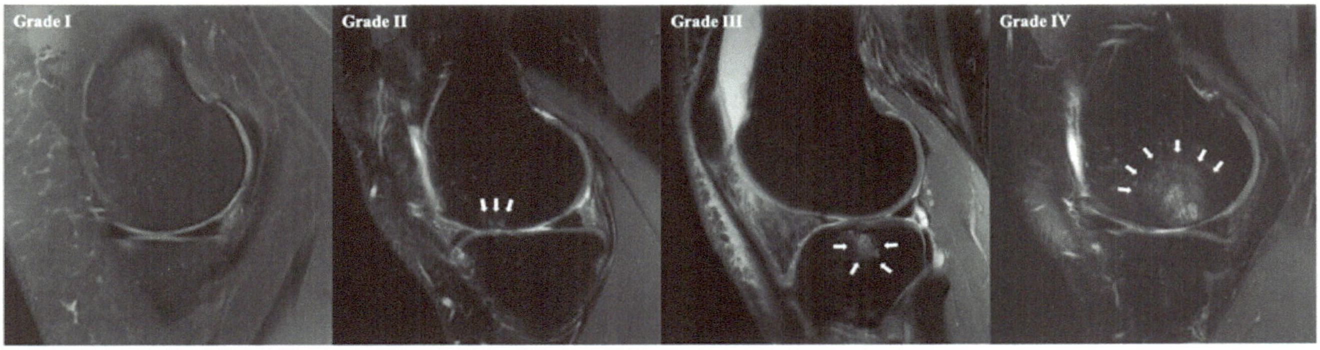

• **Fig. 3.12** Bone marrow edema. (From Henderson IJP, Tuy P, Connell D, Oakes B, Hettwer WH. Prospective clinical study of autologous chondrocyte implantation and correlation with MRI at three and 12 months. *J Bone Joint Surg Br*. 2003;85(7):1060-1066.)

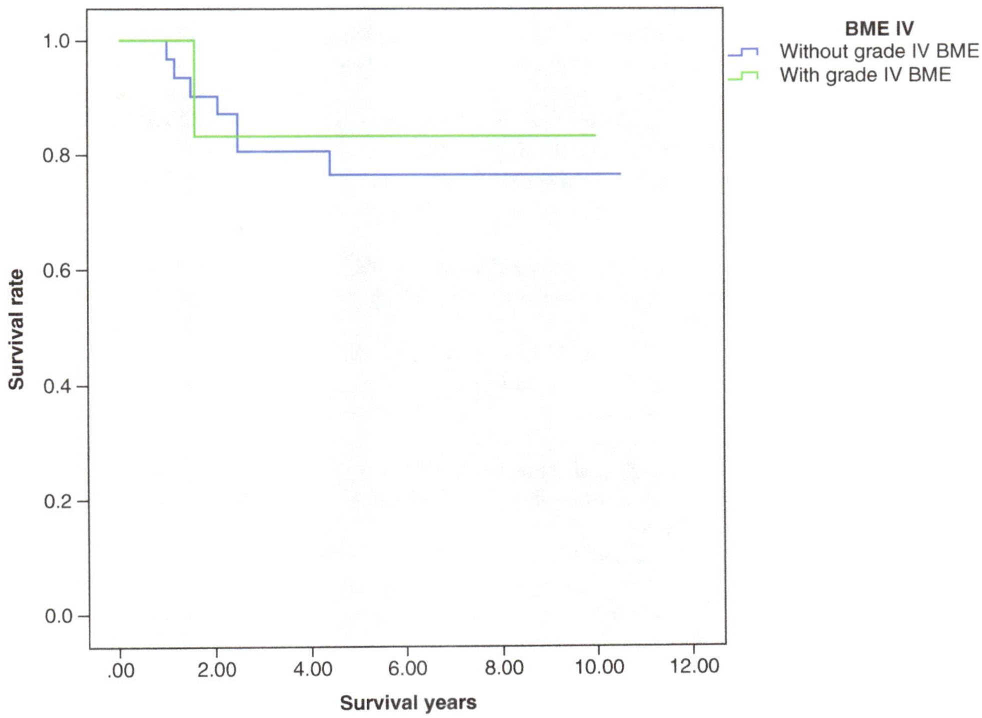

• **Fig. 3.13** Control group for the failure rate of autologous chondrocyte implantation with and without Grade IV bone marrow edema (BME). The 5-year failure rate with Grade IV BME was 21.4%.

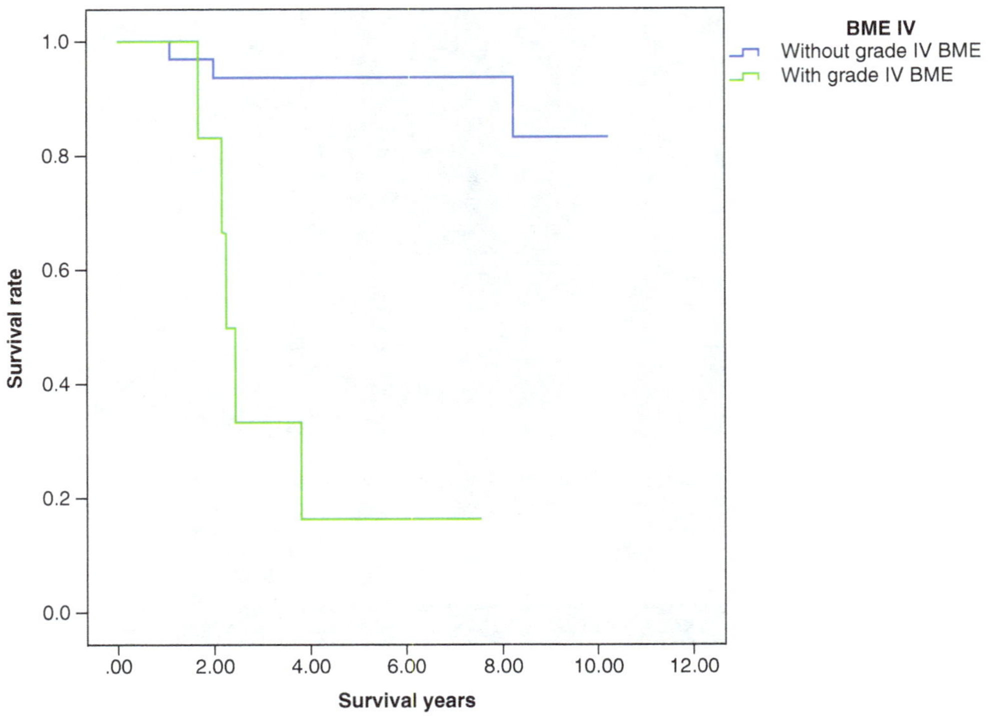

• **Fig. 3.14** Case group for autologous chondrocyte implantation failure rate after microfracture with and without Grade IV bone marrow edema (BME). The 5-year failure rate with Grade IV BME was 83.7%.

References

1. Rosenberg T, Paulos L, Parker RD, et al. The forty-five-degree posteroanterior flexion weight bearing radiograph of the knee. *J Bone Joint Surg Am*. 1988;70(10):1479–1483.
2. Ahlback S. Osteoarthrosis of the knee: a radiographic investigation. *Acta Radiologica*. 1968;Suppl 277:7–72.
3. Harmon MK, Marcovich GD, Banks SA, Hodge W. Wear patterns on tibial plateaus from varus and valgus osteoarthritic knees. *Clin Orthop Relat Res*. 1998;352:149–158.
4. Dejour H, Walch G, Nove-Josserand L, Guier C. Factors of patellar instability: an anatomic radiographic study. *Knee Surg Sports Traumatol Arthrosc*. 1994;2:19–26.
5. Recht M, Bobic V, Burstein D. Magnetic resonance imaging of articular cartilage. *Clin Orthop*. 2001;391:S379–S396.
6. Alparslan L, Minas T, Winalski CS. Magnetic resonance imaging of autologous chondrocyte implantation. *Semin Ultrasound CT MR*. 2001;22(4):341–351.
7. Winalski CS, Minas T. Evaluation of chondral injuries by magnetic resonance imaging: repair assessments. *Op Tech Sports Med*. 2000;8(2):108–119.
8. Potter HG, Linklater JM, Allen AA, Hannafin JA, Haas SM. Magnetic resonance imaging of articular cartilage in the knee. An evaluation with use of fast-spin-echo imaging. *J Bone Joint Surg Am*. 1998;80(9):1276–1284.
9. Recht MP, Kramer J, Marcelis S, et al. Abnormalities of articular cartilage in the knee: analysis of available MR techniques. *Radiology*. 1993;187(2):473–478.
10. Disler DG, Peters TL, Muscoreil SJ, et al. Fat-suppressed spoiled GRASS imaging of knee hyaline cartilage: technique optimization and comparison with conventional MR imaging. *AJR*. 1994;163(4):887–892.
11. Rubin DA, Harner CD, Costello JM. Treatable chondral injuries in the knee: frequency of associated focal subchondral edema. *AJR*. 2000;174(4):1099–1106.
12. Winalski CS, Aliabadi P, Wright RJ, Shortkroff S, Sledge CB, Weissman BN. Enhancement of joint fluid with intravenously administered gadopentetate dimeglumine: technique, rationale, and implications. *Radiology*. 1993;187(1):179–185.
13. Kramer J, Recht MP, Imhof H, Stiglbauer R, Engel A. Postcontrast MR arthrography in assessment of cartilage lesions. *J Comput Assist Tomogr*. 1994;18(2):218–224.
14. Kramer J, Stiglbauer R, Engel A, Prayer L, Imhof H. MR contrast arthrography (MRA) in osteochondrosis dissecans. *J Comput Assist Tomogr*. 1992;16(2):254–260.
15. Bashir A, Gray M, Boutin RD, Burstein D. Glycosaminoglycan in articular cartilage: in vivo assessment with delayed Gd(DTPA)(2-)-enhanced MR imaging. *Radiology*. 1997;205(2):551–558.
16. Gillis A, Bashir A, McKeon B, Scheller A, Gray ML, Burstein D, et al. Magnetic resonance imaging of relative glycosaminoglycan distribution in patients with autologous chondrocyte transplants. *Invest Radiol*. 2001;36(12):743–748.
17. Azer N, Winalski CS, Minas T. MR imaging for surgical planning and postoperative assessment in early osteoarthritis. *Arthritis Imaging*. 2004;42(1):43–60.
18. Potter HG, Rodeo SA, Wickiewicz TL, Warren RF. MR imaging of meniscal allografts: correlation with clinical and arthroscopic outcomes. *Radiology*. 1996;198(2):509–514.
19. Alparslan L, Winalski CS, Boutin RD, Minas T. Postoperative magnetic resonance imaging of articular cartilage repair. *Semin Musculoskelet Radiol*. 2001;5(4):345–363.
20. Gold GE, Bergman AG, Pauly JM. Magnetic resonance imaging of knee cartilage repair. *Top Magn Reson Imaging*. 1998;9(6):377–392.
21. Henderson I, Tuy B, Connell D, Oakes B, Hettwer W. Prospective clinical study of autologous chondrocyte implantation and correlation with MRI at three and 12 months. *J Bone Joint Surg Br*. 2003;85(7):1060–1066.
22. Merkely G, Ogura T, Bryant T, Minas T. Severe bone marrow edema among patients who underwent prior marrow stimulation technique is a significant predictor of graft failure after autologous chondrocyte implantation. *Am J Sports Med*. 2019;47(8):1874–1884.

4

Patient Evaluation, Cartilage Defect, and Evidence: Putting It All Together

TOM MINAS MD, MS

CHAPTER OUTLINE

The Decision to Proceed with Joint Preservation

The History

To have a successful relationship with a patient, the desires, needs, and expectations of the patient must be balanced with what is possible. The surgeon must use his best judgment and draw upon the best available evidence, his own experience, and skills to match these goals. This is sometimes not possible and the patient should be referred to someone expert in the condition. Patients often present with pain and limitation of function. They are often anxious and have different reasons for the appointment. Determining the pathology and considering surgical options may not necessarily be what the patient is seeking.

An opening question such as "What is your goal by coming to see me today?" usually helps to direct the surgeon's line of questioning and treatment options offered to the patient. The patient may respond;

"I have knee pain and I want to know what it is and if it can be treated with physical therapy"

"I have knee pain and a family history of osteoarthritis and I wanted to avoid knee replacement surgery"

"I have been referred to Dr. X for a specific knee reconstructive procedure"

"I have no pain, but I was sent here because I have a cartilage defect."

Alternatively, the patient may be self-referred based on his own ambitions. This is becoming more commonplace in the day of the World Wide Web. This is especially true in the modern age of the Internet where patients are often well-informed and wish to take matters into their own hands: "empowerment of the patient". The cartoon (Fig. 4.1) illustrates this. A useful tool in developing a healthy relationship with the patient are the 5 Es (Fig. 4.2).

Cartilage repair and joint preservation are relatively new topics in the orthopedic management of young patients without large cohorts of patients having been treated or long-term follow-up. Internet information is not always reliable, is not peer-reviewed, may be market-driven, and it is therefore up to the orthopedic surgeon to know the evidence as it exists and present this to the patient as an educator, patient advocate, and doctor.

Patient Characteristics

The surgeon's recommendation of treatment options may very well depend on patient characteristics. A patient who has a high sense of vitality and optimistic outlook with strong social supports has demonstrated a good clinical outcome with almost any surgical procedure. We have reviewed our clinical outcome data using the Short Form 36 questionnaire[1] and had noted that vitality and social supports played strongly into a positive clinical outcome with physical pain relief and well-being (paper presented at the

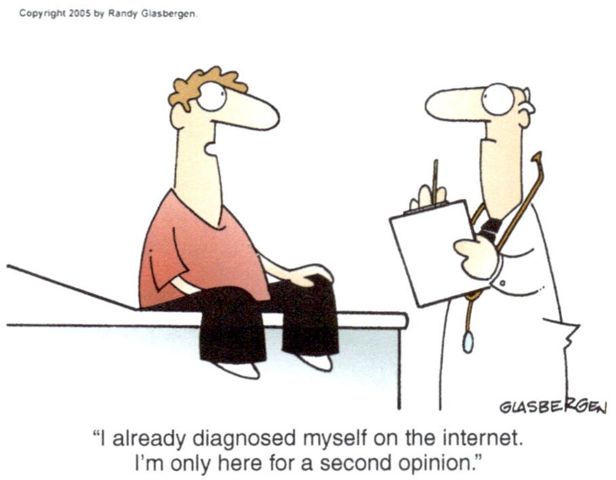
Copyright 2005 by Randy Glasbergen.
GLASBERGEN
"I already diagnosed myself on the internet.
I'm only here for a second opinion."

• **Fig. 4.1** Empowerment of the patient. (Copyright Randy Glasbergen, 2005)

International Cartilage Repair Society 2002). I have also found that patients who are athletic at baseline and had a relatively acute injury less than 1 year before, do better clinically after surgery.[2–4] It is suspected that if the athlete becomes deconditioned, the injury becomes chronic with thickened subchondral bone and expanding margins such that both the patient and the lesion require more extensive rehabilitation. Obesity is also a factor that faces us as surgeons. It is approaching epidemic proportions in the United States with approximately 30% of the population being considered obese. It has been demonstrated in the osteotomy literature that body weight greater than 1.32 times normal adversely affects the outcome and survivorship of osteotomy surgery.[5] Obesity has also been shown to correlate with an increased incidence of osteoarthritis, which presumably corresponds to enlargement of an existing cartilage defect, or factors adversely towards a cartilage repair procedure because of the force across the regenerative tissue. Counseling about weight loss prior to a biologic repair procedure may actually prevent the need for the procedure based on symptom relief with weight loss. For the morbidly obese patient with a BMI greater than 40 or Class III obesity, gastric bypass surgery may be necessary. Some insurance carriers in the United States will not allow cartilage repair in patients with a BMI greater than 30; for other carriers, the cutoff is a BMI of 35. Further research into the correlation between weight and progression of cartilage damage is necessary.

However, patients who are on medications for depression or anxiety or have addictive baseline behavior patterns such as the use of alcohol, smoking, narcotic usage for pain outside the postoperative setting, tend to demonstrate difficult postoperative patient management patterns. These factors must be delineated preoperatively and addressed individually. When discussing with patients who have depression or anxiety, preoperative counseling and maximizing medications to improve postoperative sense of well-being and compliance are important. I do not operate on patients who are taking narcotics for baseline pain management for their chondral defect or osteoarthritis until they are weaned off to a minimum baseline amount of narcotics that will allow good postoperative pain management. Smoking has demonstrated an adverse event with regard to bone healing and spinal fusions, long bone fractures and trauma, and also with the proteoglycan formation during cartilage healing. For this reason we do not offer biologic repair to smokers until they have completed a smoking cessation program. If they are unwilling or unable to follow the program and if they are at the transition age for a prosthetic reconstruction, a unicompartmental, bicompartmental, or total knee arthroplasty is recommended.

Injured Knee

As mentioned in the first chapter on characteristics that predispose to progression of cartilage injuries to arthritic change, a thorough evaluation to assess the background factors to cartilage loss is critical to the potential success of a biological preserving procedure. Radiographic studies to delineate long axial alignment of the limb relative to the knee joint, weight-bearing x-ray examination in extension and flexion to assess joint space narrowing or complete obliteration (a good screening tool to rule out the possibility of cartilage repair and recommend osteotomy or arthroplasty in isolation) must be performed.

A careful physical examination will identify the patient's gait pattern, varus or valgus thrust of the leg, atrophy of the musculature, range of motion of the tibiofemoral joint, effusion in the knee, status of the patellofemoral joint with regard to quadriceps angle, presence or absence of a J-sign from extension into flexion, mobility of the patella medial lateral proximal or distal and possible contracture of the patellofemoral articulation, crepitus in the patellofemoral or tibiofemoral joint, instability of the collateral and cruciate ligaments. The physical examination is also very important in determining whether the pain is in the medial tibiofemoral, lateral tibiofemoral, patellofemoral, or a combination thereof.

At this juncture, a tentative diagnosis is made based on the patient's history, x-ray studies, and physical examination. An MRI scan at this time is very helpful in making the diagnosis accurately without proceeding to arthroscopy.

If a cartilage injury is suspected, a high-resolution MRI scan is performed. Excellent resolution with orthogonal 1-mm cuts and longer acquisition times with a dedicated knee coil on either a 1.5 Tesla magnet or a 3 Tesla magnet give excellent resolution. Intra-articular dye enhancement (either indirect IV Gadolinium arthrogram[6] or direct intra-articular arthrogram) will maximize the information but is rarely needed with the newer MRI scanners. In this way the leg alignment and normal cartilage space are assessed, cartilage defect or defects are delineated, underlying bone marrow edema or cysts are identified, the volume and status of the menisci and preservation of the anterior cruciate

PATIENT FIRST TIP

To consistently provide excellent customer service always remember to use the 5 E's in interactions with every patient or family member, whether in person on the phone

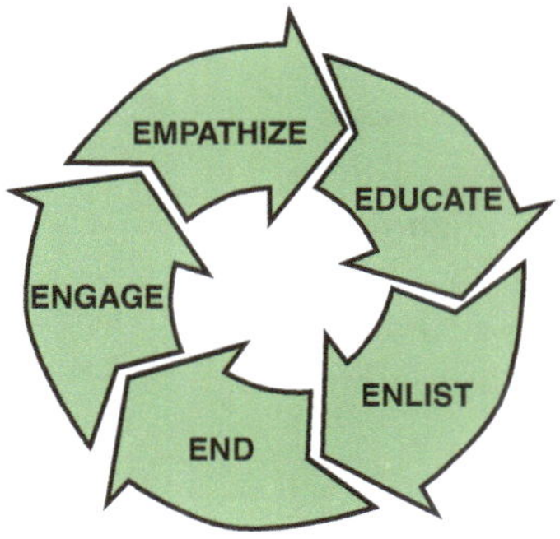

Step 1: ENGAGE

Build a relationship with the patient!

- Sit/stand straight keep your body relaxed
- Make eye contact
- Give the patient your attention
- Have an appropriate rate and volume of speech
- Speak clearly and pronunciate

Step 2: EMPATHIZE

Assure the patient feels seen, heard and accepted!

- Step into the patient's shoes to view their situation and try to understand their feelings
- Refrain from attaching your own judgment or feelings to the situation
- Offer a gesture of empathy (provide a tissue, nod your head to show you are listening, offer a blameless apology)

Step 3: EDUCATE

Inform the patient and answer questions/concerns!

- Define the problem, separating it from its emotional content try to understand their feelings
- Check continually for understanding so that you remain on the same page
- Describe what you can do and what your limitations are (use positive language)

Step 4: ENLIST

Invite the patient to collaborate as a decision maker on their plan of care!

- Invite the patient to discuss their situation
- Explain the available options
- Let the patient choose what they think/feel is best
- Support two-way conversations to empower the patient
- Agree on a solution

Step 5: END

Insure you have made a positive connection with the patient!

- Summarize the key points and what has been agreed upon
- Review next steps (ensure you follow-up on what it is promised)
- Ask if the patient has any remaining questions
- End with your own personal touch and 'goodbye and thank you'

Adapted from Carroll, J. & Keller, V., 'E4 Model'
Bayer Institute of Healthcare Communication, 1992

• **Fig. 4.2** A useful tool in developing a healthy relationship with the patient are the 5 Es.

ligament (ACL) and posterior cruciate ligament (PCL) are noted. Contracture of Hoffa's fat pad may be identified as well as intra-articular adhesions, loose bodies, synovitis, and effusion.

If the patient has been referred from another orthopedist, prior arthroscopic photographs and operative notes may be very valuable in accurately making a diagnosis and treatment plan. At this stage the diagnosis is usually made. After a thorough history and physical examination, alignment and standing x-ray examinations, high resolution MRI scans, and once the background factors are known and the cartilage damage understood, the only thing left to confirm the findings would be an arthroscopy.

Critical Cartilage Defect Size

Cartilage defects may be present and minimally symptomatic if either the defect is small or the activity level is insufficient to cause progression of disease. Previous studies will have identified lesions that are 2 cm^2 to coexist without degenerative changes in the knee up to 4 years after onset of symptoms.[7,8] More recent studies[9] have shown that there were no differences in clinical outcomes in ACL injured and stabilized knees with chondral defects of 2.1 cm^2 at 15 years compared with controls in 36 knees. This also supports the finding that lesions less than 2 cm^2 are unlikely to progress and this may represent a critical defect size. Based on these studies, early algorithms identified 2 cm^2 as a small defect.[10–12]

A critical size defect is considered a defect that shoulders the subchondral bone well from stimulus, hence reducing symptoms from subchondral bone nerve stimulation and lessening the abrasive effects of the subchondral bone on the opposing articular cartilage and therefore preventing bipolar changes from developing. However, a larger defect that is poorly shouldered will damage the opposing articular surface, developing progressive joint space cartilage loss, remaining symptomatic, and enlarging quickly based on the excessive force on the edges of the defect. Fig. 4.3 demonstrates this principle, which I described in an earlier publication.[12]

A relatively small defect that is symptomatic may be treated by either arthroscopic debridement of unstable margins and left alone or stabilized with a repair tissue that is fibrocartilaginous or hyaline cartilage. However, a larger poorly shouldered chondral defect will require a repair tissue with the same or nearly the same viscoelastic and mechanical properties as normal hyaline cartilage (Fig. 4.4). Procedures that may produce hyaline-like cartilage for this situation will be the topic of the remainder of this chapter (Fig. 4.5).

Prevalence of Articular Cartilage Injury

In making a recommendation to the patient, it is important to recognize defects that are causing symptoms.

Damage to the articular cartilage comprises a spectrum of disease entities ranging from single, focal chondral defects to more advanced degenerative disease. Focal

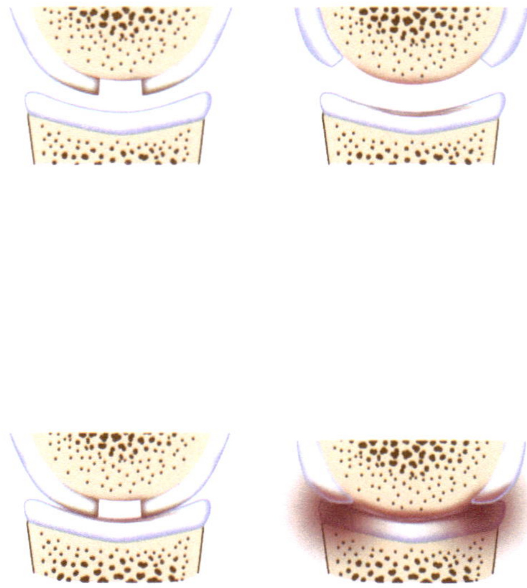

• **Fig. 4.3** A small well-shouldered chondral defect on the left prevents damage to the opposing surface; the shoulders of the defect support the subchondral bone. However, the defect on the right excessively overloads the shoulders, leading to premature breakdown of the supporting surface with abrasive changes developing on the opposing tibial surface. Persistent symptoms and degenerative changes are likely in this situation. A repair tissue that stabilizes the small defect is usually adequate; however, a repair tissue that simulates the normal viscoelastic mechanical properties of hyaline cartilage in the larger defect is necessary if the repair is to allow high-demand activities and be durable.

chondral defects result from various etiologies. Patients are approximately evenly split in reporting a traumatic versus an insidious onset of symptoms; athletic activities are the most common inciting event associated with the diagnosis of a chondral lesion.[13] Traumatic events and developmental etiologies such as osteochondritis dissecans (OCD) predominate in younger age groups. Several large studies have found high-grade chondral lesions (Fig. 4.6; Outerbridge grade III and IV) in 5% to 11% of younger patients (less than 40 years) and up to 60% of older patients.[13–15] The most common locations for these defects are the medial femoral condyle (up to 32%) and the patella,[14,15] and most are detected incidentally during meniscectomy or anterior cruciate ligament reconstruction.[13,16] Many of these defects are incidental in nature and asymptomatic.

The Asymptomatic Defect

The patient may have a known cartilage defect that is relatively asymptomatic; the question then becomes whether the lesion will progress over time. I have counseled patients in this situation to modify their activities to avoid impact and torsional sports and to cross-train with activities such as cycling, swimming, elliptical trainer, and upper body weight training. I then follow the patient with annual high-resolution MRI scans to determine whether the defect size is enlarging (Fig. 4.7) and if there is no enlargement, continue with annual weight-bearing x-ray examinations to determine joint space loss or the onset of symptoms, which

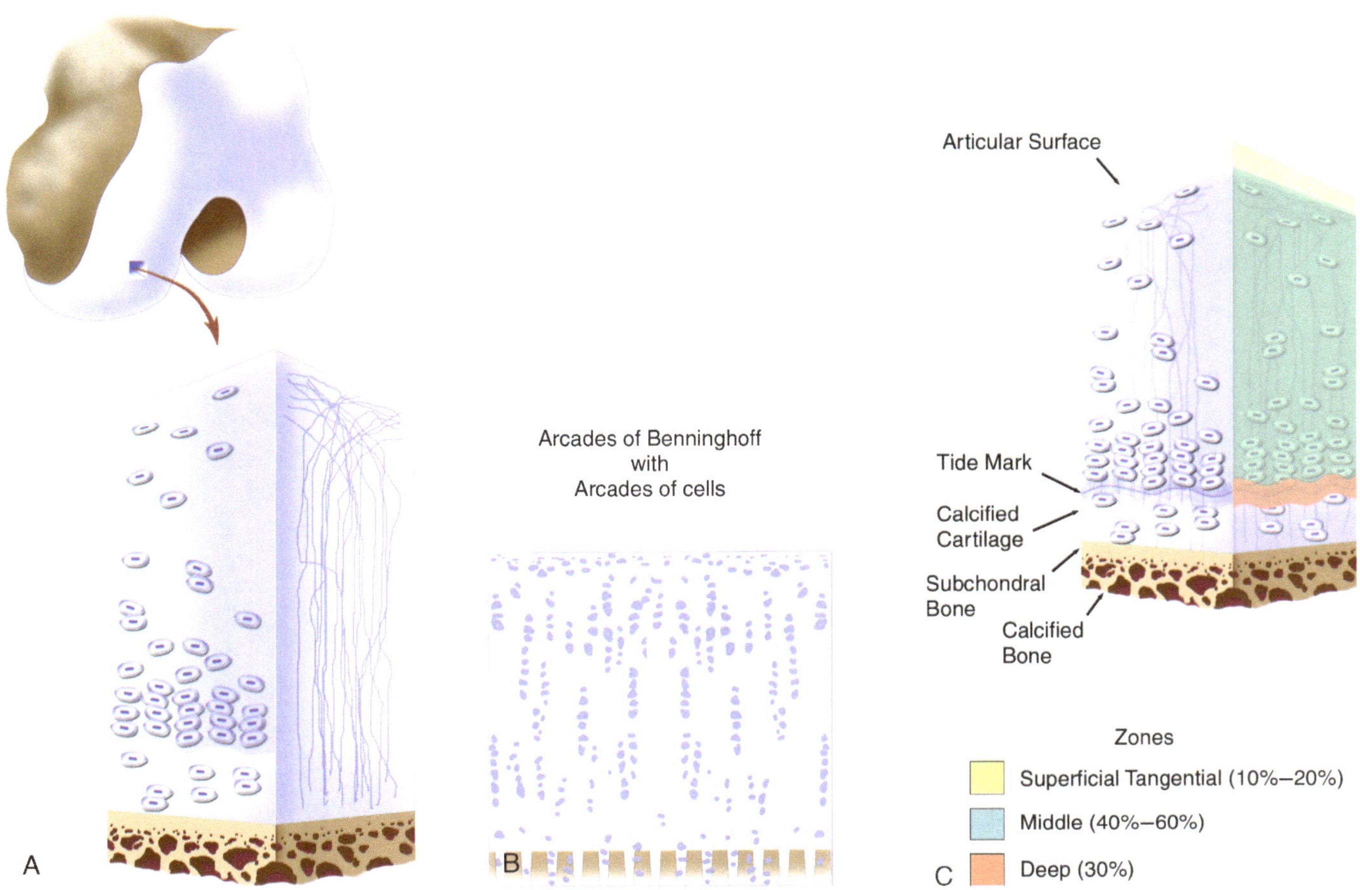

• **Fig. 4.4** (A) Articular cartilage can be thought of as a viscoelastic mechanical tissue that integrates into the subchondral bone allowing force transmission through an osteochondral unit. Restoration of the osteochondral unit via cartilage repair is the goal we are trying to achieve. (B) Type II collagen, unique to articular cartilage, is vertically arranged anchoring to the subchondral bone at the level of the tidemark of articular cartilage and running parallel to the articular surface forming a regularly arranged scaffold that is well bonded to the bone and produces the framework for articular cartilage (arcades of Benninghoff). Characteristic deep, middle, and superficial layers of cartilage cells with their distinct behavioral properties are shown on the right. (C) Schematic of cartilage layers.

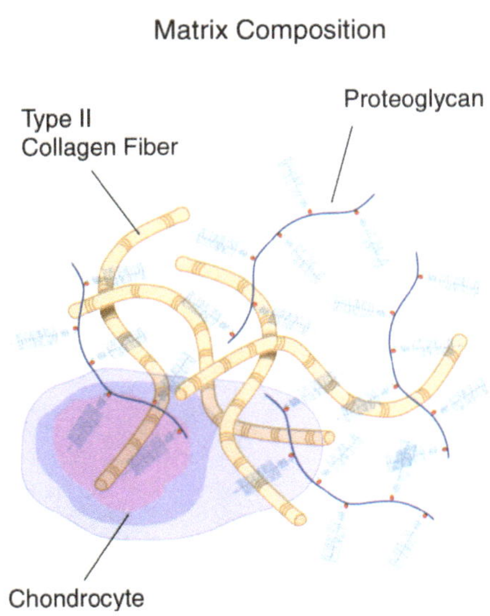

• **Fig. 4.5** The proteoglycans that are produced by the articular chondrocytes are highly negatively charged attracting and binding to positively charged water molecules forming a very resilient and unique visco elastic mechanical tissue. In order for a tissue to withstand large mechanical compressive, torsional, and shearing forces, a hyaline-like reparative tissue is required. This is the goal of cartilage repair for large lesions.

includes activity-related effusions of the knee despite an absence of pain, indicating a degenerative response of the joint symptoms. If there is progression of disease and the patient is concerned about the loss of opportunity for cartilage repair and preservation of their joint, a treatment-based discussion ensues. The discussion is based on the defect size, existing background factors, and the treatment options available surgically versus nonoperative intervention and the possibility of a prosthesis.

Treatment of Symptomatic Defects

The field of cartilage repair is a recent development within orthopedic surgery with techniques that continue to evolve. Although no formal treatment algorithms have been agreed upon and validated by prospective comparative trials of the emerging techniques, practice-based algorithms have been recommended based upon existing evidence and by matching patient characteristics to treatment efficacy and risks. High-quality outcomes research is necessary to provide a better understanding of the efficacy of these procedures and to enable physicians to identify appropriate treatment.

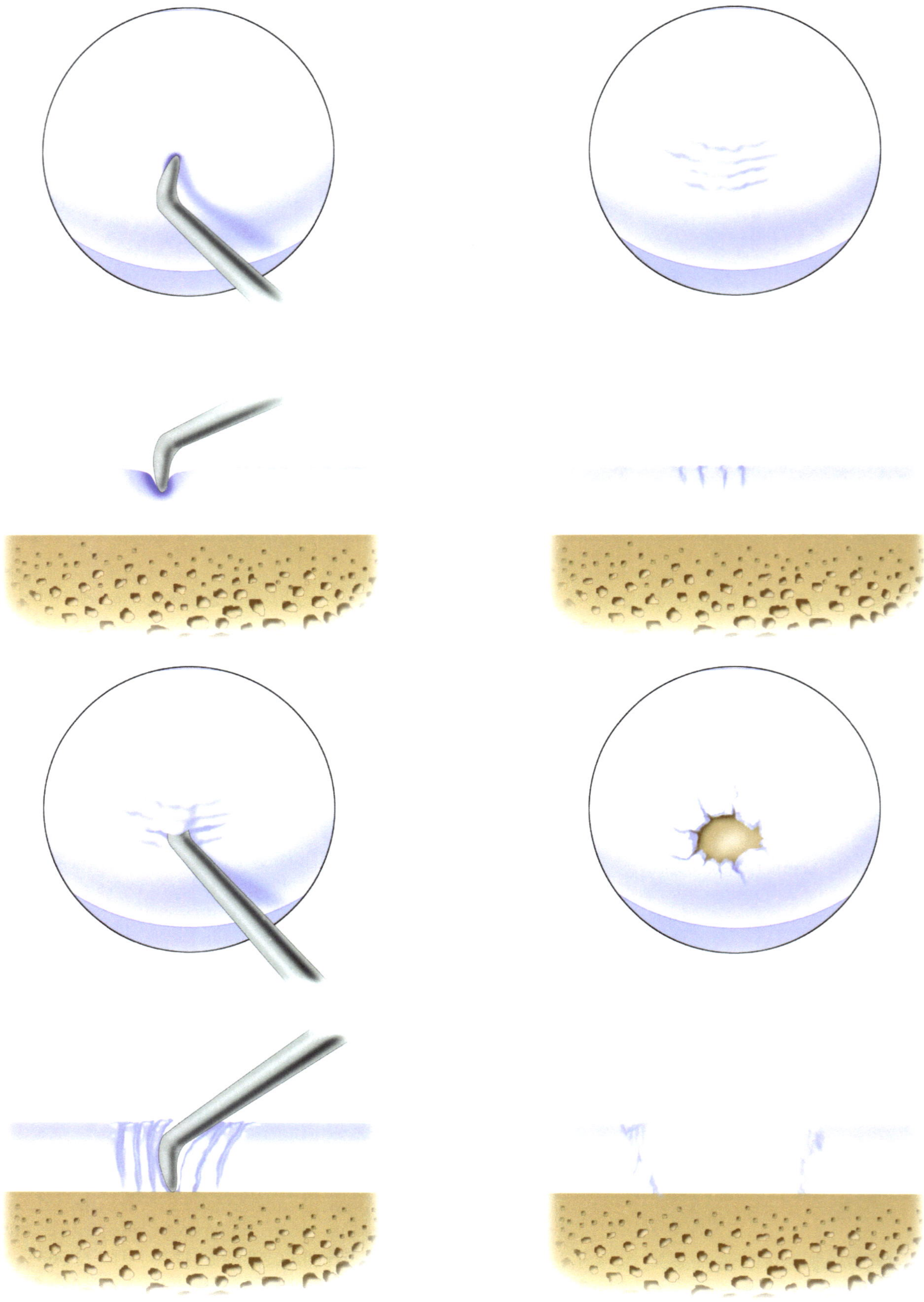

• **Fig. 4.6** Modified Outerbridge Classification. Grade 1: intact articular cartilage with softening of the surface. Grade 2: fissuring of the surface up to 50% of the thickness of the articular cartilage. Grade 3: fissuring to the subchondral bone. Grade 4: exposed bone with undermining of cartilaginous tissue. (From Outerbridge RE. The etiology of chondromalacia patellae. *J Bone Joint Surg Br*. 1961;43-B:752-757.)

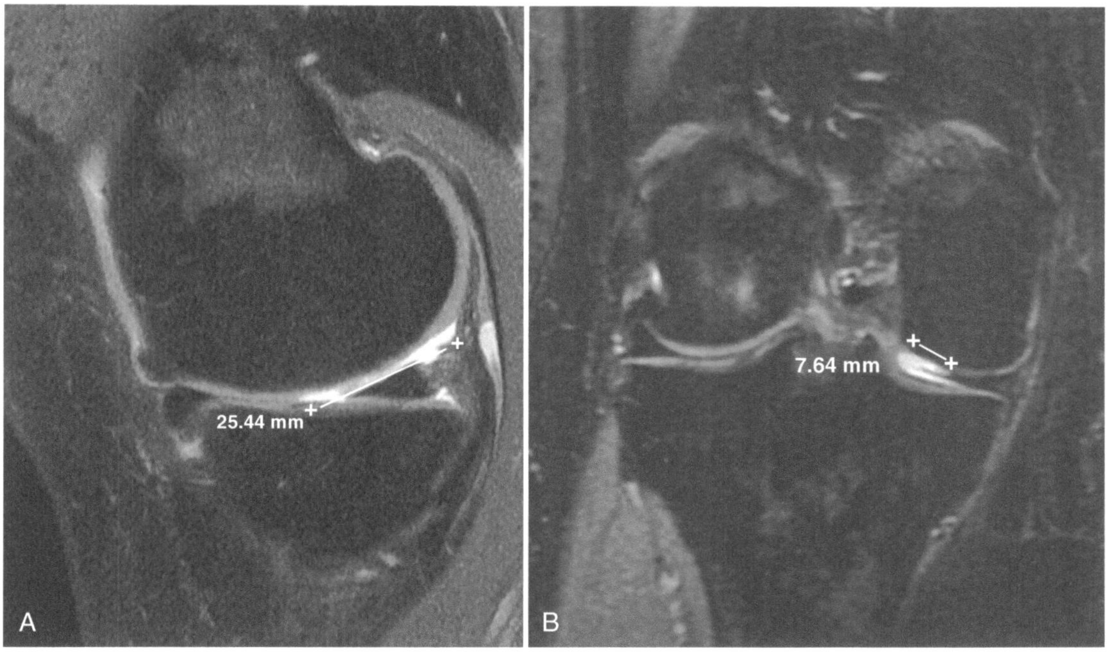

• **Fig. 4.7** High-resolution MRI scan with 20 cc of intravenous Gadolinium in a 32-year-old woman who has an asymptomatic medial femoral condyle, Outerbridge grade 4 cartilage defect. The patient has been followed for 3 years with consecutive MRI scans to assess articular cartilage degeneration and progression of disease. (A) The contrast-enhanced fat-suppressed sagittal image notes the defect is 25 mm long and (B) in the coronal image, the defect is 8 mm wide. This long and narrow lesion is in a slim patient with slight valgus to their knee and can be followed nonoperatively. If the patient were to develop symptoms or effusions, or progression of an enlarging cartilage defect, a discussion regarding cartilage repair would ensue.

When treating symptomatic defects, a thorough discussion and informed consent of what is involved postoperatively for the patient is essential. Patients can be made worse with a failed treatment. For an unexpected coincidental defect, a gentle chondroplasty is a treatment that will not make someone worse and if it fails, a formal discussion of the next step can be taken electively with all options available.

An overview of the existing techniques and supporting data will ensue in an attempt to guide surgeons in their indications for the treatment of cartilage defects of the knee. In the end, however, the practical realities prevail and surgeons will use what they are technically comfortable with and will take into consideration the availability of the techniques and the cost associated with the treatment and the health care system in which they practice.

Options

Until the 1990s, orthopedists were restricted to procedures that aimed to palliate the effects of chondral lesions or attempted to stimulate a healing response initiated from the subchondral bone resulting in the formation of fibrocartilage to fill the defect.[17] Simple arthroscopic lavage and debridement of lesions has been used since the 1940s in an effort to reduce symptoms resulting from loose bodies and cartilage flaps and is a common first-line treatment, especially for coincidental defects. Arthroscopic debridement on its own has been demonstrated to produce measurable symptomatic improvement. Hubbard[18] noted that grade 4 femoral condyle defects randomized to arthroscopic lavage versus debridement did better when debrided. The Lysholm score increased to 28 points at 1 year and 21 points at 5 years in over 50% of patients, however, without defect repair. The defect size was not measured and radiographic evidence of progression or follow-up arthroscopy was not performed in this study.

Levy[19] noted that debridement for acute small lesions (average 42 mm^2) in 15 young soccer players allowed all players to return to soccer at 10.8 weeks postoperatively, with 6 excellent and 9 good results. One player developed extensive continued delamination. Follow-up was after 1 year.

In a study evaluating Return to Play (RTP) for National Football League (NFL) athletes,[20] 52 patients (54 procedures) over a 10-year period were reviewed after isolated chondroplasty. Of these players 67% (36) were able to RTP on an average of 8.2 months after arthroscopy. With an average follow-up of 5.9 years, 24% (24%) were still actively playing. Players who underwent microfracture were 4.4 (95% CI, 1.3–15.5) times less likely to RTP.

The natural history of an untreated chondral injury is yet to be established, although most agree that even small lesions, less than 1 cm^2, are likely to progress very slowly,[21] with over 50% developing osteoarthritis over a 14-year follow-up.

Marrow stimulation techniques (MST), such as drilling, abrasion arthroplasty, and microfracture attempt to induce a reparative response by perforation of the subchondral bone after radical debridement of damaged cartilage and removal of the tide mark "calcified" zone to enhance the integration of repair tissue. The resultant blood clot and the primitive mesenchymal cells contained within may differentiate into a fibrocartilaginous repair tissue that fills the defect. Unlike hyaline cartilage, this fibrocartilage largely consists of type I collagen and is mechanically less stable and less durable.[22] The pluripotential marrow-derived cells may also form bone, another mode of MST-related failure that is increasingly becoming recognized.[23]

Restorative cartilage repair techniques such as autologous chondrocyte implantation (ACI) introduce chondrogenic cells into the defect area, resulting in the formation of a repair tissue that more closely resembles the collagen type-II rich hyaline cartilage. The original technique of ACI was developed over 20 years ago[8] and has been used in the United States to treat 30,266 patients since 1995 (Vericel database, Vericel, Cambridge, MA—formerly Genzyme Tissue Repair). ACI is indicated for the treatment of medium to large chondral defects with no or shallow associated osseous deficits. It originally received FDA approval for application in the femoral condyle (medial, lateral, and trochlea) but has also been used successfully to treat patellar defects. ACI in its current form is a two-stage procedure with an initial arthroscopic cartilage biopsy, followed by a staged reimplantation through an arthrotomy. The next generation ACI-c (collagen covered) technique was developed to reduce the re-operation rate caused by hypertrophy of the periosteal patch used to cover the defect. This was achieved by substitution of periosteum with a collagen membrane, frequently consisting of a porcine type-I/III collagen bi-layer membrane. The latest generation of ACI, termed MACI (matrix-induced autologous chondrocyte implantation), cultures the chondrocytes directly on the aforementioned collagen membrane for 2–3 days prior to implantation, which is then implanted arthroscopically or through a mini-open approach with fibrin glue or limited suturing. MACI has been FDA-approved and available in the United States since December 2017. In 2019, 2270 MACI cases were performed in the United States (Vericel database).

Cartilage replacement techniques include osteochondral auto- and allograft transfers, such as the osteochondral allograft transfer system (OATS) (Arthrex, Naples, FL), mosaicplasty (Smith & Nephew, Andover, MA), and mega-OATS allograft techniques. OATS is used to address small to medium defects (1–4 cm^2), often with associated bone loss. Osteochondral cylinders are harvested from lesser marginal weight-bearing areas of the knee joint and press-fitted into the prepared defect. Commonly, multiple cylinders have to be transplanted to fill larger defects. Osteochondral autografting is limited by the amount of cartilage that can be harvested without violating the weight-bearing articular surface,[24] "taking from Peter to pay Paul." The main advantage lies in its autogeneity, avoidance of disease transmission, immediate graft availability through harvesting of the patient's own tissue, and decreased cost of this single-stage procedure.

The treatment of chondral defects with fresh osteochondral allografts has garnered significant attention because of its potential to restore and resurface even extensive areas of damaged cartilage and bone. Osteochondral allograft transplantation is used predominantly in the treatment of large and deep osteochondral lesions resulting from osteochondritis dissecans, osteonecrosis, and traumatic osteochondral fractures, but can also be used to treat peripherally uncontained cartilage and bone defects. Furthermore, osteochondral allografting presents a viable salvage option after failure of other cartilage resurfacing procedures. The main advantages over autograft transplantation are the ability to match very closely the curvature of the articular surface by harvesting the graft from a corresponding location in the donor condyle, the ability to transplant large grafts, and the avoidance of donor site morbidity. The main concerns with allograft transplantation are failure to incorporate with subchondral collapse and the risk of disease transmission (estimated at 1 in 1.6 million for the transmission of HIV[25]).

Evidence

The following is a review of the published reports on techniques for cartilage repair evaluating the indications, defect size, locations within the joint, and efficacy of the technique with the levels of evidence of the studies reviewed. The findings are summarized in Tables 4.1, 4.2, and 4.3.[26]

Microfracture

Most studies show good outcomes in 60% to 80% of patients. Several studies have tried to define the indications for microfracture with regard to patient and defect characteristics. In an early study,[27] Steadman reported that 67% of patients were able to return to sports or heavy manual labor, 20% were unchanged by the treatment, and 13% were made worse. Kreuz and Erggelet have demonstrated improved results in patients younger than 40 years of age, in regard both to validated scores and to MRI findings of better fill and quality.[28] They also demonstrated a worsening between the 18- and 36-month follow-up scores for all patients in the older age group and for younger patients with patellofemoral defects.[28] In another study, the same authors reported the association between outcomes and defect locations and found the best outcomes in femoral condyle lesions, while those in the patella fared worst.[29] Other authors have described better results in cases with smaller lesions, BMI of less than 30, and shorter duration between onset of symptoms and treatment.[30–32]

TABLE 4.1 Summary of Published Reports on Techniques for Cartilage Repair

Study	Design; (Level of Evidence/ LoE)	Follow-up interval; (number of cases)	Patient population	Patient age; (Defect Size)	Treatment groups	Results
Kreuz[28] 2006	Prospective (LoE 2)	3 years (70 patients)	Grade 3 and 4 chondral defects treated with microfracture	30 and 39 years (average 2.2 cm^2)	Patient age: <40 years, >40 years	All groups improved significantly; younger patients improved more. Older patients and patellofemoral lesions in younger patients worsened between 18 and 36 months
Kreuz[29] 2006	Prospective (LoE 2)	3 years (70 patients)	Grade 3 and 4 chondral defects treated with microfracture	40 years (average 2.2 cm^2)	Defect locations: Femoral condyle, trochlea, tibia, patella	All groups improved significantly, most in the femoral condyle group; results decreased between 18 and 36 months
Mithoefer[30] 2005	Case series (LoE 4)	41 months (48 patients)	Grade 3 and 4 chondral defects treated with microfracture	41 years (median 2.8 cm^2)	N/A	Significant improvement until 24 months post-op, then deterioration. Poor fill on MRI correlated with poor outcome. BMI >30 associated with poor fill and outcome.
Blevins[32] 1998	Case series (LoE 4)	3.7 years (140 patients)	Grade 3 and 4 chondral defects treated with microfracture	26 and 38 years (average 2.2 cm^2)	Activity status: High-level versus recreational athletes	Both groups with significant improvements. On second-look arthroscopy no improvement in lesion grade in 8% of high-level and 35% of recreational athletes
Bartlett[36] 2005	RCT (LoE 1)	12 months (91 patients)	Grade 3 and 4 chondral defects	34 years (average 6 cm^2)	ACI technique: ACI-c, MACI	No statistically significant differences between groups. Better outcomes in patients younger than 35 years and with symptoms for less than 50 months. Reoperation rate for graft hypertrophy in 9% of ACI-c and 6% of MACI.
Gooding[35] 2005	RCT (LoE 1)	24 months (68 patients)	Grade 3 and 4 chondral defects	31 years (average 4.5 cm^2)	ACI technique: ACI-p, ACI-c	Good and excellent results (Cincinnati score) in 74% of ACI-c and 67% of ACI-p, but dissimilar defect locations: 61% of lesions treated with ACI-p were patellar, while only 20% of those treated with ACI-c were in this location. Reoperation rate for graft hypertrophy was 36% in ACI-p and 0% for ACI-c.
Bentley[33] 2003	RCT (LoE 1)	19 months (100 patients)	Grade 3 and 4 chondral defects	31 years (average 4.7 cm^2)	Cartilage repair technique: ACI-c, mosaicplasty	Good and excellent results (Cincinnati score) in 88% of ACI and 69% of mosaicplasty patients. All 5 patellar mosaicplasties failed. No graft hypertrophy in ACI patients (collagen membrane used).

Continued

TABLE 4.1 Summary of Published Reports on Techniques for Cartilage Repair—cont'd

Study	Design; (Level of Evidence/ LoE)	Follow-up interval; (number of cases)	Patient population	Patient age; (Defect Size)	Treatment groups	Results
Knutsen[37] 2004	RCT (LoE 1)	2 years (80 patients)	Grade 3 and 4 chondral defects	33 years (average 5 cm^2)	Cartilage repair technique: ACI, microfracture	No statistically significant differences between the groups at 2 years, except SF-36, which was better in microfracture group. Patients younger than 30 years and more active (Tegner >4) did better, regardless of treatment. Defects larger than 4 cm^2 fared worse with microfracture, no similar effect was seen with ACI.
Gudas[40] 2005	RCT (LoE 1)	37 months (57 patients)	Grade 3 and 4 chondral defects	24 years (average 2.8 cm^2)	Cartilage repair technique: Microfracture, OATS	Good and excellent results in 96% of OATS and 52% of microfracture patients. Return to sports in 93% of OATS and 52% of microfracture patients. Microfracture significantly worse in lesions >2 cm^2, and results deteriorated after 12 months. Both groups showed better results in patients <30 years.
Gross[41] 2005	Case series (LoE 4)	10 years (127 patients)	Osteochondral defects of the femur and tibia	27 years (femur) 43 years (tibia)	N/A	Survivorship of 95% at 5 years, 80%–85% at 10 years, and 65%–74% at 15 years.
Gortz[42] 2007	Case series (LoE 4)	4.5 years (43 patients)	Osteochondral defects of the femur	35 years (average 5.9 cm^2)	N/A	88% good and excellent results

ACI, autologous chondrocyte implantation; *OATS*, osteochondral allograft transfer system.

TABLE 4.2 Updated High-Quality Studies since 1st Edition, 2010–2020

Study	Design; (Level of Evidence/ LoE)	Follow-up interval; (no. of cases)	Patient population	Patient age; (mean defect size)	Treatment groups	Results
Brittberg[48] 2018	RCT (LoE I)	5 years (128 patients)	Grade 3 and 4 chondral defects, femoral condyle or trochlea	Medians 34 and 38 years (5.0 cm^2)	Cartilage repair technique: Microfracture, MACI	Cartilage defects 3 cm^2 or larger treated with MACI were clinically and statistically significantly improved at 5 years compared with microfracture treatment.
Volz[49] 2017	RCT (LoE I)	5 years (34 patients)	Grade 3 and 4 chondral defects, all surfaces	37 years (3.6 cm^2)	Cartilage repair technique: Microfracture, AMIC glued, AMIC sutured	Clinical outcome improvement was seen for the first 2 years in all subgroups. After 2 years, a progressive and significant outcome score decline was evident in the microfracture group. All functional scores were sustained for at least five years in the AMIC groups.
Knutsen[50] 2016	RCT (LoE I)	15 years (80 patients)	Grade 3 and 4 chondral defects, femoral condyle	32.2 years (4.8 cm^2)	Cartilage repair technique: Microfracture, ACI	Of the retained grafts, all clinical outcome scores improved significantly. No significant differences were observed between groups with respect to outcome measurements. At the 15-year evaluation, the failure rate was 42.5 % in the ACI group and 32.5% in the microfracture group ($P = .356$).
Clave[51] 2016	RCT (LoE 1)	2 years (55 patients)	Grade 3 and 4 chondral defects, femoral condyle	28.8 years (3.4 cm^2)	Cartilage repair technique: Mosaicplasty, MACI with CARTIPATCH	IKDC results were significantly better in the mosaicplasty-treated patients. There was a 12.6-point overall difference in IKDC scores between groups and a 20.2-point difference in defects ≥3.5 cm^2.
Shive[52] 2015	RCT (LoE I)	5 years (80 patients)	Grade 3 and 4 chondral defects, femoral condyle	36.1 years (2.25 cm^2)	Cartilage repair technique: Microfracture, Microfracture + BST-CarGel	BST-CarGel-treated patients showed a significantly greater improvement in defect filling over 5 years. Significant increases in clinical outcome parameters were observed in both groups. No significant difference in clinical outcomes between treatment groups.
Bentley[53] 2012	RCT (LoE 1)	10 years (100 patients)	Grade 3 and 4 chondral defects, all surfaces	31.3 years (4.4 cm^2)	Cartilage repair technique: Mosaicplasty, ACI	Of the retained grafts, clinical and functional outcomes were significantly better in the ACI group. Ten (17%) patients' grafts failed in the ACI group and 23 (55%) failed in the mosaicplasty group ($P < .001$).

Continued

TABLE 4.2 Updated High-Quality Studies since 1st Edition, 2010–2020—cont'd

Study	Design; (Level of Evidence/ LoE)	Follow-up interval; (no. of cases)	Patient population	Patient age; (mean defect size)	Treatment groups	Results
Crawford[54] 2012	RCT (LoE 1)	2 years (30 patients)	Grade 3 chondral defect, femoral condyle	40 years (2.70 cm^2)	Cartilage repair technique: Microfracture, NeoCart	Clinical outcome improvement was significantly better in the NeoCart group at 6, 12, and 24 months postoperatively, with a significantly greater net score improvement. More NeoCart-treated patients responded to therapy at 6 and 12 months ($P = .0125$).
Niethammer[55] 2018	Prospective (LoE 2)	2 years (91 patients)	Grade 3 and 4 chondral defects, all surfaces treated with NOVOCART 3D	34.5 years (5.55 cm^2)	Graft appearance: Hypertrophic grafts, nonhypertrophic grafts	No significant difference was found in T2-weighted relaxation times between hypertrophic and nonhypertrophic grafts over 4 years. IKDC scores did not differ between groups.
Minas[46] 2018	Case control (LoE 3)	7.8 years (41 patients)	Deep osteochondral defects, secondary to OCD or AVN	31.5 years (7.0 cm^2)	Cartilage repair technique: ACI sandwich + ABG (autologous bone grafting), ABG alone	ACI sandwich + ABG-treated patients had greater improvement in clinical, functional, and satisfaction results, with more than 90% of patients reporting their knees as good or excellent.
Ebert[56] 2017	Retrospective (LoE 3)	2 years (194 patients)	Grade 3 and 4 chondral defects, all surfaces treated with MACI	37.8 years (3.0 cm^2)	Defect location: tibiofemoral, patellofemoral	All patients experienced significant improvement in clinical results. The PF group had lower baseline reported clinical outcomes than the TF group. However, the PF-treated (with concurrent correction of PF maltracking) experienced a greater net improvement, resulting in near equivalent scores at final follow-up.
Niethammer[57] 2017	Case-control (LoE 3)	3 years (40 patients)	Grade 3 and 4 chondral defects, all surfaces treated with NOVOCART 3D	16 years and 36.7 years (5.2 cm^2)	Patient age: <20, >20 years	All patients had significantly improved clinical outcomes throughout the postoperative timeline. IKDC and VAS scores were significantly better in children and adolescents (<20 years) than adults.
Ogura[47] 2019	Case series (LoE 4)	7.8 years (15 patients)	Deep osteochondral defects, all surfaces treated with ACI segmental sandwich technique	31 years (6.0 cm^2)	N/A	All clinical and functional scores significantly and clinically meaningfully improved, with a 93% satisfaction rate. Complete or near-complete defect filling was evident in 83% of the patients at 3 years postoperative.

TABLE 4.2 Updated High-Quality Studies since 1st Edition, 2010–2020—cont'd

Study	Design; (Level of Evidence/LoE)	Follow-up interval; (no. of cases)	Patient population	Patient age; (mean defect size)	Treatment groups	Results
Lopez-Alcorocho[58] 2018	Case series (LoE 4)	2 years (50 patients)	Grade 3 and 4 chondral defects, all surfaces treated with high density ACI (HD-ACI with Chondro-Gide)	Median 35 years ($3.7 cm^2$)	N/A	Mean IKDC scores showed statistically significant increases and clinically meaningful improvement at 12 and 24 months postoperative, with reduced pain and swelling.
Siebold[59] 2018	Case series (LoE 4)	3 years (30 patients)	Grade 3 and 4 chondral defects, all surfaces treated with arthroscopic ACI using chondrospheres (ACT3D)	35.5 years ($6.0 cm^2$)	N/A	Significant increases in all clinical outcome parameters were observed, with parallel improvement in MOCART scores.
Anderson[60] 2017	Case series (LoE 4)	5 years (29 patients)	Grade 3 chondral defect, femoral condyle	41.0 years ($2.08 cm^2$)	MOCART analysis of Neocart repair tissue	Significant ($P < .001$) improvement in the quality of repair tissue was observed from 3 to 12 months with moderate progression in MOCART parameters to 24 months ($P < .05$). MOCART composite scores correlated with the IKDC and KOOS-Pain scores at 6 months. All primary clinical outcome scores significantly improved from baseline to the mean final follow-up.
Ogura[61] 2017	Case series (LoE 4)	20 years (23 patients)	Grade 3 and 4 chondral defects, all surfaces treated w/ first-generation ACI (ACI-P)	35.4 years ($5.6 cm^2$)	N/A	All 15 knees with retained grafts showed significant improvement in all clinical outcome scores, apart from WOMAC subscore for stiffness and SF-36 mental component score. Survival rate was 63% at 10 and 20 years after ACI surgery.
Minas[62] 2014	Case series (LoE 4)	10 years (210 patients)	Grade 3 and 4 chondral defects, all surfaces treated w/ first-generation ACI (ACI-P)	36 years (4.9 cm^2)	N/A	At 10 years, the survivorship of ACI-P was 71% with 75% of patients reporting improved function. All clinical outcome scores improved significantly at final follow-up.

MACI, matrix autologous chondrocyte implantation; *AMIC*, autologous matrix-induced chondrogenesis; *MOCART*, magnetic resonance observation of cartilage repair tissue.

TABLE 4.3 Treatment Recommendations and Respective Level of Evidence

Level of Evidence	Recommendation
B	Microfracture treatment shows better results in smaller defects (<2–4 cm^2)
B	Microfracture treatment shows best results in femoral condyle lesions
B	Microfracture treatment results in better outcomes in younger patients (<30–40 years)
C	Microfracture treatment results in better outcomes in patients with BMI <30
I	ACI, microfracture, or mosaicplasty result in outcomes superior to each other
B	Shorter duration of symptoms prior to cartilage repair results in better outcomes
A	The use of a collagen membrane in place of a periosteal patch for ACI reduces the re-operation rate for graft hypertrophy
A	ACI-c and MACI have comparable outcomes
B	Osteochondral defects are amenable to osteochondral allograft transplantation

A: Good evidence (Level I Studies with consistent finding) for or against recommending intervention. B: Fair evidence (Level II or III Studies with consistent findings) for or against recommending intervention. C: Poor-quality evidence (Level IV or V with consistent findings) for or against recommending intervention. I: There is insufficient or conflicting evidence not allowing a recommendation for or against intervention. *ACI*, Autologous chondrocyte implantation; *MACI*, matrix-induced autologous chondrocyte implantation.

Autologous Chondrocyte Implantation

Several long-term case series have reported good to excellent results in 70% to 90% of patients after ACI in the knee, depending on the location (patella and femoral condyle) or the clinical series.[2,11] Bentley compared ACI-c with mosaicplasty in a prospective RCT, showing good and excellent results (Cincinnati score) in 88% of ACI patients, but only 69% of mosaicplasties. All five patellar mosaicplasties were considered failures.[33] In a similar study by Horas, mosaicplasty performed significantly better than ACI. Biopsies were obtained from a sub group of patients and uniformly revealed fibrous tissue in all defects treated with ACI. This study, however, was limited by the use of non standard cell-culturing facilities.[34]

In a prospective RCT comparing ACI-p with ACI-c, Gooding found no statistically significant differences in the clinical outcome, but a re-operation rate for symptomatic graft hypertrophy of 36% in the periosteal covered group versus 0% with the collagen membrane.[35] Bartlett recently presented a prospective RCT comparing the advanced techniques ACI-c and MACI and reported no statistically significant differences between the groups. He also found improved outcomes in patients younger than 35 years and with preoperative symptoms for less than 50 months.[36] Knutsen compared ACI with microfracture and found no significant differences. The SF-36 improved more in the microfracture group and the author hypothesized whether this could be due to the more invasive nature of ACI. Furthermore, he observed better results in younger (less than 30 years) and more active (Tegner >4) patients. Defects larger than 4 cm^2 fared worse than smaller lesions after microfracture treatment; no such effect was seen after ACI.[37]

Graft hypertrophy resulting in mechanical symptoms such as clicking and popping occurs in up to 25%–30% of patients, typically 7 to 9 months after the procedure,[38] and can be addressed with arthroscopic debridement of the hypertrophic tissue. Newer techniques such as ACI-c and MACI have decreased the rate of symptomatic graft hypertrophy to less than 10%.[36]

Osteochondral Autograft Transplantation

Patients treated with osteochondral autograft transplantation experienced good to excellent results in approximately 90% of condylar lesions, 80% of tibial defects, and 70% of trochlear lesions.[39] The technique is technically demanding arthroscopically, more reproducible by open or mini open techniques. The treatment of patellar defects remains controversial with some groups reporting almost universal failure in this location.[33] Gudas compared OATS with microfracture in a group of athletes and demonstrated good and excellent results in 96% of patients treated with OATS versus 52% with microfracture. Return to sports was 93% with OATS and 52% with microfracture. Microfracture performed significantly worse in lesions larger than 2 cm^2 and results started to deteriorate after the 12-month examination. Both groups showed better results in patients younger than 30 years.[40]

Osteochondral Allograft Transplantation

Gross reported on a large series of fresh osteochondral allografts for the treatment of predominately traumatic distal femoral and proximal tibial defects. Survivorship analysis demonstrated intact and well-functioning grafts (HSS score greater than 70) in 95% of patients at 5 years, which decreased to 80%–85% at 10 years and 65%–74% at 15 years.[41] Gortz reported good and excellent results in 88% of 43 fresh osteochondral allografts of the distal femur at an average follow-up of 4.5 years.[42]

Areas of Uncertainty

Study Design and Indications

Symptomatic chondral defects are relatively rare in a clinical practice; therefore, a surgeon must have a large tertiary referral practice to develop clinical expertise in this area. In order to compare treatments for a rare problem such as a chondral defect, there must be a large difference in the treatment outcomes to have an adequately statistically powered study. However, the time endpoints must also be established in this field as any fibrocartilage repair may do well in the first 3 years and then the tissue and the clinical results will deteriorate. Hence, not only is an adequately powered study necessary, but an appropriate length of follow-up to determine durability of the repair and the prevention of degenerative joint disease. Therefore, a multicenter prospective randomized study is necessary in order to recruit adequately.

Several authors have conducted studies comparing different repair techniques such as microfracture, mosaicplasty, and ACI with conflicting results. These studies are often compromised by the very nature of the procedures they were designed to investigate; for example, ACI as a cell-based therapy is dependent on a sophisticated cell-culturing process. The cell-culturing process requires phenotypic validation, cell viability assessment, and sterility process validation according to USFDA (US Food and Drug Administration), GLP (Good Laboratory Practices), and GMP (Good Manufacturing Practices) to ensure sterile, safe, phenotypically stable cell implantation; however, not all authors utilize standardized and approved laboratory facilities.

The technical skill factor and learning curve for the ACI procedure and multiple osteochondral grafting technique is crucial. These procedures are challenging. Some studies have used multiple surgeons performing few surgeries, which may compromise the clinical outcomes. This is another appealing facet of the microfracture technique—its technical ease of performance to most parts of the knee joint, which may bias against a comparative study using ACI or mosaicplasty where technical perfection is a must in order to obtain a good clinical result.

Furthermore, it is unlikely that every chondral defect is amenable to every available treatment, but rather that there will be differences depending on the exact defect size and location. Therefore, even well-designed prospective randomized controlled trials attempting to compare treatment options for a wide range of defects are bound to yield conflicting results.

In order to formulate better treatment guidelines, each treatment option will first have to be investigated on its own to ascertain which type of defect it is most efficacious in. The success rates and clinical outcomes may then be established from these well-performed prospective clinical cohorts. A range of patient characteristics, defect location, and size will thus be established. Each defect will have one or several associated treatment options. We will then be able to conduct well-designed, adequately powered, ethically sound, comparative studies. These will be true Level 1 Evidence-Based Outcome studies that will help guide treatments for our patients and provide data for evidence-based treatment algorithms. Only then will we be able to design trials that compare the efficacy of treatment options for the same type of defect.

Engebretsen evaluated the quality of cartilage repair studies in a recent update[43] to a previous publication[44] and commented on this subject: "The increased focus on methodology in major journals by marking original articles with a level-of-evidence is highly appreciated. However, we would like to emphasize the fact that randomized controlled trials can have serious design flaws (i.e., not using independent reviewers, no statistical power analysis, not using an adequate randomization procedure, not accounting for eligible subjects not included in study), and therefore be rated as level-of-evidence II. We would also like to draw the reader's attention to the fact that several well performed case series (level-IV evidence) score very well on the CMS. These studies largely take into consideration multiple aspects of good methodological quality such as independent investigator, sufficient number of patients, well-described rehabilitation protocol, validated outcome measures and so forth, and are mainly lacking in not having a control group. We therefore recommend the reader to not entirely dismiss articles marked level-IV evidence, yet themselves assess the methodological quality of the paper when interpreting the results (for example using a grading system like the CMS)." We agree with their recommendation that inclusion and exclusion criteria should be well established, validated outcome measures for cartilage injuries should be used, and outcome assessment should be made by an independent investigator, ideally by the patient without assistance.

Background Factors

The presence of these associated abnormalities introduces an additional layer of variability into studies because the reproducibility of assessing background factors between surgeons and treating these prior to or concomitantly with the treatment of the chondral defect varies. To date, this correlation has not been firmly established. The disappointing early results of cartilage repair have been explained by the failure to diagnose and correct these associated bony and ligamentous abnormalities. For example, in early studies of patellar defects treated with ACI alone, good and excellent results were found in only one-third of patients.[8] Later studies, however, identified patellar maltracking as an important associated abnormality and concurrent use of a corrective osteotomy led to 71% good or excellent results[45] and improved the initial poor results in the Peterson series to 79%[2] excluding the early cohort when tracking of the patella was also treated. These reports emphasize the importance of a thorough patient evaluation to correctly identify and treat all associated abnormalities to ensure the long-term success of chondral repair.

Guidelines

There are no established societal (International Cartilage Repair Society [ICRS], American Academy of Orthopedic Surgeons [AAOS], Arthroscopy Association of North America [AANA], International Society of Arthroscopy, Knee Surgery, and Orthopedic Sports Medicine [ISAKOS], etc.) guidelines based on comparative trials for the treatment of articular cartilage. An updated evidence-based treatment algorithm that I have published[11] in the past is shown in Figs. 4.8 and 4.9. My personal treatment preferences are described in the following section.

Recommendations

I do not treat asymptomatic chondral defects at this time because of the possibility of worsening the patient's condition. Existing techniques do not report excellent results greater than 90% and the natural history and progression of a chondral defect remains unknown for a given individual. Careful

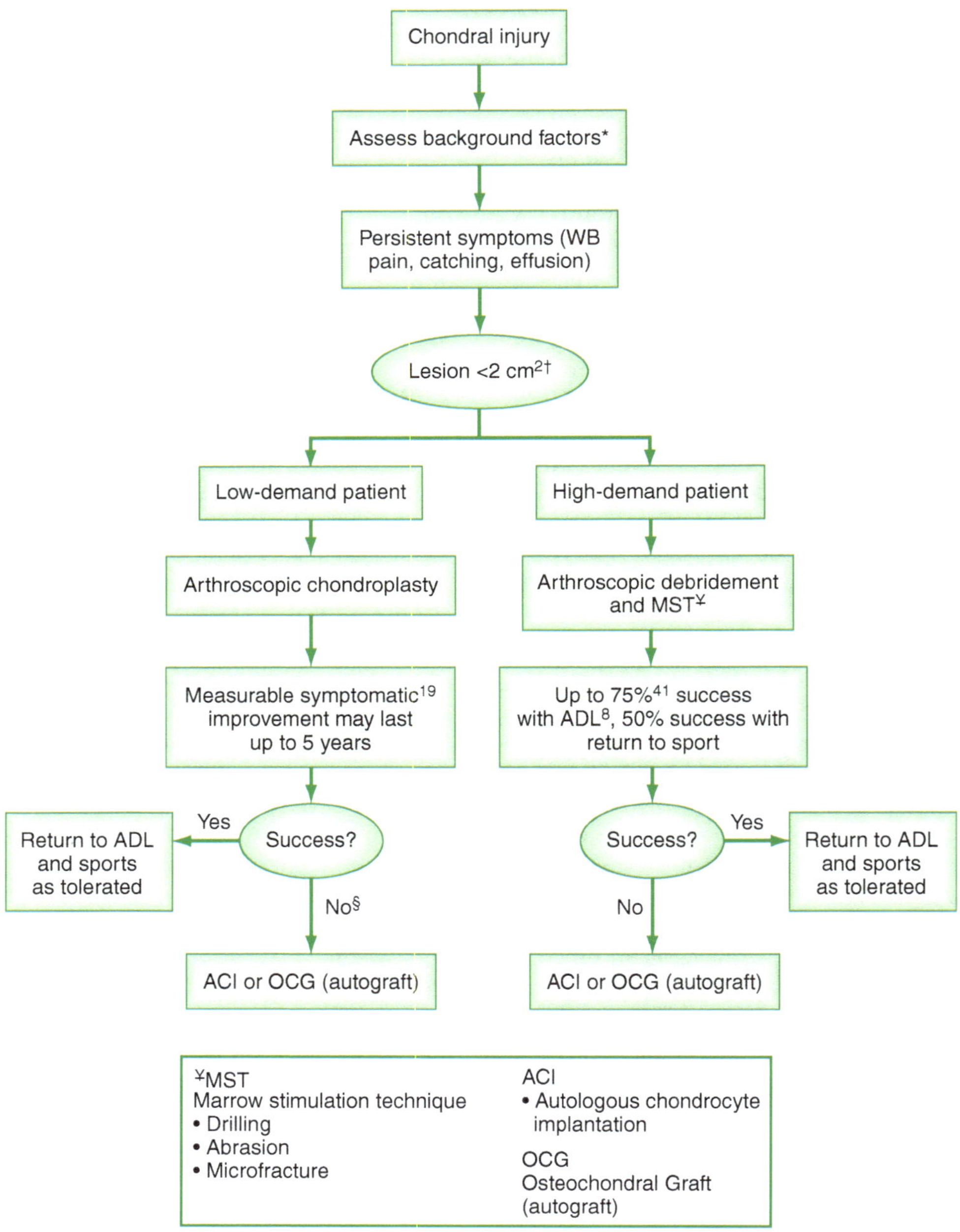

• **Fig. 4.8** Modified and updated clinical algorithm for the management of symptomatic cartilage defects of the femoral condyle when the defect of small, <2 cm^2, based on patient activity level, after assessing background factors.

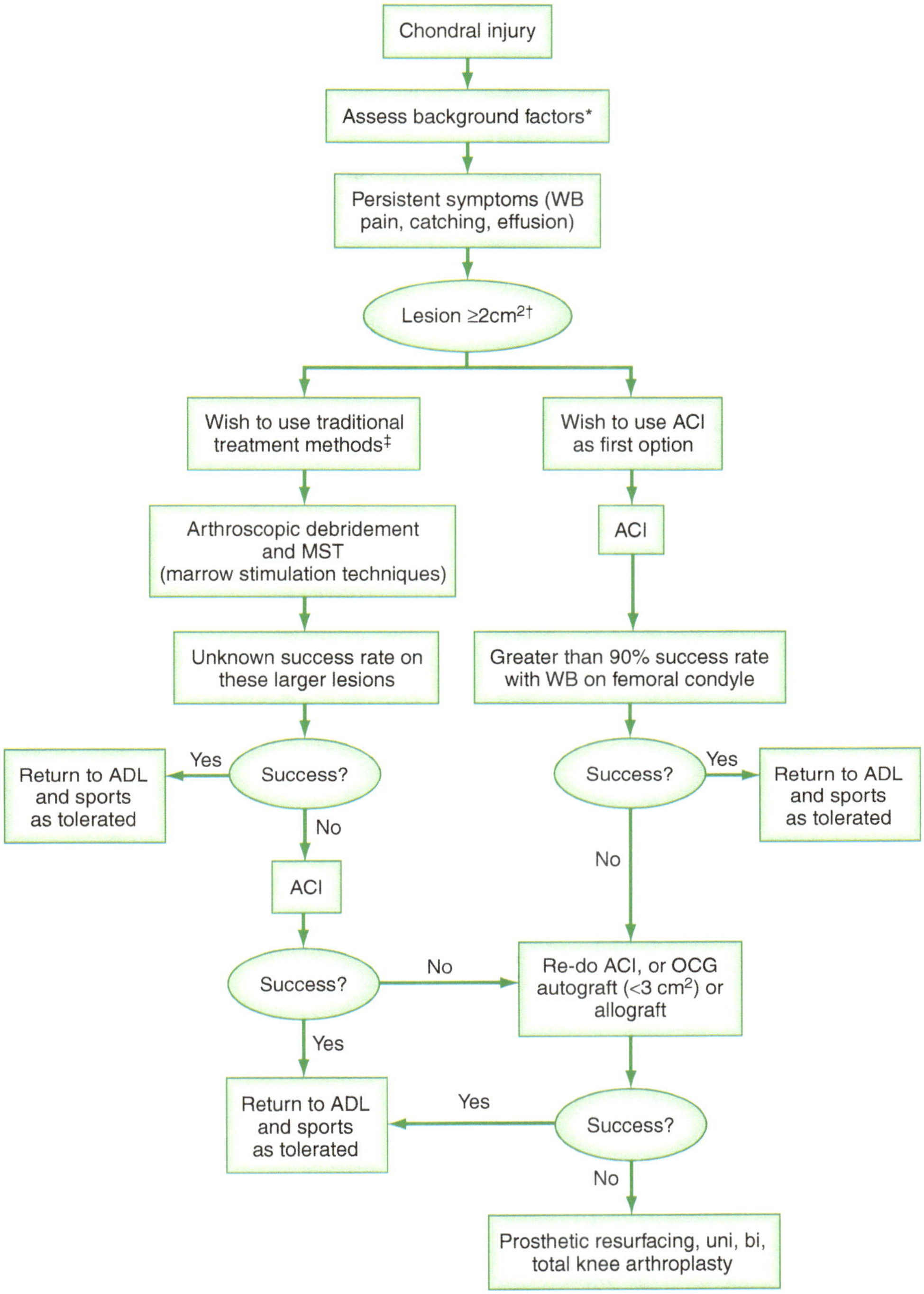

ACI, autologous chondrocyte implantation
ADL, activities of daily living
DJD, degenerative joint disease
WB, weight bearing
*For tibiofemoral or patellofemoral malalignment, consider realignment osteotomy. For ligamentous or bone insufficiency, consider grafting. If family predisposition to DJD exists, examine for Heberden's and Bouchard's nodes.

†Homminga[17] and Brittberg[5] noted that lesions greater than or equal to 2 cm are symptomatic and Messner[26] noted radiographic narrowing at 14-year follow-up.
‡Drilling and microfracture may make later ACI difficult/increased failure[32] due to increased bone stiffness due to intralesional osteophytes.

§Persistent symptoms 1–2 years post-op

• **Fig. 4.9** Modified and updated clinical algorithm for the management of symptomatic cartilage defects of the femoral condyle when the defect is large, >2 cm^2, based on patient activity level, after assessing background factors.

longitudinal follow-up in this situation is recommended to the patient with clinical evaluation annually by physical examination for progressive crepitus and effusion. High-resolution MRI scan is also performed to measure whether the defect size has progressed and standing AP and flexion PA radiographs help to assess the overall cartilage space. Counseling regarding weight gain and avoidance of impact-loading sports is recommended. If the patient becomes symptomatic or there is progression in size of the defect(s), then surgery is recommended after the risks and benefits are discussed with an informed consent. This is based on the most appropriate treatment from the guidelines that follow.

The background factors for the cartilage defect are evaluated with clinical examination and long alignment radiographs. The authors perform corrective osteotomy to mechanical neutral, and without overcorrection, for defects larger than 2 cm^2 at the time of cartilage repair if there are 2 degrees or more of mechanical varus or valgus and any patellar maltracking through an anteromedialization of the tibial tubercle.

Single full-thickness chondral defects of the weight-bearing femoral condyles and trochlea of less than 10 mm in diameter are amenable to osteochondral autograft transfer (OATS or mosaicplasty). Occasionally in a large knee two plugs will be used to repair a lesion of 15 mm diameter. This technique has the advantages of a single-stage procedure, transfer of mature hyaline cartilage into the defect, and a comparatively uncomplicated post surgical recovery. Donor site morbidity is acceptable with use of a single plug. The donor sites were frequently backfilled with synthetic calcium sulfate PLA/PGA copolymer (OBI TruFit plugs, Smith & Nephew); however, these are no longer available because there has been a recall. Instead, sites are usually backfilled with morselized allograft chips impacted into the donor site using the OATS chisels for delivery. Drains are used after surgery to prevent hemarthrosis and arthrofibrosis. Defects of the patella and tibial plateau should not be managed with this technique because the cartilage thickness mismatch between donor site (average 2 mm) and patella (average 5–7 mm) results in incongruities, resorption, and failure. Osteochondral autograft transfer may be performed arthroscopically but must be a precise fit—flush to the surface and orthogonally placed; hence mini-arthrotomy for accurate placement should be considered if there is any concern for graft placement by arthroscopy.

Defects of the weight-bearing condyles and tibia for defects 1–2 cm^2 in size are also amenable to microfracture with acceptable long-term results, but the results for trochlea and patella deteriorate over time. The recovery and return to sports is longer than osteochondral autografting and the success rate is lower. However, microfracture is easier for all locations within the knee. Long-term follow-up is necessary because the durability is less predictable and recurrent symptoms are common at 2.5–5 years after surgery.

I personally do not use microfracture in my practice but prefer to use chondroplasty, OATS, ACI, and allografts depending on the defect size, small to large, and the characteristics of the patient and background factors. I have found the lack of durability and intralesional osteophytes that occur with microfracture, as well as incomplete pain relief, to be problematic. Chondroplasty for small defects offers good relief of symptoms, does not make someone symptomatically worse (as can happen with microfracture), and if symptoms return, a repair technique can be performed without prior injury to the subchondral bone as occurs with marrow stimulation that can jeopardize ACI.

We prefer to treat defects larger than 2 cm^2 with autologous chondrocyte implantation and now MACI because of the good and predictable long-term results of this technique. Associated osseous defects deeper than 6 to 8 mm have to be addressed with a bone and cartilage procedure. For many years I performed this in a staged fashion, with bone grafting followed by ACI 9 to 12 months later. Now, with the excellent results of the ACI Sandwich Technique[46,47] a single-stage bone and cartilage repair is my preference or with single-stage osteochondral allograft transplantation (mega-OATS).

Our preference for allograft is for a large peripherally bony uncontained defect or an ACI that has failed by fibrous repair. Otherwise, bone deficiency is not a contraindication for ACI if the defect is first bone grafted or treated by the sandwich ACI technique with autologous bone graft. The long-term results of ACI are superior to allograft and for this reason in a young person our preference is autologous bone graft with ACI.

The field of cartilage repair is evolving. The relative efficacies of the various techniques and their limitations are being elucidated via carefully performed prospective cohorts that are not at the highest levels of evidence to determine the best cartilage technique per defect. However, these studies will afford us success and failure rates to design comparative, statistically well-powered, ethically just randomized controlled trials that will answer the question "What is the best repair technique for this defect?"

At that time we will be able to advocate an evidence-based algorithm for treatment based on patient and defect characteristics that will be cost-effective and sound.

References

1. Ware Jr. JE, Sherbourne CD. The MOS 36-item short-form health survey (SF-36). I. Conceptual framework and item selection. *Med Care.* 1992;30(6):473–483.
2. Peterson L, Minas T, Brittberg M, Nilsson A, Sjogren-Jansson E, Lindahl A. Two- to 9-year outcome after autologous chondrocyte transplantation of the knee. *Clin Orthop Relat Res.* 2000;374:212–234.
3. Mithofer K, Peterson L, Mandelbaum BR, Minas T. Articular cartilage repair in soccer players with autologous chondrocyte transplantation: functional out-come and return to competition. *Am J Sports Med.* 2005;33(11):1639–1646.
4. Mithofer K, Minas T, Peterson L, Yeon H, Micheli LJ. Functional outcome of knee articular cartilage repair in adolescent athletes. *Am J Sports Med.* 2005;33(8):1147–1153.

5. Coventry MB, Ilstrup DM, Wallrichs SL. Proximal tibial osteotomy. A critical long-term study of eighty-seven cases. *J Bone Joint Surg Am.* 1993;75(2):196–201.
6. Winalski C, Aliabadi P, Wright R. Enhancement of joint fluid with intravenously administered gadopentetate dimeglumine: technique, rationale, and implications. *Radiology.* 1993;187:179–185.
7. Homminga GN, Bulstra SK, Bouwmeester PSM, et al. Perichondral grafting for cartilage lesions of the knee. *J Bone and Joint Surg [Br].* 1990;72:1003–1007.
8. Brittberg M, Lindahl A, Nilsson A, Ohlsson C, Isaksson O, Peterson L. Treatment of deep cartilage defects in the knee with autologous chondrocyte transplantation. *N Engl J Med.* 1994;331(14):889–895.
9. Widuchowski W, Koczy B, Szyluk K. Untreated asymptomatic deep cartilage lesions associated with anterior cruciate ligament injury. *Am J Sports Med.* 2009;37(4):688–692.
10. Minas T. *Treatment of chondral defects in the knee.* Orthopedic Special Edition: Summer/Fall; 1997:69–74.
11. Minas T. The role of cartilage repair techniques, including chondrocyte transplantation, in focal chondral knee damage. *Instr Course Lect.* 1999;48:629–643.
12. Minas T, Nehrer S. Current concepts in the treatment of articular cartilage defects. *Orthopedics.* 1997;20(6):525–538.
13. Aroen A, Loken S, Heir S, et al. Articular cartilage lesions in 993 consecutive knee arthroscopies. *Am J Sports Med.* 2004;32(1):211–215.
14. Curl WW, Krome J, Gordon ES, Rushing J, Smith BP, Poehling GG. Cartilage injuries: a review of 31,516 knee arthroscopies. *Arthroscopy.* 1997;13(4):456–460.
15. Hjelle K, Solheim E, Strand T, Muri R, Brittberg M. Articular cartilage defects in 1,000 knee arthroscopies. *Arthroscopy.* 2002;18(7):730–734.
16. Piasecki DP, Spindler KP, Warren TA, Andrish JT, Parker RD. Intraarticular injuries associated with anterior cruciate ligament tear: findings at ligament reconstruction in high school and recreational athletes. An analysis of sex-based differences. *Am J Sports Med.* 2003;31(4):601–605.
17. Dzioba RB. The classification and treatment of acute articular cartilage lesions. *Arthroscopy.* 1988;4(2):72–80.
18. Hubbard MJ. Articular debridement versus washout for degeneration of the medial femoral condyle. A five-year study. *J Bone Joint Surg Br.* 1996;78(2):217–219.
19. Levy AS, Lohnes J, Sculley S, et al. Chondral delamination of the knee in soccer players. *Am J Sports Med.* 1996;24:634–639.
20. Scillia AJ, Aune KT, Andrachuk JS, et al. Return to play after chondroplasty of the knee in National Football League athletes. *Am J Sports Med.* 2015;43(3):663–668.
21. Messner K, Maletius W. The long-term prognosis for severe damage to weight-bearing cartilage in the knee: a 14-year clinical and radiographic follow-up in 28 young athletes. *Acta Orthop Scand.* 1996;67(2):165–168.
22. Nehrer S, Spector M, Minas T. Histologic analysis of tissue after failed cartilage repair procedures. *Clin Orthop Relat Res.* 1999;365:149–162.
23. Minas T, Gomoll AH, Rosenberger R, Royce RO, Bryant T. Increased failure rate of autologous chondrocyte implantation after previous treatment with marrow stimulation techniques. *Am J Sports Med.* 2009;37(5):902–908.
24. Garretson 3rd RB, Katolik LI, Vernma N, Beck PR, Bach BR, Cole BJ. Contact pressure at osteochondral donor sites in the patellofemoral joint. *Am J Sports Med.* 2004;32(4):967–974.
25. Gitelis S, Cole BJ. The use of allografts in orthopaedic surgery. *Instr Course Lect.* 2002;51:507–520.
26. Minas T, Gomoll AH *What is the best treatment for chondral defects in the knee?* In: Wright JG, ed. Evidence-based Orthopaedics: The Best Answers to Clinical Questions. Philadelphia, PA: Saunders/Elsevier; 2009:640–647.
27. Steadman J, Rodkey W, Singleton S, Briggs K. Microfracture technique for full-thickness chondral defects: technique and clinical results. *Oper Tech Orthop.* 1997;7(4):300–304.
28. Kreuz PC, Erggelet C, Steinwachs MR, et al. Is microfracture of chondral defects in the knee associated with different results in patients aged 40 years or younger? *Arthroscopy.* 2006;22(11):1180–1186.
29. Kreuz PC, Steinwachs MR, Erggelet C, et al. Results after microfracture of full-thickness chondral defects in different compartments in the knee. *Osteoarthr Cartil.* 2006;14(11): 1119–1125.
30. Kreuz PC, Williams RJ 3rd, Warren RF, et al. The microfracture technique for the treatment of articular cartilage lesions in the knee. A prospective cohort study. *J Bone Joint Surg Am.* 2005;87(9):1911–1920.
31. Steadman JR, Briggs KK, Rodrigo JJ, Kocher MS, Gill TJ, Rodkey WG. Outcomes of microfracture for traumatic chondral defects of the knee: average 11-year follow-up. *Arthroscopy.* 2003;19(5):477–484.
32. Blevins FT, Steadman JR, Rodrigo JJ, Silliman J. Treatment of articular cartilage defects in athletes: an analysis of functional outcome and lesion appearance. *Orthopedics.* 1998;21(7):761–767, discussion 767–768.
33. Bentley G, Biant LC, Carrington RW, et al. A prospective, randomised comparison of autologous chondrocyte implantation versus mosaicplasty for osteochondral defects in the knee. *J Bone Joint Surg Br.* 2003;85(2):223–230.
34. Horas U, Pelinkovic D, Herr G, Aigner T, Schnettler R. Autologous chondrocyte implantation and osteochondral cylinder transplantation in cartilage repair of the knee joint. A prospective, comparative trial. *J Bone Joint Surg Am.* 2003;85-A(2):185–192.
35. Gooding CR, Bartlett W, Bentley G, Skinner JA, Carrington R, Flanagan A. A prospective, randomised study comparing two techniques of autologous chondrocyte implantation for osteochondral defects in the knee: periosteum covered versus type I/III collagen covered. *Knee.* 2006;13(3):203–210.
36. Bartlett W, Skinner JA, Gooding CR, et al. Autologous chondrocyte implantation versus matrix-induced autologous chondrocyte implantation for osteochondral defects of the knee: a prospective, randomised study. *J Bone Joint Surg Br.* 2005;87(5):640–645.
37. Knutsen G, Engebretsen L, Ludvigsen TC, et al. Autologous chondrocyte implantation compared with microfracture in the knee. A randomized trial. *J Bone Joint Surg Am.* 2004;86-A(3):455–464.
38. Micheli LJ, Browne JE, Erggelet C, et al. Autologous chondrocyte implantation of the knee: multicenter experience and minimum 3-year follow-up. *Clin J Sport Med.* 2001;11(4):223–228.
39. Hangody L, Fules P. Autologous osteochondral mosaicplasty for the treatment of full-thickness defects of weight-bearing joints: ten years of experimental and clinical experience. *J Bone Joint Surg Am.* 2003;85-A Suppl 2:25–32.
40. Gudas R, Kalesinskas RJ, Kimtys V, et al. A prospective randomized clinical study of mosaic osteochondral autologous transplantation versus microfracture for the treatment of

osteochondral defects in the knee joint in young athletes. *Arthroscopy*. 2005;21(9):1066–1075.
41. Gross AE, Shasha N, Aubin P. Long-term followup of the use of fresh osteochondral allografts for posttraumatic knee defects. *Clin Orthop Relat Res*. 2005;435:79–87.
42. Gortz S, Bugbee WD. Allografts in articular cartilage repair. *Instr Course Lect*. 2007;56:469–481.
43. Jakobsen RB, Engebretsen L. *An analysis of the quality of cartilage repair studies - an update, in ISAKOS Current Concepts Winter 2007*. ISAKOS; 2007.
44. Jakobsen RB, Engebretsen L, Slauterbeck JR. An analysis of the quality of cartilage repair studies. *J Bone Joint Surg Am*. 2005;87(10):2232–2239.
45. Minas T, Bryant T. The role of autologous chondrocyte implantation in the patellofemoral joint. *Clin Orthop Relat Res*. 2005;436:30–39.
46. Minas T, Ogura T, Headrick J, Bryant T. Autologous chondrocyte implantation "sandwich" technique compared with autologous bone grafting for deep osteo-chondral lesions in the knee. *Am J Sports Med*. 2018;46(2):322–332.
47. Ogura T, Merkely G, Bryant T, Winalski CS, Minas T. Autologous chondrocyte implantation "segmental-sandwich" technique for deep osteochondral defects in the knee: clinical outcomes and correlation with magnetic resonance imaging findings. *Orthop J Sports Med*. 2019;7(5): 2325967119847173.
48. Brittberg M, Recker D, Ilgenfritz J, Saris DBG, Group SES. Matrix-applied characterized autologous cultured chondrocytes versus microfracture: five-year follow-up of a prospective randomized trial. *Am J Sports Med*. 2018;46(6): 1343–1351.
49. Volz M, Schaumburger J, Frick H, Grifka J, Anders S. A randomized controlled trial demonstrating sustained benefit of autologous matrix-induced chondrogenesis over microfracture at five years. *Int Orthop*. 2017;41(4):797–804.
50. Knutsen G, Drogset JO, Engebretsen L, et al. A randomized multicenter trial comparing autologous chondrocyte implantation with microfracture: long-term follow-up at 14 to 15 years. *J Bone Joint Surg Am*. 2016;98(16):1332–1339.
51. Clave A, Potel JF, Servien E, Neyret P, Dubrana F, Stindel E. Third-generation autologous chondrocyte implantation versus mosaicplasty for knee cartilage injury: 2-year randomized trial. *J Orthop Res*. 2016;34(4):658–665.
52. Shive MS, Stanish WD, McCormack R, et al. BST-CarGel(R) treatment maintains cartilage repair superiority over microfracture at 5 years in a multicenter randomized controlled trial. *Cartilage*. 2015;6(2):62–72.
53. Bentley G, Biant LC, Vijayan S, Macmull S, Skinner JA, Carrington RW. Minimum ten-year results of a prospective randomised study of autologous chondrocyte implantation versus mosaicplasty for symptomatic articular cartilage lesions of the knee. *J Bone Joint Surg Br*. 2012;94(4):504–509.
54. Crawford DC, DeBerardino TM, Williams 3rd RJ. NeoCart, an autologous cartilage tissue implant, compared with microfracture for treatment of distal femoral cartilage lesions: an FDA phase-II prospective, randomized clinical trial after two years. *J Bone Joint Surg Am*. 2012;94(11):979–989.
55. Niethammer TR, Loitzsch A, Horng A, et al. Graft hypertrophy after third-generation autologous chondrocyte implantation has no correlation with reduced cartilage quality: matched-pair analysis using T2-weighted mapping. *Am J Sports Med*. 2018;46(10):2414–2421.
56. Ebert JR, Schneider A, Fallon M, Wood DJ, Janes GC. A comparison of 2-year outcomes in patients undergoing tibiofemoral or patellofemoral matrix-induced autologous chondrocyte implantation. *Am J Sports Med*. 2017;45(14):3243–3253.
57. Niethammer TR, Holzgruber M, Gulecyuz MF, Weber P, Pietschmann MF, Muller PE. Matrix based autologous chondrocyte implantation in children and adolescents: a match paired analysis in a follow-up over three years post-operation. *Int Orthop*. 2017;41(2):343–350.
58. Lopez-Alcorocho JM, Aboli L, Guillen Viciente I, et al. Cartilage defect treatment using high-density autologous chondrocyte implantation: two-year follow-up. *Cartilage*. 2018;9(4):363–369.
59. Siebold R, Suezer F, Schmitt B, Trattnig S, Essig M. Good clinical and MRI outcome after arthroscopic autologous chondrocyte implantation for cartilage repair in the knee. *Knee Surg Sports Traumatol Arthrosc*. 2018;26(3):831–839.
60. Anderson DE, Williams RJ 3rd, DeBerardino TM, et al. Magnetic resonance imaging characterization and clinical outcomes after neocart surgical therapy as a primary reparative treatment for knee cartilage injuries. *Am J Sports Med*. 2017;45(4):875–883.
61. Ogura T, Mosier BA, Bryant T, Minas T. A 20-year follow-up after first-generation autologous chondrocyte implantation. *Am J Sports Med*. 2017;45(12):2751–2761.
62. Minas T, Von Keudell A, Bryant T, Gomoll AH. The John Insall Award: A minimum 10-year outcome study of autologous chondrocyte implantation. *Clin Orthop Relat Res*. 2014;472(1):41–51.

5

Preclinical Evidence for Biologics in Cartilage Repair and Early Osteoarthritis

BRENDAN MALONEY BS, BRIDGETTE NIXON BS, JOHN G. KENNEDY MD, FRCS AND LISA A. FORTIER DVM, PHD

CHAPTER OUTLINE

Introduction

Numerous biologics have been investigated in vitro and in preclinical animal models and show significant promise as methods of cartilage repair or as treatments for osteoarthritis (OA). Although there is mounting preclinical and clinical evidence for the use of certain biologics in treating articular disease, data for each biologic should be carefully weighed against where and how the drug has been tested. In the laboratory, it is not uncommon for biologics to be applied to chondrocytes isolated from their native matrix environment to test their effect. Similarly, in animal models of cartilage repair or OA, it is also not uncommon for outcome measures to focus on the articular cartilage surfaces alone. Although chondrocyte and cartilage homeostasis are undoubtedly important, it should be remembered that these biologics will affect the whole joint including the synovial membrane, meniscus, any exposed subchondral bone, and intra-articular ligaments in addition to their notable effects on chondrocytes. Furthermore, any chondrogenic or chondroprotective effect mediated by these biologic adjuncts are only of benefit if there is mechanical stability and alignment in the joint.

Biologics are often promoted as therapeutics based on the presence of growth factor and/or as stem cell therapies containing mesenchymal stromal cells (MSCs). Despite recent advances in our understanding of the role of MSCs in producing secretome with trophic effects on the local immune response, antiinflammatory, and regenerative effects, the precise mechanism of these actions is not yet fully elucidated. Similarly, it is nearly impossible to identify the precise mechanisms of action of growth factors contained within autologous biologic adjuncts because they all contain mixtures of growth factors, pro- and antiinflammatory cytokines, and chemokines that have direct and indirect effect on local cells to effectuate tissue restoration. This combination of bioactive factors will have pleiotropic effects on the complex disease processes associated with loss of joint homeostasis.

By understanding the integration of biologic agents into treatment paradigms that respect the biomechanics, and variability due to disease stage and patient physiology, we can provide better integrated patient care. Ultimately, continued research will guide patient protocols regarding the optimal dose and timing of biologic treatment for each specific disease stage.

Platelet-Rich Plasma

Platelet-rich plasma (PRP) is autologous plasma that contains more platelets than the starting blood sample. Growth factors such as platelet-derived growth factor (PDGF), transforming growth factor-B (TGF-β), vascular endothelial growth factor (VEGF), and other growth factors within platelet alpha granules are commonly cited as responsible for the anabolic and reparative effects of PRP.[1–3] White blood cells or leukocytes (lymphocytes, granulocytes, and monocytes) are also abundant in PRP and are typically associated with catabolic or pro-inflammatory effects of PRP.[4] This "growth factor = good, leukocyte = bad" paradigm is an oversimplification given that there are also red blood cells and over 1500 proteins in PRP. Nonetheless, platelet and leukocyte concentrations still form the basis for PRP classification schemes.

There are numerous commercial devices marketed for generation of PRP and several classification systems for PRP products, resulting in lack of standardization in classification and treatment protocols.[5–7] Very broadly, PRP preparations can be divided into leukocyte-rich (LR-PRP), leukocyte-poor (LP-PRP), and platelet-rich fibrin (PRF). To answer the important and prevailing clinical questions of dosing, timing, and type of PRP (LP or LR) that is indicated for each musculoskeletal injury, it is critical that investigators of basic science, preclinical, and clinical studies analyze and report the contents of PRP used in studies. This can be done with automated machine counting or equally as accurately with simple, inexpensive manual direct smear analysis.[8]

Once administered, the cellular and soluble contents of PRP including growth factors, chemokines, and cytokines will have direct and indirect effects on local tissue cells. Although the intent might be to treat a focal cartilage defect or to enhance repair of an anterior cruciate ligament, it should be remembered that any injection will affect all the tissues of the joint including the synovial membrane, cartilage, meniscus, exposed subchondral bone, and peri- or intra-articular structures.[4] Growth factors in PRP will directly affect local fibroblasts, endothelial, and articular cartilage cells resulting in cell proliferation, angiogenesis, synthesis of collagens types I and II, extracellular matrix formation, migration, and facilitated recruitment of cells including mesenchymal stromal cells and macrophages (Fig. 5.1). This will often culminate in decreased inflammation and pain restoring joint homeostasis.[9–12]

Growth factor signaling pathways have both positive and negative feedback mechanisms that are critical for regulating their activity.[13–16] Ex vivo studies on several tissues of the musculoskeletal system suggest that a negative feedback loop also exists for PRP where there is a plateau effect of matrix synthesis occurring beyond which further increased platelet concentration is of no further benefit.[16] The optimal log dose response curve is not yet known, but it is unlikely that repeated administration of PRP into a joint will have a cumulative beneficial effect on joint homeostasis.

Leukocyte subtypes are commonly grouped together when defining PRP and have been negatively correlated

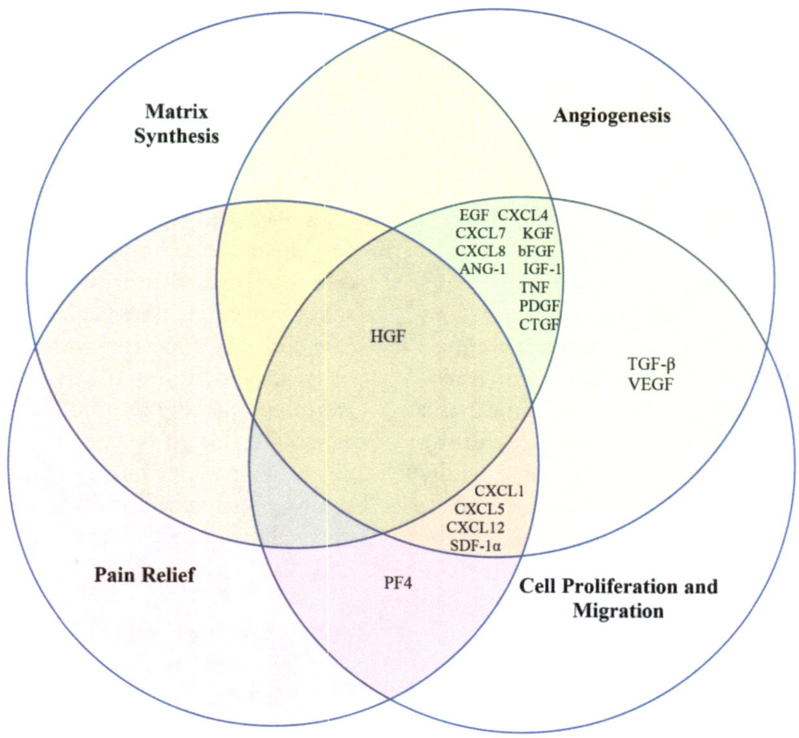

• **Fig. 5.1** The bioactive factors in biologics used for cartilage repair or for treatment of osteoarthritis have overlapping physiologic effects on target tissues. Bioactive factors: epidermal growth factor (EGF), chemokine ligand (CXCL), keratinocyte growth factor (KGF), basic fibroblast growth factor (bFGF), angiopoietin 1 (ANG-1), insulin-like growth factor (IGF-1), tumor necrosis factor (TNF), platelet-derived growth factor (PDGF), connective tissue growth factor (CTGF), hepatocyte growth factor (HGF), transforming growth factor beta (TGF-β), vascular endothelial growth factor (VEGF), stromal derived factor 1α (SDF-1α), platelet factor 4 (PF4).

with in vitro and in vivo results.[17] However, the preponderance of evidence indicates that it is the neutrophils that impart inflammatory and catabolic characteristics to a PRP preparation.[18–20] Neutrophil concentrations have been shown to correlate with catabolic cytokines interleukin-1 and matrix metalloproteinase-9.[21,22] In contrast, monocytes appear to be beneficial in a PRP preparation.[9,23,24] Peripheral blood monocytes are divided into three subsets based on phenotype and function[25] with the heterogeneity and phenotypic plasticity of these cells having implications in several human diseases.[26] Although monocyte subsets have not been studied in relation to PRP, monocyte-enriched PRP can be generated by two commercial systems: Arthrex Angel System (Arthrex Inc., Naples, FL) and EmCyte PurePRP (EmCyte Corp., Fort Myers, FL). In both of these commercial systems, within the leukocyte population monocytes are enriched and neutrophils are relatively decreased in concentration. Further basic and clinical research will guide development of commercial systems with the ability to generate personalized PRP depending on donor and patient variabilities.

Identifying patient- and donor-related factors associated with successful PRP treatment are probably as important as defining and standardizing PRP formulations for achieving predictable outcomes. Differences in clinical response have been attributed to patient donor factors and disease state of the patient (Table 5.1). More recently, a focus on the physiology of the donor has identified several variables that negatively affect the quality of resultant PRP independent of the disease state targeted for therapy. Growth factor concentrations in PRP have been reported to be negatively affected by daily low-dose aspirin, naproxen, antiplatelet drugs, diabetes mellitus, age, and female compared with male gender.[27–31] Increased age has been associated with an increase in the pro-inflammatory cytokines interleukin-1β and tumor-necrosis-factor alpha,[30] and in another study, age, but not gender, was negatively correlated with growth factors in PRP.[28] In contrast, platelet and TGF-β concentrations in PRP were significantly increased after a burst of high-intensity exercise but neither RBC nor WBC concentrations were affected.[32,33] There are other, not yet identified, donor-related factors that can alter the biological effect of PRP. One study reported that PRP generated from older patients with knee osteoarthritis suppressed chondrocyte matrix synthesis, and promoted macrophage inflammation in vitro independent of the concentration of inflammatory mediators interleukin-1β and tumor-necrosis-factor alpha, or the growth factors insulin-like growth factor 1 or transforming growth factor-β1.[3] This might suggest that autologous PRP from patients with OA could accentuate the disease process, but it should be cautioned that the OA patients in this study had end-stage OA and the PRP was generated at the time of knee arthroplasty, which might not reflect the clinical scenario.[30]

Although there is sufficient evidence that PRP is an effective treatment for OA, to improve the ability of PRP to restore joint homeostasis, basic science and preclinical studies need to continue to go beyond measuring bulk cellular contents and common growth factors in PRP. Further refinement of donor factors including monocyte subtypes and other donor factors reflecting the physiology of the patient need to be identified so that the quality of a PRP preparation can be defined prior to use in a patient.

TABLE 5.1 Donor Variables Affecting Platelet-Rich Plasma Characteristics

Donor variable	Influence on PRP quality (+, −, ND)	Reference
Age	−	Taniguchi[28], O'Donnell[30], Tian[31]
Gender	ND	Taniguchi[28], Anz[33]
	−	Xiong[69]
Exercise	+	Baria[32]
Aspirin, naproxen, anti-platelet drugs	−	Jayaram[27], Mannava[29], Tian[31]
End-stage osteoarthritis	−	O'Donnell[30]
Diabetes mellitus	−	Tian[31]

The influence of donor demographic or physiology is classified as positive (+), negative (−), or no difference (ND).
PRP, platelet-rich plasma.

Mesenchymal Stromal Cells

Mesenchymal stromal cells (MSCs) can be found in various adult tissues such as bone marrow, adipose tissue, and peripheral blood as well as from neonatal tissues such as amniotic fluid and amniotic membrane. Culture expanded MSCs and MSC retained within their resident niches, such as micronized adipose tissue and bone marrow aspirate concentrate, have been extensively studied in the laboratory and in numerous clinical studies for their use in autologous and allogeneic tissue repair.[34] The originally ascribed benefit of MSC was to differentiate into functional cells and engraft into and regenerate damaged tissue. Although MSCs can differentiate into various cell types including chondrocytes in vitro, this chondrogenic capacity has not been validated in vivo, turning attention to the paracrine effects of MSC to understand their mechanism of action. This paracrine effect of MSCs has been observed in the laboratory since the 1970s in hematopoietic stem cells and is now accepted as the mechanism of action of MSCs.[35] MSCs exert their paracrine reparative effects through secretion of immunomodulatory cytokines and chemokines collectively known as the secretome.

The collective secretome promotes functional changes in monocytes/macrophages, dendritic cells, T cells, B cells, and natural killer cells and culminating in immunomodulation, recruitment of endogenous MSCs, and angiogenesis (Fig. 5.2A). For example, MSC-secreted interleukin-1 receptor antagonist protein (IL-1RA, IRAP), which is a component of the MSC secretome, has been shown to enhance polarization of macrophages toward the M2, antiinflammatory and tissue reparative phenotype (Fig. 5.2B).[36] Another proposed mechanism of MSC-mediated immunomodulation is through phagocytosis of MSCs by M1 monocytes promoting cell differentiation into M2 monocytes (Fig. 5.2C). Although it is an oversimplification of macrophage polarization, the M1/M2 ratio and activation state of monocytes and macrophages is important in many diseases and has been highly associated with severity of disease in OA. The paracrine-mediated function of MSCs can be enhanced by cell activation[37] or priming. Activation can occur naturally in vivo as a result of signals from the local stem cell niche[38,39] or be achieved ex vivo to optimize generation of an MSC secretome for a particular therapy.

In clinical studies, bone marrow and adipose tissue-based therapies are the most commonly used MSC-based therapies because of their accessibility; and excellent outcomes have been achieved in augmenting chondrogenic repair in focal defects as well as altering joint homeostasis in arthritic joints. When commercially available as a treatment for patients, MSC secretome will have the distinct advantage of being an off-the-shelf product, imparting the paracrine effects of MSC while not being subject to patient–patient variability currently inherent in PRP and bone marrow aspirate concentrate (BMC).

Secretome or MSC Extracellular Vesicles as a Therapeutic

The paracrine effects of MSCs are mediated by what they secrete, collectively termed the secretome. Secretome is composed of numerous chemokines, cytokines, growth factors, and extracellular vesicles (EV) (Figure 5-2B). It is the cargo within the MSC extracellular vesicles (MSC-EV) that is thought to impart the paracrine and immunomodulatory effects of MSCs.[40] MSC-EV enhance M1 polarization to a M2 reparative phenotype.[41] Both isolated MSC-EV and unfractionated secretome from bone marrow or adipose-derived MSCs have proven effective in vitro and in rodent models of arthritis.[42–45] While no secretome or MSC-EV products has regulatory approval, the distinct advantage of this MSC-based approach compared with all of the other biologic approaches discussed is the ability to generate and scale-up a uniform biologic that would be manufactured like a drug, without the confounding patient/donor factors affecting efficacy.

Micronized Adipose Tissue

Micronized adipose tissue (MAT), or micro-fragmented fat, is a point-of care biologic that retains MSCs in their native niche and has been used to address several musculoskeletal injuries including cartilage defects and OA.[46–48] Autologous lipoaspirate material is mechanically disaggregated to produce cell clusters while removing blood and fat residue. Several cell types including MSCs, endothelial cells, and pericytes[49] are retained in the product. Similar to MSC, these cells secrete numerous bioactive factors resulting in angiogenesis, immunomodulation, decreased inflammation,

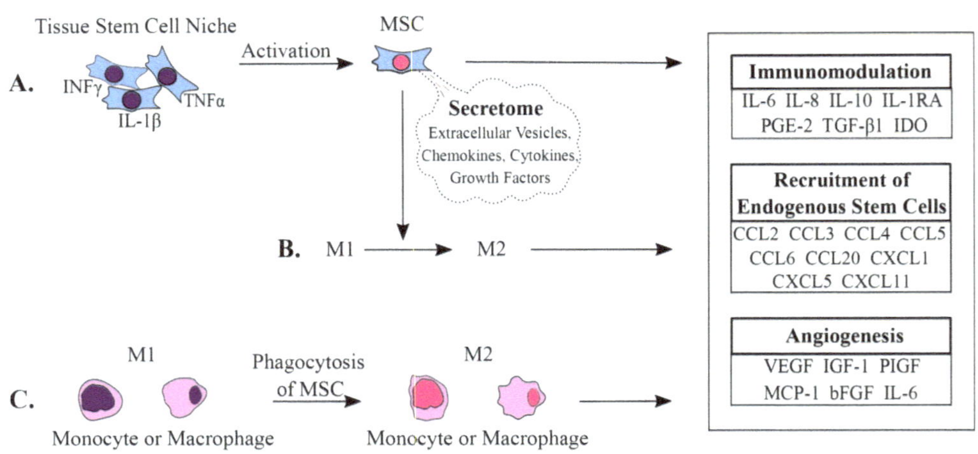

• **Fig. 5.2** Three proposed mechanisms for mesenchymal stromal cell (MSC)-mediated mechanisms of action culminating in immunomodulation, recruitment of endogenous stem cells, and angiogenesis. (A) MSCs in their resident tissue niche become activated and produce secretome containing extracellular vesicles, growth factors, chemokines, and cytokines. (B) Secretome promotes polarization of pro-inflammatory M1 monocytes/macrophages to reparative M2 macrophages/monocytes. (C) Phagocytic M1 monocytes or macrophages engulf MSCs and are polarized to regenerative M2 monocytes/macrophages. Bioactive factors in MSC-secretome: interferon gamma (INFγ), interleukin-1 beta (IL-1β), tumor necrosis actor alpha (TNFα), mesenchymal stromal cell (MSC), extracellular vesicles (EV), interleukin-6 (IL-6), prostaglandin E_2 (PGE-2), interleukin-1 receptor antagonist protein (IL-1RA), indoleamine 2,3-dioxygenase (IDO), chemokine ligand (CCL), chemokine ligand (CXCL), vascular endothelial growth factor (VEGF), insulin-like growth factor (IGF-1), placental growth factor (PIGF), monocyte chemoattractant protein-1 (MCP-1), basic fibroblast growth factor (bFGF).

and tissue restoration.[48,50,51] In a rat cartilage defect model, histologic scores using the International Cartilage Repair Society (ICRS) scoring system were not different between MAT and saline control-treated limbs.[52] This might suggest that MAT is better suited for OA than as an approach for cartilage repair. Although not investigated for MAT at this time, similar to other autologous MSC-based biologics, donor-related variability such as age, body mass index, and cardiovascular disease will remain a challenge for consistent success of MAT therapies.[53]

Bone Marrow Aspirate Concentrate

Bone marrow aspirate concentrate (BMC) has been used as an adjunct for cartilage repair and as an intra-articular injection for OA.[54,55] Uniquely, compared with the other biologics available, BMC contains MSCs and significant quantities of regenerative bioactive factors including growth factors, chemokines, and cytokines similar to, but not identical with, PRP. Most notably, BMC has a significantly higher concentration of IL-1RA than any other biologic.[56,57] IL-1RA has been shown in vitro and in preclinical and clinical studies to modify the disease process of OA by competitively binding and inhibiting the effects of the pro-inflammatory cytokine IL-1.[58] Further, as stated earlier, IL-1RA secreted from MSCs promotes the switching of macrophage from M1 to reparative M2 phenotypes (Fig. 5.2B) making BMC unique in its mechanism compared with other biologics.

The concentration of MSCs in BMC is low and therefore difficult to quantify accurately: only one publication has identified MSCs using multicolor flow cytometry for simultaneous measurement of validated cell surface marker.[59] A more simplified flow cytometry protocol for $CD45^{low}CD271^{high}$ cells has been reported as a method for quantifying MSC in BMC.[60] Even more simple to perform in the laboratory are colony-forming unit (CFU) assays, which have been used as a surrogate marker for MSC in BMC,[61,62] but there is no meaningful correlation between CFU and MSC in BMC.[63] Although the number of MSCs in BMC is often cited as a concern for BMC in orthobiologics, there is currently no study indicating an optimal dose of MSCs for cartilage repair or for treatment of OA. With the contemporary understanding of the immunomodulatory function of MSCs and that both MSC secretome and BMC can recruit MSCs,[10] the literal quantity of MSC in BMC is unlikely to be of significant consequence. More concerning for consistent quality of repair is the considerable literature on donor–donor and site variability.[55,56,64]

Amnion and Other Birth Tissue-Derived Products

There are numerous neonatal, birth tissue-related products promoted for use in the musculoskeletal system including those derived from amniotic fluid, amniotic membrane, umbilical cord, and combinations thereof. Similar to the other biologics, they contain hundreds of proteins with potential beneficial effects, but few growth factors in low concentrations. Furthermore, no stem cells have been identified in any product investigated to date.[65,66] In vitro, amniotic fluid had similar antiinflammatory effects as corticosteroids on IL-1β-stimulated cartilage and synovium.[67] An amniotic suspension allograft that has good clinical data has also been investigated in a rat model of OA. Joints treated with amnion product had increased concentrations of IL-10 and decreased pain, but no difference in joint tissue histology.[68] In a rat medial meniscus transection OA induction study, an amnion/chorion product mitigated the development of OA. These treatments suggest that amnion might mitigate morbidity associated with OA but does not modify the disease process.

Conclusion

There is no doubt that the evidence exists in the basic science literature that biologics have a positive effect in the treatment of focal cartilage defects and early OA. The translation of that evidence to good quality and level of evidence in clinical studies has not been linear, but an increasing number of clinical studies support the continued use of biologics in these conditions. Just as importantly, the clinical studies are underscoring that biologics do no harm in these conditions.

Because of the financial incentive for boutique stem cell clinics to offer magical cures for arthritic conditions, it is critical that orthopedic practitioners provide evidence-based medical advice to their patients. That evidence exists now both in basic science and in clinical studies. Collaboration between industry, translational scientists, and practitioners is critical to develop clinical algorithms using appropriate biologics to direct future practice guidelines. Regulatory oversight will be essential to control this ever-expanding industry but the future for biologics augmentation in cartilage is as exciting as it is inevitable.

References

1. Filardo G, Previtali D, Napoli F, Candrian C, Zaffagnini S, Grassi A. PRP injections for the treatment of knee osteoarthritis: a meta-analysis of randomized controlled trials [published online June 19, 2020]. *Cartilage*. 2020. doi:10.1177/1947603520931170.
2. Dai WL, Zhou AG, Zhang H, Zhang J. Efficacy of platelet-rich plasma in the treatment of knee osteoarthritis: a meta-analysis of randomized controlled trials. *Arthroscopy*. 2017;33(3):659–670.
3. Sundman EA, Cole BJ, Karas V, et al. The anti-inflammatory and matrix restorative mechanisms of platelet-rich plasma in osteoarthritis. *Am J Sports Med*. 2014;42(1)
4. Boswell SG, Cole BJ, Sundman EA, Karas V, Fortier LA. Platelet-rich plasma: a milieu of bioactive factors. *Arthroscopy*. 2012;28(3):429–439.
5. Kon E, Di Matteo B, Delgado D, et al. Platelet-rich plasma for the treatment of knee osteoarthritis: an expert opinion and proposal for a novel classification and coding system. *Expert Opin Biol Ther*. 2020;20(12):1447–1460.

6. Rossi LA, Murray IR, Chu CR, Muschler GF, Rodeo SA, Piuzzi NS. Classification systems for platelet-rich plasma. *Bone Joint J.* 2019;101-B(8):891–896.
7. Dohan Ehrenfest DM, Rasmusson L, Albrektsson T. Classification of platelet concentrates: from pure platelet-rich plasma (P-PRP) to leucocyte- and platelet-rich fibrin (L-PRF). *Trends Biotechnol.* 2009;27(3):158–167.
8. Wilson BH, Cole BJ, Goodale MB, Fortier LA. Short-term storage of platelet-rich plasma at room temperature does not affect growth factor or catabolic cytokine concentration. *Am J Orthop (Belle Mead NJ).* 2018;47(4). doi:10.12788/ajo.2018.0022.
9. Everts P, Onishi K, Jayaram P, Lana JF, Mautner K. Platelet-rich plasma: new performance understandings and therapeutic considerations in 2020. *Int J Mol Sci.* 2020;21(20):1–36.
10. Holmes HL, Wilson B, Goerger JP, et al. Facilitated recruitment of mesenchymal stromal cells by bone marrow concentrate and platelet rich plasma [published online March 22, 2018]. *PLoS One.* 2018;13(3). doi:10.1371/journal.pone.0194567.
11. Blair P, Flaumenhaft R. Platelet α-granules: basic biology and clinical correlates. *Blood Rev.* 2009;23(4):177–189.
12. Nishio H, Saita Y, Kobayashi Y, et al. Platelet-rich plasma promotes recruitment of macrophages in the process of tendon healing. *Regen Ther.* 2020;14:262–270.
13. Miyazono K. Positive and negative regulation of TGF-β signaling. *J Cell Sci.* 2000;113(7):1101–1109.
14. Coleman SJ, Bruce C, Chioni AM, Kocher HM, Grose RP. The ins and outs of fibroblast growth factor receptor signalling. *Clin Sci.* 2014;127(4):217–231.
15. Karaman S, Leppänen VM, Alitalo K. Vascular endothelial growth factor signaling in development and disease. [published online July 20, 2018]. *Development.* 2018;145(14). doi:10.1242/dev.151019.
16. Boswell SG, Schnabel LV, Mohammed HO, Sundman EA, Minas T, Fortier LA. Increasing platelet concentrations in leukocyte-reduced platelet-rich plasma decrease collagen gene synthesis in tendons. *Am J Sports Med.* 2014;42(1):42–49.
17. McCarrel T, Fortier L. Temporal growth factor release from platelet-rich plasma, trehalose lyophilized platelets, and bone marrow aspirate and their effect on tendon and ligament gene expression. *J Orthop Res.* 2009;27(8):1033–1042.
18. Pifer MA, Maerz T, Baker KC, Anderson K. Matrix metalloproteinase content and activity in low-platelet, low-leukocyte and high-platelet, high-leukocyte platelet rich plasma (PRP) and the biologic response to PRP by human ligament fibroblasts. *Am J Sports Med.* 2014;42(5):1211–1218.
19. Assirelli E, Filardo G, Mariani E, et al. Effect of two different preparations of platelet-rich plasma on synoviocytes. *Knee Surg Sports Traumatol Arthrosc.* 2015;23(9):2690–2703.
20. Dragoo JL, Braun HJ, Durham JL, et al. Comparison of the acute inflammatory response of two commercial platelet-rich plasma systems in healthy rabbit tendons. *Am J Sports Med.* 2012;40(6):1274–1281.
21. Sundman EA, Cole BJ, Fortier LA. Growth factor and catabolic cytokine concentrations are influenced by the cellular composition of platelet-rich plasma. *Am J Sports Med.* 2011;39(10):2135–2140.
22. Oudelaar BW, Peerbooms JC, Huis In 't Veld R, Vochteloo AJH. Concentrations of blood components in commercial platelet-rich plasma separation systems: a review of the literature. *Am J Sports Med.* 2019;47(2):479–487.
23. Yoshida R, Murray MM. Peripheral blood mononuclear cells enhance the anabolic effects of platelet-rich plasma on anterior cruciate ligament fibroblasts. *J Orthop Res.* 2013;31(1):29–34.
24. Lana JF, Huber SC, Purita J, et al. Leukocyte-rich PRP versus leukocyte-poor PRP - the role of monocyte/macrophage function in the healing cascade. *J Clin Orthop Trauma.* 2019;10(Suppl 1):S7–S12.
25. Kapellos TS, Bonaguro L, Gemünd I, et al. Human monocyte subsets and phenotypes in major chronic inflammatory diseases. *Front Immunol.* 2019;10(Aug):2035. doi:10.3389/fimmu.2019.02035.
26. Wong KL, Yeap WH, Tai JJY, Ong SM, Dang TM, Wong SC. The three human monocyte subsets: implications for health and disease. *Immunol Res.* 2012;53(1-3):41–57.
27. Jayaram P, Yeh P, Patel SJ, et al. Effects of aspirin on growth factor release from freshly isolated leukocyte-rich platelet-rich plasma in healthy men: a prospective fixed-sequence controlled laboratory study. *Am J Sports Med.* 2019;47(5):1223–1229.
28. Taniguchi Y, Yoshioka T, Sugaya H, et al. Growth factor levels in leukocyte-poor platelet-rich plasma and correlations with donor age, gender, and platelets in the Japanese population. *J Exp Orthop.* 2019;6(1). doi:10.1186/s40634-019-0175-7.
29. Mannava S, Whitney KE, Kennedy MI, et al. The influence of naproxen on biological factors in leukocyte-rich platelet-rich plasma: a prospective comparative study. *Arthroscopy.* 2019;35(1):201–210.
30. O'Donnell C, Migliore E, Grandi FC, et al. Platelet-rich plasma (prp) from older males with knee osteoarthritis depresses chondrocyte metabolism and upregulates inflammation. *J Orthop Res.* 2019;37(8):1760–1770.
31. Tian J, Lei XX, Xuan L, Tang JB, Cheng B. The effects of aging, diabetes mellitus, and antiplatelet drugs on growth factors and anti-aging proteins in platelet-rich plasma. *Platelets.* 2019;30(6):773–792.
32. Baria MR, Miller MM, Borchers J, et al. High intensity interval exercise increases platelet and transforming growth factor-β yield in platelet-rich plasma. *PM R.* 2020;12(12):1244–1250.
33. Anz AW, Parsa RS, Romero-Creel MF, et al. Exercise-mobilized platelet-rich plasma: short-term exercise increases stem cell and platelet concentrations in platelet-rich plasma. *Arthroscopy.* 2019;35(1):192–200.
34. Fortier LA, Lintz M. Basic science of resident stem cells. *Oper Tech Sports Med.* 2020;28(4):150776.
35. Dexter TM, Wright EG, Krizsa F, Lajtha L. Regulation of haemopoietic stem cell proliferation in long term bone marrow cultures. *Biomedicine.* 1977;27(9-10):344–349.
36. Luz-Crawford P, Djouad F, Toupet K, et al. Mesenchymal stem cell-derived interleukin 1 receptor antagonist promotes macrophage polarization and inhibits B cell differentiation. *Stem Cells.* 2016;34(2):483–492.
37. Cassano JM, Schnabel LV, Goodale MB, Fortier LA. Inflammatory licensed equine MSCs are chondroprotective and exhibit enhanced immunomodulation in an inflammatory environment. *Stem Cell Res Ther.* 2018;9(1):82.
38. Cassano JM, Schnabel LV, Goodale MB, Fortier LA. The immunomodulatory function of equine MSCs is enhanced by priming through an inflammatory microenvironment or TLR3 ligand. *Vet Immunol Immunopathol.* 2018:195.
39. Kadle RL, Abdou SA, Villarreal-Ponce AP, et al. Microenvironmental cues enhance mesenchymal stem cell-mediated immunomodulation and regulatory T-cell expansion [published online March 7, 2018]. Camussi G, ed. *PLoS One.* 2018;13(3): e0193178. doi:10.1371/journal.pone.0193178.

40. Nooshabadi VT, Mardpour S, Yousefi-Ahmadipour A, et al. The extracellular vesicles-derived from mesenchymal stromal cells: a new therapeutic option in regenerative medicine. *J Cell Biochem*. 2018;119(10):8048–8073.
41. Wang J, Xia J, Huang R, et al. Mesenchymal stem cell-derived extracellular vesicles alter disease outcomes via endorsement of macrophage polarization. *Stem Cell Res Ther*. 2020;11(1):424.
42. Khatab S, van Osch GJVM, Kops N, et al. Mesenchymal stem cell secretome reduces pain and prevents cartilage damage in a murine osteoarthritis model. *Eur Cell Mater*. 2018;36:218–230.
43. Wang J, Cen P, Chen J, et al. Role of mesenchymal stem cells, their derived factors, and extracellular vesicles in liver failure. *Stem Cell Res Ther*. 2017;8(1):137.
44. Giannasi C, Niada S, Magagnotti C, Ragni E, Andolfo A, Brini AT. Comparison of two ASC-derived therapeutics in an in vitro OA model: secretome versus extracellular vesicles. *Stem Cell Res Ther*. 2020;11(1):521.
45. Ijsselsteijn ME, van der Breggen R, Sarasqueta AF, Koning F, de Miranda NFCC. A 40-marker panel for high dimensional characterization of cancer immune microenvironments by imaging mass cytometry. *Front Immunol*. 2019;10(Oct):2534. doi:10.3389/fimmu.2019.02534.
46. Shimozono Y, Fortier LA, Brown D, Kennedy JG. Adipose-based therapies for knee pain—fat or fiction. *J Knee Surg*. 2019;32(1):55–64.
47. Schroeder A, Rubin JP, Kokai L, Sowa G, Chen J, Onishi K. Use of adipose-derived orthobiologics for musculoskeletal injuries: a narrative review. *PM R*. 2020;12(8):805–816.
48. Bianchi F, Maioli M, Leonardi E, et al. A new nonenzymatic method and device to obtain a fat tissue derivative highly enriched in pericyte-like elements by mild mechanical forces from human lipoaspirates. *Cell Transplant*. 2013;22(11):2063–2077.
49. Crisan M, Corselli M, Chen WCW, Péault B. Perivascular cells for regenerative medicine. *J Cell Mol Med*. 2012;16(12): 2851–2860.
50. Ceserani V, Ferri A, Berenzi A, et al. Angiogenic and anti-inflammatory properties of micro-fragmented fat tissue and its derived mesenchymal stromal cells. *Vasc Cell*. 2016;8(1):3.
51. Polancec D, Zenic L, Hudetz D, et al. Immunophenotyping of a stromal vascular fraction from microfragmented lipoaspirate used in osteoarthritis cartilage treatment and its lipoaspirate counterpart. *Genes (Basel)*. 2019;10(6):474.
52. Xu P, Yang X. The efficacy and safety of mesenchymal stem cell transplantation for spinal cord injury patients: a meta-analysis and systematic review. *Cell Transplant*. 2019;28(1):36–46.
53. Mastrolia I, Foppiani EM, Murgia A, et al. Challenges in clinical development of mesenchymal stromal/stem cells: concise review. *Stem Cells Transl Med*. 2019;8(11):1135–1148.
54. Kim GB, Seo MS, Park WT, Lee GW. Bone marrow aspirate concentrate: its uses in osteoarthritis. *Int J Mol Sci*. 2020;21(9):3224.
55. Chahla J, Dean CS, Moatshe G, Pascual-Garrido C, Serra Cruz R, LaPrade RF. Concentrated bone marrow aspirate for the treatment of chondral injuries and osteoarthritis of the knee: a systematic review of outcomes. *Orthop J Sports Med*. 2016;4(1). doi:10.1177/2325967115625481.
56. Cassano JM, Kennedy JG, Ross KA, Fraser EJ, Goodale MB, Fortier LA. Bone marrow concentrate and platelet-rich plasma differ in cell distribution and interleukin 1 receptor antagonist protein concentration. *Knee Surg Sports Traumatol Arthrosc*. 2018;26(1):333–342.
57. Ziegler CG, Van Sloun R, Gonzalez S, et al. Characterization of growth factors, cytokines, and chemokines in bone marrow concentrate and platelet-rich plasma: a prospective analysis. *Am J Sports Med*. 2019;47(9):2174–2187.
58. Dinarello CA. The IL-1 family of cytokines and receptors in rheumatic diseases. *Nat Rev Rheumatol*. 2019;15(10):612–632.
59. Wells K, Klein M, Hurwitz N, et al. Cellular and clinical analyses of autologous bone marrow aspirate injectate for knee osteoarthritis: a pilot study. *PM R*. 2021;13(4):387–396.
60. El-Jawhari JJ, Cuthbert R, McGonagle D, Jones E, Giannoudis PV. The $CD45^{low}$ $CD271^{high}$ cell prevalence in bone marrow samples may provide a useful measurement of the bone marrow quality for cartilage and bone regenerative therapy. *J Bone Joint Surg Am*. 2017;99(15):1305–1313.
61. Schäfer R, Debaun MR, Fleck E, et al. Quantitation of progenitor cell populations and growth factors after bone marrow aspirate concentration. *J Transl Med*. 2019;17(1):115.
62. Dragoo JL, Guzman RA. Evaluation of the consistency and composition of commercially available bone marrow aspirate concentrate systems. *Orthop J Sports Med*. 2020;8(1):2325967119893634. doi:10.1177/2325967119893634.
63. Gaul F, Bugbee WD, Hoenecke HR, D'Lima DD. A review of commercially available point-of-care devices to concentrate bone marrow for the treatment of osteoarthritis and focal cartilage lesions. *Cartilage*. 2019;10(4):387–394.
64. Siegel G, Kluba T, Hermanutz-Klein U, Bieback K, Northoff H, Schäfer R. Phenotype, donor age and gender affect function of human bone marrow-derived mesenchymal stromal cells. *BMC Med*. 2013;11(1):146.
65. Panero AJ, Hirahara AM, Andersen WJ, Rothenberg J, Fierro F. Are amniotic fluid products stem cell therapies? A study of amniotic fluid preparations for mesenchymal stem cells with bone marrow comparison. *Am J Sport Med*. 2019;47(5):1230–1235.
66. Becktell L, Matuska AM, Hon S, et al. Proteomic analysis and cell viability of nine amnion, chorion, umbilical cord, and amniotic fluid–derived products. *Cartilage*. December 2020; 1947603520976767. doi:10.1177/1947603520976767.
67. O'Brien D, Kia C, Beebe R, et al. Evaluating the effects of platelet-rich plasma and amniotic viscous fluid on inflammatory markers in a human coculture model for osteoarthritis. *Arthroscopy*. 2019;35(8):2421–2433.
68. Kimmerling KA, Gomoll AH, Farr J, Mowry KC. Amniotic suspension allograft modulates inflammation in a rat pain model of osteoarthritis. *J Orthop Res*. 2020;38(5):1141–1149.
69. Xiong G, Lingampalli N, Koltsov JCB, et al. Men and women differ in the biochemical composition of platelet-rich plasma. *Am J Sports Med*. 2018;46(2):409–419.

6

PRP, BMAC, Stem Cells, and Other Adjuvants and How They Affect Repair: Clinical Outcome Studies

ANGELO BOFFA MD, LUCA ANDRIOLO MD, ALESSANDRO DI MARTINO MD AND GIUSEPPE FILARDO MD, PHD

CHAPTER OUTLINE

Introduction

Biological-based therapies are emerging as a promising alternative for treating articular cartilage degenerative defects and early osteoarthritis (OA). These treatments can reduce symptoms, restore joint function, and possibly prevent the progression of OA by delaying the need for metal resurfacing. Numerous biologic agents are currently used in clinical practice, ranging from platelet concentrates to minimally manipulated mesenchymal stromal cells (MSCs). These have been mostly successful for the intra-articular treatment of degenerative joint disease, in particular knee OA. However, because of their potential to improve cartilage healing, biologics are also being used for augmentation in cartilage repair techniques, to enhance clinical outcomes and possibly improve cartilage repair tissue quality.

Platelet-Rich Plasma

Platelet-rich plasma (PRP) is being used to improve the healing of tissues with low healing potential, such as cartilage. There has been growing interest in PRP because of the high content of cytokines, growth factors, and bioactive molecules stored in platelet α-granules, which play a role in the homeostasis, healing process, and immunoregulation of articular cartilage. PRP is widely used in clinical practice because of its safety, low cost, and the simple preparation technique needed to obtain its biologically active content and it has given promising results as a treatment for several orthopedic diseases, in particular cartilage degeneration and OA.[1]

Until now, research has focused on the effectiveness of delivering PRP through intra-articular injections in the treatment of knee OA, a minimally invasive approach that seems to provide increased functional improvement and reduced pain-related symptoms for up to 12 months.[2–4] Moreover, some evidence suggests that some patients notice a clinical improvement provided by PRP beyond 24 months, although this benefit gradually wanes over time.[5] Despite the placebo effect of intra-articular injections, in particular when dealing with new orthobiologics such as PRP,[6] a recent meta-analysis on 34 randomized controlled trials (RCTs) concluded that PRP injections offered a statistically and clinically significant improvement in patients with knee OA compared with saline injections at 12-month follow-up, without increasing the risk of adverse events.[7] Moreover, PRP injections provided better results than other commonly used injectable options such as corticosteroids or hyaluronic acid. Although this benefit was not significant at earlier follow-ups, it increased over time and was clinically significant after 6–12 months. However, this improvement (greater than what is considered to be the minimal clinically important difference [MCID]) was partial and is supported by a low level of evidence.[7] This partial improvement has also recently been highlighted in a study by Altamura et al.[4] in a cohort of sport-active patients suffering from knee cartilage degeneration and OA. In this relatively young population (mean age 41 years), PRP injective treatment provided good clinical outcomes, but results were less satisfactory in terms of return to sport since only half of the patients achieved the same competitive level as before the onset of symptoms. Other authors underlined the potential of PRP for the injective treatment of hip OA and some investigated the potential of intra-articular PRP injections as a conservative treatment for patients with focal osteochondral lesions of the talus and ankle OA. The ability of PRP to reduce pain and improve function for up to 12 months has also been documented in these patients, although more data are needed to elucidate the real effects of these PRP applications.[8–11]

The use of PRP has also been extended to cartilage repair procedures, with the aim of exploiting its potential to improve repair tissue quality. Indeed, growth factors released by the activated platelets can support the proliferation of chondrocytes and the production of extracellular matrix.[12,13] Several preclinical studies have confirmed that PRP can promote chondrocyte proliferation and the differentiation of MSCs from subchondral bone into the chondrogenic line after microfracture surgery.[14,15] These preclinical results prompted researchers to evaluate the effect of PRP augmentation to microfracture in clinical practice. A recent meta-analysis on seven clinical comparative studies revealed that PRP augmentation improved the clinical outcome offered by microfractures in patients affected by knee or ankle cartilage defects for up to 24 months of follow-up.[16] Although PRP augmentation was safe and showed the potential to improve the results of microfractures, the comparative analysis also showed that this improvement did not reach the MCID and thus was not clinically perceivable by all patients. Besides the clinical results, Papalia et al.[17] provided a magnetic resonance imaging (MRI) evaluation of patients with knee cartilage lesions treated with microfractures alone or combined with PRP or platelet-rich fibrin (PRF) in a retrospective comparative study at 5-year follow-up. The authors reported better results in terms of the Magnetic Resonance Observation of Cartilage Repair Tissue (MOCART) score for the groups treated with platelet concentrates compared with the microfracture alone group, thus confirming the possible role of PRP in improving cartilage repair.

PRP-augmented scaffolds have also been investigated for cartilage defects. In particular, scaffolds can be soaked in PRP with the aim of supplying localized growth factors that facilitate cell infiltration, proliferation, and differentiation.[18] Several preclinical studies have reported that PRP-augmented scaffolds are beneficial in the articular cartilage repair process.[19,20] Thus, different scaffolds have been used in clinical practice combined with PRP to treat articular cartilage defects and have shown promising clinical results.[18,21] In autologous matrix-induced chondrogenesis (AMIC), a porcine collagen type I/III membrane has been used with fibrin glue and autologous serum or PRP to cover the microfractured defect: Dhollander et al. reported the successful clinical combination of PRP and AMIC for the treatment of patellar cartilage defects in a small number of patients at 24-month follow-up.[22] Newer approaches favor the use of synthetic scaffolds, such as textile polyglycolic acid–hyaluronan (PGA-HA) implants for covering microfractured defects. Siclari et al.[18] evaluated 52 patients treated with PRP-augmented PGA/HA scaffolds for articular cartilage defects of the knee. They reported a statistically significant clinical improvement at 12-month follow-up, with histological evaluation showing a homogenous hyaline-like cartilage repair tissue.

Overall, PRP research seems promising for cartilage repair, but many questions remain unanswered. In particular, the most suitable type of concentrate is still being debated. Different preparation methods for PRP can yield products with different compositions and characteristics, and different features in terms of content of platelets and leukocytes, volume of whole blood harvested, storage procedures, exogenous activation of platelets, and formation of a fibrin matrix.[23] All this makes it very difficult to merge and analyze clinical results from different studies and gain a full understanding of the actual benefits of this biological approach. Further studies will be required to investigate these aspects to gain a better understanding of the potential and limitations of PRP for the treatment of cartilage defects and OA.

Bone Marrow Aspirate Concentrate

Bone marrow aspirate concentrate (BMAC) has been proposed as a promising alternative for the treatment of cartilage lesions. It is a combination of biologically active cells and proteins obtained through a technically easy and minimally invasive procedure.[24] BMAC exploits the rich content of cells, growth factors, cytokines, and chemokines, which are involved in several crucial pathways for cell maintenance and function, differentiation, extracellular matrix production, and for the regulation of cell catabolic/anabolic activity.[25,26] Since the use of BMAC has been introduced recently as an injective approach, its clinical evidence is still limited. Few clinical studies have focused on the injective treatment in knee OA. They show the safety and effectiveness of this intra-articular approach and give promising clinical results in terms of pain relief and knee function improvement, which need to be confirmed by high-level studies.[27,28] A new application has recently been proposed to exploit the potential of BMAC by targeting the subchondral bone, which is commonly affected by the OA processes.[29] In particular, Hernigou et al.[30,31] supported the effectiveness of subchondral BMAC injections for the treatment of knee OA by showing the superiority of this approach in terms of clinical improvement and MRI findings compared with the intra-articular treatment.

For cartilage repair, BMAC has been used either as augmentation to microfracture surgery or combined with scaffolds. Murphy et al.[32] compared the clinical outcomes of microfractures alone with microfractures augmented with BMAC in the treatment of ankle osteochondral lesions (101 patients) for a minimum of 36 months. Both groups showed a statistically significant improvement in pain scores, quality of life scores, participation in sport and activities of daily living, but a lower revision rate in patients treated with BMAC (12% vs. 29%). Hannon et al.[33] retrospectively evaluated 34 patients who underwent arthroscopic bone marrow stimulation with and without BMAC for osteochondral lesions of the talus. Although they reported no differences between the groups in terms of clinical improvement at mid-term follow-up, patients treated with microfractures combined with BMAC showed better MRI findings evaluated through the MOCART score, thus suggesting a better quality of the repair tissue.

BMAC has also been used as scaffold augmentation in clinical practice (Fig. 6.1) to increase multipotent cell levels that can differentiate into local cell types and improve the healing of the target region.[34] Numerous studies have described the clinical efficacy of scaffolds augmented with BMAC in the treatment of chondral lesions of the knee. Gobbi et al.[35] evaluated BMAC in combination with a collagen I/III matrix in large focal cartilage defects (average size of 8.3 cm^2) and found a significant improvement in clinical scores for up to 3 years. In this study MRI also revealed a complete filling of the defects in 80% and less than 50% filling in 20% of the cases and a complete integration of cartilage in 88% of cases. In another study,[36] the same authors compared microfracture surgery with a BMAC-augmented hyaluronic acid scaffold for knee chondral defects. At 5-year follow-up, clinical assessments showed higher scores in the BMAC group compared with the microfracture group. More recently,[37] they reported a significant improvement also in patients over 45 years with focal ICRS grade IV articular cartilage lesions of the knee treated with the hyaluronic scaffold soaked in BMAC. Enea et al.[38] evaluated nine patients with knee chondral lesions treated with microfractures supplemented with a collagen membrane soaked in BMAC. At 1-year follow-up, four patients underwent second-look arthroscopy and cartilage biopsy and macroscopic cartilage assessment showed that all the repairs appeared to be almost normal. Moreover, histological analysis showed a hyaline-like cartilage repair in one lesion, a fibrocartilaginous repair in two lesions, and a mixture of both in one lesion, thus suggesting that BMAC is an effective adjunct treatment for creating a more hyaline-like cartilage repair tissue. In a comparative study, Krych et al.[39] followed 46 patients with MRI for 1 year after treating knee cartilage defects with a Trufit BGS scaffold, a scaffold with PRP, or a scaffold with BMAC. The PRP-treated and BMAC-treated scaffolds had superior cartilage fill compared with that of the control group and the BMAC group showed better results with mean T2 values closer to those of the superficial native hyaline cartilage. De Girolamo et al.[40] conducted a comparative study by assessing long-term outcomes after AMIC in the treatment of focal knee chondral lesions and any improvements achieved by the combination of this technique with BMAC (AMIC+). This study showed that AMIC and AMIC+ were effective treatments for focal chondral lesions with a beneficial effect lasting up to 9 years. The authors concluded that AMIC+ enabled faster recovery from injury and was thus better indicated for patients requiring a prompt return to activity (see Fig. 6.1).

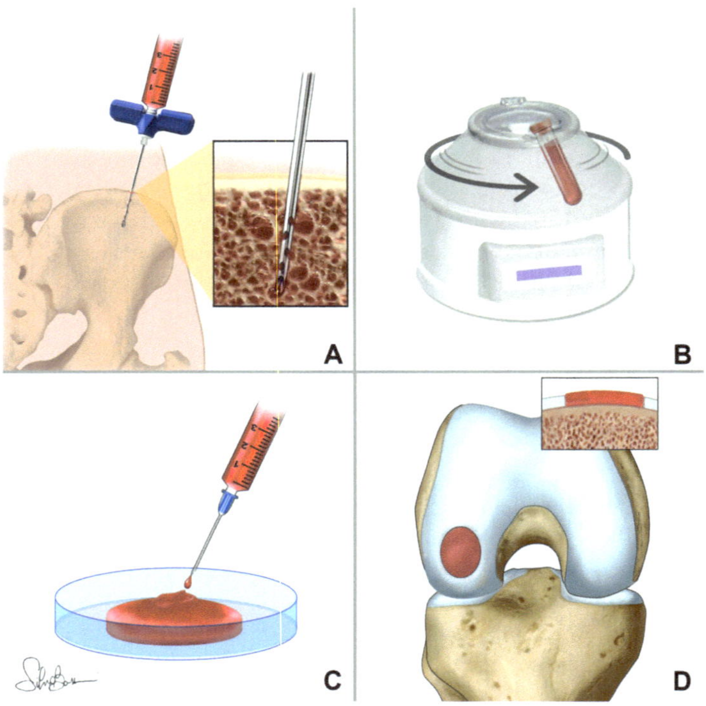

• **Fig. 6.1** Scaffolds can be combined with biologic agents, including bone marrow aspirate concentrate (BMAC). In a one-step technique, (A) bone marrow is harvested from the iliac crest and (B) then centrifuged. (C) The BMAC obtained is applied to the scaffold and (D) the BMAC-augmented matrix is placed on the defect. (Courtesy Silvia Bassini.)

The clinical efficacy of scaffolds augmented with BMAC has been investigated for the treatment of chondral lesions of the ankle in some clinical studies. In a prospective study by Giannini et al. on 48 patients with talar osteochondral lesions, a one-step arthroscopic technique was used by combining BMAC with collagen powder or hyaluronic acid membrane as a scaffold for cell support and platelet gel.[41] At 24-month follow-up, clinical scores improved in all patients and the histologic evaluation showed regenerated tissue in various degrees of remodeling although none showed complete hyaline cartilage. In another study, the same authors compared this one-step arthroscopic technique with two cartilage procedures (open ACI and arthroscopic ACI) and reported a similar clinical improvement in all groups, with good restoration of the cartilaginous layer, as seen by MRI and histological analysis, which resembled hyaline cartilage.[42]

BMAC has also recently been investigated as augmentation to osteochondral allograft transplantation to enhance osseous integration of the allograft. Oladeji et al.[43] performed a cohort study to evaluate the effect of BMAC on the integration of femoral condyle osteochondral allografts. Grafts were saturated in BMAC for a minimum of 2 minutes before implantation (compared with no BMAC). Radiography showed graft incorporation was significantly increased in the BMAC group at 6 weeks, 3 months, and 6 months. The BMAC group also showed significantly less sclerosis at 6 weeks and 3 months. Conversely, in a retrospective comparative MRI study with 12-month follow-up, Wang et al.[44] showed that osteochondral allografts augmented with BMAC did not produce improved osseous integration, decreased cystic changes, or other bone, cartilage, or ancillary feature changes compared with osteochondral allografts alone. Together, these studies suggest the inconsistent clinical results of BMAC as osteochondral allograft augmentation. On the other hand, BMAC-augmented scaffolds showed promise for the single-stage management of chondral defects in both knee and ankle, although further high-level studies with long follow-up are needed.

Mesenchymal Stromal Cells

MSCs are heterogeneous populations of cells that can exhibit variable growth potential and distinct morphologic, phenotypic, and functional characteristics.[45,46] They all have chondrogenic potential and potent immuno suppressive or modulatory characteristics and thus represent a powerful tool for treating cartilage defects and OA.[45] MSC-based therapy has become the focus of attention because MSCs are relatively easy to handle in terms of tissue harvest, rapid proliferation and cell expansion, and present a high chondrogenic differentiation potential. Among the available sources of MSCs, two have taken the spotlight for the augmentation of cartilage repair procedures: adipose-derived mesenchymal stromal cells (ADSCs) and bone marrow-derived MSCs (BMSCs).[47] Positive results have been shown both in animal models and in human treatment. Some clinical trials have recently shown that MSC injections yield beneficial outcomes for patients with OA.[46,48] In particular, a meta-analysis on nine RCTs described increased clinical improvement from baseline to 24 months in patients with knee OA compared with the control group (saline, hyaluronic acid, steroids), with no difference in terms of adverse events.[49] These treatments might be difficult to manage from a legal point of view, because these cell types might be considered a pharmacological agent administration and studies, albeit promising, are still heterogeneous and need stronger data.

For cartilage repair, MSCs have been used either as augmentation to microfracture or combined with scaffolds. In a study on 30 patients with medial condylar cartilage defects, Qiao et al.[50] assessed the effect of ADSC injections to enhance microfractures and found a significantly increased clinical improvement up to 24 months in patients treated with microfractures followed by intra-articular ADSCs and HA injections compared with patients who were treated by microfractures with the adjunct of HA or normal saline. Kim et al. provided more evidence of the benefits of ADSCs in the treatment of osteochondral lesions of the talus in several clinical studies.[51–53] These authors compared the clinical and MRI outcomes of patients treated with one intra-articular ADSC injection and microfractures with patients treated by microfractures alone at short-term follow-up. They reported better clinical and MRI findings in the ADSCs group and concluded that ADSC injections as augmentation to microfractures should be considered as a treatment for osteochondral lesions of the talus, even when poor prognostic factors, including older age, large-sized lesion, or subchondral cysts are present. In an RCT on 80 patients,[51] the same authors reported the effectiveness of ADSCs loaded in fibrin glue as augmentation to microfractures. The 40 patients treated with the combined approach showed better clinical results compared with patients treated with microfractures alone at 24-month follow-up, although second-look arthroscopy showed good repair tissue quality in both groups without a significant intergroup difference.

Regarding scaffold augmentation with MSCs, BMSCs have been the most widely studied in clinical practice. Haalem et al.[54] used BMSCs on a platelet fibrin glue scaffold for the treatment of articular knee cartilage defects in five patients: the symptoms in all patients improved at 12 months and MRI revealed complete defect filling and complete surface congruity with native cartilage in three patients, although two showed incomplete congruity. Kasemkijwattana et al.[55] showed good defect filling and repair tissue stiffness with cultured BMSCs on a collagen scaffold in two patients with knee OA and reported good incorporation with the adjacent cartilage and a significant clinical improvement. Nejadnik et al.[56] compared BMSC implantation with the first-generation ACI technique in a study on 72 patients affected by full-thickness knee cartilage defects. These authors reported similar clinical results in both treatment groups and highlighted the advantages of the BMSC technique that was as effective as using chondrocytes for cartilage repair but required one less knee operation, cost less, and minimized donor-site morbidity. Despite these promising results on small cohorts, the biological properties of cultured MSCs and their effects on cartilage healing still remain uncertain in clinical practice. Moreover, considering the strict regulations and the problems related to cell manipulation and expansion, the use of cultured MSCs remains extremely limited.

Other Adjuvants and Future Perspectives

Over the last few years, researchers have tested novel treatments for cartilage lesions and OA. Among these, some authors assessed the role of placental tissue extracts in the treatment of cartilage defects and OA. Different parts of the placenta may be of clinical importance, because it contains numerous soluble factors and MSCs that can differentiate along a fibroblastic lineage.[57] Research into the clinical efficacy of placental tissue extracts is still in its early stages and very few studies have been published to date reporting clinical outcomes. Vines et al.[58] tested a single intra-articular injection of amniotic suspension allograft, containing cryopreserved particulated human amnion and amniotic fluid cells in six patients with Kellgren-Lawrence grades 3 and 4 tibiofemoral knee OA. At 1-year follow-up, the authors found an overall trend of improvement in clinical scores, with no significant adverse events. Alden et al.[59] conducted a retrospective review of 100 knees treated for symptomatic OA with an injection of 100 mg of micronized dehydrated human amnion/chorion membrane and found a clinical improvement at up to 6-month follow-up. A recent RCT on 200 patients with knee OA compared the injection of an amniotic suspension allograft with hyaluronic acid or saline injection, with subjects blinded to their allocation. Patients receiving amniotic treatment had significantly greater clinical improvement from baseline up to 6 months compared with patients treated with hyaluronic acid or saline, and had a lower clinical failure rate at 3 months.[60]

Other researchers have investigated the role of MSC secretome, because it has been shown that the therapeutic ability of MSCs is mainly related to their secretion of biologically active factors, rather than their differentiation properties.[61] All these paracrine factors, with the addition of a broad variety of nucleic acid and different lipids, can also be found within cell-secreted vesicles (extracellular vesicles), a key part of the secretome that is gaining increasing attention by the scientific community.[61] A recent systematic review suggested that the use of secretome and extracellular vesicles for the treatment of cartilage pathology and knee OA had pleiotropic effects and overall positive results. In vitro, both secretome and extracellular vesicles showed anti-catabolic, immunomodulatory, and regenerative properties, and in vivo animal studies confirmed their effectiveness as a minimally invasive treatment, with positive effects on the whole joint.[62] Nevertheless, more research is required to translate the promising preclinical findings into clinical trials to confirm the potential of secretome and extracellular vesicles as a minimally invasive biological treatment to address cartilage diseases.

Conclusion

Overall, several new solutions are emerging and show promise. However, all the new approaches need to be better studied and their role investigated in cartilage repair in large, high-level studies specifically to define potential and limitations of each treatment. Moreover, it will be important to identify which patients may benefit most from these procedures and to determine the factors that influence their response to a specific treatment, ranging from baseline clinical characteristics to biomarker profiles.[63] Only after a proper characterization of the biologics has been applied and solid data supporting their clinical safety and efficacy have been gathered will it be possible to extend these promising biological approaches to clinical practice for the treatment of cartilage lesions and OA degeneration.

References

1. Ayhan E, Kesmezacar H, Akgun I. Intraarticular injections (corticosteroid, hyaluronic acid, platelet rich plasma) for the knee osteoarthritis. *World J Orthop*. 2014;5:351–361. 10.5312/wjo.v5.i3.351.
2. Southworth TM, Naveen NB, Tauro TM, Leong NL, Cole BJ. The use of platelet-rich plasma in symptomatic knee osteoarthritis. *J Knee Surg*. 2019;32:37–45.
3. Dai WL, Zhou AG, Zhang H, Zhang J. Efficacy of platelet-rich plasma in the treatment of knee osteoarthritis: a meta-analysis of randomized controlled trials. *Arthroscopy*. 2017;33:659–670.
4. Altamura SA, Di Martino A, Andriolo L, et al. Platelet-rich plasma for sport-active patients with knee osteoarthritis: limited return to sport. *Biomed Res Int*. 2020;2020:8243865.
5. Di Martino A, Di Matteo B, Papio T, et al. Platelet-rich plasma versus hyaluronic acid injections for the treatment of knee osteoarthritis: results at 5 years of a double-blind, randomized controlled trial. *Am J Sports Med*. 2019;47:347–354.
6. Previtali D, Merli G, Di Laura Frattura G, Candrian C, Zaffagnini S, Filardo G. The long-lasting effects of "placebo injections" in knee osteoarthritis: a meta-analysis. *Cartilage*. 2020;1947603520906597.
7. Filardo G, Previtali D, Napoli F, Candrian C, Zaffagnini S, Grassi A. PRP injections for the treatment of knee osteoarthritis: a meta-analysis of randomized controlled trials. *Cartilage*. 2020;1947603520931170.
8. Mei-Dan O, Carmont MR, Laver L, Mann G, Maffulli N, Nyska M. Platelet-rich plasma or hyaluronate in the management of osteochondral lesions of the talus. *Am J Sports Med*. 2012;40:534–541.
9. Akpancar S, Gul D. Comparison of platelet rich plasma and prolotherapy in the management of osteochondral lesions of the talus: a retrospective cohort study. *Med Sci Monit*. 2019;25:5640–5647.
10. Dallari D, Stagni C, Rani N, et al. Ultrasound-guided injection of platelet-rich plasma and hyaluronic acid, separately and in combination, for hip osteoarthritis: a randomized controlled study. *Am J Sports Med*. 2016;44:664–671.

11. Boffa A, Previtali D, Di Laura Frattura G, Vannini F, Candrian C, Filardo G. Evidence on ankle injections for osteochondral lesions and osteoarthritis: a systematic review and meta-analysis. *Int Orthop*. 2020;45:509–523.
12. Anitua E, Andia I, Ardanza B, Nurden P, Nurden AT. Autologous platelets as a source of proteins for healing and tissue regeneration. *Thromb Haemost*. 2004;91:4–15.
13. Eppley BL, Woodell JE, Higgins J. Platelet quantification and growth factor analysis from platelet-rich plasma: implications for wound healing. *Plast Reconstr Surg*. 2004;114:1502–1508.
14. Akeda K, An HS, Okuma M, et al. Platelet-rich plasma stimulates porcine articular chondrocyte proliferation and matrix biosynthesis. *Osteoarthritis Cartilage*. 2006;14:1272–1280.
15. Kruger JP, Hondke S, Endres M, Pruss A, Siclari A, Kaps C. Human platelet-rich plasma stimulates migration and chondrogenic differentiation of human subchondral progenitor cells. *J Orthop Res*. 2012;30:845–852.
16. Boffa A, Previtali D, Altamura SA, Zaffagnini S, Candrian C, Filardo G. Platelet-rich plasma augmentation to microfracture provides a limited benefit for the treatment of cartilage lesions: a meta-analysis. *Orthop J Sports Med*. 2020;8(4): 2325967120910504.
17. Papalia R, Diaz Balzani L, Torre G, et al. Intraoperative application Platelet rich fibrin, postoperative injections OF PRP or microfracture only for osteochondral lesions of the knee: a five-year retrospective evaluation. *J Biol Regul Homeost Agents*. 2016;30:41–49.
18. Siclari A, Mascaro G, Gentili C, Kaps C, Cancedda R, Boux E. Cartilage repair in the knee with subchondral drilling augmented with a platelet-rich plasma-immersed polymer-based implant. *Knee Surg Sports Traumatol Arthrosc*. 2014;22:1225–1234.
19. Qi YY, Chen X, Jiang YZ, et al. Local delivery of autologous platelet in collagen matrix simulated in situ articular cartilage repair. *Cell Transplant*. 2009;18:1161–1169.
20. Titan A, Schar M, Hutchinson I, Demange M, Chen T, Rodeo S. Growth factor delivery to a cartilage-cartilage interface using platelet-rich concentrates on a hyaluronic acid scaffold. *Arthroscopy*. 2020;36:1431–1440.
21. Sermer C, Devitt B, Chahal J, Kandel R, Theodoropoulos J. The addition of platelet-rich plasma to scaffolds used for cartilage repair: a review of human and animal studies. *Arthroscopy*. 2015;31:1607–1625.
22. Dhollander AA, De Neve F, Almqvist KF, Verdonk R, Lambrecht S, Elewaut D, Verbruggen G, Verdonk PC. Autologous matrix-induced chondrogenesis combined with platelet-rich plasma gel: technical description and a five pilot patients report. *Knee Surg Sports Traumatol Arthrosc*. 2011;19:536–542.
23. Arnoczky SP, Sheibani-Rad S. The basic science of platelet-rich plasma (PRP): what clinicians need to know. *Sports Med Arthrosc Rev*. 2013;21:180–185.
24. Fortier LA, Strauss EJ, Shepard DO, Becktell L, Kennedy JG. Biological effects of bone marrow concentrate in knee pathologies. *J Knee Surg*. 2019;32:2–8.
25. Fortier LA, Barker JU, Strauss EJ, McCarrel TM, Cole BJ. The role of growth factors in cartilage repair. *Clin Orthop Relat Res*. 2011;469:2706–2715.
26. Mariani E, Pulsatelli L, Facchini A. Signaling pathways in cartilage repair. *Int J Mol Sci*. 2014;15:8667–8698.
27. Cavallo C, Boffa A, Andriolo L, et al. Bone marrow concentrate injections for the treatment of osteoarthritis: evidence from preclinical findings to the clinical application. *Int Orthop*. 2020;45(2):525–538.
28. Di Matteo B, Vandenbulcke F, Vitale ND, et al. Minimally manipulated mesenchymal stem cells for the treatment of knee osteoarthritis: a systematic review of clinical evidence. *Stem Cells Int*. 2019;2019:1735242.
29. Hernigou P, Auregan JC, Dubory A, Flouzat-Lachaniette CH, Chevallier N, Rouard H. Subchondral stem cell therapy versus contralateral total knee arthroplasty for osteoarthritis following secondary osteonecrosis of the knee. *Int Orthop*. 2018;42:2563–2571.
30. Hernigou P, Delambre J, Quiennec S, Poignard A. Human bone marrow mesenchymal stem cell injection in subchondral lesions of knee osteoarthritis: a prospective randomized study versus contralateral arthroplasty at a mean fifteen year follow-up. *Int Orthop*. 2020;45(2):365–373.
31. Hernigou P, Bouthors C, Bastard C, Flouzat Lachaniette CH, Rouard H, Dubory A. Subchondral bone or intra-articular injection of bone marrow concentrate mesenchymal stem cells in bilateral knee osteoarthritis: what better postpone knee arthroplasty at fifteen years? A randomized study. *Int Orthop*. 2020;45(2):391–399.
32. Murphy EP, McGoldrick NP, Curtin M, Kearns SR. A prospective evaluation of bone marrow aspirate concentrate and microfracture in the treatment of osteochondral lesions of the talus. *Foot Ankle Surg*. 2019;25:441–448.
33. Hannon CP, Ross KA, Murawski CD, et al. Arthroscopic bone marrow stimulation and concentrated bone marrow aspirate for osteochondral lesions of the talus: a case-control study of functional and magnetic resonance observation of cartilage repair tissue outcomes. *Arthroscopy*. 2016;32:339–347.
34. Gigante A, Cecconi S, Calcagno S, Busilacchi A, Enea D. Arthroscopic knee cartilage repair with covered microfracture and bone marrow concentrate. *Arthrosc Tech*. 2012;1:e175–e180.
35. Gobbi A, Karnatzikos G, Sankineani SR. One-step surgery with multipotent stem cells for the treatment of large full-thickness chondral defects of the knee. *Am J Sports Med*. 2014;42:648–657.
36. Gobbi A, Whyte GP. One-stage cartilage repair using a hyaluronic acid-based scaffold with activated bone marrow-derived mesenchymal stem cells compared with microfracture: five-year follow-up. *Am J Sports Med*. 2016;44:2846–2854.
37. Gobbi A, Scotti C, Karnatzikos G, Mudhigere A, Castro M, Peretti GM. One-step surgery with multipotent stem cells and Hyaluronan-based scaffold for the treatment of full-thickness chondral defects of the knee in patients older than 45 years. *Knee Surg Sports Traumatol Arthrosc*. 2017;25:2494–2501.
38. Enea D, Cecconi S, Calcagno S, Busilacchi A, Manzotti S, Gigante A. One-step cartilage repair in the knee: collagen-covered microfracture and autologous bone marrow concentrate. A pilot study. *Knee*. 2015;22:30–35.
39. Krych AJ, Nawabi DH, Farshad-Amacker NA, et al. Bone marrow concentrate improves early cartilage phase maturation of a scaffold plug in the knee: a comparative magnetic resonance imaging analysis to platelet-rich plasma and control. *Am J Sports Med*. 2016;44:91–98.
40. de Girolamo L, Schönhuber H, Viganò M, et al. Autologous matrix-induced chondrogenesis (AMIC) and AMIC enhanced by autologous concentrated bone marrow aspirate (BMAC) allow for stable clinical and functional improvements at up to 9 years follow-up: results from a randomized controlled study. *J Clin Med*. 2019;8:392.
41. Giannini S, Buda R, Vannini F, Cavallo M, Grigolo B. One-step bone marrow-derived cell transplantation in talar osteochondral lesions. *Clin Orthop Relat Res*. 2009;467:3307–3320.

42. Giannini S, Buda R, Cavallo M, et al. Cartilage repair evolution in post-traumatic osteochondral lesions of the talus: from open field autologous chondrocyte to bone-marrow-derived cells transplantation. *Injury*. 2010;41:1196–1203.
43. Oladeji LO, Stannard JP, Cook CR, et al. Effects of autogenous bone marrow aspirate concentrate on radiographic integration of femoral condylar osteochondral allografts. *Am J Sports Med.* 2017;45:2797–2803.
44. Wang D, Lin KM, Burge AJ, Balazs GC, Williams 3rd RJ. Bone marrow aspirate concentrate does not improve osseous integration of osteochondral allografts for the treatment of chondral defects in the knee at 6 and 12 months: a comparative magnetic resonance imaging analysis. *Am J Sports Med.* 2019;47:339–346.
45. Harrell CR, Markovic BS, Fellabaum C, Arsenijevic A, Volarevic V. Mesenchymal stem cell-based therapy of osteoarthritis: current knowledge and future perspectives. *Biomed Pharmacother.* 2019;109:2318–2326.
46. Robinson PG, Murray IR, West CC, et al. Reporting of mesenchymal stem cell preparation protocols and composition: a systematic review of the clinical orthopaedic literature. *Am J Sports Med.* 2019;47:991–1000.
47. Filardo G, Madry H, Jelic M, Roffi A, Cucchiarini M, Kon E. Mesenchymal stem cells for the treatment of cartilage lesions: from preclinical findings to clinical application in orthopaedics. *Knee Surg Sports Traumatol Arthrosc.* 2013;21:1717–1729.
48. Roffi A, Nakamura N, Sanchez M, Cucchiarini M, Filardo G. Injectable systems for intra-articular delivery of mesenchymal stromal cells for cartilage treatment: a systematic review of preclinical and clinical evidence. *Int J Mol Sci.* 2018;99:3322.
49. Huang R, Li W, Zhao Y, Yang F, Xu M. Clinical efficacy and safety of stem cell therapy for knee osteoarthritis: a meta-analysis. *Medicine (Baltimore).* 2020;99:e19434.
50. Qiao Z, Tang J, Yue B, et al. Human adipose-derived mesenchymal progenitor cells plus microfracture and hyaluronic acid for cartilage repair: a Phase IIa trial. *Regen Med.* 2020;15:1193–1214.
51. Koh YG, Kwon OR, Kim YS, Choi YJ, Tak DH. Adipose-derived mesenchymal stem cells with microfracture versus microfracture alone: 2-year follow-up of a prospective randomized trial. *Arthroscopy.* 2016;32:97–109.
52. Kim YS, Park EH, Kim YC, Koh YG. Clinical outcomes of mesenchymal stem cell injection with arthroscopic treatment in older patients with osteochondral lesions of the talus. *Am J Sports Med.* 2013;41:1090–1099.
53. Kim YS, Lee HJ, Choi YJ, Kim YI, Koh YG. Does an injection of a stromal vascular fraction containing adipose-derived mesenchymal stem cells influence the outcomes of marrow stimulation in osteochondral lesions of the talus? A clinical and magnetic resonance imaging study. *Am J Sports Med.* 2014;42:2424–2434.
54. Haleem AM, Singergy AA, Sabry D, et al. The clinical use of human culture-expanded autologous bone marrow mesenchymal stem cells transplanted on platelet-rich fibrin glue in the treatment of articular cartilage defects: a pilot study and preliminary results. *Cartilage.* 2010;1:253–261.
55. Kasemkijwattana C, Hongeng S, Kesprayura S, Rungsinaporn V, Chaipinyo K, Chansiri K. Autologous bone marrow mesenchymal stem cells implantation for cartilage defects: two cases report. *J Med Assoc Thai.* 2011;94:395–400.
56. Nejadnik H, Hui JH, Feng Choong EP, Tai BC, Lee EH. Autologous bone marrow-derived mesenchymal stem cells versus autologous chondrocyte implantation: an observational cohort study. *Am J Sports Med.* 2010;38:1110–1116.
57. Roubelakis MG, Trohatou O, Anagnou NP. Amniotic fluid and amniotic membrane stem cells: marker discovery. *Stem Cells Int.* 2012;2012:107836.
58. Vines JB, Aliprantis AO, Gomoll AH, Farr J. Cryopreserved amniotic suspension for the treatment of knee osteoarthritis. *J Knee Surg.* 2016;29:443–450.
59. Alden KJ, Harris S, Hubbs B, Kot K, Istwan NB, Mason D. Micronized dehydrated human amnion chorion membrane injection in the treatment of knee osteoarthritis—a large retrospective case series. *J Knee Surg.* 2019. 10.1055/s-0039-3400951.
60. Farr J, Gomoll AH, Yanke AB, Strauss EJ, Mowry KC. A randomized controlled single-blind study demonstrating superiority of amniotic suspension allograft injection over hyaluronic acid and saline control for modification of knee osteoarthritis symptoms. *J Knee Surg.* 2019;32:1143–1154.
61. Madrigal M, Rao KS, Riordan NH. A review of therapeutic effects of mesenchymal stem cell secretions and induction of secretory modification by different culture methods. *J Transl Med.* 2014;12:260.
62. D'Arrigo D, Roffi A, Cucchiarini M, Moretti M, Candrian C, Filardo G. Secretome and extracellular vesicles as new biological therapies for knee osteoarthritis: a systematic review. *J Clin Med.* 2019;8:1867.
63. Boffa A, Merli G, Andriolo L, Lattermann C, Salzmann GM, Filardo G. Synovial fluid biomarkers in knee osteoarthritis: a systematic review and quantitative evaluation using bipeds criteria. Cartilage. 2020:1947603520942941.

7

Debridement, Microfracture, and Osteochondral Autograft Transfer for the Treatment of Cartilage Defects

TOM MINAS, MD, MS AND ANDREAS H. GOMOLL, MD

CHAPTER OUTLINE

All three techniques discussed in this chapter are treatment options for small articular cartilage defects, predominately because of their low invasiveness. Debridement is mostly indicated for the treatment of (1) incidental lesions discovered during surgery directed at other joint pathology, such as meniscectomy and ACL reconstruction; and (2) lesions in lower demand patients who are reluctant to undergo other cartilage repair procedures that are more invasive and/or require long rehabilitation. Debridement is also a good initial treatment option for lesions that are deemed borderline or too large for microfracture or osteochondral autograft transfer (OAT) because it does not appear to compromise later treatment with autologous chondrocyte implantation (ACI).

Microfracture is a minimally invasive option whose indications have been refined in the last few years through multiple investigations. However, unlike chondroplasty, patients can be made worse in up to 13% of cases[1] and it should only be used for incidental lesions after an informed discussion with the patient and obtaining their consent. It has a high success rate when used appropriately for the treatment of small (< 2–4cm^2) defects in the femoral condyles of younger (< 35–40 years) patients with acute defects.[2]

Larger defects and those located in the patellofemoral joint deteriorate after 24–36 months.[3] Not all defect sizes, whether small or large, have the same clinical improvement nor responsiveness as ACI as demonstrated in the Summit Trial.[4,5]

OAT is generally indicated for the treatment of small (< 2–4 cm^2) defects in the femoral condyles and trochlea, but not the patella.[6] The recommendation for size is based on the limited availability of cartilage elsewhere in the knee (donor site morbidity); and to minimize the complication of plug necrosis, which is seen more frequently in central plugs that are completely surrounded by other plugs and therefore have no direct contact with native bone for integration. Although lesions up to 4 cm^2 have been indicated for OAT, it is our preference to use this technique for active, fit individuals as a first-line treatment with lesions 1–1.5 cm^2 because it does not cause donor-site symptoms in these small lesions and results in a rapid return to sport (4–8 months) with a mature hyaline cartilage repair.

Planning

Standard radiographic and magnetic resonance imaging examinations should be performed preoperatively to determine the size and number of lesions to be treated, because both microfracture and OAT have upper size limitations. Similar to the more invasive cartilage repair techniques, long-leg films are crucial to determine alignment. Any significant malalignment should be corrected through neutralization osteotomy to maximize the success rate of cartilage repair.

Surgical Technique

Debridement and Chondroplasty

Debridement is performed arthroscopically, mainly for the treatment of incidental lesions found during treatment of other issues in the joint. Although removal of loose flaps with the motorized shaver is considered debridement, which is our preference, true chondroplasty requires a more thorough treatment of the defect with removal of degenerated tissue. Thermal chondroplasty may create extensive chondrocyte death and should be avoided. We do not create vertical shoulders similar to the process outlined for microfracture because it removes existing remaining cartilage. The purpose of chondroplasty is to alleviate mechanical symptoms. There is also evidence that it can affect repair tissue with the cell source arising from synovial tissue or endothelial stem cells in Hoffa's fat pad.[7–9] There has never been a head-to-head comparison of microfracture with chondroplasty for small defects.

Patients return to activities postoperatively as tolerated with no specific precautions or restrictions.

Microfracture

Microfracture is performed arthroscopically; set-up and patient positioning is that of routine knee arthroscopy. However, especially for very posterior defects, the leg should be positioned so that knee hyperflexion can be achieved.

After routine diagnostic arthroscopy to evaluate the defect (Fig. 7.1) and the rest of the joint for potential other comorbidities, loose flaps and degenerated tissue are debrided with a motorized shaver. Subsequently, a curette is used to trim any soft and fissured cartilage along the rim to create stable vertical shoulders (Fig. 7.2). The debridement also includes the calcified cartilage layer (Fig. 7.3) but should not violate the subchondral plate. Rarely, accessory portals have to be created depending on the exact defect size and location.

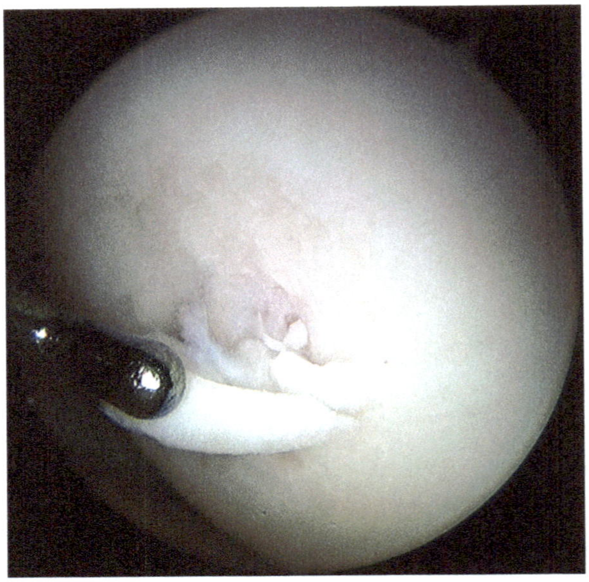

• **Fig. 7.1** Arthroscopic probe demonstrating a loose flap in a chondral defect of the femoral condyle.

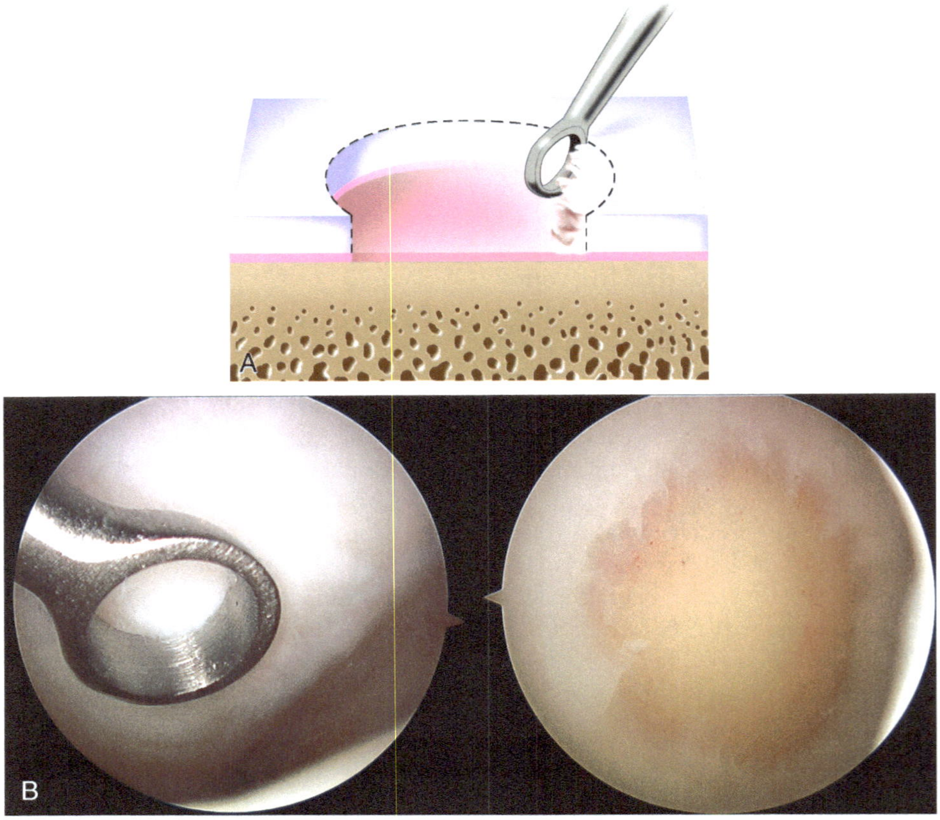

• **Fig. 7.2** Defect preparation (A) shown in sketch and (B) arthroscopic images. *Left*, Sharp ring curette for the debridement of cartilage; *Right*, defect after thorough debridement of degenerated tissue and creation of stable shoulders.

After thorough debridement, multiple holes are created in the subchondral plate with a microfracture awl (Fig. 7.4). This step should be performed last if multiple procedures are planned in the same setting, such as concomitant meniscal debridement or ACL reconstruction, because otherwise the marrow elements are washed away by the prolonged arthroscopy irrigation. When placing the microfracture holes, care should be taken not to destabilize the subchondral plate when holes become confluent or break into each other, which can occur when holes are placed too closely. Ideally, the microfracture holes should be spaced approximately 3 to 4 mm apart, resulting in 3 to 4 holes per cm^2. Also, if the microfracture awl is placed at a low angle to the bone, there is a tendency to skive off or create a hole that is not round but oblong, further destabilizing the bone. In an effort to remain perpendicular to the chondral surface, it may be necessary to flex and extend the knee to rotate the articular surface in line with the awl or create accessory portals. Stability of the transition zone between surrounding cartilage and regenerate fibrocartilage can be improved by placing holes as close as possible to the surrounding cartilage. After completion of the microfracture, the tourniquet (if used) is deflated and pump pressure is lowered. Bleeding should be observed from all holes, eventually filling the defect with a clot (Fig. 7.5).

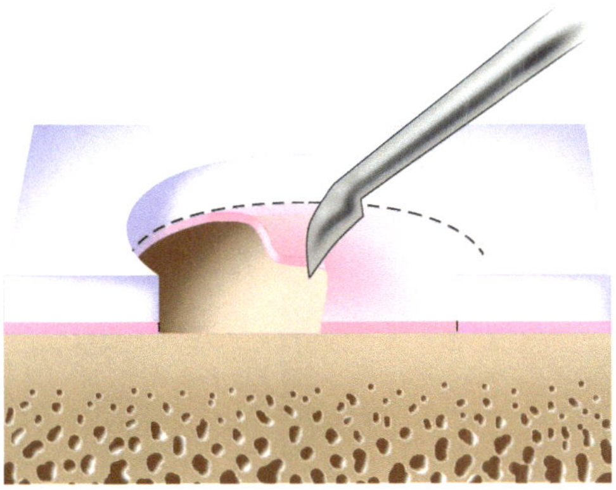

• **Fig. 7.3** Debridement of the zone of calcified cartilage.

Postoperatively, patients are placed on touch-down weight-bearing restrictions for 6 weeks and start a continuous passive motion (CPM) machine on POD no. 1 for 6 weeks, 6 to 8 hours per day. Return to athletic activities is based on the size of the defect but should be delayed for 6 to 9 months to allow for tissue maturation.

Intralesional osteophytes can develop in up to 30% of treated lesions,[10] which may make revision cartilage repair

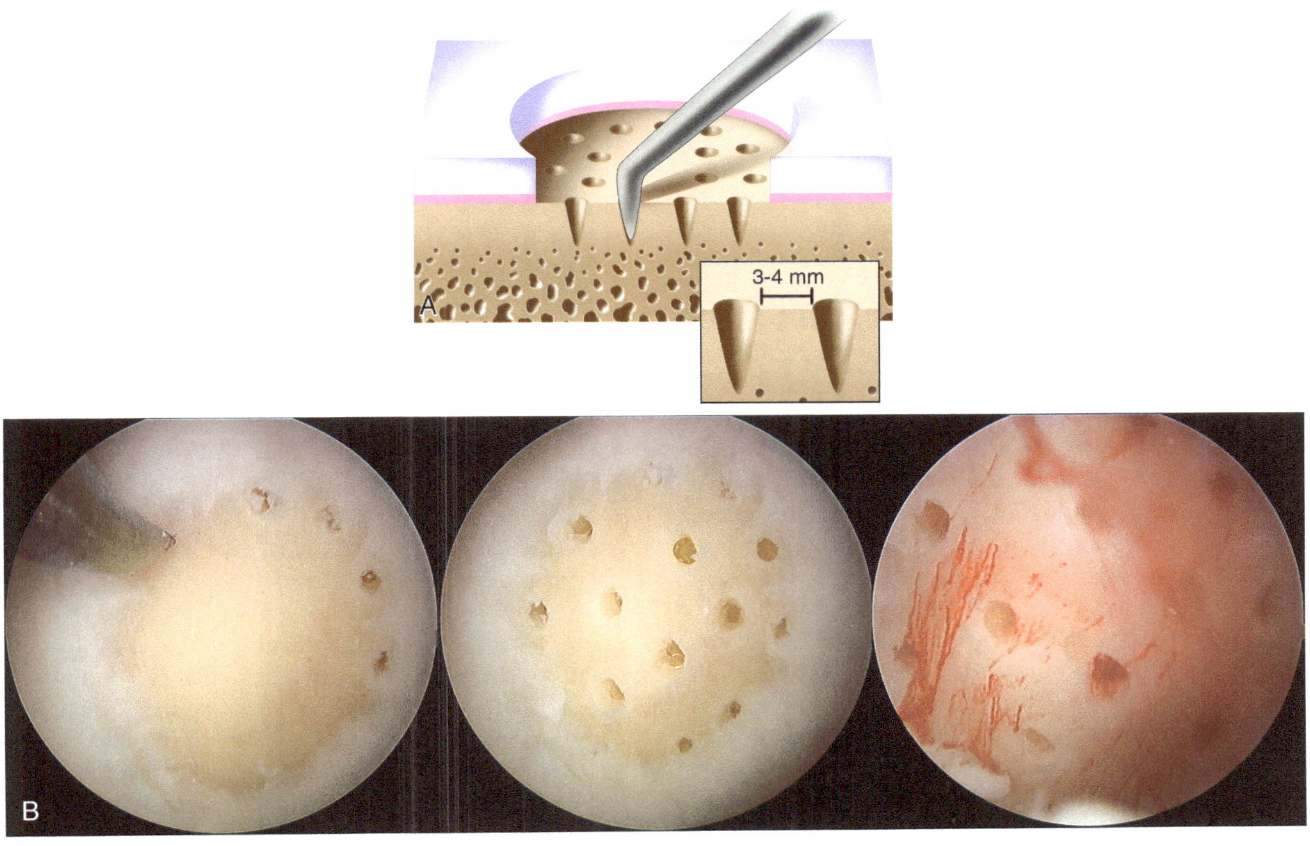

• **Fig. 7.4** Microfracture shown in: (A) sketch and (B) arthroscopic images. *Left*, Multiple microfracture holes are placed directly adjacent to the defect shoulders to improve integration. *Middle*, The defect is evenly filled with microfracture holes. *Right*, After release of the tourniquet, bleeding is observed from the microfracture holes.

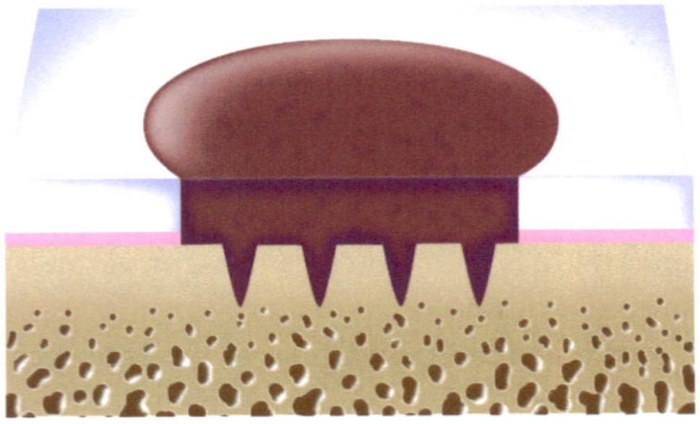

• **Fig. 7.5** A blood clot fills the defect, eventually forming a fibrocartilaginous repair tissue.

treatments such as ACI more prone to fail.[11] In an attempt to lessen the subchondral bone response, marrow stimulation techniques (MSTs) have been developed.

In addition, adjuvants that enhance the repair response are being marketed such as chitosan-derived products (BST-CarGel).[12] In a multicenter randomized controlled trial, microfracture augmented with BST-CarGel (Piramal Life Sciences, Bio-Orthopaedic Division, Aurora, Ontario, Canada) had superior fill and patient-reported outcomes compared to conventional microfracture at 1-year and 5-year follow-up.[13,14] Other emerging MST-augmented techniques include GelrinC (Regentis Biomaterials, Or Akiva, Israel)[15] and BioCartilage (Arthrex, Inc., Naples, FL).[16] Further studies are needed to evaluate long-term radiographic and clinical outcomes. As with conventional microfracture, augmentation strategies following microfracture are warranted for small, contained focal chondral injuries on the femoral condyle.

Osteochondral Autograft Transfer

OAT can be performed either arthroscopically or through an open approach, based on the exact defect size and location, and surgeon's preference.

The lesion is evaluated arthroscopically and accessory portals are created through spinal needle localization to allow perpendicular orientation of the instrumentation to the articular surface, for both the donor and recipient sites. Horizontal skin portals are preferred for an arthroscopic approach because this allows transverse enlargement of a portal to ensure orthogonal placement of the grafts. Occasionally, a central, transpatellar tendon approach is required. In this case, the patellar tendon should be split in line with its fibers and repaired at the end of the procedure. First, sizing guides are used to determine the size and number of grafts required to fill the defect (Fig. 7.6). Subsequently, an appropriately sized harvesting tube is selected and an osteochondral plug is obtained, usually approximately 10 mm long, being mindful to introduce the harvester perpendicular to the articular surface (Fig. 7.7). Several sites have been identified in the knee joint as suitable for osteochondral plug harvest. Although the superior lateral trochlear ridge (Fig. 7.8B) is considered a lesser weight-bearing area of the knee, it is an important load-bearing portion of the patellofemoral joint in 40–70 degrees of flexion and may cause significant symptoms if harvested. We prefer to harvest two or three plugs from the area of the sulcus terminalis on the distal lateral trochlea, just proximal to the sulcus terminalis, the transition zone between the tibiofemoral and patellofemoral weight-bearing areas (Fig. 8A), or the lateral intercondylar notch. After a plug has been obtained, the length and any potential angulation is noted (Fig. 7.9). A defect-harvesting tube is used to remove an appropriately sized and angled plug from the defect and the depth is checked with a sizing rod to ensure that the defect is approximately 1 mm deeper than the length of the graft. The graft is then advanced within the harvesting tube so that the end is just visible. The harvester is introduced into the joint, oriented perpendicularly to the articular surface, and the graft is slowly advanced into the recipient site (Fig. 7.10).

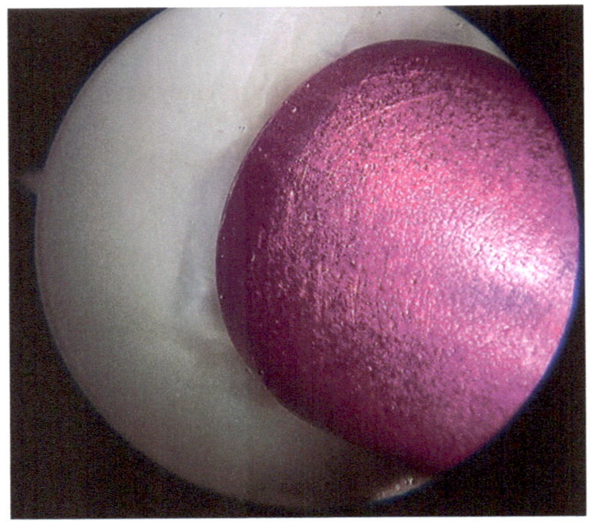

• **Fig. 7.6** The defect is measured using sizing rods to estimate the size and number of plugs required to fill the area.

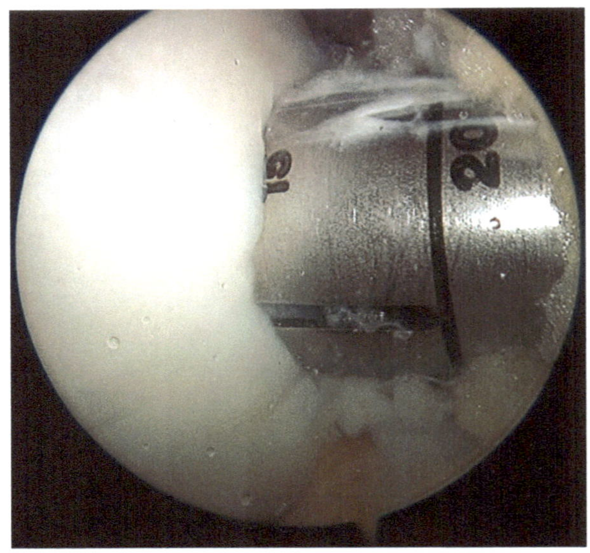

• **Fig. 7.7** An osteochondral plug is retrieved with a harvesting tube.

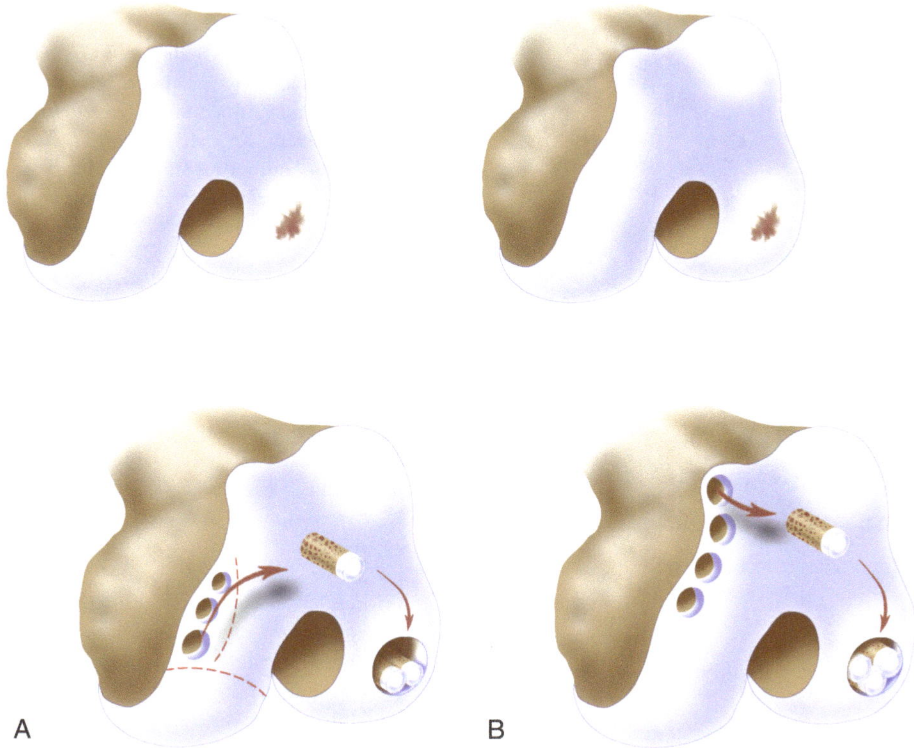

A B

• **Fig. 7.8** (A) The distal lateral trochlear ridge above the sulcus terminalis is the preferred harvest site for the plug. The lateral intercondylar notch proximal to the sulcus terminalis is also a suitable site. (B) Although the superior lateral trochlear ridge is considered a lesser weight-bearing area of the knee, it is an important load-bearing portion of the patellofemoral joint in 40–70 degrees of flexion, which may cause significant symptoms if harvested and therefore should be avoided.

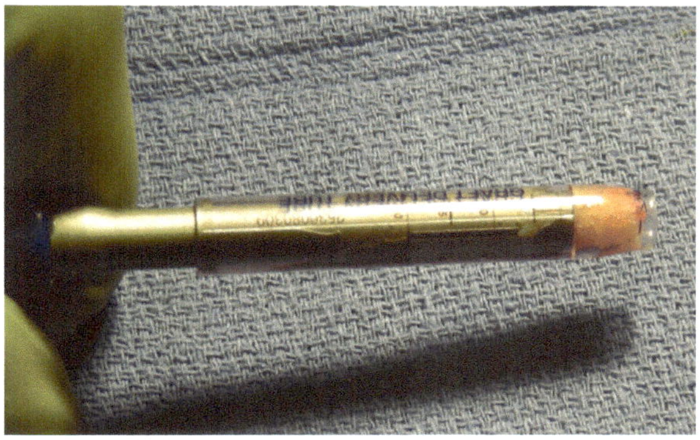

• **Fig. 7.9** The harvesting tube with the osteochondral plug ready for use.

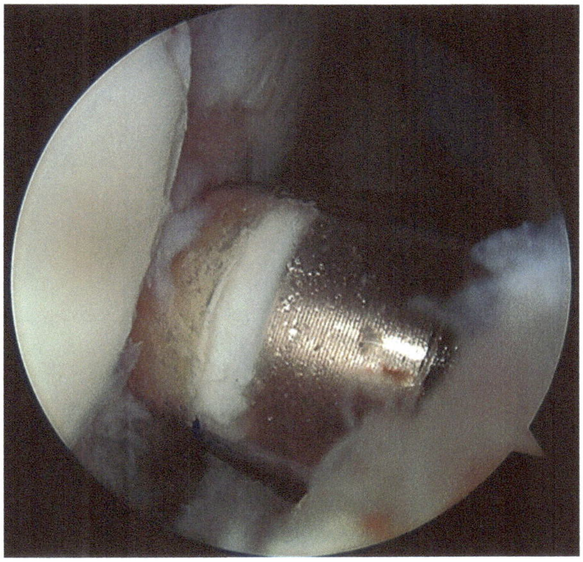

• **Fig. 7.10** Introduction of the plug into the recipient defect with gentle pressure.

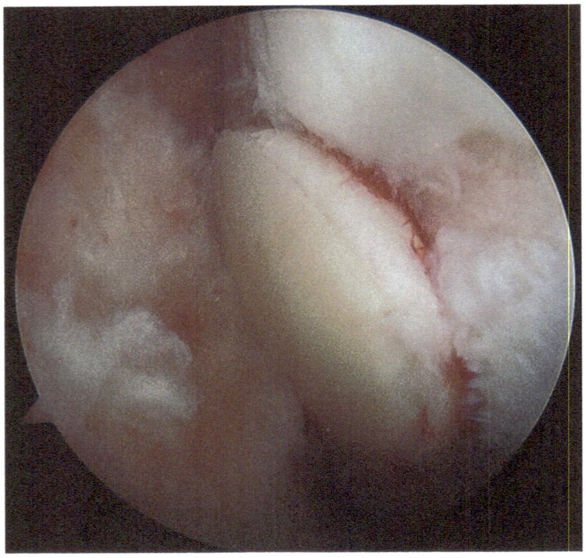

• **Fig. 7.11** Plug slightly proud prior to final seating.

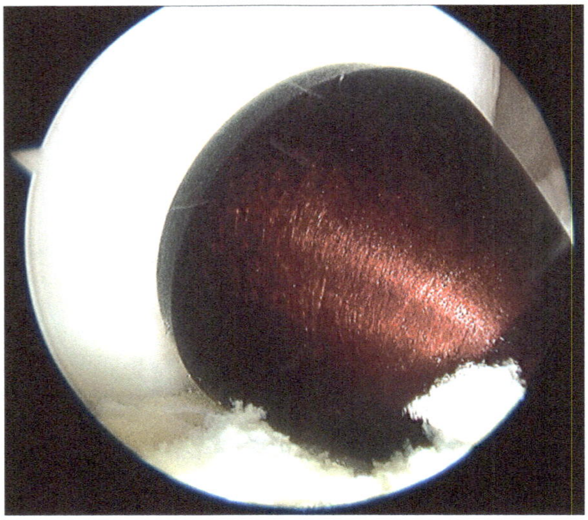

• **Fig. 7.12** Seating of the plug with the oversize tamp.

Subsequently, the harvester is removed (Fig. 7.11) and the graft fully seated and made flush by gentle pressure with an oversized tamp (Fig. 7.12). It is preferable to recess the graft slightly rather than leaving it proud to reduce contact forces. The process is then repeated until the defect is filled.

Postoperatively, patients are placed on touch-down weight-bearing restrictions for 6 weeks, but do not routinely require the use of a CPM machine because the mature hyaline cartilage was transferred. If there are concerns about postoperative stiffness, CPM can be utilized for 2 to 3 weeks as needed. Return to athletic activities is based on the size and location of the defect but should be delayed for 4 to 6 months to allow quadriceps strength and proprioception to return.

References

1. Steadman JR, Rodkey WG, Singleton SB, Briggs KK. Microfracture technique for full-thickness chondral defects: technique and clinical results. *Oper Tech Orthop.* 1997;7(4):300–304.
2. Mithoefer K, McAdams T, Williams RJ, Kreuz PC, Mandelbaum BR. Clinical efficacy of the microfracture technique for articular cartilage repair in the knee: an evidence-based systematic analysis. *Am J Sports Med.* 2009;37(10):2053–2063.
3. Kreuz PC, Steinwachs MR, Erggelet C, et al. Results after microfracture of full-thickness chondral defects in different compartments in the knee. *Osteoarthritis Cartilage.* 2006;14(11): 1119–1125.
4. Saris D, Price A, Widuchowski W, et al. Matrix-applied characterized autologous cultured chondrocytes versus microfracture: two-year follow-up of a prospective randomized trial. *Am J Sports Med.* 2014;42(6):1384–1394.
5. Brittberg M, Recker D, Ilgenfritz J, Saris DBF, Group SES. Matrix-applied characterized autologous cultured chondrocytes versus microfracture: five-year follow-up of a prospective randomized trial. *Am J Sports Med.* 2018;46(6):1343–1351.
6. Bentley G, Biant LC, Carrington RW, et al. A prospective, randomised comparison of autologous chondrocyte implantation versus mosaicplasty for osteochondral defects in the knee. *J Bone Joint Surg Br.* 2003;85(2):223–230.
7. Hunziker E, Rosenberg L. Repair of partial-thickness defects in articular cartilage: cell recruitment from the synovial membrane. *J Bone Joint Surg Am.* 1996;78-A:721–733.
8. Hunziker E. Articular cartilage repair: basic science and clinical progress. A review of the current status and prospects [comment]. *Osteoarthritis Cartilage.* 2002;10(6):432–463.
9. Nakamura N, Horibe S, Toritsuka Y, et al. The location-specific healing response of damaged articular cartilage after ACL reconstruction: short-term follow-up. *Knee Surg Sports Traumatol Arthrosc.* 2008;16(9):843–848.
10. Mithoefer K, Williams RJ, Warren RF, et al. The microfracture technique for the treatment of articular cartilage lesions in the knee. A prospective cohort study. *J Bone Joint Surg Am.* 2005;87(9):1911–1920.
11. Minas T, Gomoll AH, Roseberger R, Royce RO, Bryant T. Increased failure rate of autologous chondrocyte implantation after previous treatment with marrow stimulation techniques. *Am J Sports Med.* 2009;37(5):902–908.
12. Shive MS, Hoemann CD, Restrepo A, et al. BST-CarGel: in situ chondroinduction for cartilage repair. *Oper Tech Orthop.* 2006;16(4):271–278.
13. Shive WD, Stanish WD, McCormack R, et al. BST-CarGel® treatment maintains cartilage repair superiority over microfracture at 5 years in a multicenter randomized controlled trial. *Cartilage.* 2015;6(2):62–72.
14. Stanish MS, McCormack R, Forriol F, et al. Novel scaffold-based BST-CarGel treatment results in superior cartilage repair compared with microfracture in a randomized controlled trial. *J Bone Joint Surg Am.* 2013;95(18):1640–1650.
15. Schreiner MM, Raudner M, Szomolanyi P, et al. Chondral and osteochondral femoral cartilage lesions treated with GelrinC: significant improvement of radiological outcome over time and zonal variation of the repair tissue based on T_2 mapping at 24 months. *Cartilage.* 2020;1947603520926702.
16. Brusalis CM, Greditzer HG IV, Fabricant PD, Stannard JP, Cook JL. BioCartilage augmentation of marrow stimulation procedures for cartilage defects of the knee: two-year clinical outcomes. *Knee.* 2020;27(5):1418–1425.

8

Use of Fresh Osteochondral Allograft for Chondral and Osteochondral Defects in the Knee

TOM MINAS, MD, MS

CHAPTER OUTLINE

Introduction

Fresh osteochondral allografts are composite grafts consisting of a living mature hyaline cartilage portion anchored to a nonliving subchondral bone portion, forming an intact osteochondral functional unit that replaces a damaged corresponding tissue in the recipient joint.

Increasing demand for allografts has been met with advancements in tissue procurement and increased availability of fresh donor tissue from commercial entities as opposed to university-based specialized transplantation centers, which in the past had limited availability to orthopedists in the community.[1–3]

The advantage of fresh osteochondral allografting is the transplantation of mature hyaline cartilage with viable chondrocytes,[4] which survive hypothermic storage and transplantation while maintaining their metabolic activity and sustaining the surrounding collagen matrix.[5] Investigations have focused on extending the storage interval of fresh human osteochondral allograft tissue. Ball et al.[6] compared the effects of different storage media on human osteochondral allograft tissue when stored hypothermically in either lactated Ringer's solution or a standard culture media containing amino acids, glucose, and inorganic salts. The standard culture media demonstrated superior storage properties as measured by chondrocyte density, viability, and metabolic activity. Biomechanical properties of the matrix remained relatively intact in both media. Chondrocyte viability essentially remained unchanged from baseline for up to 14 days in the standard media, at which time viability was 90.5% in standard media versus 80% in lactated Ringer's solution.

Graft Procurement and Storage

Availability of suitable graft tissue remains the limiting factor. Fresh osteochondral allografting is associated with inherent challenges related to tissue recovery, storage, and timely delivery for treatment.

Recovery, processing, and testing of donor tissue follow guidelines established by the American Association of Tissue Banks (AATB)[7,8] and is under the authority of the US Food and Drug Administration (FDA).[9] Most tissue banks have a 24-hour time limit for retrieval of tissue from refrigerated cadaveric donors in a sterile operating room environment following strict sterile technique. Donors between the ages of 15 and 40 years are generally considered for inclusion in the donor pool if their articular surfaces pass direct inspection for cartilage quality.

It is the policy of tissue banks to hold transplants for a minimum of 14 days to allow completion of microbiologic and serologic testing prior to release. Hence the actual surgical implantation is delayed by 3 to 6 weeks after procurement compared with university center clinical practice of implanting allografts usually within 1 week of harvest. Although results using this traditional fresh tissue protocol have been good even in mid-term follow-up,[10] the effects of prolonged allograft storage on clinical outcomes have not yet been determined.

Use of fresh-frozen grafts improves graft availability, reduces immunogenicity, and may be appropriate for bulk allografting in major osseous reconstruction as encountered in musculoskeletal tumor cases. However, deep freezing of chondrocytes within their extracellular matrix (usually at −80°C) practically eliminates all viable chondrocytes in the articular cartilage portion of osteochondral grafts. Furthermore, clinical experience indicates that the articular matrix in frozen allografts deteriorates over time, presumably because insufficient surviving cells are present within the matrix to maintain tissue equilibrium.[11,12] However, retrieval studies have demonstrated that with fresh, cold-stored osteochondral allografts, viable chondrocytes are present and mechanical properties of the matrix are maintained many years after transplantation.[13,14]

Safety and Risk of Disease Transmission

Osteochondral allografts are aseptically procured, which reduces but does not eliminate the risk of graft contamination during recovery via postmortem invasion by gastrointestinal flora or occult infection in the donor. Any transplantation of allogeneic organs or tissue is associated with a residual risk of transmission of infectious disease, despite donor screening and testing, and rare allograft-associated bacterial infections have been reported. Advances in serologic testing for human immunodeficiency virus, hepatitis, and other diseases have improved safety, but a measurable risk remains. The surgeon and the patient should be well aware of the possibility of risk of transmission of serious diseases when fresh allograft tissue is used, making the discussion of the risk of bacterial or viral disease transmission part of the informed consent.[15]

Immunology

Small-fragment allografts are not human leukocyte antigen (HLA) or blood-type matched between the donor and recipient. Although hyaline cartilage appears to be relatively immunoprivileged,[16] fresh unmatched osteochondral allografts elicited a variable immune response in one study of fresh osteochondral allografts, and 50% of individuals generated serum anti-HLA antibodies.[17] The presence of anti-HLA antibodies correlated with an inferior appearance of the graft–host interface on magnetic resonance imaging (MRI) studies. Poor MRI incorporation has also been correlated with inferior clinical results[10] and may be a result of immunologic mechanisms. The issue of immune behavior may ultimately become clinically relevant and it is clearly an area where more knowledge is necessary to improve outcomes of the use of fresh osteochondral allografts.

Indications

As per other cartilage repair procedures, successful reconstruction is dependent upon careful evaluation of background factors and their treatment at the time of or prior to fresh osteochondral allografting. These factors include tibial femoral and patellofemoral malalignment, joint stability, and meniscal deficiency.

Specific conditions that are most amenable to allografting in clinical practice include osteochondritis dissecans,[18] osteonecrosis,[19,20] and posttraumatic defects, such as those occurring after periarticular fractures around the knee.[21] A particularly troublesome condition to manage is posttraumatic tibial plateau fracture, which is especially suitable to management by fresh osteochondral allograft.[22] Allografts have also proved valuable for the salvage of knees for which other cartilage resurfacing procedures, such as microfracture, autologous chondrocyte implantation (ACI), and transfer of autologous osteochondral plugs, have been unsuccessful.

Contraindications include inflammatory arthritis, chondrocalcinosis involving the cartilage articular surface, generalized osteoarthrosis of the joint, patients who are obese or noncompliant with postoperative rehabilitation, and those who are smokers or narcotic-dependent.

Common to all allografting procedures is matching donor with recipient on the basis of size.[23] In the knee, an anteroposterior radiograph with a standardized magnification marker is used and the mediolateral dimension of the tibia, just below and parallel to the joint surface, is measured. The measurement is accurately adjusted for magnification and the tissue bank makes a direct measurement on the donor tibial plateau. Alternatively, a measurement of the affected condyle can be performed. A match is considered acceptable within 2 mm.

Surgical Techniques

Surgical transplantation of a fresh osteochondral allograft requires a medial or lateral arthrotomy. Occasional meniscal takedown for very posterior lesions with possible patellar eversion may be necessary. The lesion then is inspected and palpated with a probe to determine its extent, margins, and maximum size. Two techniques commonly used for preparation and implantation of osteochondral allografts are the press-fit plug (dowel) technique (Fig. 8.1) and the shell graft technique (Fig. 8.2). Each technique has advantages and disadvantages. The press-fit plug technique is similar in principle to autologous osteochondral transfer systems. It is optimal for contained condylar lesions between 15 and 35 mm in diameter. Fixation is generally not required because of the stability achieved with the press fit. Disadvantages include the fact that many lesions, such as very posterior femoral, tibial, patellar, and trochlear lesions, are not accessible to a circular coring system. In addition, the more ovoid the lesion, the more normal cartilage must be sacrificed at the recipient site in order to accommodate a circular donor plug. Shell grafts are technically more difficult to perform and typically require fixation. However, depending on the technique used, less normal cartilage may need to be sacrificed. Also, certain lesions are more amenable to shell allografts because of their location.

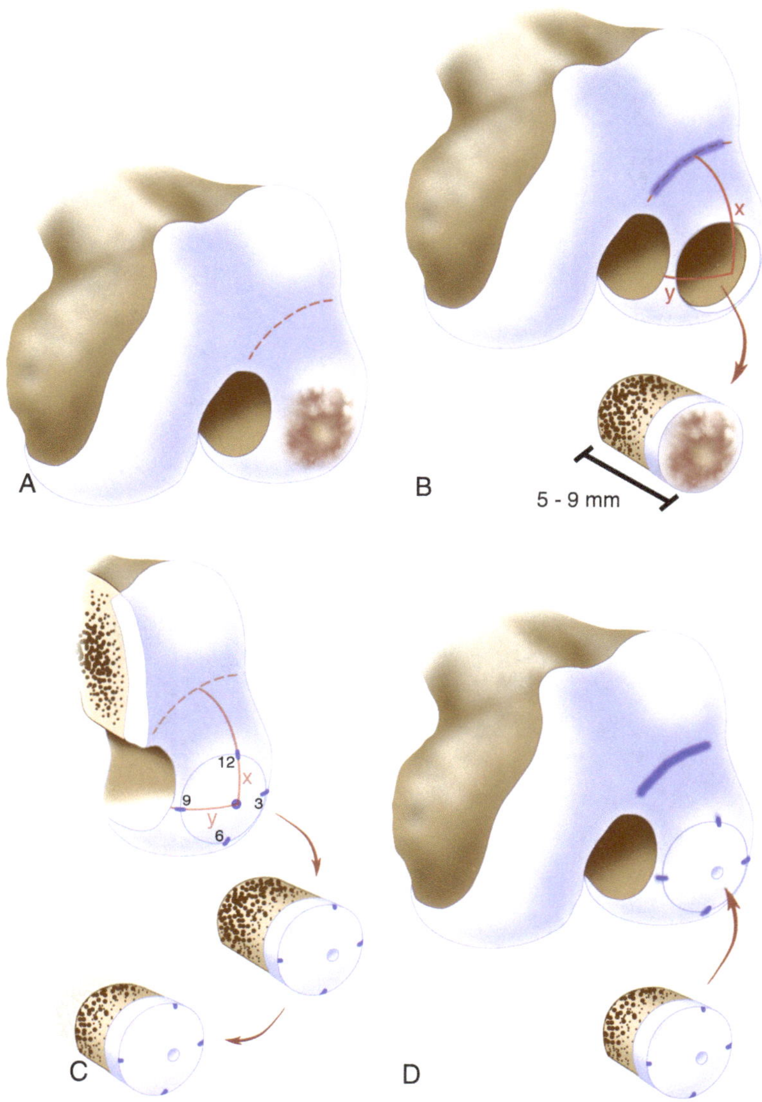

• **Fig. 8.1** Diagrammatic representation of modern-day osteochondral allograft procedure by the dowel technique. (A) Large focal chondral defect on the medial femoral condyle and its position relative to the sulcus terminalis (leading weight-bearing surface in full extension of the medial or lateral femoral condyles) is identified. (B) Chondral defect is sized and removed as an osteochondral dowel for a total depth, including cartilage, of 5 to 9 mm. The position of the osteochondral defect is measured and referenced relative to the sulcus terminalis and the intercondylar notch in order to harvest a similar healthy osteochondral dowel from the donor allograft tissue. A donor osteochondral dowel will be oversized by 1 mm to provide a press fit at the time of implantation. Some systems require the recipient site to be conically dilated to allow ease of implantation, press fit, and no need for internal fixation. (C) The donor osteochondral dowel is harvested relative to the position of the sulcus terminalis and intercondylar notch for its central coring reamer guidewire. The orientation of the dowel is marked with a sterile marking pen at the four quadrants of 12, 3, 6, and 9 o'clock to facilitate accurate placement at the recipient socket. The larger the diameter of the donor dowel, the more important it is to ensure that the quadrant marking depths are absolutely precise in order to have a flush transplant that is neither proud nor recessed below the articular surface. (D) The deep surface of the donor dowel is measured and cut to depth precisely at all four quadrants. The recipient socket is usually dilated with a conical dilator prior to a press fit of the donor osteochondral allograft dowel. Implantation is performed with hand pressure or a gel-covered impaction device so as not to injure the fresh preserved cartilage cap.

Several proprietary instrumentation systems are available for the preparation and implantation of press-fit dowel allografts up to 35 mm in diameter. Currently this technique is the most commonly used. The lesion is identified, the proposed graft is outlined, and a template is made using sizing dowels. After size determination has been made, a guidewire is driven into the center of the lesion, perpendicular to the curvature of the articular surface. If more than one dowel is required to treat the defect, one proximal to the other, a "snowman" technique can be used or a cut can be made into the graft to maximize the treated surface. The remaining articular cartilage is scored and a core reamer is used to remove that piece of cartilage and at least 3 to 4 mm of subchondral bone. When a patient has a deeper lesion, fibrous and sclerotic bone is removed up to a healthy, bleeding osseous base. When a lesion is very deep, coring should not exceed 10 mm in depth and packed morselized autologous bone graft should be used to fill any

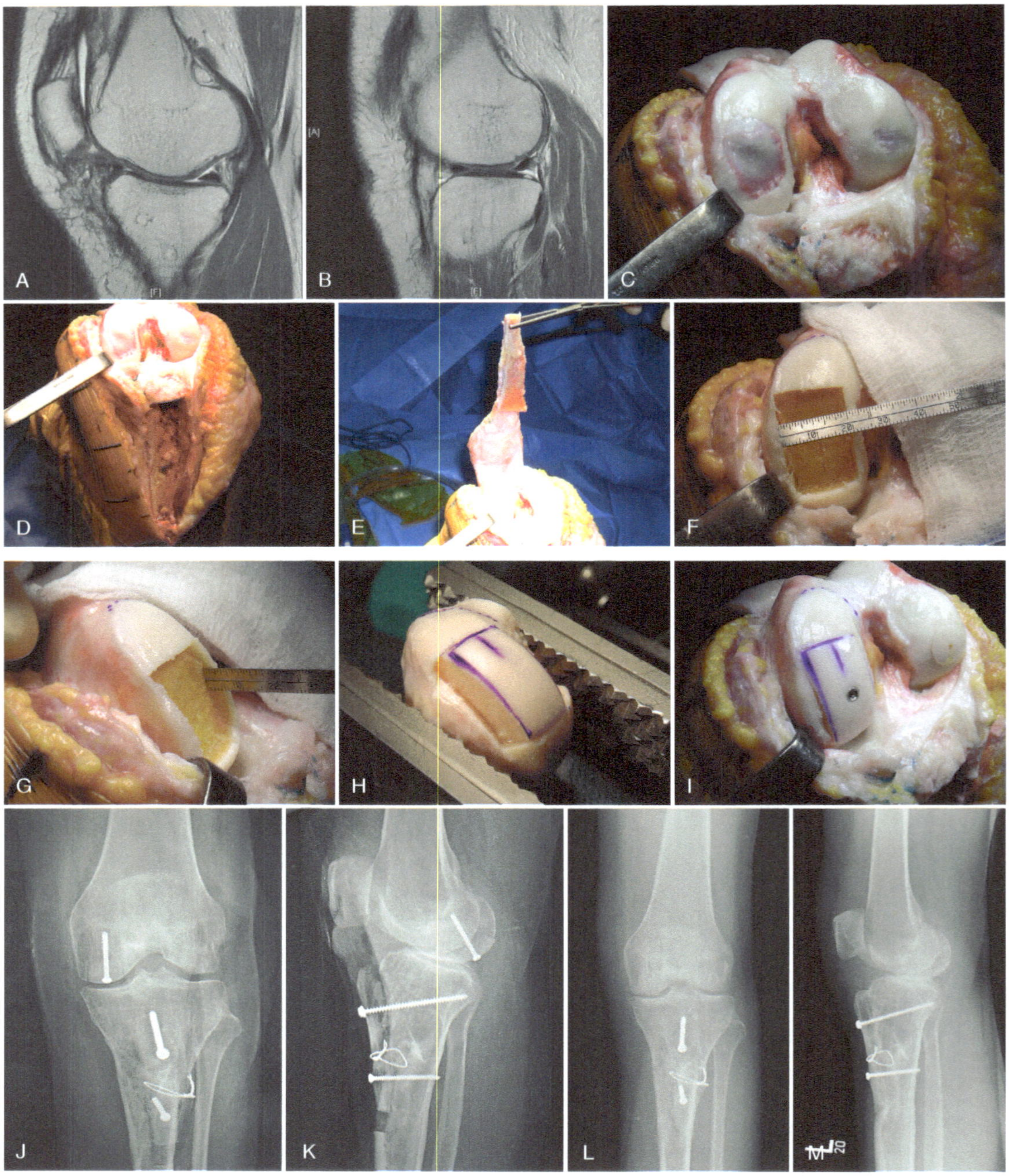

• **Fig. 8.2** A young woman in her late 20s sustained a severe tibial plateau fracture to the left knee when she was kicked by a horse. Open reduction internal fixation was performed and the fracture went on to union. However, the patient was left with disabling, medially based pain following a large articular injury to the medial femoral condyle. The patient developed patella infera with limited range of motion of the knee after the fracture. This was treated by autologous chondrocyte implantation (ACI) to medial femoral and lateral femoral condyles with lysis of adhesions by open technique. Despite early improved motion, she developed recurrent stiffness and continued weight-bearing pain. Her patella infera worsened. This case demonstrates the use of fresh shell osteoarticular allograft with an inlay technique to the medial femoral condyle and a dowel technique to the lateral femoral condyle as well as proximalization of the extensor mechanism with an extended tibial tubercle osteotomy. (A) Sagittal magnetic resonance imaging (MRI) scan demonstrates patella infera, flattening of posterior medial femoral condyles at ACI transplant site, and old screw holes in the proximal tibia from the previous fracture. (B) Sagittal MRI scan demonstrates a small lateral femoral condyle at ACI transplant site that is also somewhat flattened and incompletely filled. (C) Open appearance of left knee with large medial femoral condyle and small lateral femoral condyle incompletely filled at ACI graft sites. Extended tibial tubercle osteotomy is performed to provide excellent exposure and allow proximalization of extensor mechanism to restore motion. (D) Proximal tibia appearance after extended tibial tubercle osteotomy. (E) Tibial tubercle osteotomy with medial and lateral subvastus arthrotomies maintaining quadriceps mechanism intact. (F) Preparation of recipient bed on patient's medial femoral condyle to accept a fresh shell osteochondral allograft. (G) Exact measurements that include length, width, and depth are necessary. (H) Preparation of shell allograft on back table. (I) Final appearance of medial femoral condyle shell allograft after fixation with cannulated screw (buried screwhead). Lateral femoral condyle restoration with a dowel technique fresh osteochondral allograft. (J) Anteroposterior radiograph after allograft implantation and proximalization of tibial tubercle osteotomy. (K) Immediate postoperative lateral radiograph. (L and M) Four-year postoperative radiographs demonstrate maintenance of joint space after allograft transplantation and proper patella height. The patient has maintained full range of motion of the knee, no extensor lag, good quadriceps strength, and pain-free function.

deeper or more extensive osseous defects. The guidewire is then removed and circumferential depth measurements of the prepared recipient site are made so that the donor can be matched exactly.

The corresponding anatomic location of the recipient site is then identified on the graft, which is placed into a graft holder or is held with bone-holding forceps. A saw guide is placed in the appropriate position, again perpendicular to the articular surface, and an appropriately sized tube saw is used to core out the graft. Before the graft is removed from the condyle, an identifying mark is made to ensure proper orientation. Once the graft has been removed, the depth measurements determined from the recipient are transferred to the graft. This graft is then cut with an oscillating saw and trimmed with a rasp to the appropriate thickness in all four quadrants. The donor is then copiously pulse lavaged with bacitracin and saline to remove marrow elements from the donor. The donor is orientated appropriately and gently press-fit so that it is flush to the host articular surface. Fig. 8.3 shows the technique for a failed ACI procedure left in mechanical varus that requires fresh osteoarticular allograft with high tibial valgus-producing osteotomy. Fig. 8.4 shows the technique for a patient with osteonecrosis.

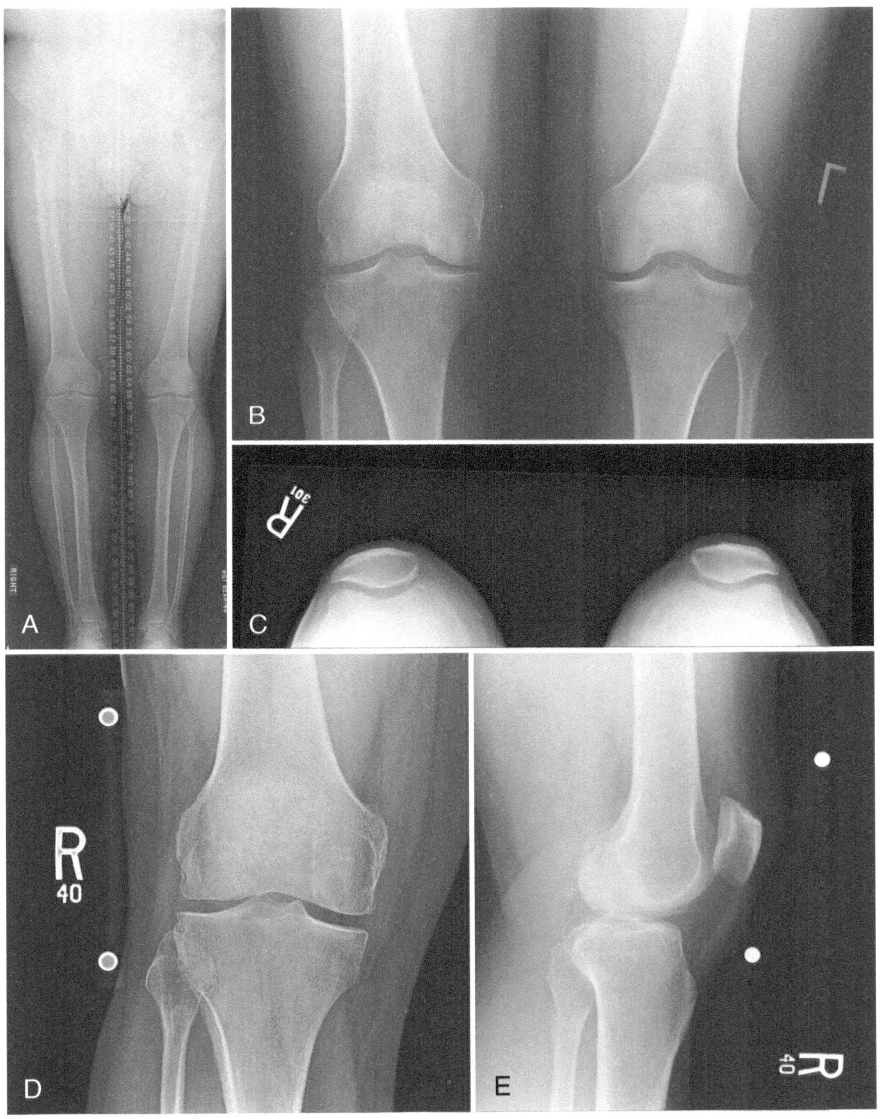

• **Fig. 8.3** Case of a 42-year-old man who has failed autologous chondrocyte implantation (ACI) to the medial femoral condyles in a knee that remains in mechanical varus. Arthroscopic evaluation of the knee demonstrated a failed fibrous repair tissue. The decision was made to treat the defects (medial femoral condyles and trochlea) and to find an alternative cartilage repair technique that did not require cellular repair (i.e., fresh osteoarticular allograft with correction of mechanical overload). (A) Long alignment radiographs demonstrate mechanical varus alignment of the right knee. (B) Flexed 45-degree posteroanterior Rosenberg views demonstrate a characteristic medial femoral condyle lesion of osteochondritis dissecans. (C) Skyline radiographs demonstrate well-preserved patellofemoral articulations. (D) In preparation for fresh osteoarticular allograft, magnification markers for radiographic sizing are performed. A 10-cm radiographic marker is noted on anteroposterior (AP) x-ray film. (E) The same procedure is performed on a lateral radiograph. The radiographic marker is measured, as are the AP and lateral dimensions of the tibia. In this way, a size match for a fresh osteoarticular allograft within 2 mm may be found.

Continued

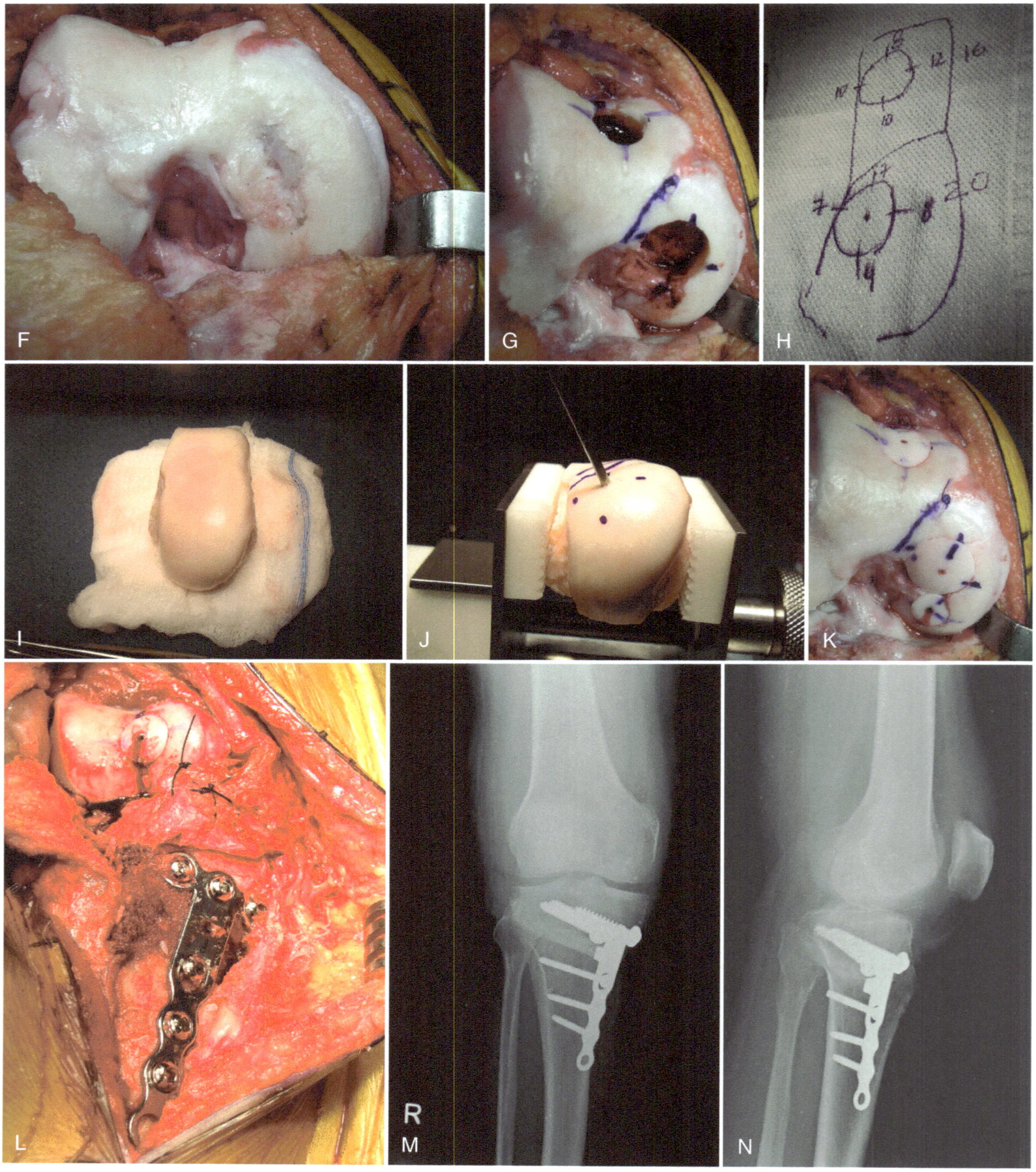

• **Fig. 8.3 Cont'd** (F) Open appearance of the failed ACI to the medial femoral condyle and trochlea. (G) Sulcus terminalis of the medial femoral condyle is marked in terminal extension with a purple marking pen shown. Circular reamers are used over a guidewire perpendicular to the articular surface to ream out the articular defects until healthy subchondral bone is noted, which is usually a total depth of 5 to 9 mm from the articular surface. Markings are then used at all four quadrants of each defect. (H) The depth of the defects are measured and noted. (I) Fresh size-matched medial femoral condyle osteoarticular allograft is taken out of its preservative. The sulcus terminalis is noted, as is the top of the intercondylar notch. (J) The central guidewire is positioned identically to the patient's defects and a coring reamer 1 mm larger than the recipient site is used. Once the osteochondral dowel is extracted from the donor allograft, the quadrant depths at all four positions are measured on the allograft and cut precisely over a clamp. The recipient site is dilated 1 mm and a donor allograft is carefully hand-fit and pressed flush with the articular surface using a gel-covered impaction device. (K) In this case, a second smaller, more posterior dowel is added to cover the defect entirely, frequently resembling a snowman (i.e., the "snowman" technique). (L) Opening wedge tibial valgus-producing osteotomy to normalize the mechanical axis to the center of the knee is performed simultaneously with the osteochondral allografts to the medial femoral condyles and trochlea. This is performed through a single midline incision. (M and N) AP and lateral radiographs, respectively, 1 year postoperatively demonstrate well-preserved tibiofemoral and patellofemoral joint spaces with neutral mechanical alignment. The patient's painful mechanical and weight-bearing symptoms are completely resolved.

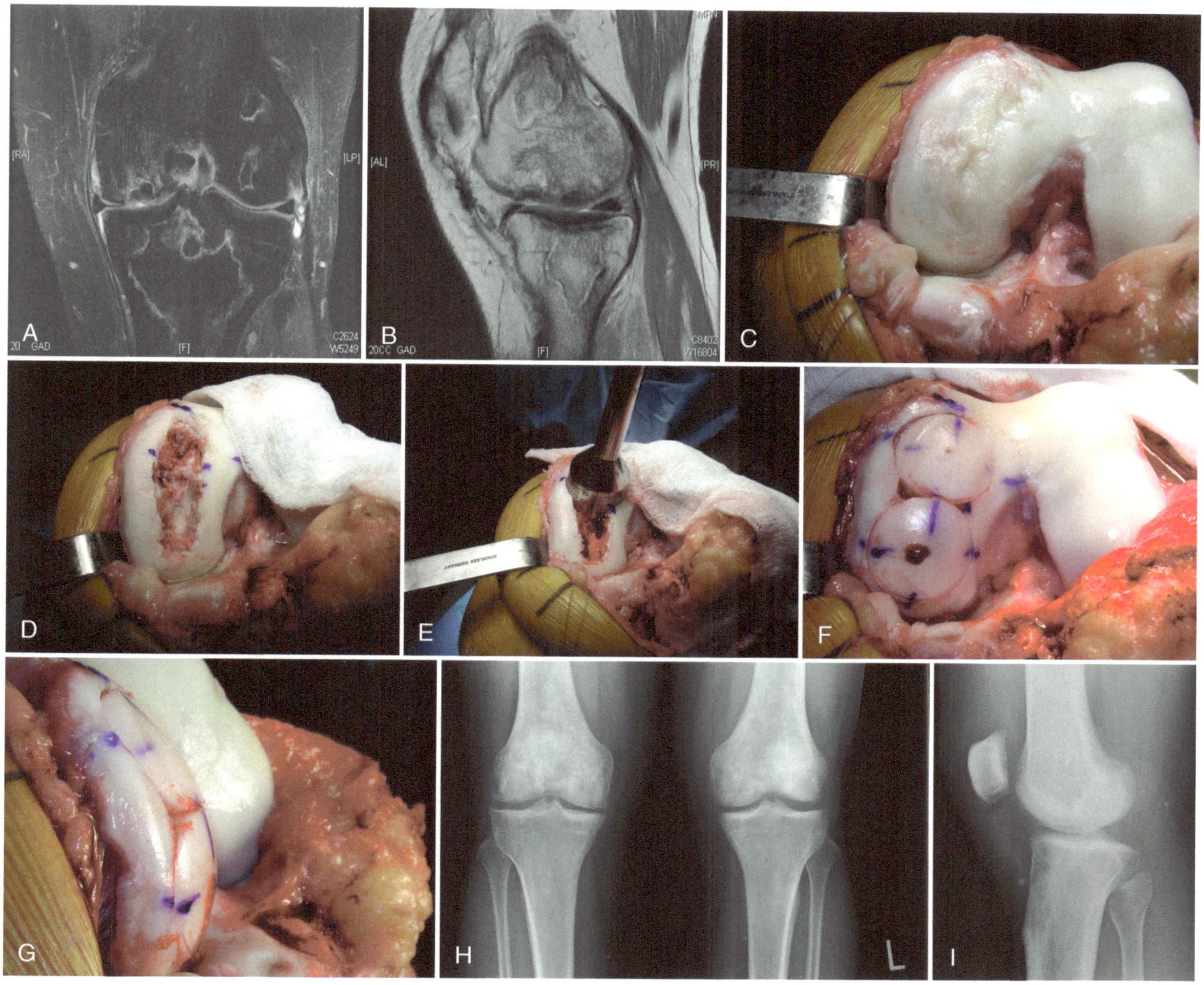

• **Fig. 8.4** Case of a 27-year-old man who had taken steroids in the past for ulcerative colitis. He has developed disabling bilateral knee pain. Magnetic resonance imaging (MRI) scan demonstrates multifocal areas of avascular necrosis in the left knee. The right knee had been treated with fresh osteoarticular allografts 2 years earlier, with excellent clinical results. The left knee is now severely painful, predominately in the medial compartment of the joint. (A) Coronal fat-suppressed MRI scan demonstrates resorption and collapse of the medial femoral condyle. In addition, avascular segments that are nonarticular in the tibia and lateral femoral condyle are present. (B) Sagittal MRI scan demonstrates resorption and collapse of the medial femoral condyle. However, the tibial articular surface and meniscus are intact. This is an appropriate case for cartilage repair by osteoarticular allograft. (C) Open appearance of medial femoral condyle at the time of arthrotomy. (D) Articular surface is easily debrided off the medial femoral condyles because the underlying bone has resorbed and collapsed. (E) Dilator is applied and impacted after coring reamer size is determined to facilitate donor graft placement. (F) Frontal appearance after placement of two fresh osteoarticular grafts in a "snowman" configuration. (G) Side profile demonstrates a sagittal curvature of the medial femoral condyles is maintained by appropriate orthogonal placement of the dowel grafts and reaming. (H and I) AP and lateral radiographs, respectively, 1 year after fresh osteoarticular allograft to the left knee, with excellent preservation of joint space and absence of symptoms for the patient.

The troublesome condition of posttraumatic collapse of the lateral tibial plateau with valgus deformity is ideally treated with fresh osteochondral allograft. My preference is to incorporate the meniscus with the allograft osteoarticular surface because its quality and its integration to the tibial plateau are perfect. The important thing to recognize after obtaining a perfect size match is that the valgus deformity cannot be corrected by the tibial plateau "stuffing the joint." This inevitably leads to premature wear and collapse of the allograft. A staged femoral osteotomy with tibial plateau allograft or simultaneous procedure, which is my preference, is appropriate. I have used an external tibial alignment guide, which is used for total knee replacement surgery, to make my sagittal and axial bone cuts to remove the damaged proximal lateral tibial plateau, leaving a perfect recipient site for the fresh osteoarticular allograft. The posterior capsule is dissected out first in preparation for passage of sutures through the capsule to anchor the posterior horn of the lateral meniscus. The anterolateral arthrotomy takes down the capsule from the diseased proximal lateral tibial plateau to the posterior lateral corner at the level of the popliteus tendon. The donor allograft is measured to

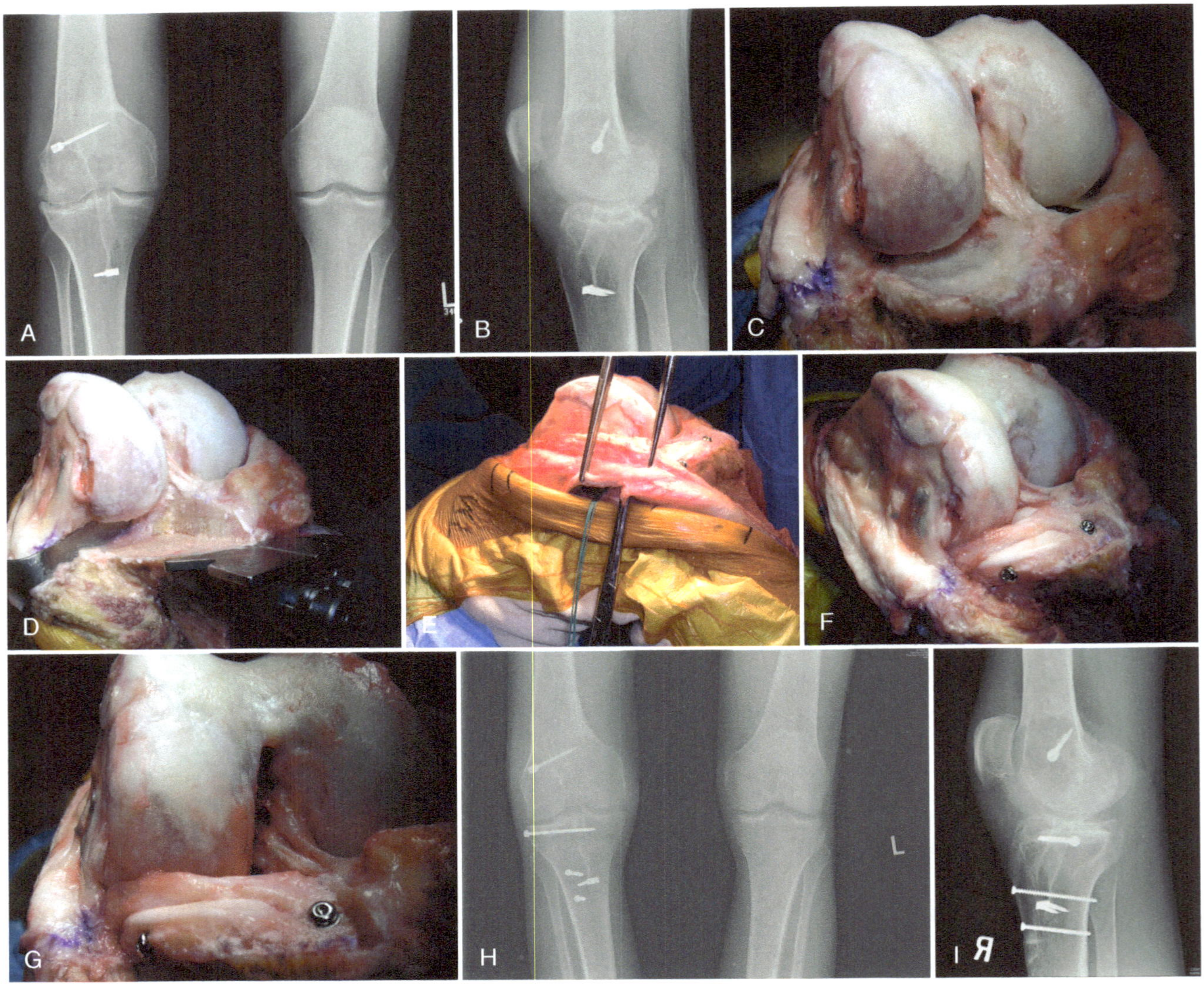

• **Fig. 8.5** Case of a 21-year-old man who sustained a lateral tibial plateau fracture with collapse and valgus deformity. It was treated by varus femoral osteotomy and debridement of the lateral tibial plateau. The patient has persistent lateral-based pain and requires the use of narcotics and single crutch ambulation in order to get around. At the time of arthroscopic assessment, grade 4 changes throughout the lateral tibial plateau and an absent meniscus were noted. The lateral femoral condyle was intact. The plan was to perform a fresh combined osteoarticular and meniscal allograft transplantation. Because of delay in approval of the transplantation and graft match availability, at the time of open transplantation, grade 4 changes to the lateral femoral condyle had also developed. The lateral tibial plateau and meniscus were transplanted, followed 3 months later by transplantation to the lateral femoral condyle by autologous chondrocyte implantation (ACI). (A) Anteroposterior (AP) radiograph demonstrates widening and irregularity, with early joint space narrowing and collapse of the lateral tibial plateau. (B) Lateral radiograph demonstrates lateral tibial plateau depression. (C) Tibial tubercle osteotomy and lateral subvastus exposure to the lateral compartment demonstrates depressed and widened lateral tibial plateau with grade 4 changes now evident on the lateral femoral condyle. (D) External tibial alignment guide used for a total knee replacement for resection of damaged lateral tibial plateau. (E) Posterior aspect of the knee has been dissected through the anterior flap for suture passage of the posterior horn of the lateral meniscal allograft through the capsule, deep to the lateral head of the gastrocnemius muscle. (F) Side view of lateral tibial plateau with internal fixation. (G) Frontal view. (H and I) AP and lateral radiographs, respectively, 1 year after reconstruction with lateral tibial plateau and meniscal allograft transplantation combined with ACI to the lateral femoral condyle. The arthritic lateral compartment has been salvaged in this young man in his early 20s. The patient has pain-free function with activities of daily living.

the recipient prepared bed, cut slightly oversized, and then trimmed as needed until a perfect fit is obtained. Fixation is generally achieved with just one or two lag screws to apply compression to the allograft, with large cancellous bony surfaces ensuring rapid osseous union (Fig. 8.5). The bony thickness of the lateral tibial plateau should be the minimal amount to allow osseous union and creeping substitution without resorption and collapse of the allograft. From 5 to 10 mm of bone is usually adequate in addition to the 4 or 5 mm of cartilage that is present on the lateral tibial plateau surface.

A new technique of transplantation of allograft articular cartilage has been devised. Fig. 8.6 illustrates the case of a young woman with advanced patellofemoral articular cartilage loss with maltracking. Minced juvenile human articular cartilage, when placed in a well-prepared articular chondral defect as per ACI, may repair the defect through migration of the juvenile chondrocytes out of the matrix into the recipient

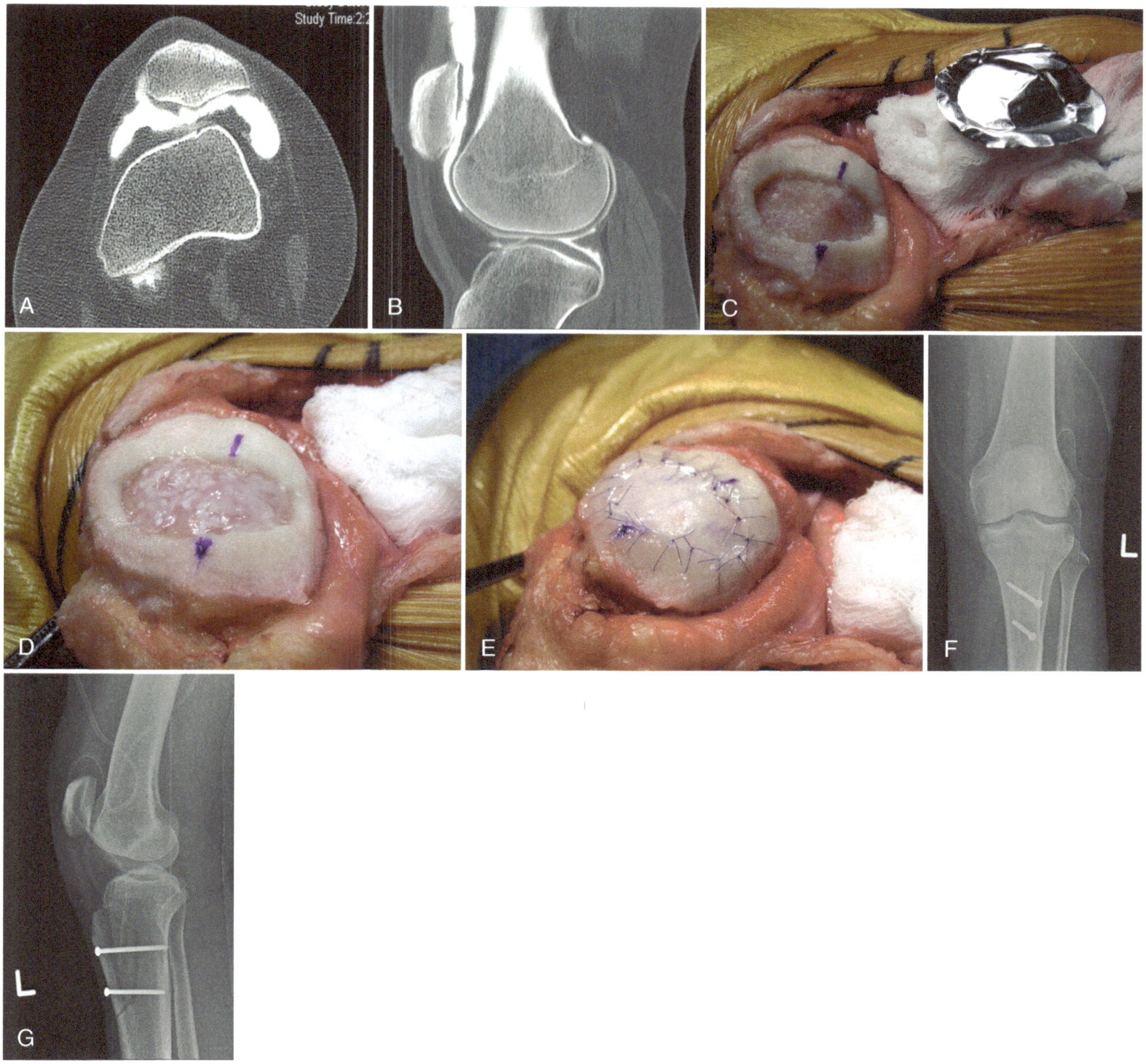

• **Fig. 8.6** Case of a 40-year-old woman with chronic patellofemoral instability, crepitus, and knee pain. She is treated with morselized juvenile articular cartilage reconstruction of the patella with realignment tibial tubercle osteotomy. (A) Axial computed tomographic (CT) arthrogram demonstrates patellar subluxation and near-pan patellar cartilage loss across the median ridge. (B) Sagittal CT arthrogram demonstrates loss of articular cartilage to the patella on the distal half of the patellar surface. (C) Open appearance of the patella after radical debridement of damaged articular cartilage. (D) Using an aluminum template of the defect, the white allogeneic morselized juvenile articular cartilage fragments are evenly spread out and admixed with fibrin glue sealant. The entire slurry is then placed into the chondral defect and a type I–III collagen membrane is sutured overtop the injured region. (E) Final appearance of transplanted morselized juvenile allograft cartilage. (F and G) AP and lateral radiographs after transplantation with tibial tubercle osteotomy.

bed, forming a chondral repair. This technology is new and represents a new paradigm of treatment. Equine research has demonstrated that this technique is effective even with xenograft species transplants. Human adolescent cartilage transplanted into horse chondral defects has demonstrated effective repair tissue originating from the human cartilage transplant. Unfortunately, the data are not yet published. Clinical human transplants at this time are demonstrating efficacy (see Chapter 16).

Results and Conclusions

Fresh osteochondral allografts demonstrate results similar to those of ACI in the short to midterm. When allografts fail, they do so by the process of incomplete incorporation of the osseous segment of the allograft or by creeping substitution with resorption and collapse of the allograft. For this reason, it is my opinion that when defects are large, it is prudent to treat surface defects that are truly isolated articular injuries by a surface repair with ACI. It is best to reserve osteoarticular allograft for failed ACI treatments or for their ideal indications of osteochondral defects, such as osteochondritis dissecans, osteonecrosis, posttraumatic osteochondral defects, and peripheral uncontained defects.

Gross et al.[21] reported Kaplan-Meier survivorship scores of 95% at 5 years and 85% at 10 years for femoral allografts. When the defects failed, it was a result of resorption and collapse necessitating prosthetic reconstruction. The graft survivorship observed by Williams et al.[10] (84% at 4 years) was lower than that reported by Gross et al. at mid-term follow-up with cold-stored commercial allografts. Nevertheless, allografts provide an excellent treatment option for osteochondral deficient lesions, which represent the ideal indication for allograft use to preserve the joint.

References

1. Gross AE, Silverstein EA, Falk J, Falk R, Langer F. The allotransplantation of partial joints in the treatment of osteoarthritis of the knee. *Clin Orthop Relat Res.* 1975;108:7–14.
2. Gross AE, McKee NH, Pritzker KP, Langer F. Reconstruction of skeletal deficits at the knee. A comprehensive osteochondral transplant program. *Clin Orthop Relat Res.* 1983;174:96–106.
3. Convery FR, Meyers MH, Akeson WH. Fresh osteochondral allografting of the femoral condyle. *Clin Orthop Relat Res.* 1991;273:139–145.
4. Czitrom AA, Keating S, Gross AE. The viability of articular cartilage in fresh osteochondral allografts after clinical transplantation. *J Bone Joint Surg Am.* 1990;72:574–581.
5. Williams SK, Amiel D, Ball ST, et al. Prolonged storage effects on the articular cartilage of fresh human osteochondral allografts. *J Bone Joint Surg Am.* 2003;85:2111–2120.
6. Ball ST, Amiel D, Williams SK, et al. The effects of storage on fresh human osteochondral allografts. *Clin Orthop Relat Res.* 2004;418:246–252.
7. *Standards for tissue banking.* Arlington, VA: American Association of Tissue Banks; 1987.
8. American Association of Tissue Banks. *Standards for Tissue Banking.* Updated November 4, 2003. Available from: http://www.aatb.org/standards-and-regulatory.
9. US Food and Drug Administration. Guidance for industry: screening and testing of donors of human tissues intended for transplantation. Available from: http://www.fda.gov/BiologicsBloodVaccines/TissueTissueProducts/Regulation-ofTissues/ucm1
10. Williams RJ, Ranawat AS, Potter HS, Carter T, Warren RF. Fresh stored allografts for the treatment of osteochondral defects of the knee. *J Bone Joint Surg Am.* 2007;89(4):718–726.
11. Ohlendorf C, Tomford WW, Mankin HJ. Chondrocyte survival in cryopreserved osteochondral articular cartilage. *J Orthop Res.* 1996;143:413–416.
12. Enneking WF, Campanacci DA. Retrieved human allografts: a clinicopathological study. *J Bone Joint Surg Am.* 2001;83:971–986.
13. McGoveran BM, Pritzker KP, Shasha N, Price J, Gross AE. Long-term chondrocyte viability in a fresh osteochondral allograft. *J Knee Surg.* 2002;15:97–100.
14. Convery FR, Akeson WH, Amiel D, Meyers MH, Monosov A. Long-term survival of chondrocytes in an osteochondral articular cartilage allograft. A case report. *J Bone Joint Surg Am.* 1996;78:1082–1088.
15. Friedlaender GE. Appropriate screening for prevention of infection transmission by musculoskeletal allografts. *Instr Course Lect.* 2000;49:615–619.
16. Langer F, Gross AE, West M, Urovitz EP. The immunogenicity of allograft knee joint transplants. *Clin Orthop Relat Res.* 1978;132:155–162.
17. Sirlin CB, Brossmann J, Boutin RD, et al. Shell osteochondral allografts of the knee: comparison of MR imaging findings and immunologic responses. *Radiology.* 2001;219:35–43.
18. Garrett JC. Fresh osteochondral allografts for treatment of articular defects in osteochondritis dissecans of the lateral femoral condyle in adults. *Clin Orthop Relat Res.* 1994;303:33–37.
19. Bugbee W, Khadavi B. *Fresh osteochondral allografting in the treatment of osteonecrosis of the knee.* Presented at: American Academy of Orthopaedic Surgeons 71st Annual Meeting; March 10–14. San Francisco, CA; 2004.
20. Gortz S, Bugbee WD. Allografts in articular cartilage repair. *J Bone Joint Surg Am.* 2006;88(6):1374–1384.
21. Gross AE, Shasha N, Aubin P. Long-term followup of the use of fresh osteochondral allografts for posttraumatic knee defects. *Clin Orthop Relat Res.* 2005;435:79–87.
22. Locht RC, Gross AE, Langer F. Late osteochondral allograft resurfacing for tibial plateau fractures. *J Bone Joint Surg Am.* 1984;66:328–335.
23. Highgenboten CL, Jackson A, Aschliman M, Meske NB. The estimation of femoral condyle size. An important component in osteochondral allografts. *Clin Orthop Relat Res.* 1989;246:225–233.

9 Autologous Chondrocyte Implantation

TOM MINAS, MD, MS

CHAPTER OUTLINE

Introduction

Historical Perspective

Autologous chondrocyte transplantation (ACT) has been known as autologous chondrocyte implantation (ACI) in North America. The technique as described by Peterson and co-workers[1] was adapted by me after several visits to Sweden in the early 1990s (Fig. 9.1). Since March 1995 after institutional review board approval in 1994, the technique of ACI was used to manage large acute and chronic focal articular cartilage injuries in knees. To date, over 1,000 treatments have been performed at our institution as of 2010, over 30,000 patients have been treated in North America with ACI. The exact number of ACI transplantations worldwide

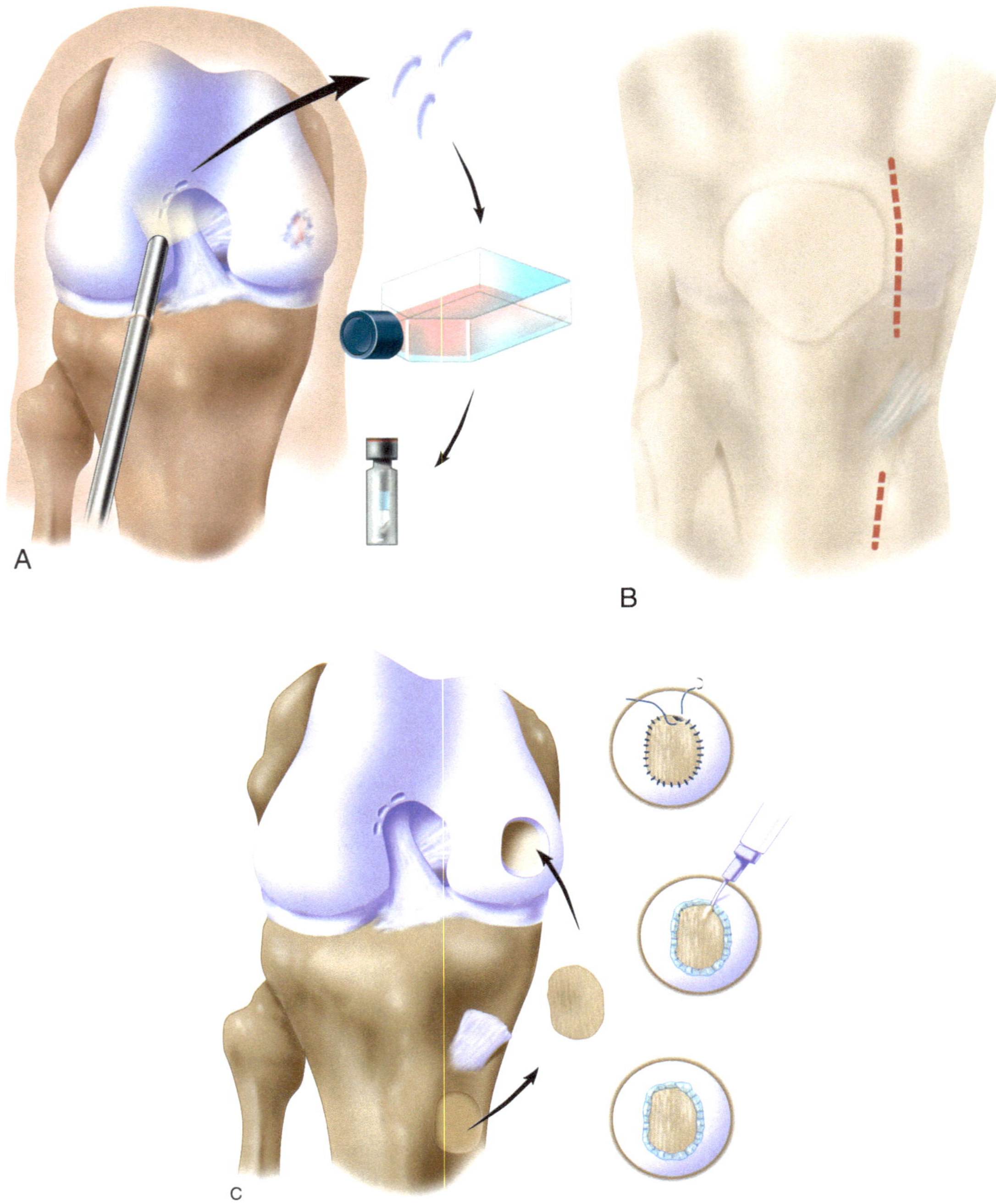

• **Fig. 9.1** Classic technique for autologous chondrocyte implantation (ACI). (A) Arthroscopic evaluation of the knee joint and identification of a full-thickness medial femoral condyle injury. A cartilage biopsy is taken from the superior intercondylar notch, digested, and cultured. Autologous chondrocyte transplantation will occur when the cells have reached a volume that can fill the articular cartilage defect. (B) A two-incision approach is made to the knee. The first is a medial arthrotomy to expose the full-thickness medial femoral condyle defect. The second is an incision distal to the pes anserinus tendon insertion to harvest periosteum templated exactly to the defect after it is debrided. (C) The technique of ACI. A periosteal patch is harvested distal to the pes anserinus tendons. It is microsutured with interrupted 6.0 Vicryl sutures flush to the articular surface and tested for water integrity tightness. It is then sealed with fibrin glue to maintain water tightness. The autologous chondrocyte suspension is injected deep to the periosteal cover to fill the defect and the opening is sutured over and sealed with fibrin glue. The knee joint is closed. The patient undergoes careful rehabilitation to restore motion and allow the graft to mature uneventfully.

is unknown due to a growing number of cell companies, including JTEC in Japan, Co.Don (ChondroSphere), B. Braun/Aesculap (NovoCart 3D) in Germany, Fidia/FAB (HyaloGraft-C) in Italy, and Tigenix (ChondroCelect) in the Benelux region.

The use of autologous chondrocytes for patient care in the United States has been carefully regulated by the Food and Drug Administration (FDA, Biologics Division) and since its introduction it has required both good laboratory practices (GLP standards) and good manufacturing practices (GMP standards). These industry standards have conseqently restricted the use of ACI to private and academic institutions. As of August 22, 1997, the FDA formally approved ACI (FDA Biologics License 1233) for the management of focal chondral defects of the femoral articular surfaces. This was based on the 1997 data of 159 patients evaluated in Sweden. Because of the early results that were unfavorable for management of the patella, tibia, or cases involving early bipolar or arthritic lesions, these defects have been considered "off-label." However, prior to FDA approval, I had gained considerable experience in the treatment of these "off-label" uses based upon patients who were sent for management of these troublesome lesions.

In my experience, the patient who is highly motivated, realistic regarding the rehabilitation protocol, is a nonsmoker, and is not using narcotics for pain management is desirable. A strong social support system and a sense of vitality as measured by the Short Form 36 has proven to be a high statistical predictor of a good physical outcome in a study conducted at our institution and presented at the International Cartilage Repair Society in Toronto, Canada, in 2001.[2] Patients under the age of 18 years also have an excellent chance of returning to full activities.[3]

This chapter will discuss the role of ACI for the treatment of full-thickness cartilage injuries in knees. Since the initial publication on this topic,[1] there has been a renewed interest in treatment and research of this clinical problem. The earlier published study indicated good and excellent results in 14 of 16 patients treated on weight-bearing femoral condyles. Only 2 of 7 patients with patellar lesions treated had similar results.

Indications

The initial early indication for ACI was for a symptomatic full-thickness weight-bearing chondral injury of the femoral articular surface in a physiologically young patient who was compliant with the rehabilitation protocol. The results of chondral injuries for the patellofemoral joint were not as consistently high as those of the femoral weight-bearing condyles. Patients with osteochondritis dissecans (OCD) have also done well.[4] The ideal indication for ACI is for treatment of a symptomatic unipolar grade III or grade IV Outerbridge classification injury, with no greater than the reciprocal articular surface having grade I to II Outerbridge classification chondromalacia.

However, these injuries are uncommon. Curl[5] in his classic review of 31,516 knee arthroscopies found that the incidence of an isolated femoral condyle defect in patients under 40 years old was less than 5%. However, the incidence of articular cartilage injuries throughout the knee was almost 60%. This has also been my experience.

Because of the heterogeneous nature of articular cartilage defects found in the knee arthroscopies that are symptomatic, yet focal in nature, I elected to classify the treatments early on in relatively homogeneous groups. The classification was Simple, Complex, and Salvage.[6,7]

Simple: An isolated grade 3 or 4 Outerbridge weight-bearing femoral condyle defect in a neutrally aligned knee that is stable with an intact meniscus.

Complex: Isolated or multiple grade 3 or 4 Outerbridge chondral defect(s) is(are) on any surface within the knee joint. As in the case of unipolar lesions, background factors may need to be corrected either prior to or at the time of the cartilage surgery.

Salvage: These patients have early osteoarthritic lesions. Radiographically there may be early joint space narrowing and intralesional or peripheral osteophyte formation. Arthroscopically, bipolar lesions may be present in the patella–trochlea or tibia–femur and generalized chondromalacia may be present. The lesions may be peripherally uncontained.

As of June 2009, 550 transplants had been performed in 500 patients (simple 35; complex 22; salvage 294). In my series, simple cases only accounted for 35 of 550 treatments (6.4%).

The management of the larger group of patients in the complex and salvage category treatments have resulted in excellent clinical outcomes despite the heterogeneous nature of the cartilage injuries.[7]

For this reason, my approach to treating young patients who are disabled with pain and poor function involves a careful assessment of long leg alignment x-ray images, a well-preserved weight-bearing joint space or early joint space narrowing, magnetic resonance imaging (MRI) scan or arthroscopic evidence of focal acute or chronic articular cartilage injury. If the lesions are focal in nature when assessed arthroscopically with identifiable borders and reasonable cartilage thickness, I consider the patient for ACI if it appears that the patient's symptoms relate to the areas of chondral damage. A cartilage biopsy is then performed, and the cells are cultured, cryopreserved, and stored awaiting second-stage implantation.

At the first postoperative visit, the proposed reconstructive surgery is discussed with the patient and the background factors that need to be corrected are addressed in addition to the transplantation to the focal articular cartilage defects. The individualized surgery, hospitalization, and rehabilitation are also discussed. The potential postoperative risk of stiffness and its management are discussed. At this visit an assessment is made of the patient's proposed goals at final clinical outcome. If the goals are unrealistic, they are further discussed with the patient and realistic expectations are set. We do not proceed with surgery if the patient remains on baseline narcotics or is a smoker or there is a concern about the patient's emotional well-being. When these issues are resolved, we can proceed with the recommended reconstruction.

Arthroscopic Assessment and Cartilage Biopsy for Cell Culturing

Arthroscopic assessment of the joint and possible biopsy for articular cartilage culturing requires a careful and systematic evaluation of the articular surfaces with an arthroscopic probe to demonstrate and determine the extent of grade III and IV chondromalacia (CM) of the symptomatic lesion. The opposing tibial articular surface must be probed throughout to ensure that the meniscus is intact, the articular surface is healthy, and with chondromalacia ideally no greater than superficial fissuring (Grade II CM), otherwise it may also be considered for repair if the radiographic joint space is intact and the defect rim healthy (Fig. 9.2). The femoral condyle lesion should be assessed for its anterior to posterior length and whether it is a contained or an uncontained lesion. The quality and thickness of the surrounding articular cartilage should also be assessed. This will determine whether healthy cartilage will be available for periosteum or collagen membrane suturing or whether an uncontained chondral injury will require suturing through synovium or small drill holes through the bone (see Fig. 9.21 technique on uncontained defects). The posterior extent of the lesion is critical and must be technically accessed at the time of open arthrotomy for periosteal suturing.

If a lesion is considered appropriate, a biopsy site for cartilage procurement must be decided upon (Fig. 9.3). In Europe, the most commonly chosen site for biopsy is the superior medial edge of the trochlea, adjacent to the medial patella (odd) facet (Fig. 9.4). In this way, a biopsy site will not be producing a reciprocal symptomatic injury because there will be no opposing articular surface to make its contact. The patellofemoral joint must be assessed carefully. If there is an overhanging patellar facet on the medial side, the superior lateral facet may be harvested. My preferred location is the superior and lateral intercondylar notch because it is convenient and known not to create problems when removed as per anterior cruciate ligament (ACL) reconstruction (Fig. 9.5). Finally, either the superior transverse trochlea margin adjacent to the supracondylar synovium or the distal lateral trochlea at the sulcus terminalis are potential biopsy sites. At the time of open implantation, the synovium may be advanced over the biopsy site via sutures through the articular cartilage.

Approximately 200–300 mg of articular cartilage are required for enzymatic digestion for cell culturing, which corresponds approximately to a cartilage surface of 5 mm wide by 1 cm in length. This contains approximately 200,000–300,000 cells, which may be enzymatically digested and grown to approximately 12 million cells per 0.4 cc of culture media per implantation vial.

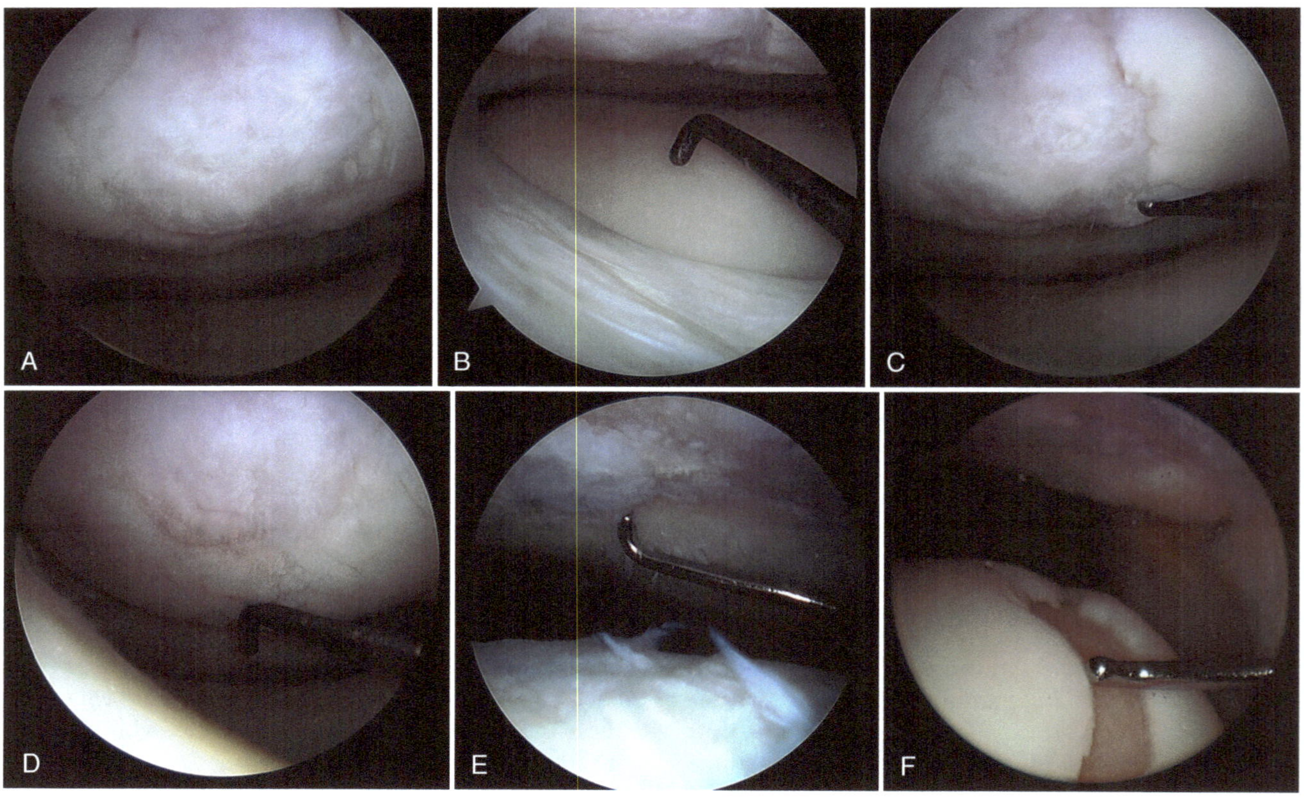

• **Fig. 9.2** Arthroscopic knee joint evaluation. (A) A focal area of cartilage damage is identified on the lateral femoral condyle. (B) The tibial plateau is carefully probed to ensure that it is intact. (C) The meniscus is also probed to ensure that it is intact. Some superficial Outerbridge grade II changes to the lateral tibial plateau are seen but are of no consequence. (D) The chondral injury is carefully probed to identify that there is only a superficial fibrous tissue cover over a large intralesional osteophyte that has developed following a previous microfracture to the lateral femoral condyle. This patient is a candidate for autologous chondrocyte implantation (ACI). (E) Another patient with arthroscopic evaluation of the patellofemoral joint. A large grade 4 defect of the patella is noted with intact margins. The trochlea has Outerbridge grade II superficial changes. Various lateral maltracking of the patella. The patient is a good candidate for ACI to the patella with tibial tubercle anteromedialization. (F) A long focal grade 4 defect of the trochlea is 4 cm long and 1 cm wide. This patient is also a candidate for ACI.

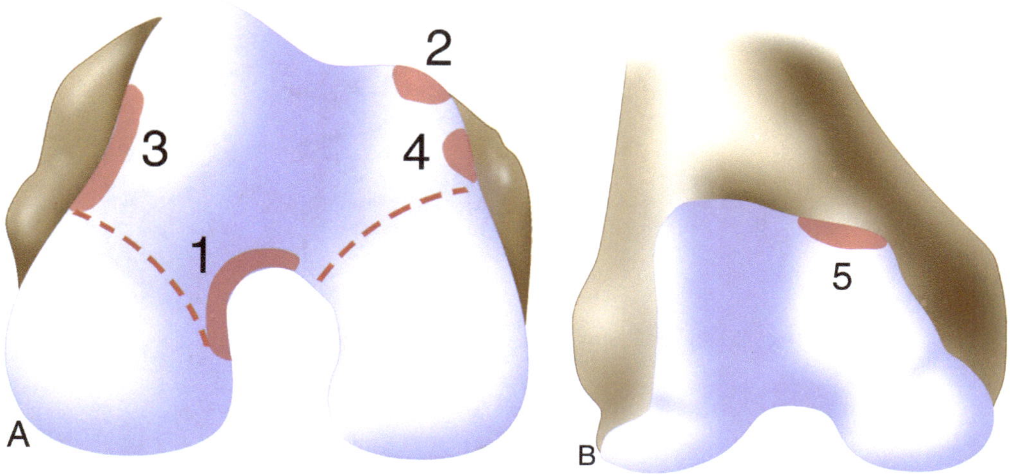

• **Fig. 9.3** Arthroscopic biopsy sites for autologous chondrocyte implantation (ACI). (A) Possible locations for biopsy performed for ACI. *Dotted lines* represent the leading weight-bearing surfaces of the femoral condyles, the sulcus terminalis both medial and lateral. Cartilage biopsies should be taken from the margins of the trochlea just proximal to the weight-bearing surfaces. When the intercondylar notch is harvested, the biopsy is taken from the superior surface to the sulcus terminalis on the lateral wall. (B) The superior portion of the trochlea on the medial corner can also be used when all other sites are not appropriate.

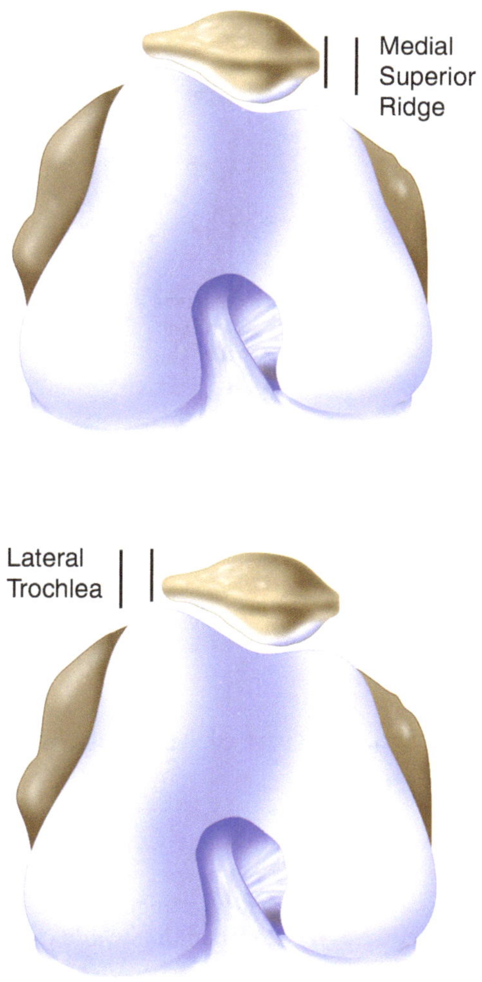

• **Fig. 9.4** Classic location for harvest of cartilage for autologous chondrocyte implantation is the superior medial corner of the trochlea adjacent to the odd facet of the patella in a nonarticulating margin. However, when the medial patellar facet overhangs this margin, another location with no engagement of the patella should be found. The distal lateral trochlea proximal to the sulcus terminalis can frequently be used.

Biopsy instruments may include ring curette or sharp gouges. It is often helpful to incise and score the area of biopsy before attempting to remove it. A whittling, side-to-side motion of the gouge or curette will then more accurately remove the desired cartilage without an unwanted slip. Full-thickness cartilage down to bone should be biopsied. It is helpful to leave an end of the articular biopsy attached so that it may be grasped with an arthroscopic grasper and torn off. This avoids an unwanted loose body in the joint, which then must be captured. Following in vitro expansion of cells 3–5 weeks later, a suitable number and volume of cells will be grown to accommodate the defect size that is required. At this time, second-stage open implantation may occur.

Surgical Correction of Background Factors Predisposing to Chondral Injury

Several predisposing factors to chondral injury must be assessed so that these may be either corrected in a staged or concomitant fashion with ACI. Tibial femoral malalignment, patellofemoral malalignment, and ligamentous, meniscal, or bone insufficiency must be assessed prior to definitive cartilage cell re-implantation.

Long leg alignment is assessed in all patients (as noted in Chapter 3) with double leg stance long alignment digital x-ray images to include hip, knee, and ankle for varus and valgus mechanical alignment assessment (clinical examination is notoriously unreliable for long leg alignment).

Patellofemoral alignment is assessed by clinical examination with localization of the tibial tubercle, determining the quadriceps angle measured with the patella in the reduced position in the trochlea, the presence of a J-sign as the patella relocates from the extended into the flexed position, and the absence or presence of crepitus of the patella with active extension of the knee. If the patient is overweight and the clinical examination is difficult, a computed tomography

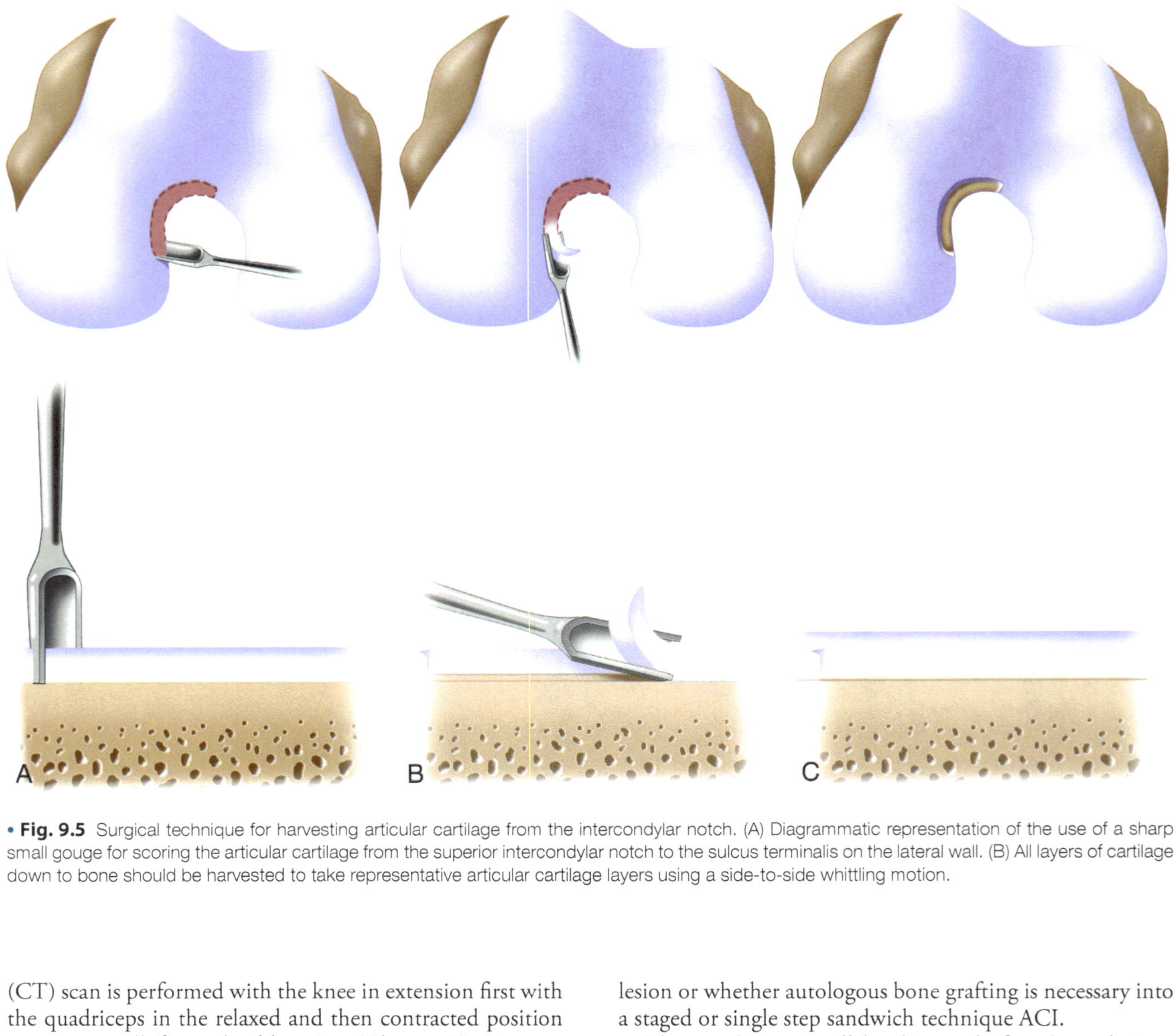

• **Fig. 9.5** Surgical technique for harvesting articular cartilage from the intercondylar notch. (A) Diagrammatic representation of the use of a sharp small gouge for scoring the articular cartilage from the superior intercondylar notch to the sulcus terminalis on the lateral wall. (B) All layers of cartilage down to bone should be harvested to take representative articular cartilage layers using a side-to-side whittling motion.

(CT) scan is performed with the knee in extension first with the quadriceps in the relaxed and then contracted position to assess patellofemoral subluxation (Chapter 8). Dye can be added within the joint to localize and measure the chondral defect(s) in the patella, trochlea, or both.

A clinical examination is best for ligamentous instability unless the patient is very muscular or obese, in which case an MRI scan may be necessary or an examination under anesthesia.

Meniscal insufficiency is difficult to quantify with an MRI scan unless the meniscus is completely absent. An arthroscopic assessment is best performed to assess the status of the meniscus and the residual hoop stress capability at the time of the arthroscopy for the cartilage biopsy for cell transplantation.

Although arthroscopy is helpful in assessing the depth and character of an osteochondral defect, CT scan is usually more useful to determine whether there are subchondral bony cysts present that cannot be visualized at the time of arthroscopy. This will help in addressing whether isolated ACI can be performed for an osteochondritis dissecans lesion or whether autologous bone grafting is necessary into a staged or single step sandwich technique ACI.

These techniques will be discussed after the technique of open surgical transplantation of autologous chondrocytes is reviewed in the case of an ideal lesion suitable for transplantation.

Surgical Implantation of Autologous Chondrocytes

The steps in open implantation include arthrotomy, defect preparation, periosteum procurement, periosteum fixation, periosteum watertight integrity testing, autologous fibrin glue sealant, chondrocyte implantation, wound closure, and rehabilitation.

For a unicondylar injury, a medial or lateral parapatellar arthrotomy is utilized, which is usually done through a midline skin incision or a longitudinal parapatellar incision. Adequate exposure is crucial to good suturing technique of periosteum and several retractors are often

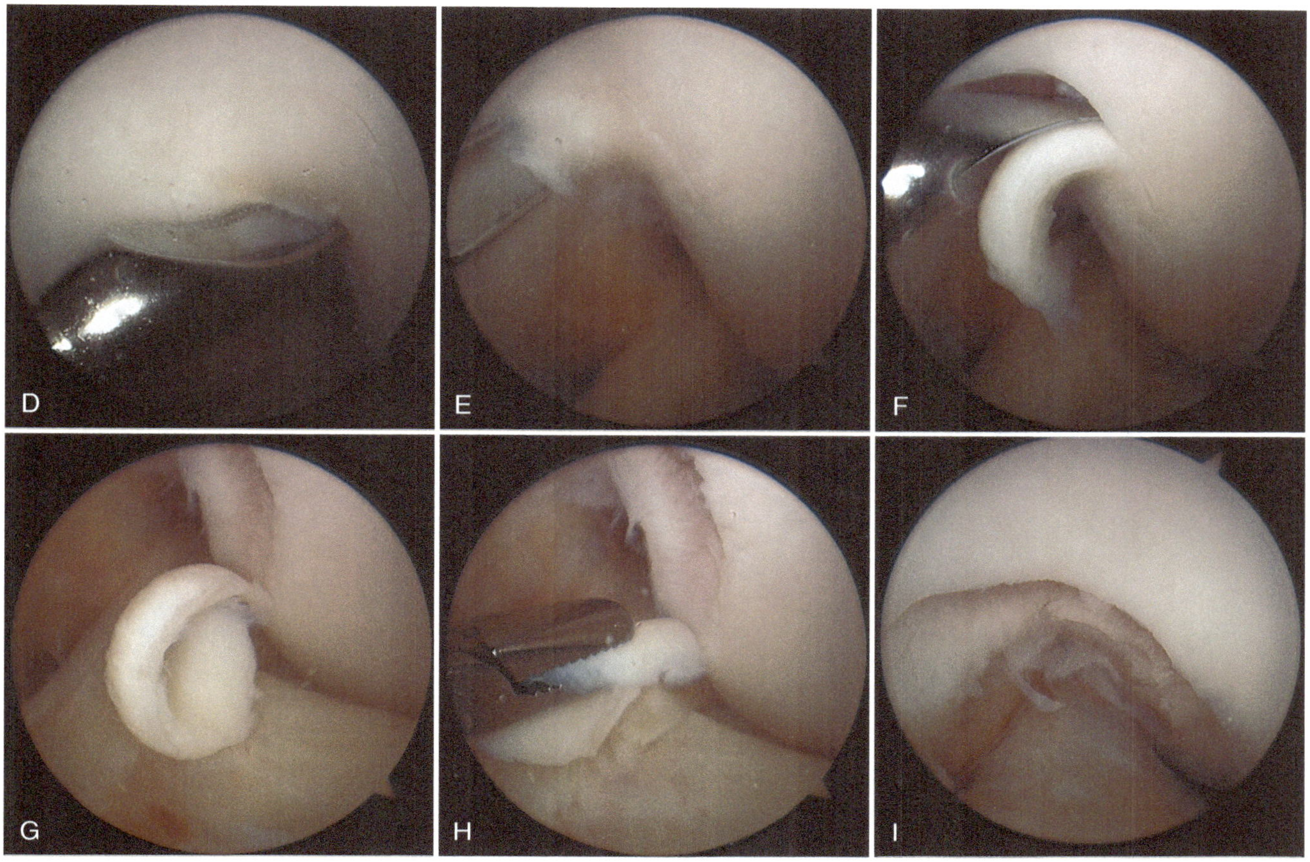

• **Fig. 9.5 —cont'd** (C) The defect left behind measures approximately 5mm wide by 1 to 1.5cm long. The full-thickness articular cartilage (usually 200–300mg) is adequate for cell culture and expansion. It represents a non-weight-bearing portion when the knee is brought into full extension and visualized. (D) Arthroscopic appearance of the intercondylar notch at the time of biopsy in the left knee. Scoring of the articular cartilage to ensure that the gouge does not stray when pressure is applied to harvest cartilage. (E) The gouge is started at the 11 o'clock position in a whittling manner. Full-thickness cartilage is engaged down to bone. (F) The cartilage is left intact as it is brought to the lateral side of the intercondylar notch. (G) The cartilage is left attached at its distal-most attachment site at the sulcus terminalis of the lateral femoral condyle. (H) It is then grasped with a grasper and brought out of the medial arthroscopic portal as one piece. (I) In full extension, no impingement of the cartilage is seen on the tibial spines or the weight-bearing surfaces.

required to achieve it. Posterior lesions on the femur will often require hyperflexion of the knee and occasional takedown of the meniscus in a subperiosteal fashion with intermeniscal ligament takedown and coronary ligament release of the tibia as the meniscus is peeled back with the entire sleeve of tissue (Fig. 9.6). A repair of these is undertaken during closure. For multiple lesions, a traditional medial parapatellar arthrotomy is often required with subluxation or dislocation and eversion of the patella with hyperflexion.

If the chondral defect is lateral, obtaining access to a posterior lesion is frequently difficult if the tibial tubercle is laterally positioned on the tibia. In this case a tibial tubercle osteotomy (TTO) and elevation is very helpful for exposing the lesion and realigning the extensor mechanism centrally (see section "ACI plus TTO for Posterior Exposure/with Patella/Trochlea ACI"). This will often allow a very posterior exposure to the femoral condyles without taking down the intermeniscal ligament with the meniscus and coronary ligament off the tibia.

Defect preparation is critical. Radical debridement of all fissured and undermined articular cartilage surrounding the full thickness chondral injury to healthy contained cartilage is desirable. Early failures occurred from inadequate debridement with poor integration to adjacent cartilage with either progression of disease in the adjacent non-debrided fissured cartilage or delamination of the repair tissue from the damaged native tissue. Oval or curvilinear excisions with a no. 15 blade are made by incising the articular cartilage vertically down to the subchondral bone plate without penetrating the bone. Small ring or closed curettes and periosteal elevators are used to debride the degenerating articular cartilage back to healthy host cartilage. Maintaining an intact subchondral bone plate without subchondral bone bleeding is important. It is essential not to perforate the subchondral bone plate such that a mixed marrow cell population does not populate the chondral defect in addition to the end-differentiated chondrocytes that have been grown in vitro. A contained lesion is desired and it is better to leave a minimally chondromalacic cartilage border than to remove the border and

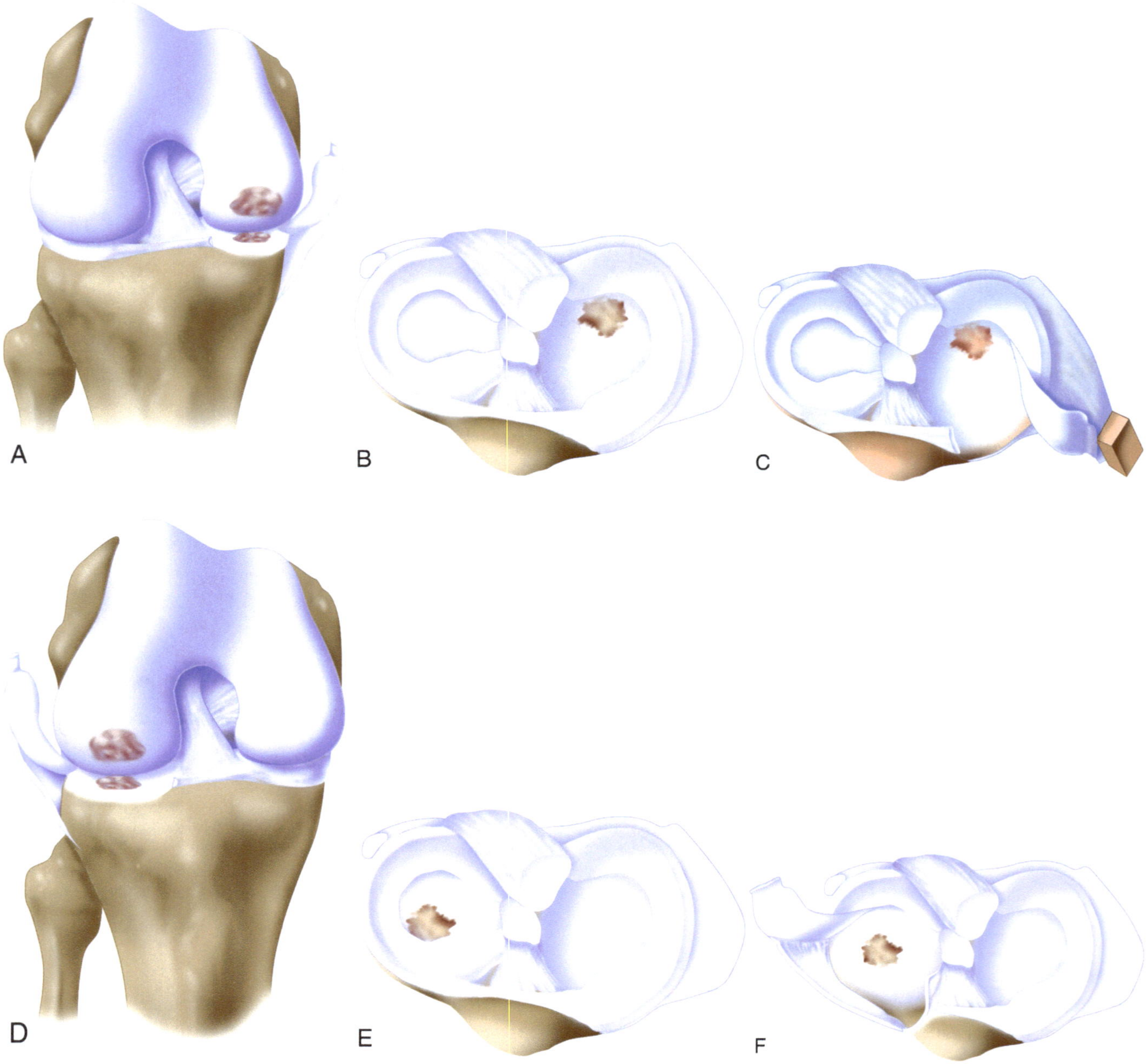

• **Fig. 9.6** Deep dissection of a medial or lateral arthrotomy to obtain exposure to the posterior medial femoral condyle or tibial plateau, or a lateral femoral condyle and lateral tibial plateau. (A) Frontal view demonstrating a medial femoral condyle defect that is posterior or a central or posterior medial tibial plateau defect. The intermeniscal ligament is taken down and the coronary meniscal attachment on the tibia is taken down to the medial meniscus. The entire soft tissue sleeve is dissected posteriorly so that it is continuous and deep to the superficial medial collateral ligaments. By hyperflexing and externally rotating the tibia, the tibial plateau can be delivered almost entirely or the medial femoral condyle posteriorly. (B) Superior view of a posterior tibial plateau chondral defect in relation to the intermeniscal ligament and the meniscus and superficial and deep medial collateral ligaments. (C) If the medial sleeve is taken down in a posterior direction off the tibia to expose the posterior tibial plateau but is still too tight, a bone block attachment to the femoral condyle origin of the medial collateral ligament will allow the entire medial side of the knee to be opened quite easily. It is then reattached with a screw and washer fixation at the end of the procedure. I have found that this is rarely required. (D) Frontal view of the lateral femoral condyle and lateral tibial plateau after dissection of a lateral sleeve of meniscus, coronary ligament, and portion of the iliotibial band insertion to gain exposure to the posterior lateral femoral condyles or lateral tibial plateau. (E) View of the lateral tibial plateau cartilage defect from above, with structures intact. (F) Superior view after release of the intermeniscal ligament and coronary ligament with lateral meniscus takedown of a lateral soft tissue subperiosteal sleeve. Upon completion of autologous chondrocyte implantation, the origins of the anterior horns of the medial or lateral menisci are reattached to their native positions using transosseous Ethibond sutures.

leave an uncontained lesion that would require suturing to synovium or micro-holes through bone drills (Fig. 9.7). Once a healthy defect bed is prepared, it is measured in its length and width, or if it is irregularly shaped, templated with sterile tracing paper (sterile glove packaging paper works well). A sterile marker can be used to template the defect and it can then be cut out to fit the defect perfectly. It can be oversized by approximately 2 mm in both length and width on the

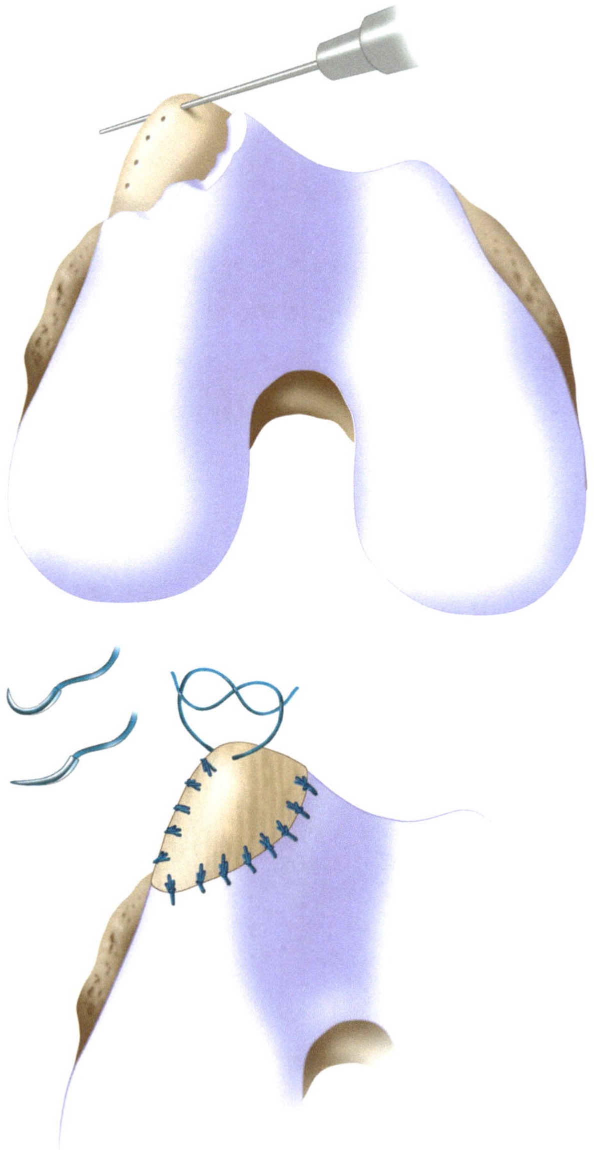

• **Fig. 9.7** Transosseous drill hole fixation for uncontained cartilage defects. A large uncontained lateral trochlear defect is demonstrated. Radical debridement of the cartilage is performed. Any sclerotic bone is removed with a sharp ring curette and possibly deepened with a high-speed bur if the bone is very sclerotic, leaving a prominent peripheral margin intact. Transosseous drill holes through the margin then allow a cavity to be formed. A small P1 cutting needle is straightened out with two heavy needle drivers. The sutures are transfixed through the membrane and the drill holes to maintain a peripheral seal to the defect. This is reinforced with fibrin glue sealant around the uncontained margins, checked for water tightness, and then injected with autologous cultured chondrocytes once the defect margins are secured and watertight.

periosteal site when it is prepared (the periosteum shrinks as it is procured). Alternatively, this can be measured and marked with a marker directly onto the periosteum if it is an uncomplicated shape and cut directly (Fig. 9.8).

If there is subchondral thickening, sclerosis or intralesional osteophyte formation at the base of the chondral defect from prior marrow stimulation technique (drilling, abrasion, microfracture), it should be taken down to the level of native subchondral bone. This can be performed with a rongeur and a high-speed bur (usually 5-mm diameter) to the level of the native subchondral bone (Fig. 9.9). This will provide a cavity for the cell suspension that is injected underneath the membrane cover and will lessen the stiffness of the subchondral bone so that the newly forming cartilage repair tissue will integrate to form a new osteochondral unit with a viscoelastic cartilage surface, a subchondral bone plate that is not overly stiff to cause premature degeneration of the tissue and a normal subchondral cancellous bone. Surprisingly this thickened and calloused bone does not bleed when a tourniquet is let down. In fact, if bleeding does occur, it is usually scant and is easily managed with a thrombin epinephrine-soaked neural patty or a drop of fibrin glue and occasionally a fine-tipped electrocautery is used.

Thickening and sclerosis of the subchondral bone is also found in cases of early osteoarthritis with chronic articular chondral defects. In these cases, the surrounding cartilage is often thinned and the periphery of the defect is marginally uncontained. A contained defect can be made by using a high-speed bur to deepen the area of bony exposure to the level of more normal subchondral bone and provide a cavity for the cartilaginous tissue repair by using transosseous drill holes around the periphery to anchor the membrane. This has been my method of repair in patients frequently seen in the salvage category of treatment.

The easiest and most suitable location for periosteum procurement is from the proximal medial tibia, distal to the pes anserinus insertion on the subcutaneous border. At this site there is a very thin fascial layer of subcutaneous fat and the periosteum is easily accessed. Once defect size has been assessed and templated, a second incision is made approximately a finger breath distal to the pes anserinus insertion, in the center of the medial subcutaneous border of the tibia. Subcutaneous fat is incised initially and then scissor dissection will reveal the shiny white proximal tibial periosteum. It is useful to use a wet sponge to sweep away loose areolar tissue. Electrocautery should not be used because it will necrose the periosteum with the very sensitive cambium layer of cells on its deep surface.

The template is then placed on the periosteum or it is marked with a ruler and a sterile marking pen. A sharp no. 15 blade is then used to incise sharply, oversizing the periosteum 1 mm in all directions down to bone. A small sharp periosteal elevator is useful in very gently advancing the periosteum from its bony bed and preventing it from under-rolling so that it does not rip. Nontoothed forceps will help to pull the periosteum upward as it is gently removed from the tibia. A gentle push/pull type of motion of the periosteal elevator from side-to-side across the periosteum will help its removal.

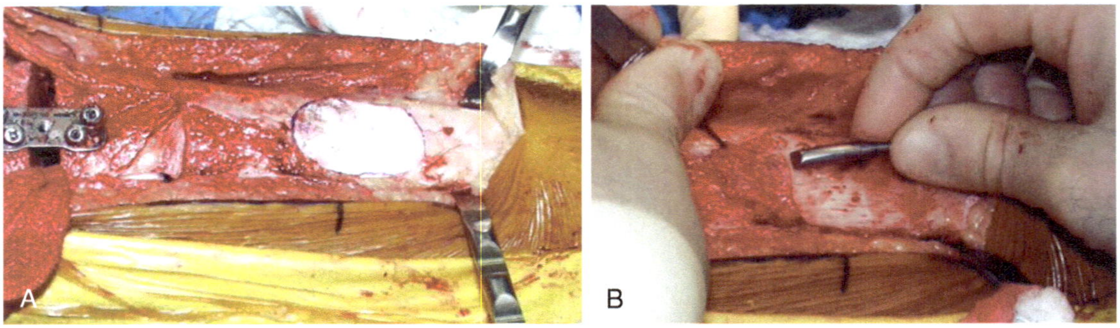

• **Fig. 9.8** Periosteal harvest. (A) Paper template is applied distal to pes anserinus tendons on the subcutaneous medial border of the tibia onto the periosteum directly. It is sharply oversized by 1 mm circumferentially using a no. 15 blade. (B) A small sharp periosteal elevator is used to remove the entire periosteal membrane from the bone, maintaining the deep cambium layer orientation. The superficial fibrous layer is marked with a sterile marking pen to ensure this orientation.

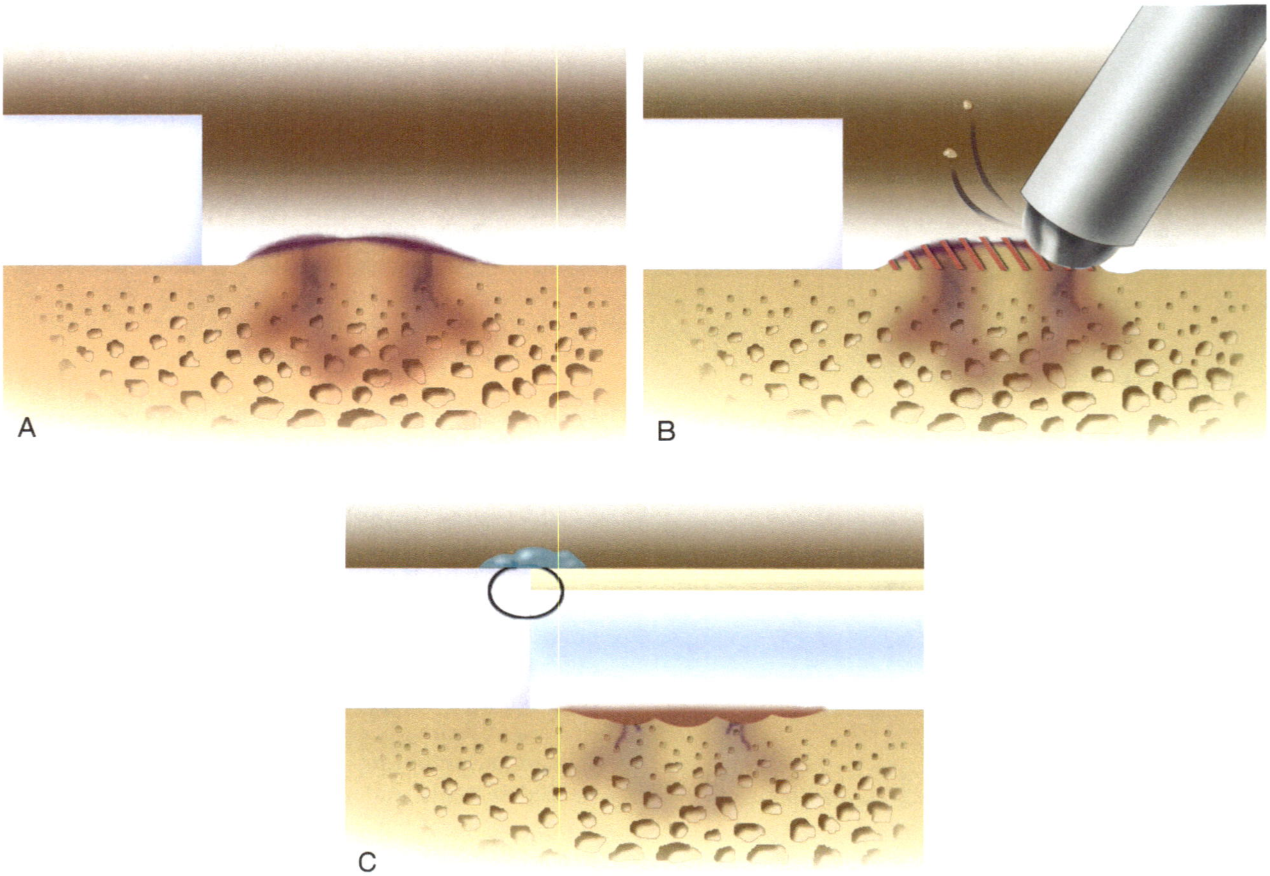

• **Fig. 9.9** Takedown of sclerotic bone/intralesional osteophytes. (A) Intralesional osteophytes may form after marrow stimulation techniques (abrasion, drilling, microfracture) or from idiopathic osteoarthritis. (B) A 5-mm high-speed bur is used under irrigation to gently take down this sclerotic cortical type bone to the level of the adjacent native subchondral bone. (C) When the tourniquet is let down, little bleeding occurs from these sites. Autologous chondrocyte implantation (ACI) may then be performed safely on a chondral defect whose depth has not been taken up by bone. Whether this technique will improve the results of ACI after marrow stimulation techniques is unknown.

Mark the outside of the periosteum so that it is not inadvertently placed upside down. This marks the superficial surface.

At this time the defect site is inspected and the tourniquet can be either let down to assess bleeding of the subchondral bone plate or let down at the end of the procedure if the surgeon is confident that the bone bed appears not to be violated. If there is any bleeding of the bony bed, it can usually be stopped by using a combination of thrombin and epinephrine soaked in a neural patty applied to the defect and gently pressed for several minutes. Upon removal, if there continues to be some bleeding, a small drop of fibrin glue will usually suffice to make the defect dry.

The goals of periosteum or collagen membrane fixation are threefold: first, to provide a watertight membrane that acts as a mechanical seal; second, to act as a semipermeable membrane for intra-articular synovial nutrition to chondrocytes; and last, to maintain a viable periosteal cambium layer of cells so that interactive growth factors between chondrocytes and periosteum may enhance chondrocyte growth. These factors have been isolated to include TGF-beta, IGF, IL-2, and IL-6 and have been found to enhance chondrocyte colony formation when separated from periosteum and delivered directly to chondrocytes in suspension. To this end, it is important to handle the periosteum delicately so that it is not perforated and to keep it moist so that it does not undergo shrinkage or cambium cell death. Its orientation is always maintained so that a cambium layer is facing in toward the subchondral bone plate as noted by a pen mark on the superficial aspect.

Periosteum may then be placed gently onto the defect in the appropriate orientation. Nontoothed forceps are used to handle the periosteum by its edges only. Suturing is usually done with a 6.0 Vicryl suture on a P-1 cutting needle that has been immersed in sterile mineral oil or glycerin. Approximately 8" of length is usually adequate and the remainder of the suture is cut and discarded. Suturing is done in an interrupted and alternating fashion. Sutures are placed through the periosteum and then the articular surface, the knots being tied on the side of the periosteum such that they remain below the level of the adjacent cartilage to avoid unraveling with motion and to evert the periosteal edge so that it may act as a washer seal on the edge of the vertical articular cartilage defect (Fig. 9.10). Hence, a watertight seal can be obtained by suture technique alone in most cases. When suturing corners, the action is like tightening a drum skin. In this way the patch is tensioned adequately throughout the entire defect and the most superior aspect of the periosteal patch is left open to accept saline and to check edge integrity and chondrocytes. Interval sutures of approximately 3–6 mm are made and these protrude through the articular surface by at least 3 mm.

Periosteum watertight integrity testing is assessed by using a plastic 18-gauge 2" angiocath with a tuberculin syringe filled with saline. This step is usually avoided when a collagen membrane cover is utilized because it tends to displace the cell suspension from being absorbed to the collagen membrane, which is the desired effect. The angiocath is placed deep to the periosteum into the defect and by gently filling the defect with saline. A meniscus should rise to the opening if the defect is watertight. Any leakage can easily be seen around the perimeter of the repair site. An additional suture may be required to aid in obtaining water integrity. The saline is then aspirated from the defect and if water integrity cannot be obtained simply by suture technique, a fibrin sealant is used.

For autologous fibrin sealant, the patient must donate 1 unit of whole blood preoperatively. This is then spun off for a pack of red blood cells and a supernatant, which is concentrated to produce cryoprecipitate by a double-spin freeze–thaw technique. This takes some 14 days of preparation prior to surgery. Following double freeze–thaw technique, a concentration of approximately of 80–100 mg/dL fibrinogen can be obtained. The fibrinogen or cryoprecipitate is activated with bovine thrombin and calcium. A double-barreled syringe is required. One barrel contains the cryoprecipitate and the other barrel contains a 50/50 admixture of 10% calcium chloride and a super concentrated bovine thrombin. Fibrinogen is cleaved into active fibrin, which is deposited along the margins of the defect to seal them. Tisseel (Tisseel, Baxter Biosurgery, Deerfield, IL) is made from pooled human serum and is commercially available in Europe and the United States.

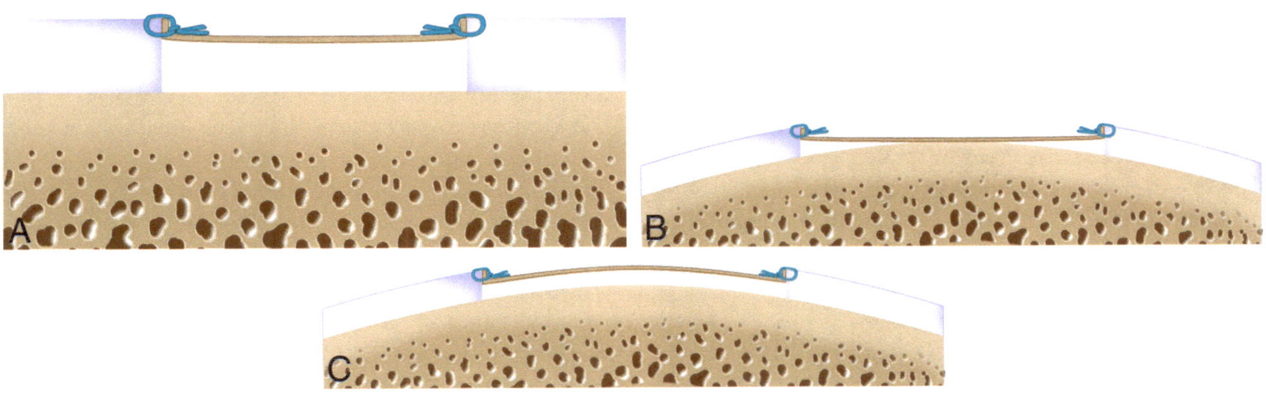

• **Fig. 9.10** Suturing techniques for large femoral condylar defects. (A) Example of good suturing technique for a cartilage defect. The suture is placed through the periosteum and then the cartilage to obtain a good purchase of both tissues. The knot is tied on the side of the periosteum to evert the periosteum flush to the cartilage side wall and make it watertight, like a washer. In this way, the suture is also below the level of the articular cartilage and is less likely to unravel once the knee starts to undergo motion. The membrane is flush with the articular surface and forms a cavity or bioactive chamber for the cells to grow to the limiting surface membrane. (B) For long femoral condylar defects in the anterior to posterior direction, suturing technique is important to maintain a uniform cavity throughout the length of the defect. If medial to lateral suturing is not performed through the length of the defect from anterior to posterior, the membrane may bottom out on the center aspect of the length of the curve. This site is more likely to undergo premature breakdown. (C) If the periosteal or collagen membrane is oversized in the anterior to posterior direction, suturing is started at the center of the defect in a medial to lateral direction, and then anterior to posterior. The chamber cavity will maintain a uniform depth and will more likely undergo full, even cartilage fill for the length of the defect.

After sealing, the defect water integrity is once more tested. The angiocath is useful underneath the periosteum to ensure that the periosteum is not inadvertently sealed to the subchondral bone. The saline is aspirated from the defect bed and the defect is now ready to accept chondrocyte implantation. The chondrocyte suspension is then sterilely aspirated in a tuberculin syringe through an 18-gauge or larger needle (smaller gauges will damage the cells); the needle is then removed and switched to a flexible 18-gauge 2" angiocath. The cells are then very gently delivered through the superior opening of the periosteal defect margin to the base of the defect. As the angiocath is withdrawn, cues are injected until a meniscus comes to the surface. When the defect is filled with cells, several sutures are used to close the defect and it is then sealed with fibrin glue.

The procedure is now complete. Drains are not generally used within the joint to avoid damaging the periosteal patch or sucking the cells from the defect. When drains are needed, it should be without suction. The wound is then closed in layers and a soft dressing applied to the knee.

Advanced Techniques for Surgical Transplantation of Autologous Chondrocytes

Exposures: Outline

Posterior Femoral Lesions and Tibial Plateaus

When attempting to approach a femoral condyle lesion that is very posterior or a tibial plateau lesion, a takedown of a soft tissue envelope to varying degrees may be necessary. This involves incising the intermeniscal ligament followed by the coronary ligament attachment to the tibial plateau with a subperiosteal peel off the tibia and in a posterior direction. It is easier to perform on the medial side with a long sleeve of medial retinaculum to the deep portion of the medial collateral ligament in the mid coronal plane. This is usually enough to access a posterior medial femoral condyle. However, to get to the midportion of the medial tibial plateau or the posterior portion, two options are available. The deep medial collateral ligament (MCL) may be further taken off in a continuous sleeve with the anterior portion until the entire tibial plateau is delivered anteriorly by externally rotating the tibia and hyperflexing the knee. At closure, transosseous sutures with no. 2 Ethibond are used to reattach the sleeve of tissue in its original position. This is relatively easy when the sutures are passed almost at the level of the joint where the metaphyseal bone is softer and the suture needle may pass directly through the bone in one easy passage. The anterior horn of the medial meniscus is then reattached using transosseous sutures to its original position. The intermeniscal ligament is repaired. The other option is to take down the origin of the medial collateral ligament with a bone block off the femoral condyles, which completely opens up the medial side of the knee. I have found that this is rarely necessary and that the first option is preferable unless a very posterior medial tibial plateau requires suturing (Fig. 9.11).

Approaching the lateral tibial plateau or posterior lateral condyles is often more difficult. A lateral parapatellar arthrotomy is performed. The intrameniscal ligament is released and the coronary ligament with the anterior horn of the lateral meniscus is peeled subperiosteally with the sleeve, which will often include some of the attachment of the iliotibial band insertion at Gerdes tubercle. The patella is subluxed into the medial parapatellar gutter and the knee is hyperflexed and internally rotated. This will usually reveal the lateral tibial plateau quite well and expose the posterior lateral femoral condyles. If the knee is stiff and there is a very laterally positioned tibial tubercle insertion, it might still not be possible. In this situation a tibial tubercle osteotomy with a subvastus lateral arthrotomy is recommended, which will easily expose the distal lateral femoral condyles and the entire tibial plateau. The meniscus may still need to be taken down and reapproximated after dealing with a tibial plateau injury (Fig. 9.12, with distal femoral varus osteotomy).

ACI Plus High Tibial Osteotomy, High Tibial Osteotomy Plus Tibial Tubercle Osteotomy, Distal Femoral Varus Osteotomy

When varus or valgus malalignment is concomitant with a medial or lateral condyle injury respectively, a corrective osteotomy is paramount to the success of the ACI. This can be done in either a staged or concomitant fashion. My preference is to do the procedure all at once. A single longitudinal incision will obtain the exposure for both procedures quite easily. However, it is imperative that if it is done concomitantly, a stable fixation must be obtained at the time of osteotomy surgery so that continuous passive motion (CPM) and early active range of motion may be pursued immediately postoperatively. Otherwise, a staged reconstruction should be performed.

A common wear pattern is a varus knee with a medial femoral condyle lesion or in combination with a trochlea or patellar injury. If there is a medial femoral condyle defect with a varus knee, a longitudinal incision is made from the superior medial pole of the patella longitudinally and distally to the inferior aspect of the tibial tubercle (Fig. 9.13). A medial parapatellar arthrotomy is then performed, the defect is debrided and templated, the template is applied to the periosteum that has been exposed distal to the past anserinus tendons and periosteum harvested. Takedown of the pes tendons and superficial MCL is then performed in preparation for the tibial valgus-producing osteotomy (see Chapter 10). The osteotomy is then performed and fixated. The tourniquet is let down and any bleeders in the soft tissue envelope or the subchondral bone plate of the area to be transplanted are dealt with. Careful suturing and transplantation to the medial femoral condyle is then performed.

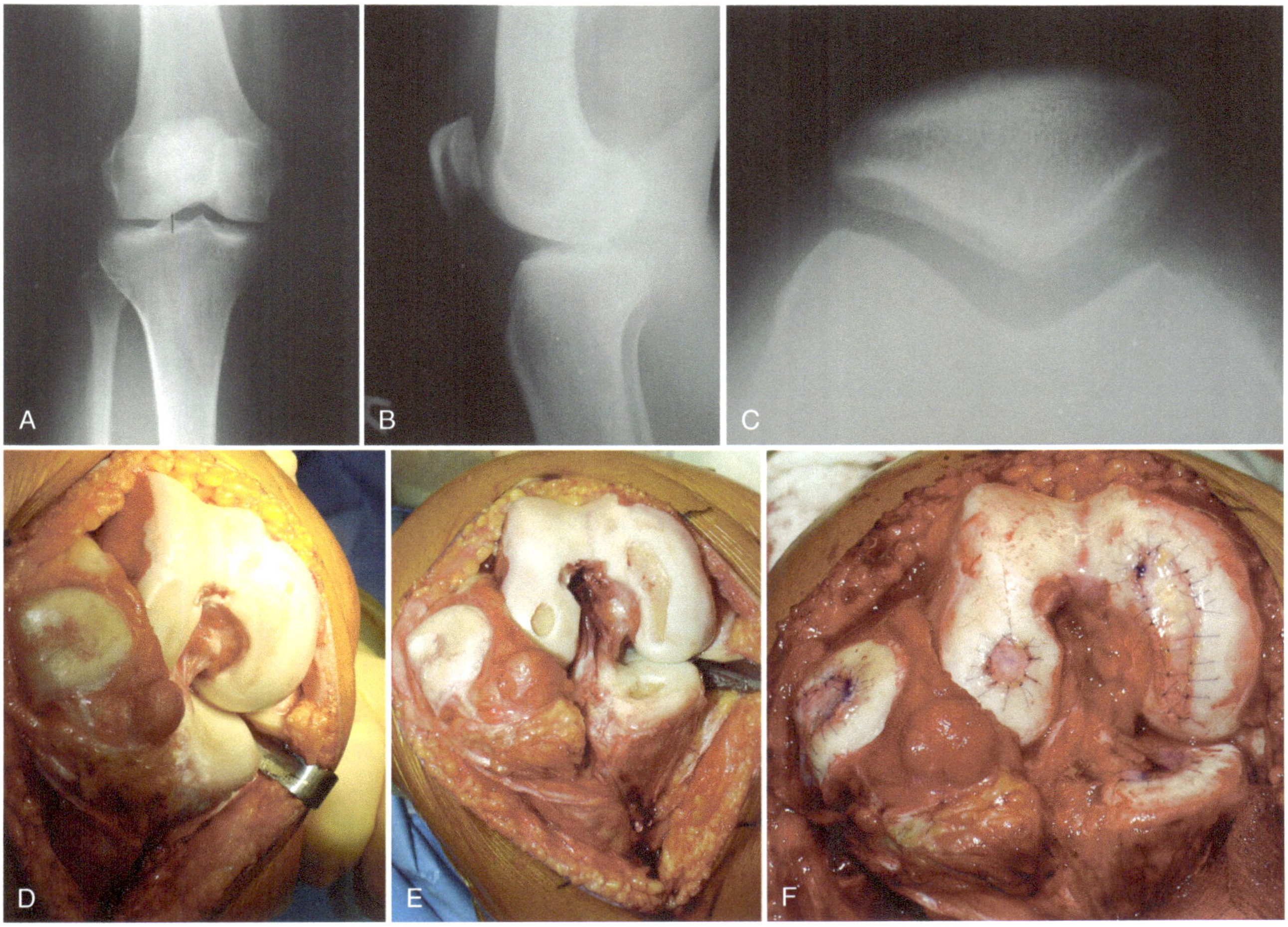

• **Fig. 9.11** Case example demonstrating exposure to posterior weight-bearing condyles and tibial plateau. (A) Weight-bearing x-ray film of a young woman involved in a motor vehicle accident who had intractable global joint pain. Her joint spaces are normal and her ligamentous examination intact. Clinical examination revealed that she has tricompartmental crepitus and joint effusions. (B) Lateral x-ray film demonstrating intact patellofemoral and tibiofemoral joints. (C) Intact skyline view of cartilage spaces. (D) Medial parapatellar arthrotomy is performed with a patellar eversion and a medial subperiosteal peel maintains the entire medial sleeve intact. This method gives excellent exposure to all the articulations, including the tibial plateau immediately in the posterior medial femoral condyles. (E) After radical debridement of the articular cartilage injuries back to intact stable cartilage, focal defects are delineated, templated, and measured. (F) Periosteal harvest from the medial subcutaneous border of the tibia is performed. The defects are microsutured, sealed with fibrin glue, and injected with autologous cultured chondrocytes. Ten years later the patient remains free of pain and discomfort and maintains normal joint spaces radiographically.

If arthroscopy revealed maltracking of the patella in addition to a chondral defect, a TTO is performed with a medial subvastus and lateral subvastus arthrotomy elevating the extensor mechanism proximally. The defects are debrided, the periosteum is harvested, the tibial valgus osteotomy is performed and fixated (see Chapter 10, combined osteotomies). The periosteal covers are then microsutured and transplanted. The tibial tubercle is repositioned and centered to normalize the extensor mechanism forces postoperatively.

ACI Plus Tibial Tubercle Osteotomy for Posterior Exposure/With Patella/Trochlea ACI

Patellofemoral maltracking combined with a trochlea or patellar chondral injury requires careful preoperative assessment with physical examination and CT or MRI imaging techniques. TTO combined with soft tissue realignment to ensure proper tracking is paramount to a successful graft healing. My preference is a longitudinal incision just off the midline laterally. In this way as the tibial tubercle is anterior medialized a skin incision is placed over the anterior muscle compartment and not over a bony prominence. If there is a wound breakdown, the bone is not exposed and the health of the wound is optimized. A lateral subvastus arthrotomy then allows visualization of the posterior femoral condyle, damaged patella, trochlea or all. An assessment of dysplasia of the trochlea can be performed at this time. The laxity of the medial soft tissue envelope can also be assessed. If the medial side of the knee is excessively lax to patellar stability, a medial arthrotomy is performed leaving a good cuff of tissue attached to the patellar portion of the extensor mechanism. The TTO can then be performed either leaving the distal hinge attached as per a classic Fulkerson-type osteotomy or making an oblique distal counter cut and elevating

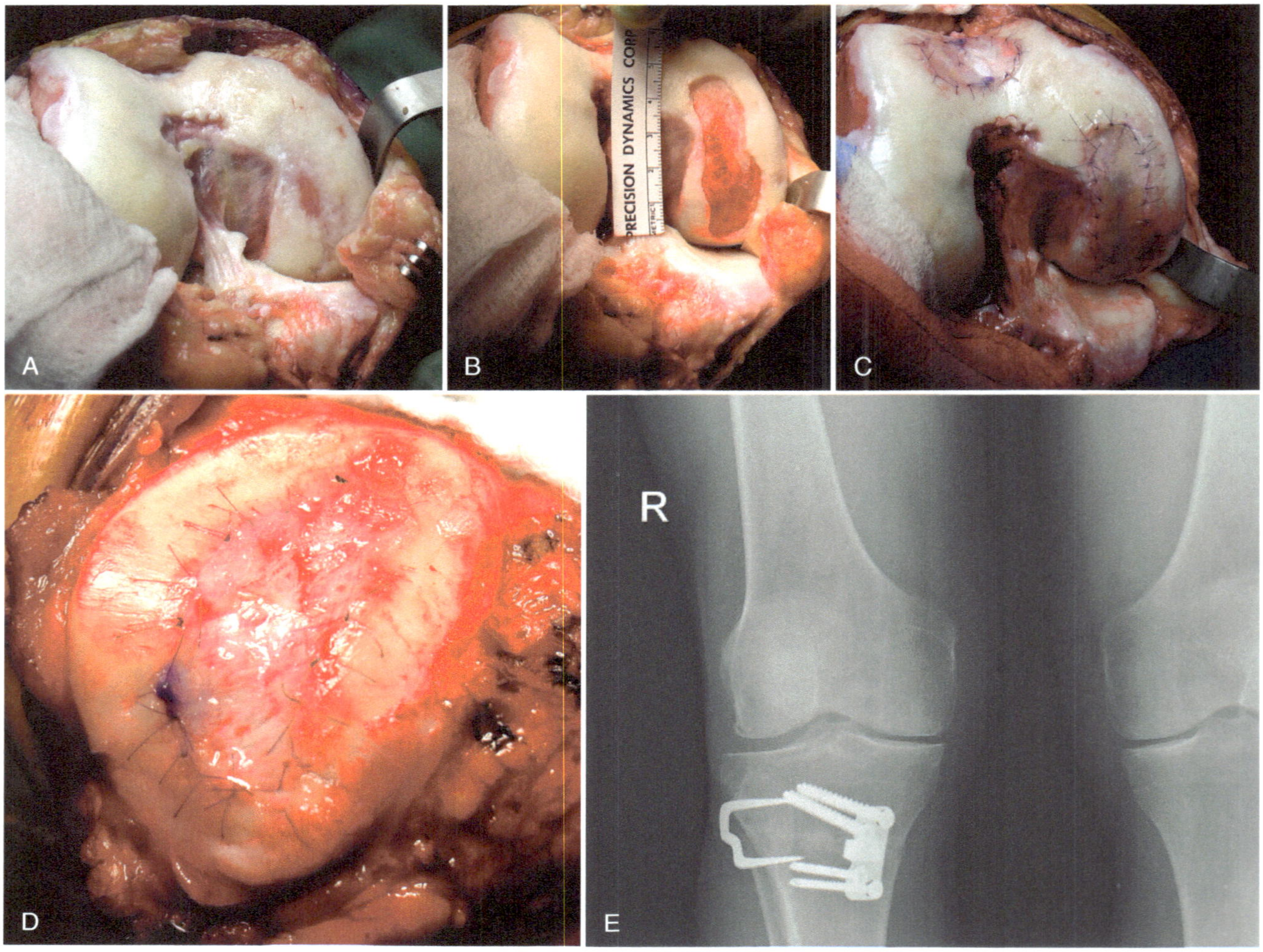

• **Fig. 9.12** Case example demonstrating exposure for osteoarthritic lesions with varus malalignment requiring open-wedge tibial valgus-producing osteotomy. (A) Open appearance of the right knee of a 48-year-old male football coach with intractable medial and anterior joint pain and effusions. A midline incision with a medial parapatellar arthrotomy is performed. The incision is continued distally and subcutaneously to the pes anserinus tendons. (B) Careful radical debridement of the joint is the most important step in the early arthritic knee undergoing autologous chondrocyte implantation. Note that a lateral intercondylar notchplasty has been performed to prevent impingement of the anterior cruciate ligament when the knee is placed into valgus. Radical debridement of the medial femoral condyle defect preserves the intercondylar osteophytes, which will be used for transosseous suture fixation of periosteum. Intralesional osteophytes are carefully taken down to increase the depth of the chondral defect to maintain a cavity throughout its entire length. (C) Periosteal microsuturing is performed throughout the length of the medial femoral condyle and the trochlear defects. Note that the final appearance of the joint appears much healthier than the initial appearance. The tibial osteotomy can easily be performed through this single midline incision after the periosteum has been harvested. (D) The periosteum on the patella is sutured by starting at the midline ridge proximal to distal to maintain the tent-like shape of the periosteum. (E) Radiographic appearance of the knee 4 years later when the patient returned for treatment of his other knee, which had become as painful as the right knee had been. He has had no pain in his right knee and he was able to return to coaching and running on the sidelines until his left knee became painful. The left knee was treated in the same way with excellent clinical outcome.

the extensor mechanism proximally (Fig. 9.14, a posterior lateral OCD lesion).

Trochlea debridement and transplantation of the surfaces can then be easily performed. Trochlea articular cartilage is generally 3 to 5 mm thick. In order for postoperative rehabilitation to be without patellofemoral catching sensations, the debridement should involve the proximal and distal or leading and trailing margins of the defect to be slightly sloped towards the subchondral bone bed, and the medial and lateral margins to be vertical. When a defect is confined to an isolated medial or lateral trochlea facet, microsuturing a periosteal or collagen membrane flush to the articular surface is easy. However, when it crosses the midline sulcus, the order of stitching is important to restore the concavity of the trochlea (Fig. 9.15), otherwise microsuturing without paying attention to this will result in a flat trochlea sulcus and abnormal forces to the membrane with possible early failure.

Similarly, after tibial tubercle proximal ionization with subvastus laterally release patella debridement and transplantation of the surfaces can then be easily performed. The patellar cartilage is generally thicker than the trochlea, 5 to 7 mm thick, and therefore similar consideration

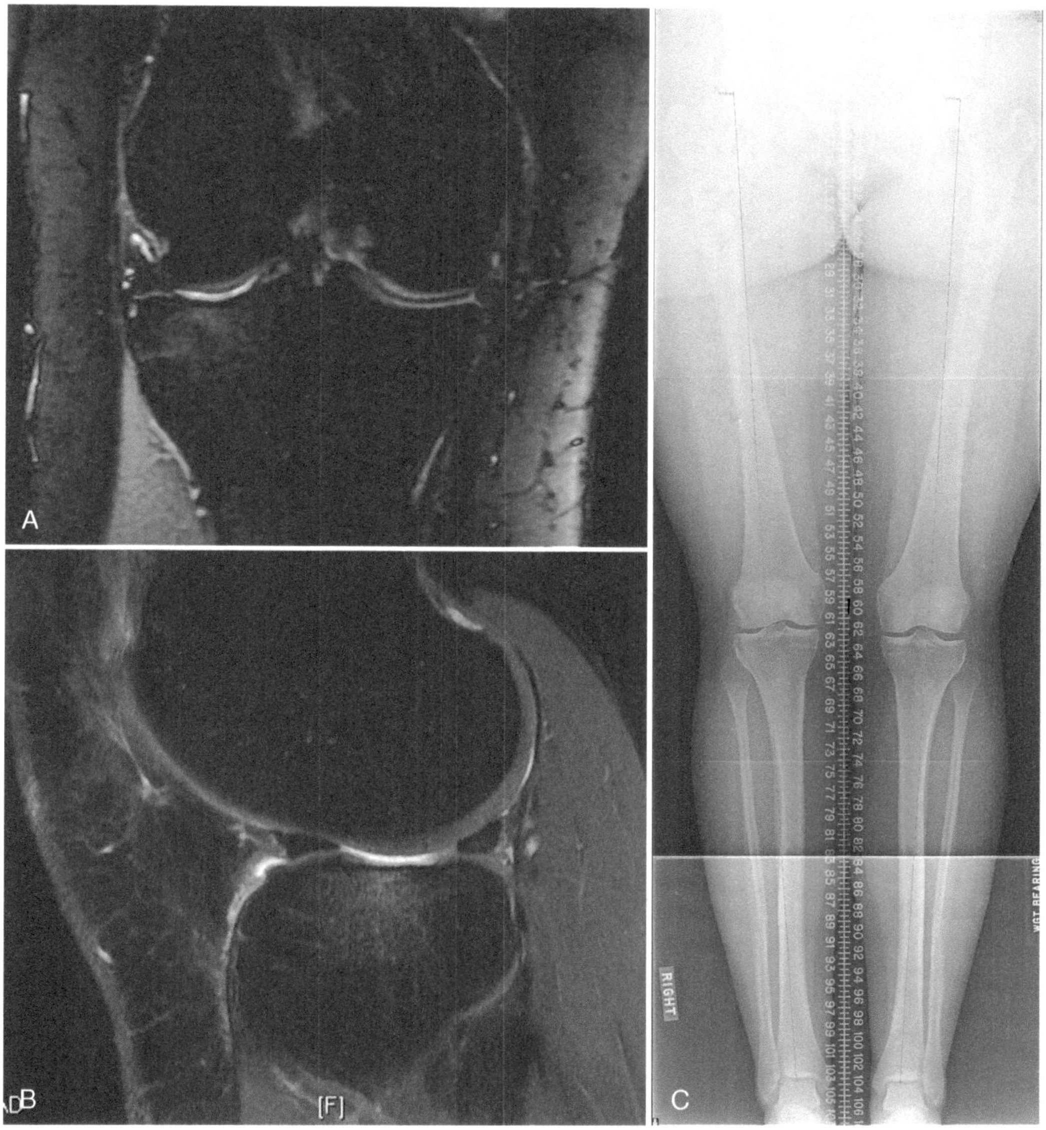

• **Fig. 9.13** Case example of a 19-year-old woman with a twisting work-related injury to the lateral compartment of her right knee. Fat-suppressed images include (A) a coronal magnetic resonance imaging (MRI) scan and (B) a sagittal MRI scan demonstrating bone marrow edema under the lateral tibial plateau with full-thickness articular cartilage loss to the lateral tibial plateau with an intact femoral surface and meniscus. (C) Long alignment weight-bearing x-ray films demonstrate valgus malalignment of the right knee with mechanical axis to the lateral tibial spine and 3 degrees of mechanical valgus.

Continued

for restoring the articular surface shape with the microsuturing technique is important (Fig. 9.16). The medial and lateral margins of the debrided defect should be vertical to the subchondral bone and the proximal and distal margins should be slightly sloped to insure that tracking is without mechanical symptoms to the patient. However, when cartilage is thin, circumferential vertical margins are necessary. The microsuture technique in this situation is even more critical to restore the normal median ridge of the patella and insure that the membrane cover is not bottomed out on the subchondral bone so that there is always a cavity for the cell suspension to grow to the membrane surface.

At completion of the transplant, the tibial tubercle is fixated in a central and normalized position for the extensor mechanism. A vastus medialis oblique (VMO) advancement is then performed bringing the VMO under the medial patellar sleeve to advance and tension the VMO such that the patella may move 30% of its width medial and lateral in full extension without subluxation completely. The VMO muscle then helps to elevate the patella away from the trochlea decompressing it further as a soft tissue sleeve in addition to the TTO elevation. This is performed with no. 2 and Ethibond sutures with a horizontal mattress stitch (see Chapter 12; Figs. 12.25 and 12.27). If there is trochlea dysplasia that is accounting for continued medial and lateral instability, the medial sleeve repair is taken down and a trochleoplasty is performed as the last step of stabilizing the patellar extensor mechanism and the soft tissue sleeve

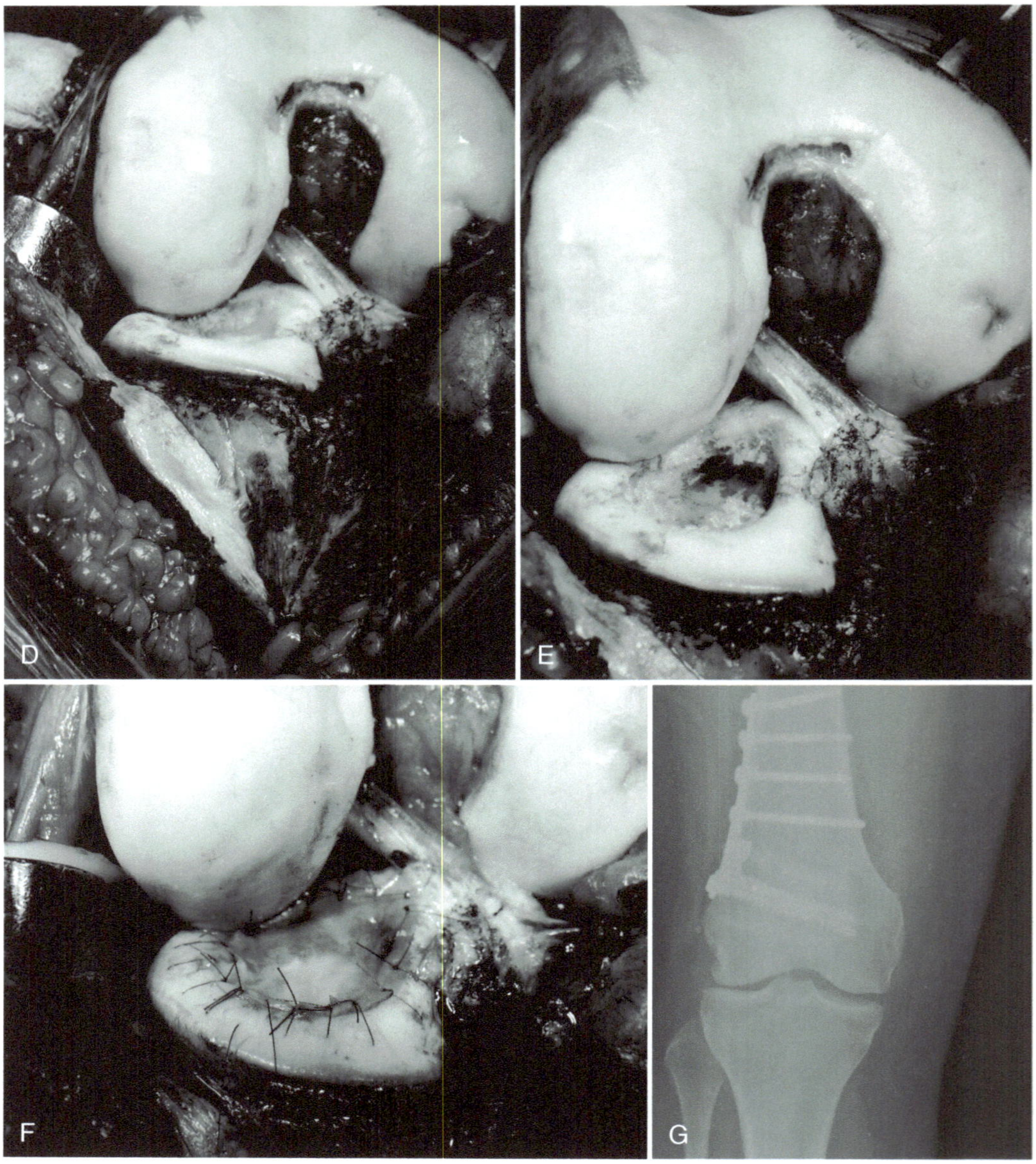

• **Fig. 9.13—cont'd** (D) Varus-producing femoral osteotomy and lateral tibial plateau autologous chondrocyte implantation (ACI) are performed through a longitudinal incision just to the lateral border of the patella and tibial tubercle. A lateral parapatellar arthrotomy is performed and the intermeniscal ligament is incised. A lateral subperiosteal peel, which includes the coronary ligament of the lateral meniscus and a portion of the iliotibial band, is performed to the posterior lateral corner of the tibia at the popliteus hiatus of the lateral meniscus. The patella is subluxed into the medial parapatellar gutter, the knee is hyperflexed, and the tibia is internally rotated to deliver the lateral tibial plateau. This technique gives excellent exposure to the entire lateral tibial plateau. Through the same incision proximally the quadriceps is split between the vastus lateralis and the rectus intermedius muscles. The vastus lateralis is dissected laterally to the posterior lateral corner of the femur and the linea aspera. A femoral varus-producing osteotomy is performed through the same dissection, which is an extensile Henry approach to the knee. (E) Radical debridement of the chondral defect of the lateral tibial plateau exposes its margins circumferentially. (F) The ACI graft is microsutured and its margins are sealed with fibrin glue. A single suture is left long laterally to allow injection of the autologous chondrocyte suspension and is easily closed and sealed. (G) Final radiographic appearance after femoral varus-producing osteotomy with lateral tibial plateau ACI graft.

is readvanced and fixated as before. Congenital trochlear dysplasia is an uncommon factor contributing to patellofemoral maltracking. It is best assessed by preoperative CT scan demonstrating a flattened or convex superior trochlear capturing entry point. Treatment is by surgical trochleoplasty, combined with patellar realignment as necessary (see Chapter 12; Figs. 12.33–12.35). Results of trochleoplasty for trochlear dysplasia have been excellent.[8]

ACI With OCD, Prior Bone Grafting, or Single-Stage Sandwich Technique ACI

In the case of bony deficiency, such as after an osteochondral fracture or osteochondritis dissecans, the depth of the bony lesion should be assessed preoperatively through radiography or CT scan. Osteochondritis dissecans defects, on average, are 6–8 mm deep including cartilage and bone. However, the margins are gradually sloped to the deepest

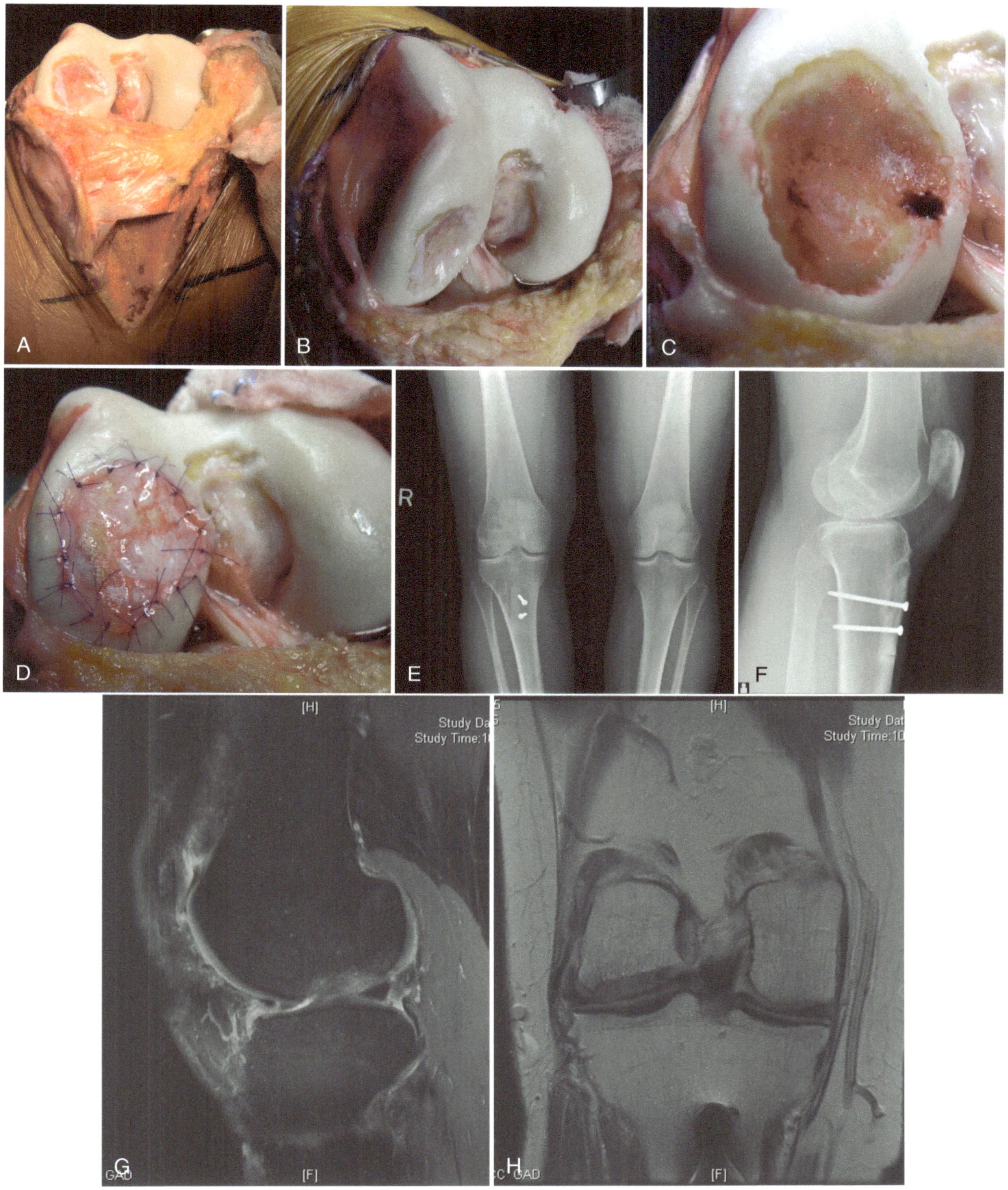

• **Fig. 9.14** Case example of a 39-year-old woman with a large osteochondritis dissecans lesion to the posterior lateral femoral condyle. This case demonstrates the use of tibial tubercle osteotomy (TTO) to expose a very posterior femoral condyle defect. (A) Tibial tubercle osteotomy is performed for a length of 6 to 7 cm in cancellous bone as an anterior medialization osteotomy. A lateral subvastus approach is performed, keeping the quadriceps entirely intact. The medial retinaculum is released to the mid-patellar pole at the level of the vastus medialis oblique insertion. Hoffa fat pad is released off the anterior tibial interval and anterior to the attachments of the menisci to the tibia. Exposure to the lateral femoral condyles is excellent. The tibial tubercle can be repositioned to a more central location to improve patellar tracking at the conclusion of the case. (B) View of lateral femoral condyle osteochondritis dissecans from the lateral aspect demonstrates just how posterior the exposure will allow you to go. It is a central lateral femoral condyle osteochondritis dissecans lesion, which is shallow at its margins and no deeper than 6 to 8 mm centrally. This defect will do well with isolated autologous chondrocyte implantation (ACI) without preliminary bone grafting or sandwich technique. (C) Close-up appearance of the defect after it is radically debrided and the tourniquet is let down to control bleeding. (D) Final appearance of the ACI graft after microsuturing of the periosteum and sealing with fibrin glue. (E) Anteroposterior and (F) lateral radiographs demonstrating well-healed TTO and well-preserved tibiofemoral joint space. (G) Two-year postoperative magnetic resonance imaging (MRI) with fat suppression demonstrating excellent cartilage repair fill to the defect. (H) Coronal MRI scan without fat suppression demonstrating complete fill. The patient remains asymptomatic.

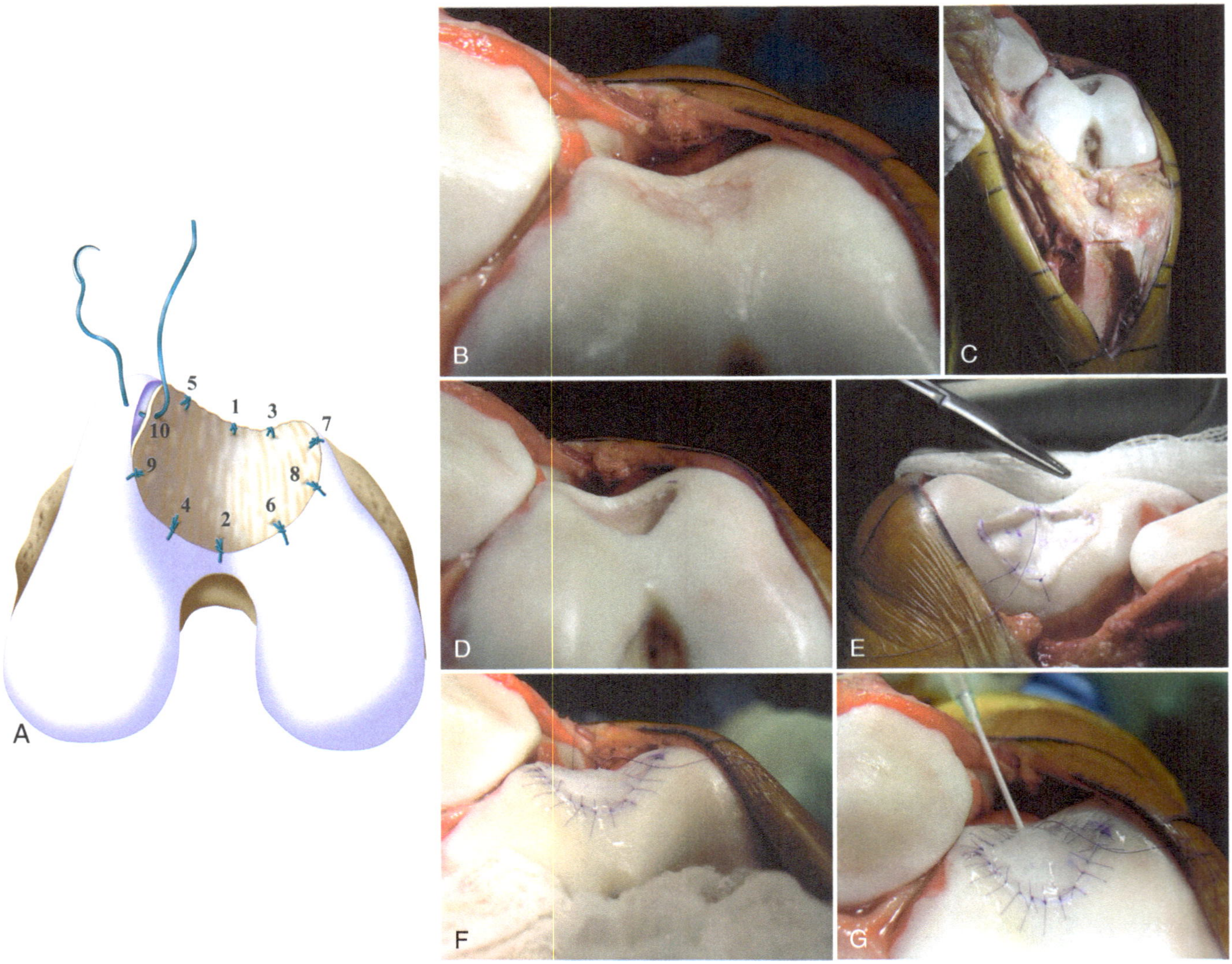

• **Fig. 9.15** Autologous chondrocyte implantation suturing technique to the trochlea, combined with tibial tubercle osteotomy. (A) When microsuturing a large defect of the trochlea across the midline sulcus, it is important to oversize the membrane in a medial to lateral direction. Suturing in a proximal to distal direction starting at the midline sulcus and working laterally and medially allows restoration of the concavity of the sulcus without undue tension on the membrane and an even depth throughout the entirety of the cartilage defect. (B) Close-up view of a trochlear defect in the left knee of a 32-year-old man who had undergone an extended tibial tubercle osteotomy. (C) The defect is clearly V shaped and will require a careful suturing technique to restore the articular topography. (D) Close-up view after debridement. (E) Microsuturing should start at the central sulcus proximal and distal (as shown) in an alternating medial and lateral pattern to restore the concavity to the trochlea. (F) Final appearance of the trochlea membranes sutured in place and sealed with fibrin glue. The superior opening sutures are left long. (G) Injection of autologous chondrocyte suspension underneath the opening, which was closed after the defect was filled.

portion. These often will do well without bone grafting, using chondrocyte implantation on its own[4] (Fig. 9.17). However, defects that are greater than 1–2 cm deep clearly need preliminary bone grafting and healing prior to cartilage resurfacing or a single-stage ACI sandwich technique. In addition, shallow defects with vertical walls, those that have cystic changes deep to the subchondral bone, and those with sclerotic bases from prior marrow stimulation techniques or osteochondral grafting should be considered for bone grafting or sandwich ACI. Autologous bone grafting may be performed either arthroscopically or by open technique (Chapter 13). An interval of 6–9 months is required before second-stage articular resurfacing is performed. This allows the cancellous bone graft to harden as it is loaded with weight bearing after an initial period of 8 weeks of protected weight bearing. In this way a new subchondral bone plate is formed and minimal, if any, bleeding occurs at the time of preparation of the defect site prior to cell implantation.

A sandwich technique ACI was so named because it involves sandwiching autologous cultured chondrocytes between two layers of periosteum (Fig. 9.18). When there is a deep defect requiring bone grafting, a radical debridement and undermining of the sclerotic or necrotic bone is performed with a high-speed bur with fluid irrigation. The base is then drilled to promote vascularization of the

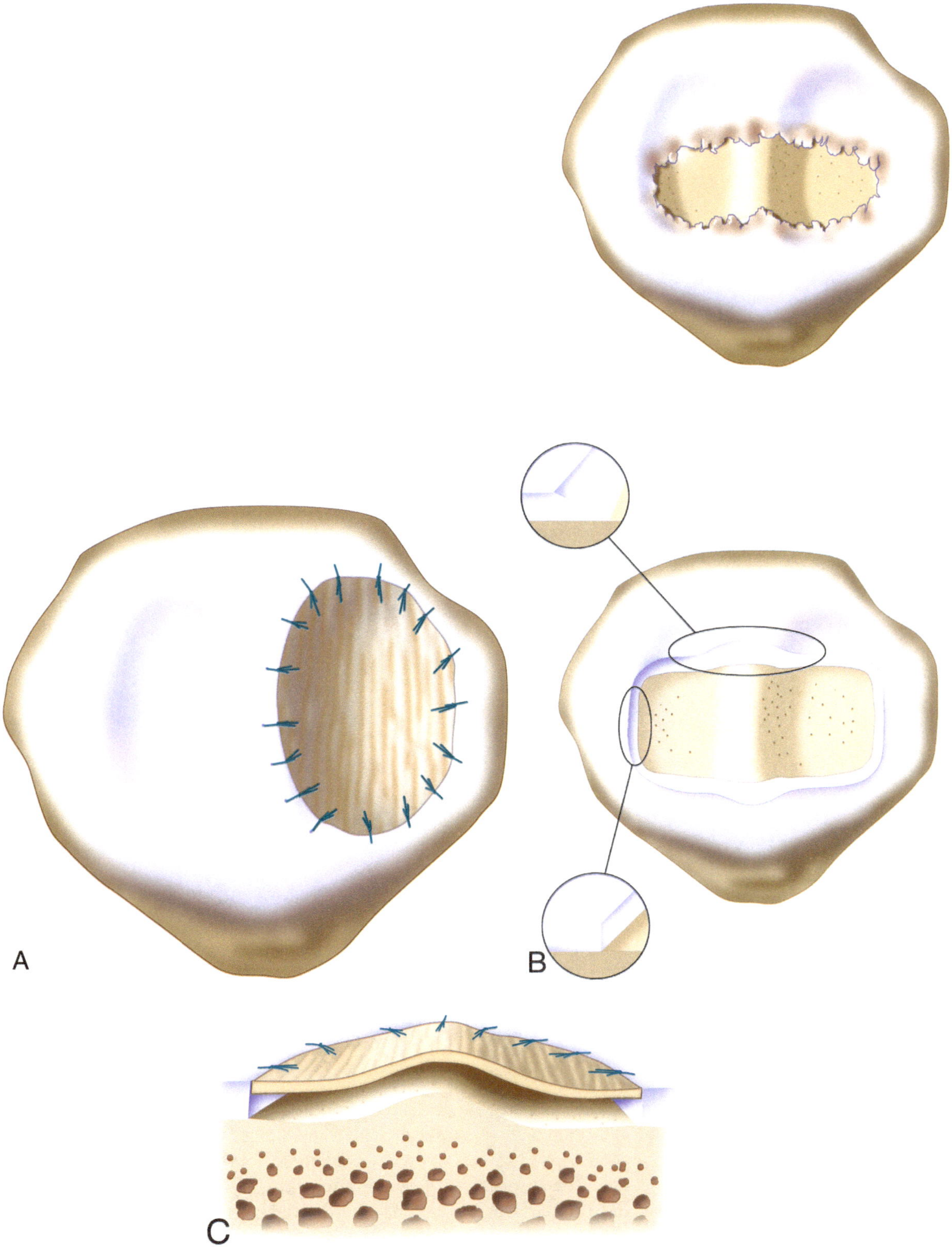

• **Fig. 9.16** Microsuturing techniques for patella defects, combined with tibial tubercle osteotomy. (A) Isolated medial or lateral patella facet is a flat surface and easy to microsuture flush with the articular surface. (B) When the defect is large, as in this Fulkerson patella type IV chondral defect (pan-patellar), a good result depends on good debridement technique as well as microsuturing. If the cartilage is thick, bleeding and trailing edge should be slightly beveled to allow easy tracking in the proximal to distal direction and vertically on the medial and lateral margins to allow maximal membrane stability. (C) As in the trochlea, microsuturing should start at the apex or median ridge of the patella to "pitch the tent" and should then alternate medially and laterally in a proximal to distal fashion to restore the articular topography of the patella. This technique will maintain a uniform cavity deep to the membrane so that articular cartilage growth develops evenly to the limiting membrane.

Continued

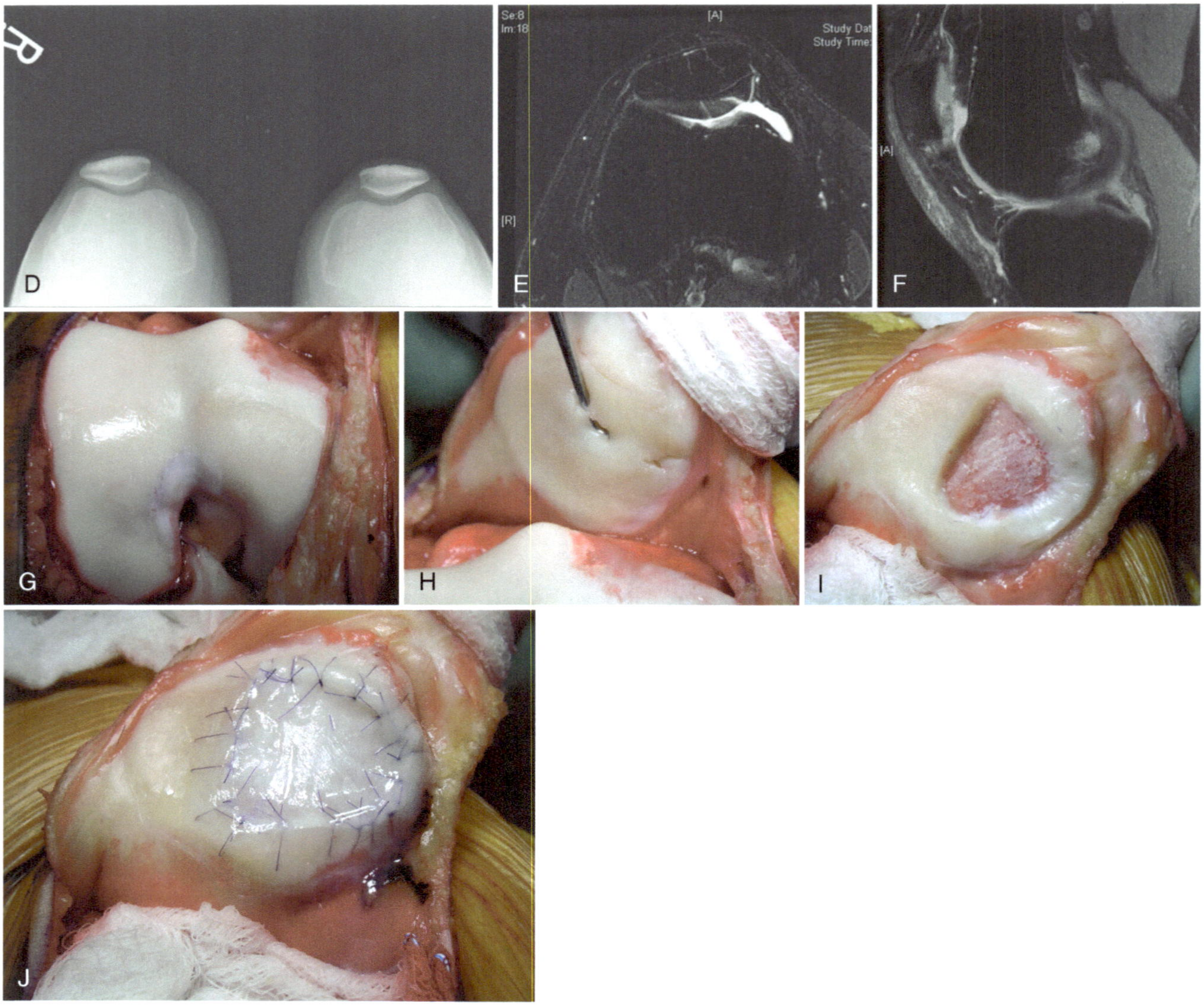

• **Fig. 9.16—cont'd** (D) Case example of a 42-year-old woman with chronic anterior knee pain bilaterally. Skyline x-ray films demonstrate well-preserved joint spaces. (E) Axial magnetic resonance imaging (MRI) scan with fat suppression demonstrates patellar tilt with fissuring and breakdown of the articular cartilage of the median ridge and medial facet of the patella. (F) Sagittal MRI scan demonstrates the same patellar damage but intact articular surfaces of the trochlea. (G) Extensile tibial tubercle exposure reveals an intact trochlea as noted by MRI. A fibrous cover over the biopsy site for autologous chondrocyte implantation is performed at the lateral intercondylar notch. (H) Metal probe demonstrates delamination and fissuring of the central and medial patellar surfaces. (I) Radical debridement of the damaged articular cartilage back to native subchondral bone and healthy cartilage margins. (J) Final appearance of microsuture collagen cover and restoration of articular topography of the patella.

defect and autologous morselized cancellous bone is used to fill the defect to the level of the subchondral bone plate. A neural patty with thrombin and fibrin glue is applied to the bone graft while the tourniquet is let down. The autologous bone graft is saturated with blood and the surface kept dry. A layer of periosteum or collagen membrane is placed and fixated with fibrin glue or additional transosseous sutures with the cambium layer facing outward toward the joint. The surface is inspected to ensure that there is no marrow-derived bleeding through the membrane and into the defect. A second periosteal layer is then sutured flush to the articular cartilage as per usual ACI procedure. It is then sealed with fibrin glue and checked for water integrity. The saline is aspirated from the defect and autologous cultured chondrocytes are injected as per ACI, the opening sutured over and sealed with fibrin glue. Hence the autologous cultured chondrocytes are in a bioactive chamber with the underlying bone deficiency having been restored and the marrow-derived cells are separated from the autologous cultured chondrocytes, which are in a watertight chamber facing the cambium layer of periosteum on both sides.

ACI Plus ACL

Cartilage repair in the face of cruciate insufficiency can jeopardize a newly regenerating cartilage graft. Staged or concomitant surgery should be performed with the goal of preventing shear forces and instability episodes from damaging a healing graft.

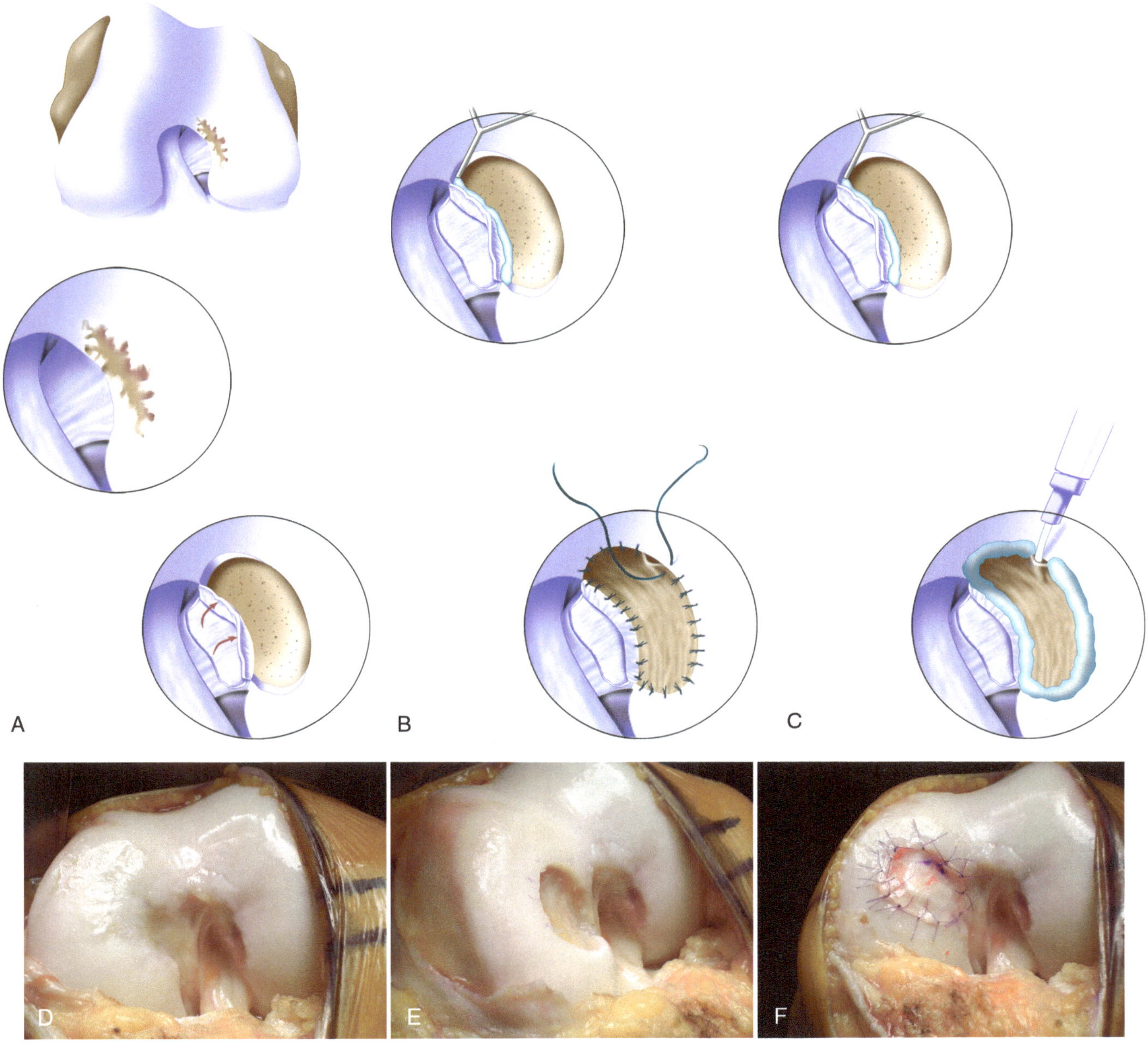

• **Fig. 9.17** Illustrations and examples of the technique for autologous chondrocyte implantation with uncontained osteochondritis dissecans and deep defects requiring a sandwich technique. (A) The intercondylar aspect of the medial femoral condyle is a classic location for osteochondritis dissecans. After debridement, the defect becomes uncontained. The technique for making this a contained defect involves releasing the synovium from the posterior cruciate ligament and leaving it attached to its intercondylar attachment, as shown in the illustration. (B) Fibrin glue is placed on the medial aspect of the synovial attachment. The periosteum can then be microsutured to the surrounding articular cartilage and synovial membrane. (C) It is then sealed with Tisseel fibrin glue and the autologous cultured chondrocytes are injected. The opening is sutured over and sealed. (D) Clinical example of a left knee medial femoral condyle osteochondritis dissecans defect. The lesion is uncontained on the synovium of the posterior cruciate ligament (PCL). (E) After radical debridement, the synovial aspect of the PCL is brought up flush with the articular cartilage off the PCL. (F) Microsuturing and sealing the defect with Tisseel fibrin glue maintains the defect in a contained fashion.

If there is any medial femoral condyle defect with ACL insufficiency, my preference is a single open incision from the superior medial pole of the patella to the inferior aspect of the tibial tubercle. A medial parapatellar arthrotomy is performed with the patella subluxed. An open technique ACL reconstruction is easily performed with only the femoral fixation having been completed with ACI to the medial femoral condyle (Fig. 9.19). Once the autologous cultured chondrocytes are injected into the medial femoral condyle and sealed with fibrin glue, the knee is brought into extension, the tibia is translated posteriorly, and the tibial fixation completes the procedure with wound closure.

For the lateral femoral condyle defect, two choices are available. If the defect is more anterior, I prefer the same approach as that used for a medial femoral condyle with hyperflexion and eversion of the patella and ACI to the

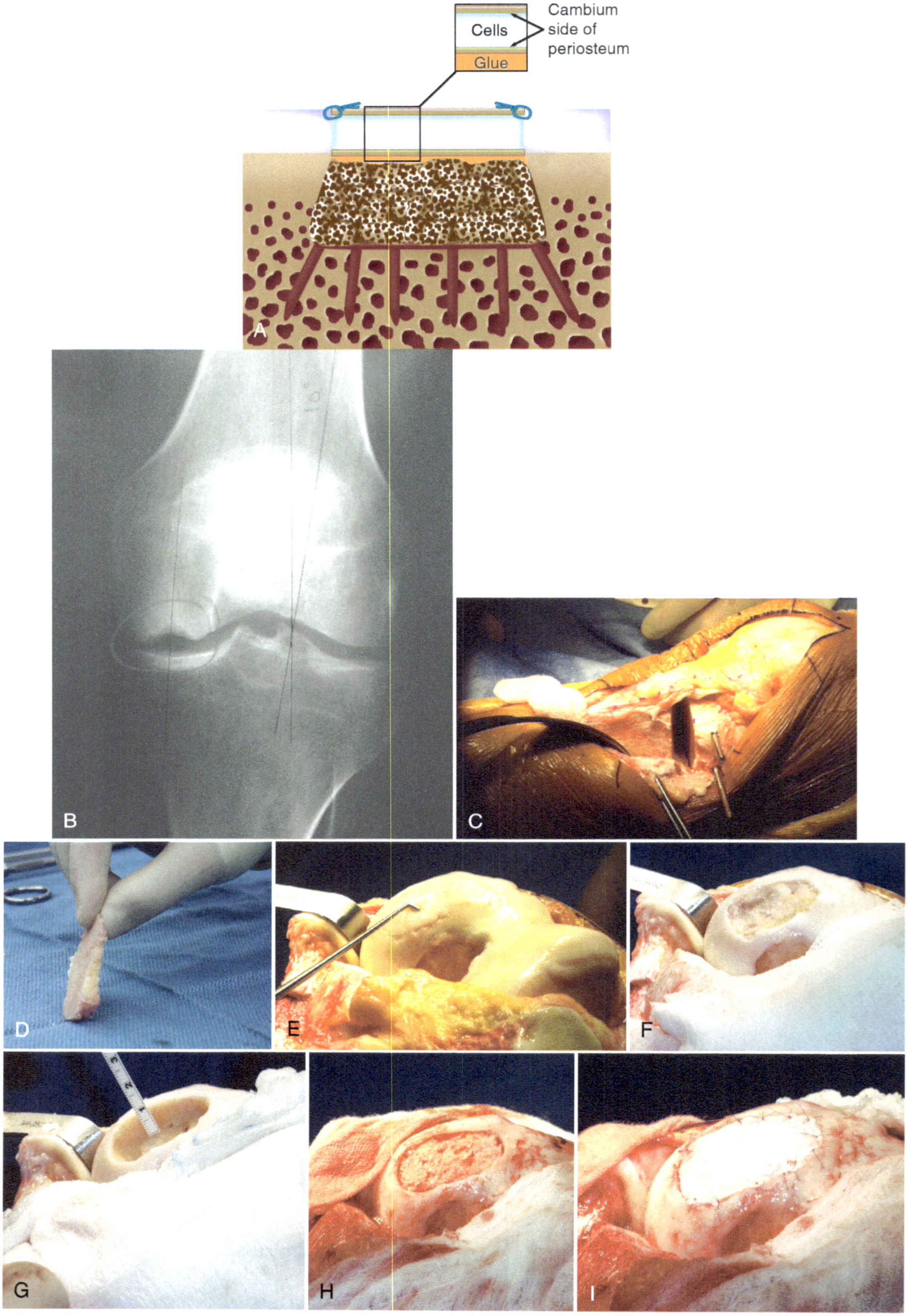

• **Fig. 9.18** Diagrammatic representation and clinical example of a sandwich technique autologous chondrocyte implantation (ACI) for an osteochondral defect. (A) Diagrammatic representation of the final appearance of an osteochondral defect treated with ACI sandwich technique. As described in Chapter 13, the osseous portion of the defect undergoes radical debridement of the necrotic or sclerotic bone, drilling deep to the osseous defect

Continued

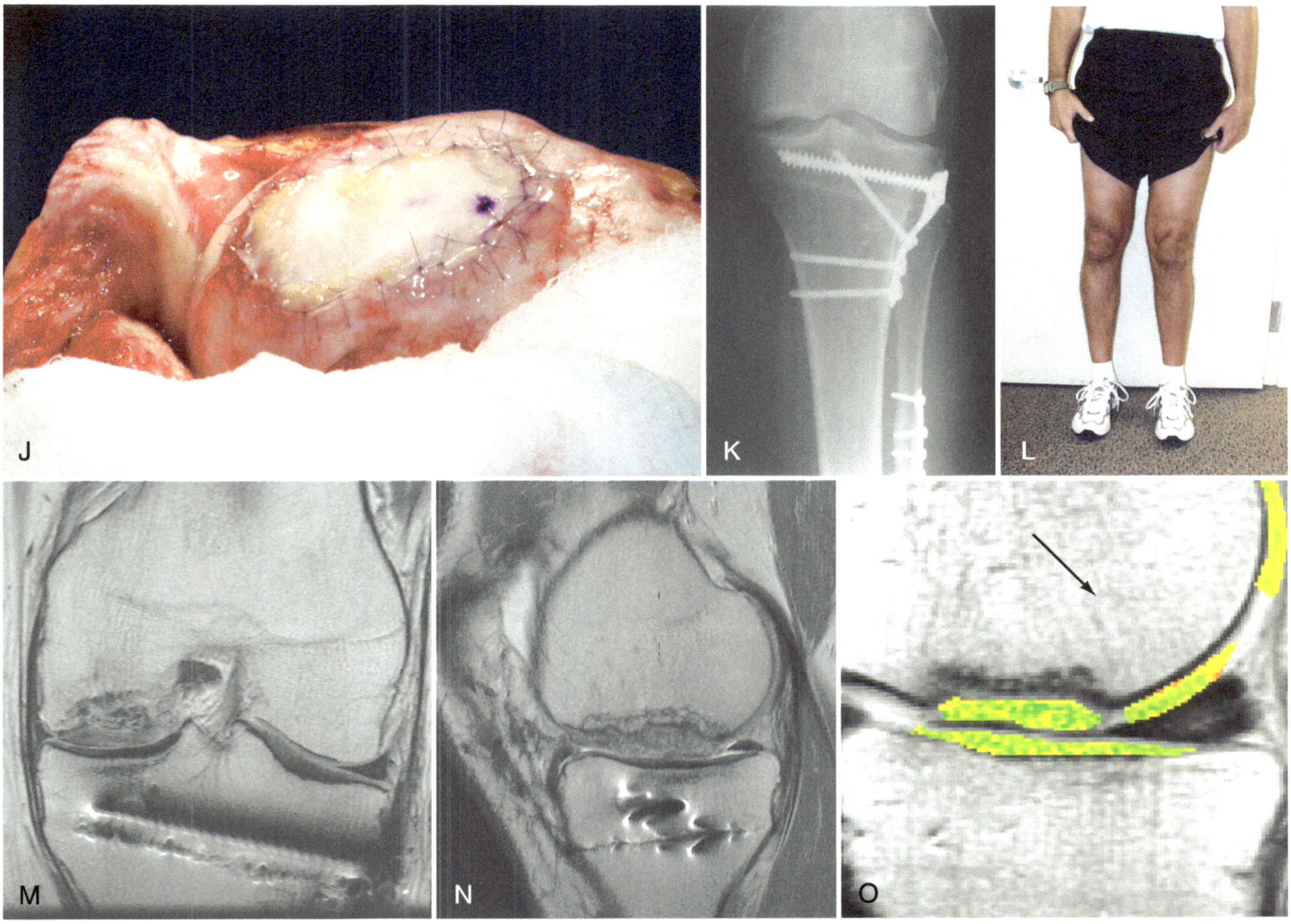

• **Fig. 9.18—cont'd** to promote revascularization, and autologous cancellous bone grafting to the level of the subchondral bone. At the level of the articular surface, a membrane or periosteum is used to contain the marrow-derived cellular response. A limiting membrane is sealed to the autologous bone graft with fibrin glue. If periosteum is used, the cambium layer faces the articular surface *(pale green)*. For the second membrane at the level of the articular surface, the cambium layer faces deep so that the two layers of cambium tissue sandwich the autologous cultured chondrocytes. The underlying marrow response is separated as a watertight separate chamber. (B) Clinical example of ACI sandwich technique in a middle-aged man with a varus knee and spontaneous osteonecrosis of the medial femoral condyle. The standing anteroposterior (AP) x-ray film demonstrates resorption and collapse of the medial femoral condyle with osteonecrosis *(circled area)*. The mechanical axis falls directly through the center of this lesion (single line). A 10-degree angular correction to the lateral tibial spine *(intersecting lines)* is required to unload the lesion by 2 degrees into mechanical valgus. (C) Lateral view of the proximal tibia bone deficiency demonstrates a 10-degree angular wedge of bone that was removed to allow performance of closing wedge osteotomy. (D) Autologous bone wedge from the closing wedge osteotomy will be morselized and used as cancellous bone graft to the medial femoral condyle avascular defect after it is radically debrided. (E) Probe demonstrates the medial femoral condyles avascular necrosis articular surface, which is ballotable and mobile. (F) Medial femoral condyles and defect after loose articular surface was easily removed. (G) Defect measured 1 cm deep after radical debridement of necrotic bony bed. (H) Appearance of medial femoral condyles after cancellous autologous bone grafting and packing to the level of the subchondral bony surface. (I) Periosteal membrane is sealed to the subchondral bone with Tisseel fibrin glue and tacked peripherally deep to the articular surface. A neural patty is applied with pressure to the periosteal cover while the tourniquet is let down to allow development of a watertight bed to the level that will undergo ACI. (J) Final appearance after the second periosteal cover, which is microsutured flush to the articular surface. *Blue dot* denotes the superficial fibrous periosteal layer surface of the membrane. The chamber between the two periosteal cambium layers is injected with autologous cultured chondrocytes and the margins are sealed with fibrin glue. (K) Standing AP radiograph 1 year after closing wedge valgus-producing osteotomy with ACI sandwich technique to the medial femoral condyle. The joint space is well maintained in the medial compartment. (L) Frontal view of the clinical appearance of left knee of the patient 1 year after closing wedge valgus osteotomy plus sandwich ACI. Note that the right knee is in slight varus and the left knee is in slight valgus. (M) Proton density magnetic resonance imaging (MRI) scan, coronal view, demonstrating excellent repair tissue cover of the medial femoral condyles. (N) Sagittal view with the same findings as shown in (M). (O) Sagittal delayed gadolinium-enhanced MRI scan of cartilage demonstrating proteoglycan content equal to adjacent nontransplanted cartilage, denoted by *arrow*. Nine years after surgery, the patient remains pain-free and is athletically active.

lateral femoral condyle (Fig. 9.20). The cells are injected and the patella is reduced with the knee extended and the tibia posteriorly translated. After femoral fixation for the ACL graft has been completed, the tibial fixation is performed and the wound closed.

If the defect is more posterior on the lateral femoral condyle, I prefer an arthroscopically performed ACL followed by a lateral arthrotomy and open ACI to the lateral femoral condyle.

Anterior cruciate rehabilitation is modified to exclude closed-chain resisted strengthening exercises until 3 months

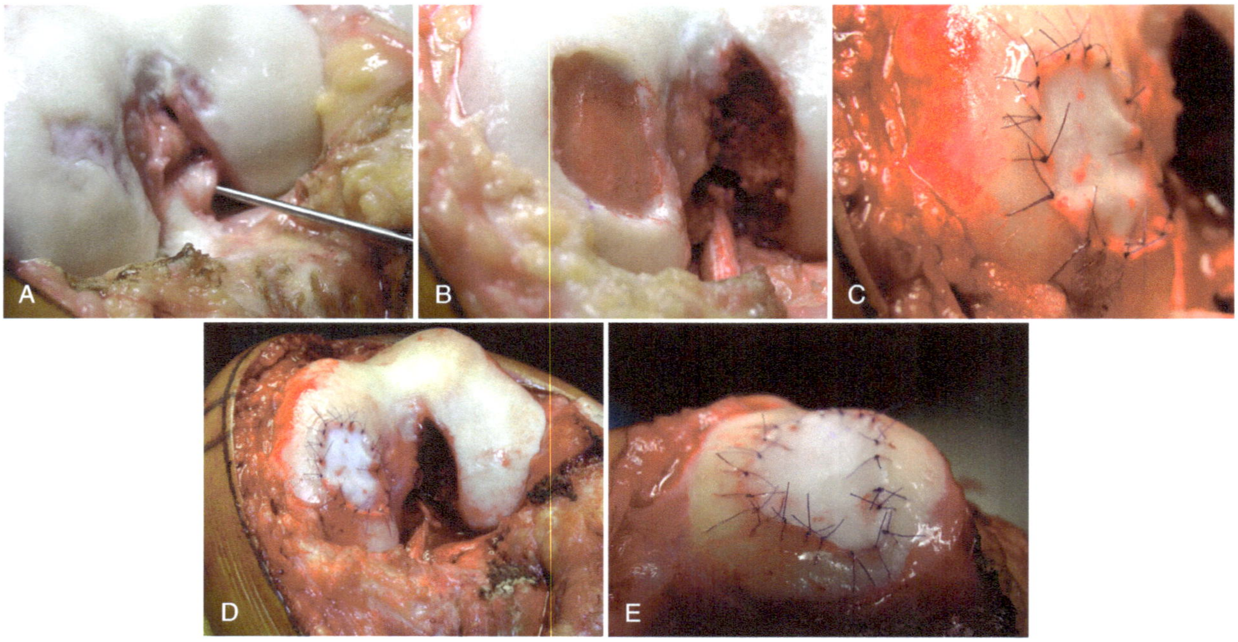

• **Fig. 9.19** Anterior cruciate ligament (ACL) reconstruction with autologous chondrocyte implantation (ACI) to the medial femoral condyle and patella in a 40-year-old man. (A) Open medial parapatellar arthrotomy, nerve hook demonstrating lax ACL torn from its femoral attachment. A medial femoral condyle defect with adjacent undermining is evident. (B) Radical debridement of the damaged articular cartilage to stable margins. When an open medial arthrotomy is performed, my preference is an open ACL reconstruction and open notchplasty. Tunnel placements are easy to acquire and perform. The same landmarks used arthroscopically are used for open technique. The femoral tunnel placement with the mini C-arm in a lateral position. (C and D) Final appearance of ACI grafts microsutured in place on the medial femoral condyle. (E) ACI appearance on the patella. Two years postoperatively, the patient has returned to pivoting sports and had no limitation.

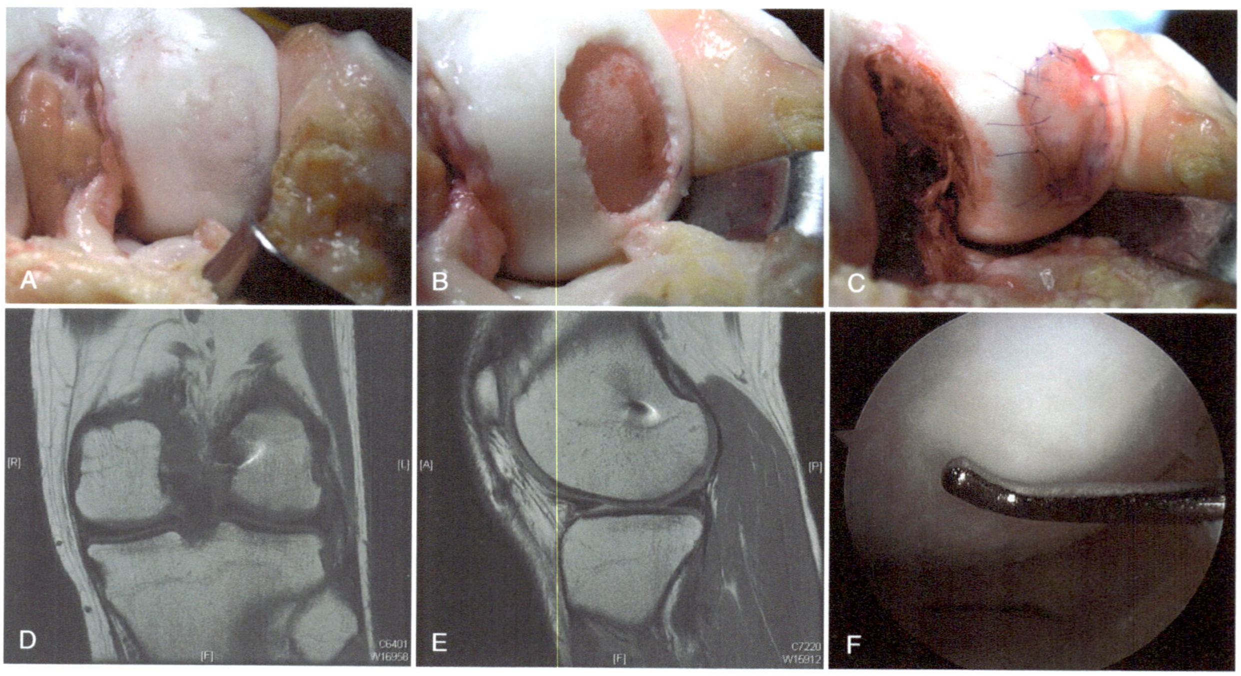

• **Fig. 9.20** Anterior cruciate ligament (ACL) reconstruction with autologous chondrocyte implantation (ACI) to the lateral femoral condyle in an 18-year-old man. (A) Clinical appearance of the lateral femoral condyles defect as viewed through a medial parapatellar arthrotomy showing a lax ACL, femoral attachment injury. The other option in this case would be an arthroscopic ACL with lateral parapatellar arthrotomy after ACL reconstruction to perform the ACI. (B) Lateral femoral condyle defect after debridement. (C) ACL reconstruction with lateral femoral condyle ACI. (D) Coronal proton density magnetic resonance imaging (MRI) scan 1 year after surgery demonstrating excellent ACI repair tissue to the lateral femoral condyle. (E) Sagittal proton density MRI scan 1 year after surgery demonstrating excellent ACI repair tissue. (F) Confirmation arthroscopy 1 year after surgery. The patient is a high-level athlete and wishes to return to sports. I frequently perform MRI and second-look arthroscopy to confirm that a patient is ready to progress to high-level activity safely.

after combined surgery to prevent excessive compressive load to the chondral repair site. Four to 6 months is required before these exercises may be started and leg presses and squats are avoided for 1 year after surgery. Rehabilitation follows that for ACI, which is the rate-limiting process in recovery.

ACI Plus Meniscal Allograft

When there is meniscal deficiency in combination with articular cartilage injury, I have found that it is much more critical on the lateral compartment of the knee than the medial to transplant the meniscus with the ACI. Medial injuries are frequently accompanied by varus malalignment. I presently have 25 years of results following valgus-producing tibial osteotomy with ACI to the medial femoral condyle in the presence of an absent meniscus with excellent clinical function and no evidence of joint space loss on standing x-ray examinations.

However, this is not always the case in the lateral compartment. Because of its meniscal dependency, the lateral compartment degenerates rapidly once the meniscus is lost even in the presence of a normal mechanical axial alignment. If there is valgus malalignment, the progression is much more rapid.

Meniscal transplantation can be performed arthroscopically using a slot technique, a posterior counterincision for posterior horn fixation followed by open arthrotomy, debridement of the chondral defects and microsuturing the periosteal membrane and ACI.

I have found it to be more straightforward to produce a slightly longer midline incision, develop a posterior deep fascial flap, and make the posterior capsular dissection for transcapsular meniscal fixation through a single open incision (Chapter 14). The defect is debrided and the periosteal suturing performed. A slot technique is easily performed with passage of the meniscus posteriorly and posterior horn fixation. The body and anterior horn of the menisci are then easily repaired to the capsule by open technique. Transosseous fixation sutures can also be placed through the body and anterior horns of the meniscus to the tibial surface preventing postoperative extrusion of the meniscus. ACI is completed when the periosteum is glued, the cells are injected, the periosteum is closed and sealed, and the wound is closed. A single set-up without arthroscopic equipment makes the procedure quite easy. Excision of any posterior meniscal remnant is usually performed arthroscopically at the time of the cartilage biopsy so that it is not necessary at the time of the open meniscal transplant with ACI.

ACI After Marrow Stimulation Techniques

We have found that alterations are common in the subchondral bone after drilling abrasion and microfracture. The bone may develop large intralesional osteophytes or just a thickened sclerotic and near cortical subchondral bone surface. Occasionally we have encountered subchondral bone cysts at the locations of the drill entry or microfracture pick. For this reason an MRI scan is useful prior to pursuing ACI after marrow stimulation technique to assess the extent of intralesional osteophyte formation, subchondral bone marrow edema, and the possibility of cyst formation.

Adequate debridement of the articular defect is the most important aspect of dealing with a previously marrow-stimulated subchondral bone. A radical cartilage debridement back to native cartilage and subchondral bone is the starting point. This identifies the level of the native subchondral bone and outlines the size of intralesional osteophyte or sclerotic subchondral bone. Large intralesional osteophytes are removed with a rongeur and a 5-mm high-speed bur is used to blend in the sclerotic or osteophytic bone to the level of the native subchondral bone. I have found that bleeding is unusual in this thickened bone surface. A template is made of the defect and the defect is prepared for microsuturing. The tourniquet is let down to assess the vascularity of the subchondral bone and deal with any excessive bleeding. Neural patties soaked in thrombin and epinephrine, fibrin glue, and judicious use of electrocautery are utilized if there is any bleeding. The periosteal cover is then microsutured in the usual fashion flush to the articular surface, sealed with fibrin glue, and the autologous chondrocyte suspension injected underneath the membrane and sutured over and sealed.

If subchondral cysts are encountered, these are burred out completely, autologous bone grafting is performed to the area of the cyst, the surface over the bone graft is sealed with Tisseel fibrin glue and a periosteal membrane, and the tourniquet is let down. If all is dry, a second periosteal cover is sutured over the entire defect, the cells injected, and the procedure completed. In this way, a segmental ACI sandwich technique is performed in which only the portion of the defect that is bone grafted is sealed watertight with fibrin glue and a periosteal cover to ensure that the entire area to be transplanted is watertight and not contaminated with marrow-derived cells.

ACI in Osteoarthritis, Uncontained Defects, and Sclerotic Subchondral Bone

When treating young patients with more advanced articular injury who have early osteoarthritis, several technically difficult situations may be presented upon open arthrotomy. Findings in the osteoarthritic knee include large ulcerative focal chondral defects with indistinct borders, chondral defects that become uncontained adjacent peripheral osteophytes, thin peripheral cartilage margins to focal defects, findings similar to post marrow stimulation techniques such as thickened subchondral bone, intralesional osteophyte formation, and subchondral cysts, and "kissing lesions" (femur on tibia and patella on trochlea and peripheral osteophytes around the patella, which may engage and produce articular injury to the trochlea).

A preoperative assessment of background factors is critical to the successful management of these complex reconstructive challenges. A decision should be made in advance of the surgery whether osteotomy of the tibiofemoral joint or tibial tubercle is required for exposure or unloading of a large defect or kissing defects. This will often make the surgical exposure easier when it is planned in advance.

The debridement of articular injuries upon exposure of the knee joint should preserve all peripheral osteophytes initially because they may be required to manage poorly contained articular cartilage injuries. Transosseous drill holes through peripheral osteophytes on the femur or tibia are commonly required in some of these larger lesions (Fig. 9.21). The subchondral bone may be sclerotic and the cartilage margins thin. In this case, I start with a ring curette and remove the sclerotic subchondral bone until the depth of the defect is 2 to 3 mm from the adjacent thinned cartilage. Articular chondrocytes will easily grow to fill these defects with articular cartilage. In this way, there is a contained defect and room for growth without undue pressure on the chondrocyte suspension. If the bone is very stiff, a 5-mm high-speed bur is useful as long as it is copiously irrigated to ensure that there is no thermal injury to the underlying bone.

Peripheral osteophytes around the patella are usually removed with a small sagittal saw obliquely to the osteophyte to avoid producing a 90-degree surface that will impinge or damage the trochlea. If there are kissing lesions in the patellofemoral joint, I routinely perform a decompressive tibial tubercle anteromedialization osteotomy.

If all is done well, at the completion of the radical debridement and preparation of the chondral defects for microsuturing of the periosteum or collagen membrane, the knee should look relatively healthy with a few large potholes. The radical debridement and preparation of the arthritic knee is the key to successful reconstruction in addition to the management of background factors. Periosteal suturing to maintain a cavity without the membrane bottoming out on the subchondral bone is essential and a suture technique for this is critical as described earlier in this chapter.

Early motion of the tibiofemoral joint and patellofemoral mobilizations are critical to success of these complex

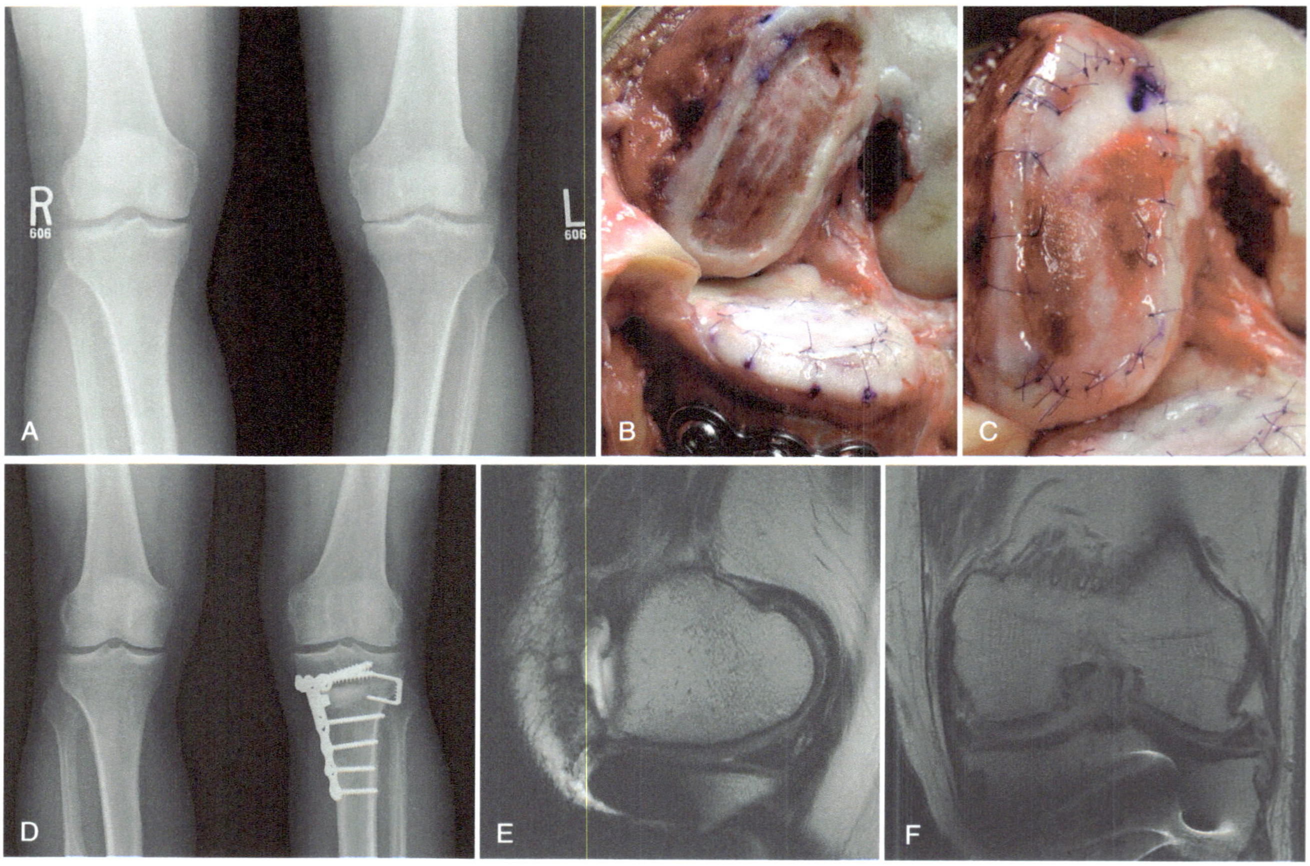

• **Fig. 9.21** Autologous chondrocyte implantation and early osteoarthritis. (A) Standing anteroposterior x-ray films of a 51-year-old former marathon runner demonstrating near bone-on-bone changes with varus malalignment of the left knee. (B) Open appearance of the medial compartment of the left knee. Uncontained defects are present on both the medial femoral condyle and tibial plateau. A medial subperiosteal peel was performed, taking down the superficial and deep medial collateral ligaments with a meniscal sleeve. This technique allows exposure of the entire medial joint compartment and concomitant opening wedge tibial valgus osteotomy. The uncontained defects were managed by maintaining the peripheral osteophytes. Transosseous drill holes were performed through the osteophytes using a small C-wire and marking the holes with a blue marking pen as noted. The 6.0 Vicryl sutures are passed through the membrane via the transosseous drill holes and anchored back to the membrane to develop a contained cavity that will accept autologous cultured chondrocytes as noted on the tibial surface. (C) The membrane on the femoral surface is microsutured using transosseous drill holes through osteophytes to anchor the defect in place. (D) One-year postoperative weight-bearing x-ray films demonstrating restoration of joint space after transplantation of "kissing" defects. (E) Sagittal proton density magnetic resonance imaging (MRI) scan showing cartilage repair on the knee or from condyle and tibial plateau. (F) Coronal MRI scan showing the same findings as in (E).

reconstructions. Adhesions and arthrofibrosis will jeopardize any good surgical reconstruction. I routinely use anti-adhesion membrane (Seprafilm, hyaluronic acid, cellulose, Genzyme Biosurgery, Cambridge, MA; FDA off-label use) on the synovial lining tissues of the joint at the end of the procedure to try to prevent this from occurring and have found it to be useful.

After Care/Rehabilitation

Prophylactic intravenous cephalosporin antibiotics are used for 24–48 hours after surgery.

There are three main goals in the postoperative period: (1) range of motion exercises to enhance chondrocyte regeneration and decrease the likelihood of intra-articular adhesions; (2) protected graft loading for 6–12 weeks after surgery to prevent the likelihood of periosteal overload and central degeneration or delamination of the graft; and (3) isometric muscle exercises to regain muscle tone and prevent atrophy.

CPM is started as soon as cell attachment has occurred after 6 hours or the next day. With bearing femoral condyles, CPM is increased to regain a full range of motion as tolerated by the patient with a very slow cycle setting of approximately 2 minutes. This is utilized for approximately 6–8 hours daily for up to 6 weeks postoperatively. This schedule is based on experimental work[9] that demonstrated an enhancement of the quality of repair tissue via this modality and clinical work[10] that demonstrated an increased repair tissue fill with CPM for 6–8 hours per day for 6–8 weeks postoperatively. At this time the exact quantity and duration of CPM for ACI has not been determined. It is clear, however, that patients are comfortable while on the machine and that it decreases the likelihood of intra-articular adhesions by motion.

CPM for defects of the trochlea is less aggressive. Initially, CPM is used for a maximum range of 0–40 degrees. The remainder of the motion is obtained by patients dangling their leg over the edge of the bed to regain further motion. CPM from 40 to 70 degrees is not recommended as maximal patellofemoral contact forces occur in this range. However, with collagen membranes this angle can be increased because it appears that these membranes are more resistant to tearing and degeneration. In addition, the surgeon must consider whether this is a large pan trochlear lesion versus a flat trochlea repair on either the medial or lateral trochlear facet. No restriction in the range of motion would be required if this were the case.

Weight-bearing for femoral condyles is protected at weight of leg-"foot flat" touch weight-bearing status for 6 weeks postoperatively on crutches. Thereafter weight-bearing is increased to full body weight by 12 weeks postoperatively. This is done as follows: weeks 7 and 8, 1/3 body weight; weeks 9 and 10, 2/3 body weight; weeks 11 and 12, full body weight on crutches. Thereafter the patient is instructed to use one crutch in the opposite arm and to switch to a cane when comfortable. Each patient's progress is individualized and guided by symptoms. If weight-bearing discomfort, catching, locking, or swelling of the knee occur, the weight-bearing status and activity level are decreased to that tolerated by the patient. These may indicate that the graft is undergoing overload, with stimulation of the subchondral bone resulting in pain. On average it is 4 to 4 1/2 months before patients discard their canes and are able to walk relatively comfortably with a small effusion. The recovery time from larger lesions is longer. At this time, non-impact activities such as long-distance walking, cycling, swimming, and cross-country skiing are encouraged. Running is not permitted until graft hardness is similar to adjacent cartilage, which takes approximately 9–12 months on a weight-bearing femoral condyle lesion. Larger lesions may take as long as 18 months. Osteochondritis dissecans may take 18–24 months. Deep lesions such as osteochondritis dissecans, large weight-bearing femoral condyle lesions, or those that are bipolar such as tibia–femur kissing lesions are usually protected with an unloader brace to allow earlier weight-bearing and recovery. For an osteochondritis dissecans lesion or a large femoral condylar lesion, the unloader brace is started approximately 3 months after transplantation. However, with kissing lesions it is started within the first week after transplant to unload the opposing membrane surfaces initially and progress as comfort allows. It is soft at 6 months postoperative before an unloader brace is discontinued in the face of kissing lesions on the tibia and femur.

Lesions of the trochlea are slower in the rehabilitation process and healing. Weight-bearing status is allowed at full weight-bearing with a knee immobilizer from the onset because the weight-bearing condyles are not affected. Isometric straight leg lifts are instituted as comfort allows. Rehabilitation at maintaining decreased patellofemoral contact pressures is encouraged. At 6–8 weeks after surgery, treadmill walking backward is encouraged and active flexion and passive extension are encouraged for the first 6 weeks. Effusion is more common with trochlea repairs for up to 6 months after surgery. Stationary bicycling with low resistance is allowed as early as 3 weeks postoperatively. Kneeling, squatting, etc. are not permitted until 12–18 months following surgery, at which time graft hardness is similar to adjacent cartilage.

Many patients and their physical therapists are interested in starting weight training in the first year after ACI. I feel that this mindset has arisen from the accelerated rehabilitation protocols following anterior cruciate ligament reconstruction. However, we believe that the first year is for restoration of functional pain-free mobility for the patient. In this regard, we focus on good tibiofemoral and patellofemoral mobilizations and muscle tone in the first 1 to 3 months postoperative and attain muscle tone and function with isometrics as well as stationary bicycling. Gait training then ensues between months 3 and 6 postoperative and we encourage distance walking as comfort allows on a treadmill or outdoors with progress to an elliptical trainer. As long as use of a stationary or outdoor bicycle does not cause pain and effusions within the knee, the resistance is increased on these devices to allow strengthening of the lower extremity without overload of the transplanted knee. Rollerblading is allowed from 6 months if this activity does not cause pain. We do not allow torque loading activities until after 12 months. These would include golfing, racquet sports, and hiking that involves descending and jumping.

After 12 months, in-line jogging is permitted if the patient responds favorably without pain or swelling. Pivoting activities such as racquet sports, soccer, and golfing are allowed from 14 to 18 months postoperative. Leg presses and squats are not encouraged at any time unless they are performed at less than the patient's body weight, and a high number of repetitions are not allowed. We emphasize to the patient that their knee is not a normal knee but a prepared knee that is now improved and better with regard to functionality compared with its preoperative condition. Patients should use symptoms other than those from the knee as a barometer to gauge their activities. We have noted that patients who maintain excellent muscle tone and strength in their quadriceps and hamstring musculature through cycling and elliptical trainer strengthening for life, do well many years thereafter. Patients with leg weakness frequently complain of aching and discomfort in the operated knee.

Strengthening for trochlea lesions should involve short arc quadriceps strengthening from 0 to 30 degrees of flexion and closed-chain strengthening from the same 0 to 30 degrees range of motion. Open-chain resisted quadriceps strengthening should not be permitted for at least 12 months following ACI to the trochlea according to symptoms. I usually recommend that patients never engage in open-change resisted quadriceps strengthening if they have a patella or trochlea lesion. Closed-chain strengthening is less traumatic and forceful on transplants in these locations and is recommended instead.

Complications

Complications related to open arthrotomy include intra-articular adhesions, arthrofibrosis of the joint, and occasional superficial wound infections. To date, I have had no patients with intra-articular joint infections after ACI.

Intra-articular adhesions are uncommon except when femoral periosteum is used from the suprapatellar pouch region or a patient has a propensity for keloid formation or arthrofibrosis. These factors may enhance intra-articular fibrosis. If arthrofibrosis with stiffness occurs, a blind manipulation is not recommended. Adhesions are best released with arthroscopic lysis of adhesions after the grafts are visualized (to ensure that there are no adhesions to the grafts) (Fig. 9.22), followed by a manipulation, a drain placement in a parapatellar gutter for 24–48 hours postoperative, and early CPM.

Periosteal problems may occur 5%–40% of the time, some of them requiring intervention. In most cases, the catching response settles and the patient remains asymptomatic. This situation probably represents graft remodeling by the patient's activity level alone without delamination. However, if the catching worsens, periosteal hypertrophy is likely. The most common problems after ACI are incomplete periosteal graft incorporation to host cartilage and hypertrophic periosteal fibrous layer response. Those not familiar with the varied appearances of periosteal hypertrophy (Fig. 9.23) might presume that a graft has failed or it is soft when in fact removing the fibrous overgrowth of the fibrous layer of the periosteum will usually result in complete relief of symptoms and ongoing maturity of the transplanted autologous cultured chondrocytes to a firm smooth repair tissue. Clinically, this usually manifests at the stage of a proliferative hypertrophic periosteal healing response between 3 and 7 months after surgery. Patients may present with new onset catching from a previously smooth tracking knee with symptoms of pain and effusion. If this occurs, the patient's activity level should be decreased to avoid the symptomatic area and an MRI evaluation followed by arthroscopic treatment is recommended.

In the worst-case scenario where a large portion of the graft has delaminated (Fig. 9.24) with the remaining portion intact and adherent to the underlying bone, an open suture repair is not recommended. Instead, arthroscopic sharp incision of the periosteum that has not attached to the subchondral bone should be performed with removal of the loose flap, leaving behind the integrated chondral graft and any repair tissue underneath the periosteal delamination.

Persistent pain after ACI in a patient who has had prior drilling or microfracture should be investigated with an MRI scan. We have seen late failures from central graft overload and breakdown, delamination and cyst formation (which would not be visible arthroscopically) (Fig. 9.25).

Of course, despite a prior history of ACI, a slip and fall can result in a new articular or meniscal injury, which is not necessarily related to the graft (Fig. 9.26).

Clinical Outcomes Using ACI

The clinical outcomes that follow include our collaborative results of the use of ACI in adolescents[3,11,12] and soccer players,[13] as well as updated results for the patellofemoral joint[11,14,15] in patients over 45 years old,[16] patients treated after marrow stimulation techniques,[17] and the osteoarthritic or salvage group[18] of patients. We have also moved on to use a collagen type I–III porcine membrane in an attempt to lessen our incidence of periosteal hypertrophy[19] and will report on this topic. We have carefully reviewed subsets in the osteoarthritic knee to include bipolar tibiofemoral[20] and bipolar patellofemoral[21] clinical outcomes. We have also looked at the first cohort of patients using periosteal ACI with survival and clinical outcome at a minimum of 20 years.[22] The cost-effectiveness of ACI remains substantiated since its early report in 1998[23,24] based on its durability.[25]

Since the first edition of this book we have also reviewed the outcomes of ACI with ACL reconstruction,[26] meniscal

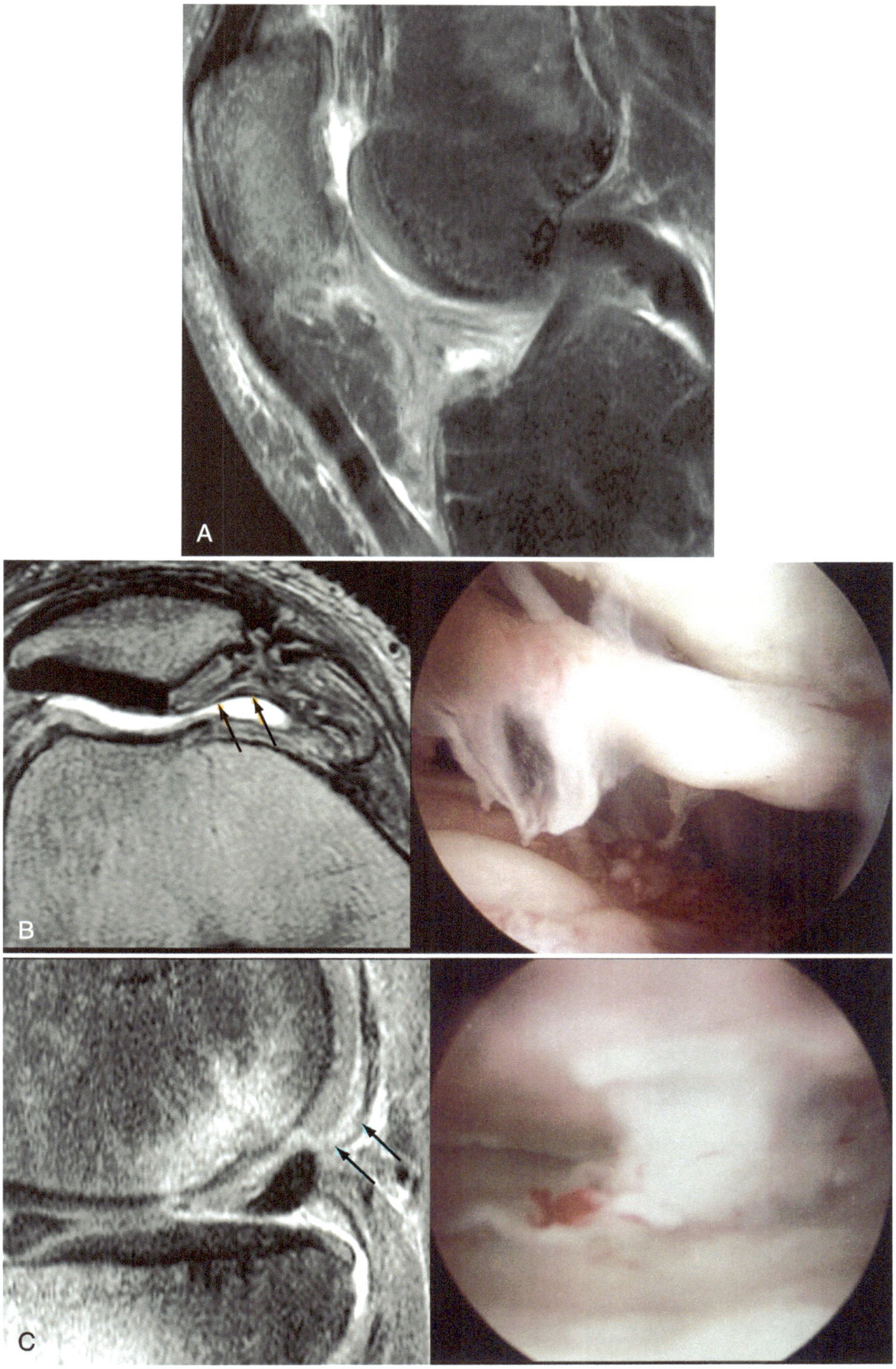

• **Fig. 9.22** Three weeks after autologous chondrocyte implantation (ACI) to the medial femoral condyles patella with tibial tubercle osteotomy, the patient's knee becomes very stiff. (A) Sagittal magnetic resonance imaging (MRI) scan demonstrating dense adhesions from Hoffa fat pad to anterior cruciate ligament. ACI to the patella appears to be intact. (B) Axial MRI scan of the patella demonstrates adhesions *(arrows)* from the medial parapatellar gutter, which is obliterated by scar tissue directly on the transplant surface, noted at the time of arthroscopy *(right)*. (C) *Arrows* indicate adhesions to the medial femoral condyle ACI transplant on sagittal MRI scan. At the time of arthroscopy, the adhesions are clearly visible attached to the graft *(right)*. A blind manipulation without arthroscopic lysis of adhesions would result in failure of both grafts by intraoperative avulsion from the subchondral bone.

allograft reconstruction,[27] and the survival of ACI in all patients after a minimum of 10 years.[28] These will be briefly summarized.

Following institutional review board approval in November 1994, from March 1995 we evaluated ACI prospectively. Initially, the expected patient clinical improvement after ACI was unknown. Patients with single articular cartilage lesions and patients with multiple lesions presented to our clinics. We wished to capture complementary clinical outcomes based on a survey to include overall quality of life and specific knee scores to include sporting activity levels as well as well-established outcome scores for arthritis improvements. Patients completed questionnaires including the Short Form-36[29] (SF-36), Knee Society Score[30] (KSS), Western Ontario MacMaster Osteoarthritis Score[31] (WOMAC), modified Cincinnati rating scale (0–10)[32] (Fig. 9.27) activity-based score, and a patient satisfaction survey (Fig. 9.28).

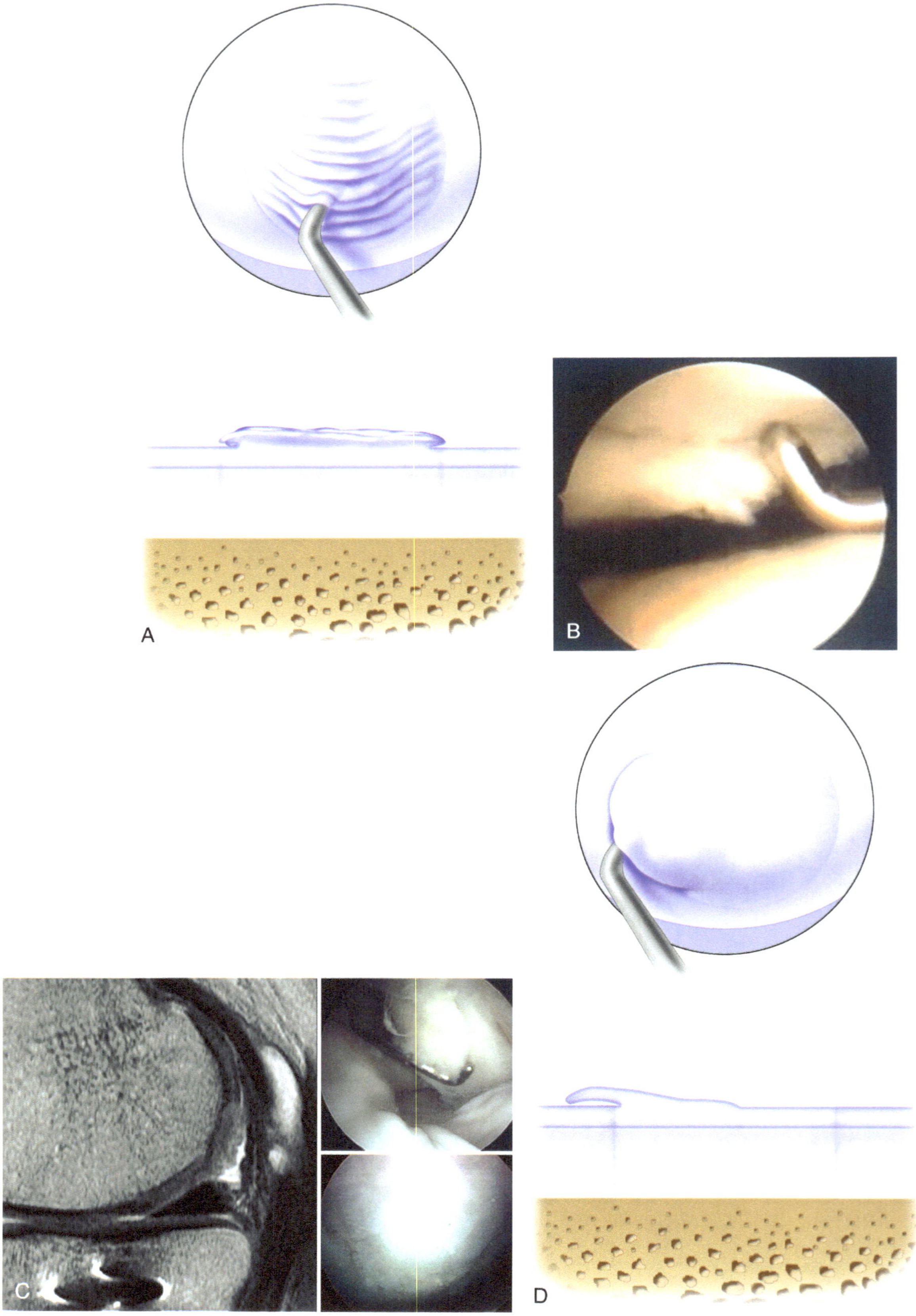

• **Fig. 9.23** Fibrous layer of the periosteum may undergo overgrowth and have varied appearances, termed onion skinning, overlapping, mounding, or superficial fibrillation. If these appearances are not recognized at the time of arthroscopic evaluation, they may be mistaken for a failed poor-quality autologous chondrocyte implantation (ACI) graft. Takedown of the overgrown fibrous layer with a motorized shaver will result in complete relief of symptoms and will demonstrate healthy repair tissue flush with the native articular surface. Magnetic resonance imaging (MRI) scan is helpful in

Continued

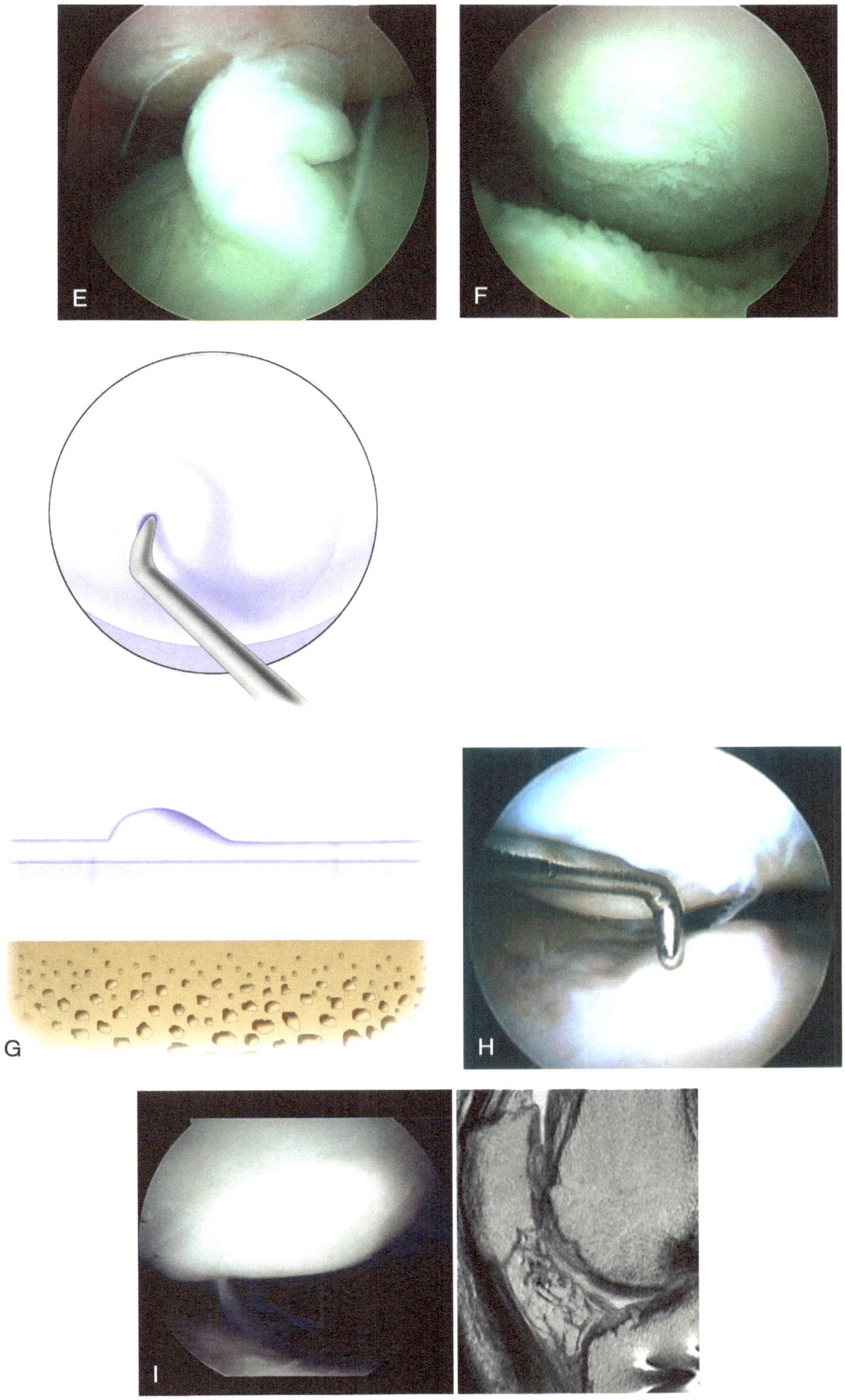

• **Fig. 9.23—cont'd** distinguishing mechanical painful symptoms of overgrowth from a delaminated failed graft. MRI scan is routinely performed prior to arthroscopic management of hypertrophy. In this way, surgical options can be discussed with the patient in advance of treatment if the graft has failed by delamination or degeneration. (A) Diagrammatic representation of onion skinning. Removing the layered fibrous tissues results in clean, shiny, hard repair tissue at the deep surface. (B) Arthroscopic appearance of onion skinning. Probe demonstrates the level of native articular cartilage adjacent to overgrown fibrous layer of periosteum. The prominent fibrous layer will be removed flush with the native tissue using a motorized shaver and will result in symptom relief. (C) Sagittal proton density MRI scan reveals a prominent hypertrophic periosteal surface on the ACI graft.

Continued

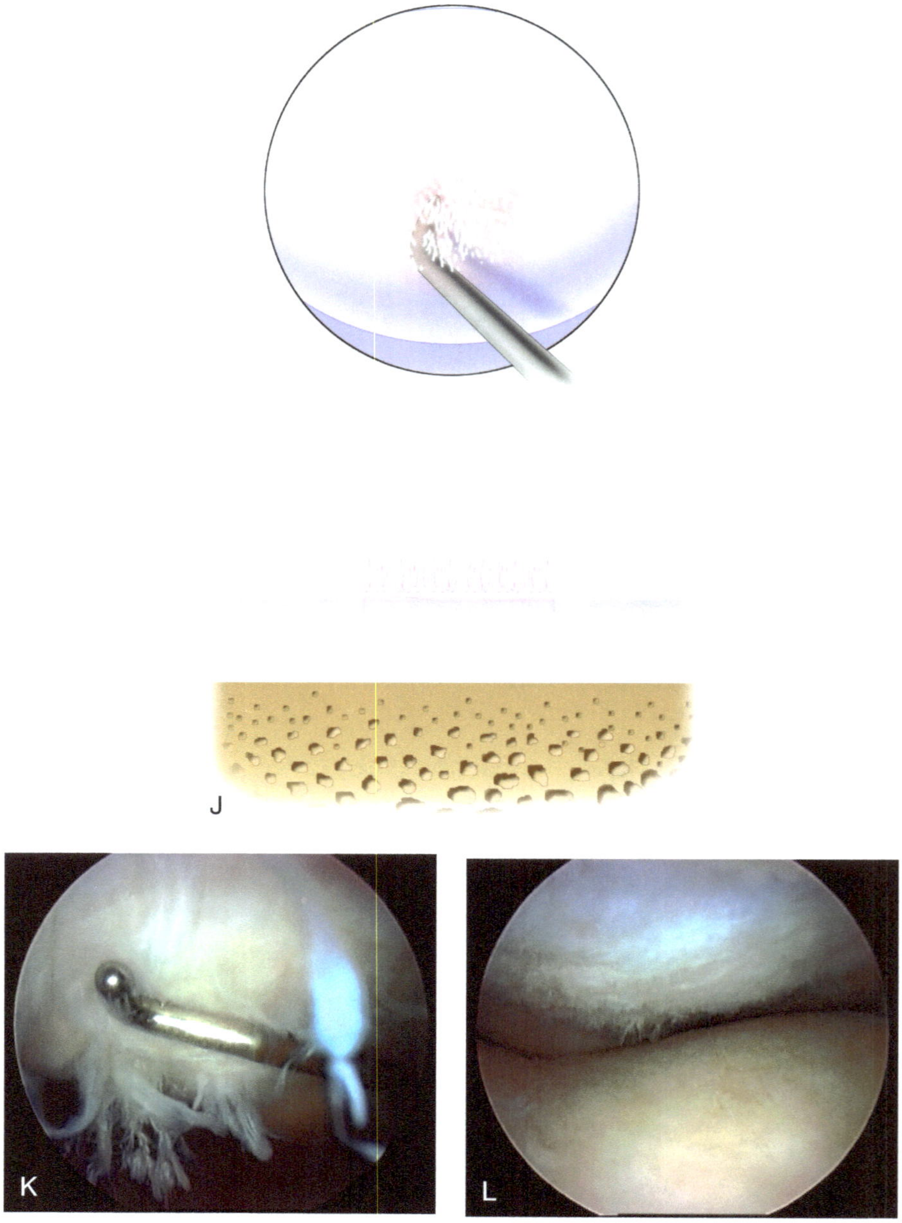

• **Fig. 9.23—cont'd** Arthroscopic photos to the *right* demonstrate onion skinning-type hypertrophy, which is removed. (D) Diagrammatic representation of overlapping hypertrophy. The flap of periosteum on top of native tissue with resulting mechanical catching sensation should be removed. (E) Arthroscopic appearance of overlapping hypertrophy on the medial femoral condyle ACI graft, which results in a painful snapping sensation in deep flexion. (F) Medial femoral condyle ACI graft appearance after removal of overlapping hypertrophy. (G) Diagrammatic representation of mounding hypertrophy. (H) Arthroscopic appearance of mounding hypertrophy to the lateral tibial plateau ACI graft. (I) Mounding hypertrophy to the patella ACI graft viewed arthroscopically *(left)* and by sagittal MRI scan *(right)*. (J) Diagrammatic representation of superficial fibrillation. (K) Arthroscopic appearance of superficial fibrillation on the patella ACI graft. Superficial fibrillation-type hypertrophy usually results in pronounced crepitus. (L) Arthroscopic appearance of ACI patellar graft after removal of superficial fibrillation hypertrophy, which results in complete resolution of crepitus, mechanical symptoms, and pain.

ACI in Adolescents[3]

Twenty patients 18 years old or younger, with 29 full-thickness articular cartilage lesions in 23 knees, were treated with ACI at Boston Children's Hospital and Brigham and Women's Hospital, between December 1995 and December 2000. All patients had failed prior conservative and surgical treatment. All patients had undergone at least one surgical procedure before ACI (mean 2.5 procedures, range 1–6 procedures). Patient demographics, defect etiology and characteristics, preoperative duration of symptoms, and surgical history were recorded. Injuries were considered chronic if the preoperative duration of symptoms was >12 months. Preoperative radiographs were obtained on every patient and demonstrated open growth plates at the time of ACI in 60% of the adolescent athletes.

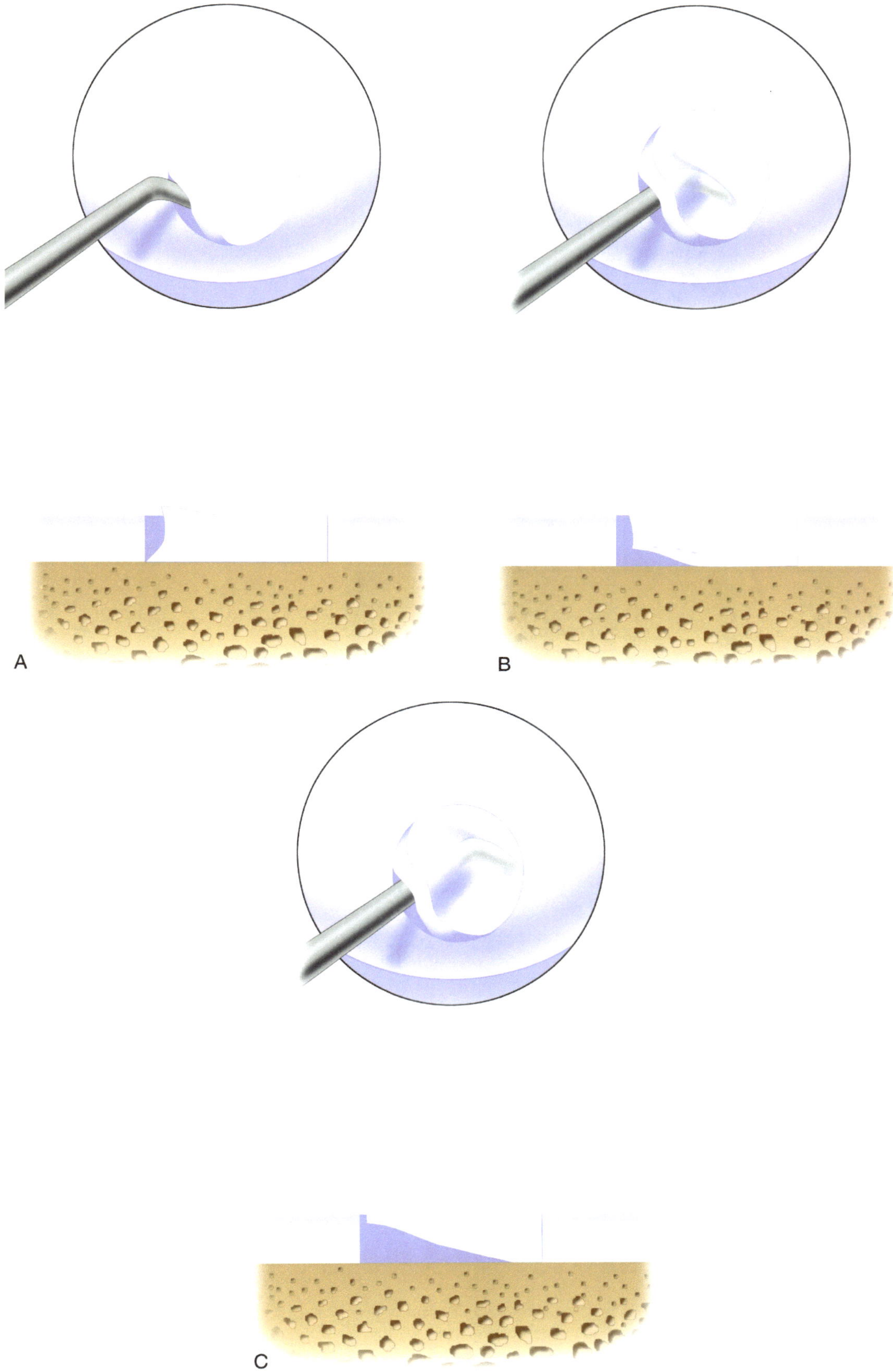

• **Fig. 9.24** Graft delamination usually results in painful symptoms of weight-bearing discomfort and catching. Severity can be marginal, partial, or complete. Treatment depends on the amount of graft that remains in the defect that ensues. Magnetic resonance imaging (MRI) scan is useful in the diagnosis of graft delamination (see text for details).

Continued

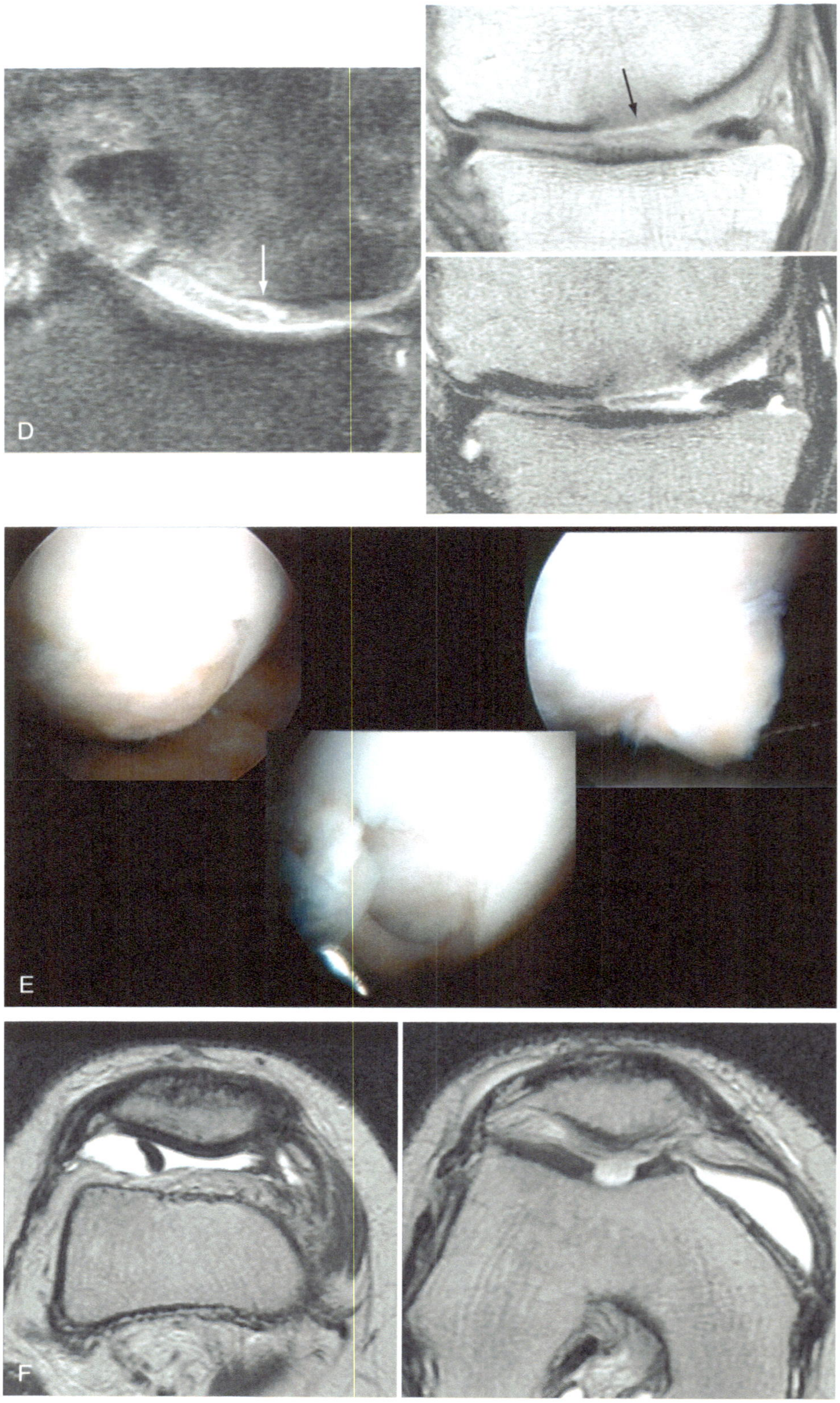

• **Fig. 9.24—cont'd** (A) Diagrammatic representation of a marginal graft delamination. This is usually managed by sharp removal of the graft edge to stabilize the defect and possible marrow stimulation to the defect edge to seal it with repair tissue. (B) Diagrammatic representation of a partial graft delamination. (C) Diagrammatic representation of complete delamination with only edge that remains attached. (D) Fat-suppressed coronal MRI scan demonstrates a fluid signal *(arrow)* deep to the autologous chondrocyte implantation (ACI) graft. Proton density MRI scans *(right)* also demonstrate a deep fluid signal indicating poor attachment of the graft to the subchondral bone. (E) At the time of arthroscopy, the graft appears to be intact *(top left)*. However, when a probe is used to assess the stability of the graft, it has become completely delaminated with only the edge attached *(center, right)*. (F) Axial proton density MRI scan demonstrates a loose body in the superior patellar pouch *(top)*. A clear defect in the trochlea at the site of a small ACI graft and the central sulcus has failed and displaced. These findings indicate complete delamination with loose body.

In two patients, the depth of the defect required autologous bone grafting in combination with ACI. Implantation of chondrocytes in these cases was performed using the sandwich technique. Reconstruction of the anterior cruciate ligament was performed in one patient at the time of chondrocyte implantation. One other patient had undergone staged ACL reconstruction before autologous chondrocyte transplantation. Meniscal repair was performed in four patients, at the time of chondrocyte implantation in two, and as part of their prior surgical procedures in two. Tibial tubercle osteotomy was performed concomitantly in one patient. Postoperatively, continuous passive motion was initiated within 6–12 hours and administered for 2 weeks. Patients remained non-weight-bearing for 6–8 weeks with gradual progression to full weight bearing by 10–12 weeks. Most patients could return to regular daily activities by 4 months, low-impact pursuits by 6 months, and progression to running at 9 months. Demanding high-impact and pivoting sports were avoided for 12 months.

Patients were evaluated preoperatively and at a mean of 47 ± 4 months postoperatively (range 23–91 months). Functional outcome was determined using established knee scoring systems including the Lysholm score and the Tegner activity score. In addition, a questionnaire was used to evaluate the patient's ability for athletic participation and subjective rating of knee function, which was graded as either excellent, good, fair, or poor. The level of athletic participation before injury was compared with the athletic ability after chondrocyte transplantation.

Twenty adolescent patients with articular cartilage lesions in 23 knees were treated with autologous chondrocyte transplantation. Seventeen patients had unilateral involvement and three patients presented with bilateral knee articular cartilage lesions. The mean age at chondrocyte transplantation was 15.9 ± 0.3 years (range 12–18 years). There were 15 male and 5 female adolescent athletes. The average duration of symptoms was 21 months and was ≤12 months in 11 knees (48%) and >12 months in 12 knees (52%). All patients had failed previous conservative and surgical treatment.

Osteochondritis dissecans was the cause of the chondral defect in 14 knees and in the remaining 9 knees the cartilage lesions resulted from acute focal trauma associated with pivoting sports such as basketball, football, and soccer. Two

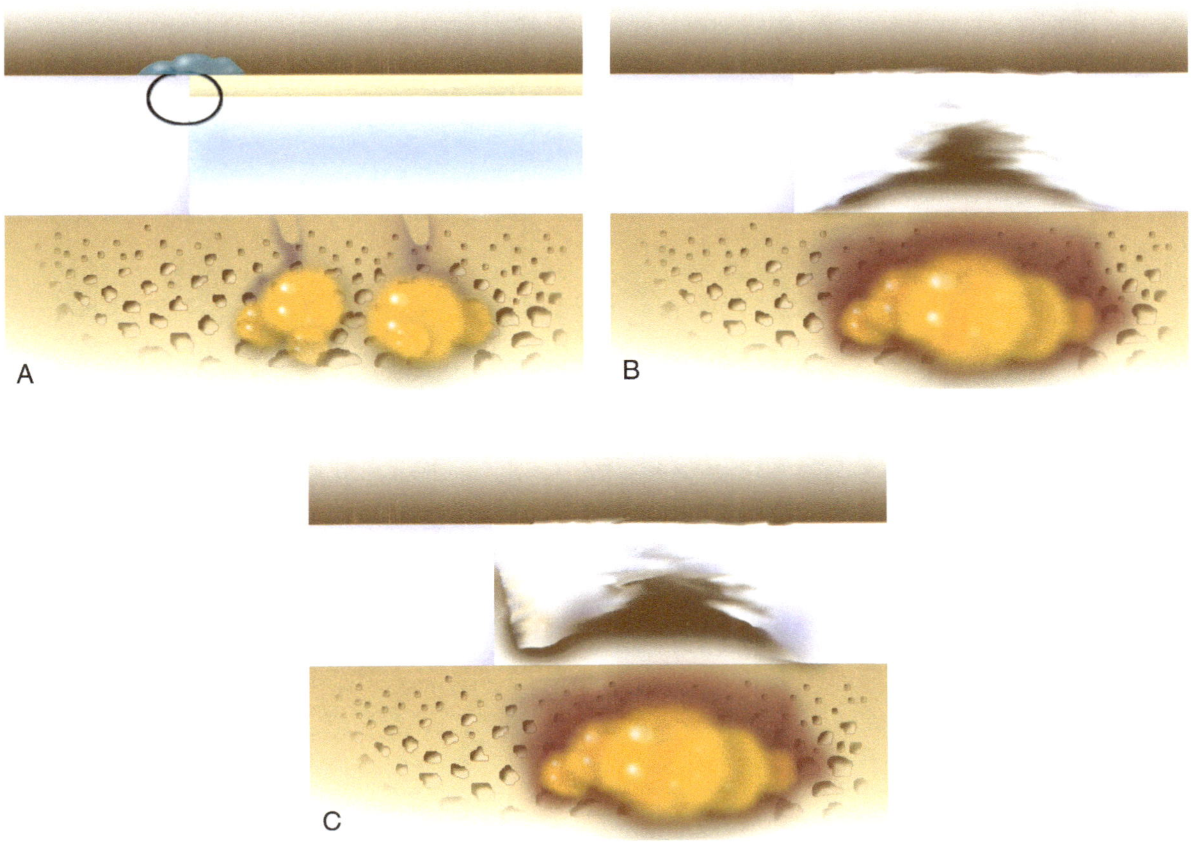

• **Fig. 9.25** Autologous chondrocyte implantation (ACI) grafts may fail because of cyst formation after prior microfracture. The cysts might expand after ACI, eventually leading to graft detachment and failure. (A) Diagrammatic representation of an ACI graft immediately after treatment with prior microfracture. Small subchondral cysts are present at the distal aspect of the pick entry sites. (B) Cysts expand over time, subchondral bone thickens, and ACI graft detaches. (C) Eventual detachment of the ACI graft from adjacent cartilage and subchondral bone.

Continued

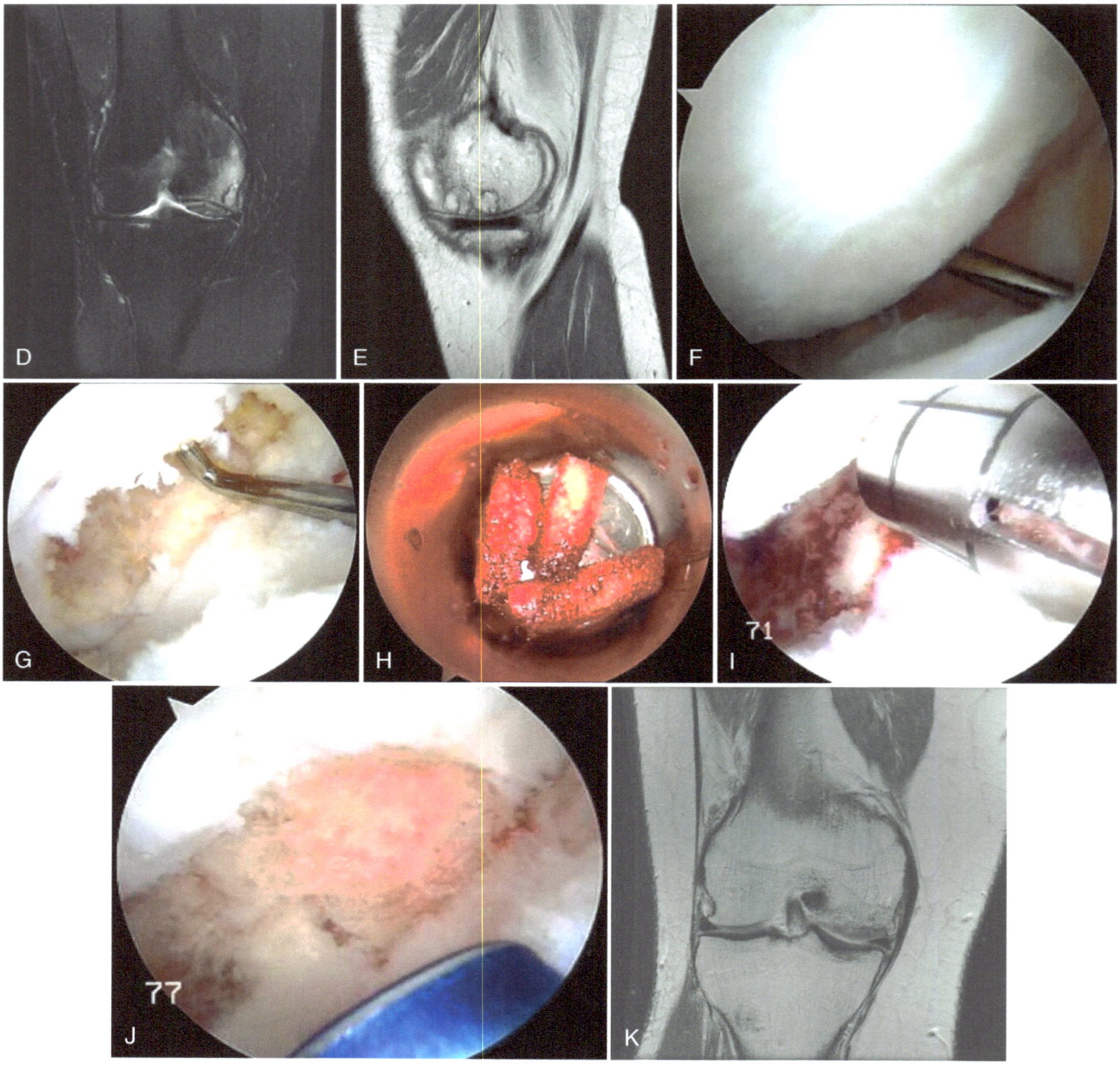

• **Fig. 9.25—cont'd** (D) Magnetic resonance imaging (MRI) scan of a 32-year-old woman 2 years after ACI to the medial femoral condyles that had been previously microfractured. Note intense subchondral edema and developing cyst formation at the margin of the ACI graft to the native articular cartilage. (E) Sagittal proton density MRI scan demonstrates large cysts in the medial femoral condyles deep to the ACI graft. (F) At the time of arthroscopy, the articular surface of the medial femoral condyles anterior cruciate ligament graft appears to be of excellent quality. However, based on the patient's painful symptoms and MRI scan, a problem is known to exist with ACI graft attachment to native cartilage and subchondral bone on the medial-most aspect of the transplant. This is carefully probed and noted to be detached. (G) Arthroscopic appearance of the defect after the delaminated articular cartilage is removed. The cysts are excavated with a curette. The bony deficiency is apparent after the cyst lining tissue is removed. (H) Autologous bone graft harvested with a 10-mm diameter osteochondral autograft transfer system (OATS) harvester from the proximal tibia near Gerdy's tubercle in a specimen cup. (I) Arthroscopic appearance of the autologous cancellous bone after it has been morselized into small chips, reloaded into the OATS harvester, and packed into the osteochondral defect on the medial femoral condyles. (J) Arthroscopic appearance of the defect completely filled to the level of the subchondral bone and packed securely with a bone tamp. The tourniquet is then let down and the patient undergoes rehabilitation as if this were a microfracture technique with 6 weeks of protected weight-bearing and continuous passive motion. (K) Coronal proton density MRI scan after 1 year shows complete resolution of the subchondral bone cysts and excellent repair tissue fill on the medial femoral condyle. The patient remains symptom-free many years later.

patients had tears of the anterior cruciate ligament (10%) and four patients (20%) had meniscal injuries. A total of 29 cartilage lesions were observed, with the majority presenting as single lesions and an average of 1.3 cartilage defects per knee. Average lesion size was 6.4 cm^2.

At latest follow-up, 96% of patients were able to participate regularly in high-impact, pivoting sports at the recreational level or higher. Sixty percent of the athletes had returned to the same or higher level of athletic activity than before their injury. Tegner activity scores increased in all

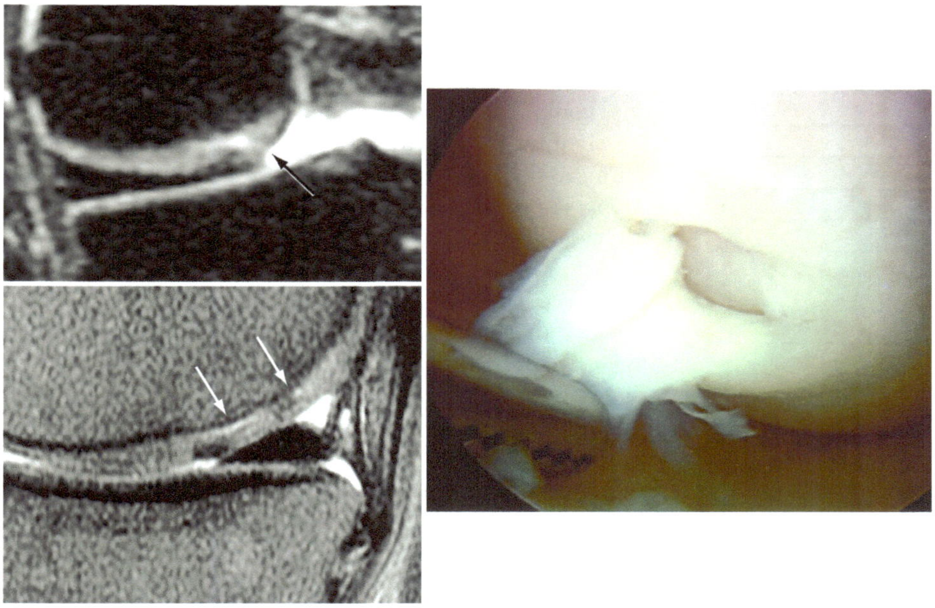

• **Fig. 9.26** Eight months after autologous chondrocyte implantation (ACI) graft to the lateral femoral condyle, the patient falls on his driveway. New-onset mechanical catching and pain ensue. The patient believes that he has damaged his transplanted knee. Magnetic resonance imaging (MRI) scan demonstrates an intact lateral femoral condyle ACI graft but a new area of subchondral bone detachment of the medial femoral condyle cartilage. Fat-suppressed MRI scan shows cartilage detachment from medial femoral condyle *(black arrow, upper left)*. Proton density sagittal image shows cartilage detachment from subchondral bone *(white arrows)*. Arthroscopic appearance demonstrates a small chondral flap to the medial femoral condyle, which is debrided and microfractured.

Modified Cincinnati rating scale
Overall condition

Rate overall condition at the present time

2	4	6	8	10
Poor	Fair	Good	Very good	Excellent

2 = Poor	Significant limitations affect activities of daily living
4 = Fair	Moderate limitations affect activities of daily living, no sports
6 = Good	Some limitations with sports but participate; I compensate
8 = Very good	Only a few limitations with sports
10 = Excellent	Able to do whatever I wish (any sport) with no problems

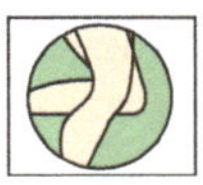

• **Fig. 9.27** Modified Cincinnati rating scale (0–10) activity-based score. Noyes FR, Barber SD, Mooar L. A rationale for assessing sports activity levels and limitations in knee disorders. *Clin Orthop Relat Res*. 1989;246:238-249.

patients compared with preoperative values. Lysholm scores were not available before injury but increased significantly from preoperative values of 64 ± 3 points to 87 ± 7 points at latest follow-up (P <.01).

Only 33% of adolescents with chronic preoperative symptoms (>12 months) returned to the same level of athletics compared with all adolescents with shorter preoperative intervals (P <.01). Postoperative Tegner scores (7.2 ± 0.3 points) and Lysholm scores (85 ± 3 points) in adolescents with chronic symptoms were lower than Tegner scores (8.7 ± 0.2 points, P <.01) and Lysholm scores (91 ± 2 points) in adolescents with symptoms ≤12 months. The average preoperative duration of symptoms of adolescents that returned to preinjury athletic levels was 15 ± 4 months and lower than in adolescents who failed to return to the same level (31 ± 6 months, P <.05). The adolescents with chronic symptoms had undergone an average of 3.2 ± 0.4 prior surgeries compared with 1.6 ± 0.2 in the adolescents with acute symptoms (P <.05). The number of prior operations also showed significant correlation with the ability to return to preinjury athletics (r = 0.453, P <.05).

Ninety-six percent of patients rated their results as good or excellent and only one patient reported a fair outcome. This patient presented with moderate genu varum and did not consent to primary realignment. He briefly returned to high-impact athletics after autologous chondrocyte transplantation to the medial femoral condyle and trochlea but developed recurrent symptoms with athletic activities and graft failures. Secondary high tibial osteotomy (HTO) was performed. The patient has not yet returned to high-impact activities at the time of last follow-up and awaits revision ACI. Other complications included graft hypertrophy, which was observed in three athletes (15%) and was successfully treated with arthroscopic chondroplasty in all cases.

ACI in adolescent patients is highly successful when used as a first-line treatment strategy for large chondral defects within the first year of injury. Multiple surgeries in an attempt to be less invasive lead to chronic dysfunction and a poor clinical outcome in those patients.

Compared to one year ago, how would you rate each operated joint now?		
Much better		
Somewhat better		
About the same		
Somewhat worse		
Much worse		
Compared to before each surgery, how would you rate each operated joint now?		
Much better		
Somewhat better		
About the same		
Somewhat worse		
Much worse		
What is your overall satisfaction level with each joint surgery?		
Very satisfied		
Somewhat satisfied		
Neutral		
Somewhat dissatisfied		
Very dissatisfied		
If you could go back in time and make the decision again, would you choose to have each joint surgery?		
Definitely yes		
Probably yes		
Completely uncertain		
Probably not		
Definitely not		
How would you rate the results of each joint surgery		
Good or excellent		
Fair		
Poor		

• **Fig. 9.28** Patient satisfaction survey for treating osteoarthritis of the knee with autologous chondrocyte implantation.

ACI in Soccer Players

Forty-five soccer players were treated with ACI at the participating institutions between March 1988 and August 2000.[13] All athletes complained about acute or chronic symptoms. Baseline evaluation included careful history and physical examination and documentation of type, onset, and duration of symptoms. Demographic data, prior surgical history, and skill level were recorded (Table 9.1). Skill level was divided into recreational and high-level competitive for athletes who participated in high school, collegiate, professional, or national team level soccer.

All patients had full-thickness Outerbridge type IV articular cartilage lesions or osteochondral lesions of the knee demonstrated at arthroscopy. The minimum follow-up duration from the time of implantation was 12 months. At follow-up the athlete's function was rated using the sports activity-based Tegner scale (Fig. 9.29). The ability and timing of return to soccer and skill level after articular cartilage repair was recorded. Successful articular cartilage repair was defined as the ability to return to soccer even if not at the patient's previous skill level. Treatment durability was defined as the percentage of players who returned to soccer and maintained this functional status at subsequent follow-up. Adverse events and complications were carefully documented.

Significant improvement of activity scores was observed in more than 80% of players, confirming the overall functional improvements described after autologous chondrocytes in previous studies. Despite the overall increased function only one-third of the players were able to return to soccer. The return rate was significantly higher in competitive than in recreational level players. A return rate of 83% was observed in competitive soccer players following autologous chondrocyte transplantation in our study. Interestingly, the return rate to recreational soccer in our study was significantly lower than at the higher skill level. Significantly prolonged preoperative morbidity was seen in players who failed to return to soccer after autologous chondrocyte transplantation in our study and could also explain the lower return rate of recreational players in the present study. Our data indicate that the longer the time between injury and chondrocyte transplantation, the lower the rate of return to competitive or recreational soccer. In fact, the success rate effectively doubled if autologous chondrocyte transplantation was performed within 1 year after the onset of the articular cartilage injury. This confirms previous observations that demonstrated a significantly better functional outcome if autologous chondrocyte transplantation was performed within 1 year of obtaining the cartilage injury as in our adolescent patients.

The average time to return to soccer in our study was 18 months and 87% of returning players were still competing at a mean of 48 months postoperatively. Although initial recovery after chondrocyte transplantation may be more prolonged, our data suggest that this cartilage repair technique provides excellent durability even under very high athletic demands. Some world-class athletes who were treated primarily with autologous chondrocyte transplantation within 4 months of their injury were able to return rapidly to their preinjury level of play and with excellent long-term durability. These excellent results under maximum demand support the use of autologous chondrocyte transplantation as a primary technique for articular cartilage repair in young active patients. In contrast, when autologous chondrocyte transplantation is used as a salvage procedure in older patients with longstanding preoperative symptoms and multiple prior operations, the results are less predictable. Adjuvant procedures, tibial osteotomy, tibial tubercle osteotomy, or ACL reconstruction did not affect the return to soccer.

The results of autologous chondrocyte transplantation in soccer athletes are encouraging. An excellent return rate to demanding athletic activity and long-term function is possible particularly in young, competitive players with short duration of symptoms and fewer prior surgical interventions. These results are comparable to those reported for microfracture or osteochondral mosaicplasty. Long-term evaluation will help to determine whether restoration of articular cartilage lesions in knees in soccer players can

TABLE 9.1 Soccer Player Demographics Undergoing ACI for Focal Chondral Defects After Knee Surgery

	All Players	Return	No Return
Gender (%male:%female)	71:29	80:20	63:37
Age (years)	26 ± 1 (14–43)	22.3 ± 1.6	27.6 ± 1.2
No. of previous surgeries	2.0 ± 0.3 (0–13)	1.5 ± 0.3	2.3 ± 0.5
Skill level (%)	–	–	–
Recreational	73	16	84
High	27	83	17
Symptom duration (months)	26 ± 3.4 (3–96)	16.7 ± 3.8	30.7 ± 4.5
Lesion size (cm^2)	5.7 ± 0.6	5.5 ± 0.8	5.6 ± 0.8
Lesion type (%)	–	–	–
Single	65	83	14
Multiple	35	30	70
Lesion location (%)	–	–	–
Medial femoral condyle	48	37	54
Lateral femoral condyle	23	21	24
Trochlea	13	16	11
Patella	11	16	8
Tibia	5	11	3
Graft failure (%)	13	6	16
Brittberg rating (%)	–	–	–
Excellent	32	60	18
Good	40	33	43
Fair	23	6	32
Poor	5	0	7

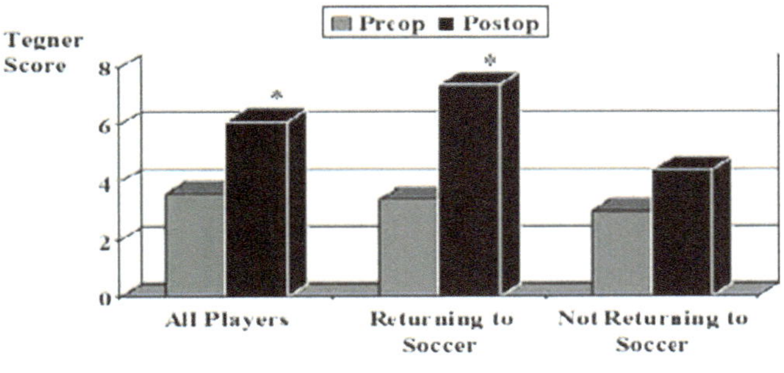

• **Fig. 9.29** Sports activity-based Tegner scale. (Mithofer K, Peterson L, Mandelbaum BR, Minas T. Articular cartilage repair in soccer players with autologous chondrocyte transplantation: functional outcome and return to competition. *Am J Sports Med*. 2005;33(11):1639–1646.)

effectively reduce the high incidence of osteoarthritis in this population.

ACI in the Patellofemoral Joint

Many factors have been implicated as contributing to abnormal pathomechanics leading to pain in the patellofemoral joint. These include patella alta, trochlea dysplasia, an increased quadriceps or Q-angle with secondary soft tissue problems, weakened or hypoplastic vastus medialis oblique quadriceps muscle with a contracted lateral retinaculum, and/or an absent redundant medial patellofemoral ligament. These pathomechanics lead to abnormal forces across the patella resulting in secondary degenerative changes or injury to the articular surfaces of the patellofemoral joint acutely or chronically. Diagnosing and correcting these underlying abnormalities when associated with cartilage injury is crucial to a successful outcome when using ACI for repair of these defects.[14] It is for these reasons that resurfacing of the patella with ACI resulted in only two good or excellent outcomes in seven patients treated (29%) in the first study introducing autologous chondrocyte transplantation from Sweden in 1994.[1] In later reports,[25,33] when patellar tracking was also addressed by realignment of the extensor mechanism at the time of transplantation, it was noted that the success rate increased at 2 years to 11 of 17 patients (65%) good or excellent[33] and at 10 years the results had improved to 13 of 17 patients (76%) good or excellent results.[25] Two

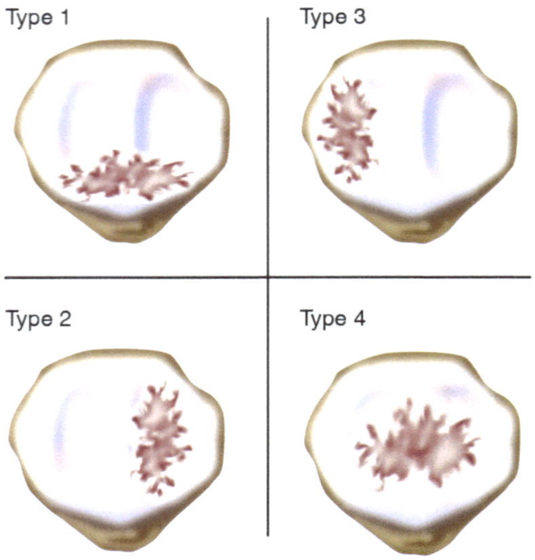

• **Fig. 9.30** Fulkerson classification for wear patterns to the patella. Type I and II defects are well managed by anteromedialization tibial tubercle osteotomy (Fulkerson osteotomy). A type 1 defect involves the inferior patellar pole. A type 2 defect involves the lateral patellar facet. A type III defect involves the medial patellar facet and is frequently associated with a trochlear defect. A type IV patellar defect is a pan-patellar defect. A variant is a proximal pole crush, which occurs in a dashboard impact-related injury. Type 3 and 4 injuries do not do well with isolated Fulkerson osteotomies but are well managed when combined with cartilage repair by autologous chondrocyte implantation.

patients who rated a fair result at 2 years had improved to good results at 3 years, improving the results over time. The importance of correcting the underlying cause for the chondral injury cannot be underestimated when attempting surgical correction with cartilage repair techniques.

Anteromedialization (AMZ) of the tibial tubercle has become a useful surgical tool for correcting maltracking and unloading an articular cartilage injury to the patella. Fulkerson and his colleagues[9] have demonstrated that the AMZ TTO successful clinical outcome correlates with the location of the patellar articular lesion (Fig. 9.30). In those patients with a type I articular cartilage lesion (inferior patellar pole) or a type II (lateral facet), the osteotomy in unloading these two locations gave 87% good to excellent subjective results and 100% of these patients said they would have the procedure done again. Type III (medial facet) lesions had a 55% good to excellent result and type IV (proximal pole or diffuse) only 20% had a good or excellent result. Patients with type I or II lesions were significantly more likely to have good or excellent results than those with type III or IV lesions. Central trochlea lesions were associated with medial patellar lesions and all patients with central trochlea lesions have poor results. Workers' compensation issues diminish the likelihood of this satisfactory outcome by 19%. Fulkerson and colleagues concluded that the location of the articular patellar cartilage lesion was significantly correlated to the success of an AMZ TTO.

Localization of the articular cartilage injury at the time of reconstruction is therefore important to determine whether osteotomy surgery alone may result in a successful outcome. Theoretically, cartilage repair to patellar type III and IV lesions as well as the trochlea may improve the clinical outcome for these difficult lesions when associated with patellar maltracking or in the absence of abnormal tracking when no other options exist.

Between March 1995 and July 2002, 248 patients had been treated. One hundred and seventy patients had a minimum of 2 years of follow-up as of July 2002. Of these 170 patients treated, 45 patients had treatments involving the patella, trochlea, in isolation or combination with other lesions with a minimum of 2 years of follow-up. These patients were followed up in this study.

Baseline patient demographics were captured and outcomes assessed by several validated outcomes instruments. In addition at the time of surgery, all patients had their surgeries photographed to assess the appearance of the native chondral injury, the debrided chondral injury, and after the completion of the suturing of the periosteal patch and injection with autologous cultured chondrocytes. These photographs are kept on a digital file. These photographs were used to classify the patellar defect location as per the Fulkerson Classification.[34]

There were 27 men and 18 women. The average patient age at surgery was 36.9 years (range 15–54). The average follow-up was 47.5 months (range 24–86 months). The average number of prior surgeries was 2.5 per patient on the affected knee. Of patients 24% (11 of 45) had been treated while on workers' compensation. There was an average of 2.2 defects per knee with an average of 2.18 vials containing 12 million cells per vial (26.16 million cells) used to treat each knee. The lesions treated were large with an average surface area per knee joint of 10.45 cm^2.

Technical issues specific to the surgical procedure of ACI in the patellofemoral joint include a suture technique that restores the surface articular shape of the patella (Fig. 9.16A–C) and the trochlea (Fig. 9.15A) as well as a soft tissue tensioning at the end of the procedure that allows the normal medial to lateral and proximal to distal patellar glide without over-constricting the patellofemoral joint. An AMZ TTO as preferred by me is discussed in Chapter 12 (Figs. 12.16–12.28). If patellar instability secondary to a dysplastic trochlea remains after the AMZ TTO and soft tissue stabilization, a trochleoplasty is added to the procedure as described by Peterson[8] and illustrated in Chapter 12 (Figs. 12.33 and 12.34).

Osteotomy was frequently performed in this series: 29 of 45 patients (64%) had tibiofemoral, patellofemoral malalignment, or both. It is felt that the success of cartilage repair includes normal alignment and tracking. Hence if 2 degrees or more of mechanical malalignment from a neutral mechanical axis in the tibiofemoral joint is noted in combination with a large chondral defect, a varus- or valgus-producing osteotomy is performed with cartilage repair on the weight-bearing condyles. If there is evidence of patellar subluxation and tilt with regards to patellar tracking as noted by clinical examination and/or CT scan assessment, an AMZ TTO is performed in combination with resurfacing of the patella or trochlea or both.

Failures were defined as poor clinical outcomes accompanied by evidence of graft failure caused by delamination from adjacent cartilage and subchondral bone, poor biomechanical properties indicative of fibrous, fibrocartilage repair as evidenced by arthroscopy, or evidence of graft detachment confirmed by MRI or arthroscopy despite a good clinical outcome.

When assessing the first 45 patients in whom the patellofemoral joint was treated by ACI with a minimum 2 years of follow-up, we found patient satisfaction to be high. Using a patient satisfaction questionnaire, patient overall satisfaction was 71% satisfied, 16% neutral, and 13% dissatisfied. Compared with before surgery 76% were better, 18% the same, and 6% were worse; 87% of patients said they would choose the surgery again and 13% said they would not. Overall patients rated their results 71% good or excellent, 22% fair, and 7% poor. Large clinical improvements and statistical significance were seen using the SF-36, the Knee Society Score, WOMAC score, and the modified Cincinnati activity score.

Our series notes that chondral defects on the patella and the trochlea have a successful clinical outcome when ACI is used to treat the chondral defect in addition to the realignment when needed, where other series have not.[34] In this series, 31 of 34 (91%) patellar lesions treated were type III or type IV. The other defects were trochlea ($n = 11$) or kissing patella and trochlea ($n = 20$). Sixty-four percent of the cases involved osteotomy of the tibial tubercle alone or in combination with a valgus-producing tibial osteotomy. The osteotomy alone would not account for the high success rate based on Fulkerson's results[34] because of the size and location of these chondral defects.

Three subgroups in our series had a small sample size and the statistics were not very meaningful: patella plus trochlea ($n = 4$), weight-bearing condyles plus patella ($n = 2$), and weight-bearing condyles plus trochlea ($n = 2$). However, the groups of patella ($n = 8$), trochlea, ($n = 9$), and weight-bearing condyles plus patella plus trochlea ($n = 20$) demonstrated a marked improvement in pain relief and functionality.

The SF-36 physical component summary demonstrated a highly significant improvement in physical well-being after ACI. Emotional well-being as measured by the SF-36 mental component summary was also significant for the larger group of weight-bearing condyle plus patella plus trochlea ($n = 20$). The WOMAC scores, which indicates relief in pain stiffness and swelling, were also significant for these three groups as was the Knee Society Score for the knee rating component of this scoring system. The highest improvement in sports activity rating, surprisingly, was in the most severely injured knees. This treatment group had the largest surface area of transplantation for knees, 15.31 cm^2.

When assessing the overall size of the defects treated, we noted that 35 trochleas were treated with an average surface area of 5.22 cm^2 and 34 patellas were treated with an average surface area of 4.86 cm^2.

Of 45 patients, 11 were defined as having failed (24%). Three of these were a result of failures of the weight-bearing condyle ACI graft. There were therefore eight failures (18%) caused by a patella or a trochlea graft failure. Of the 11 patients treated through the Workman's Compensation Program, 5 failed (45%). Three patients underwent prosthetic reconstruction. Two patients went on to total knee replacement, one patient who failed his patella transplant underwent an isolated patellofemoral prosthesis. Three patients who had partial graft failures underwent arthroscopic debridement. Five patients who had failed grafts underwent revision ACI procedure. Two were for trochlea, two were for patella, and one was for a medial femoral condyle. They have all had successful revision ACI procedures.

In our series of ACI in the patellofemoral joint, 91% of patients with chondral injuries to the patella were of type III or IV. Thirty-our patients underwent ACI to the patella with average defect size 4.86 cm^2. There were 35 patients who underwent ACI to the trochlea with defects of 5.22 cm^2. Overall the average surface transplanted per knee was 10.45 cm^2. Patient satisfaction overall was 87% for patients to choose the surgery again; 71% felt their clinical outcome was good or excellent, 22% fair, and 7% poor.

Three patients required prosthetic replacement: two for patellar failures, one for a medial femoral condyle failure. When failures occurred, they were readily managed by revision ACI when the source of the failure was a robust repair tissue that did not integrate well. If the repair tissue was of poor quality, we recommended either an osteochondral allograft or a prosthetic reconstruction. Hence despite initial failure, the final good result was usually obtained by biologic means and preserved the patient's function and joint.

We feel that ACI offers a complementary role, not previously available, to offer symptomatic pain relief and improved functionality in young patients for whom osteotomy is unsuccessful and prosthetic reconstruction is not desired. Based on the clinical outcomes presented in this study we have found the following algorithm to be useful in the clinical management of patients with patellofemoral disease. A successful treatment is based on identification of: (1) patellar tilt, (2) patellar subluxation, and (3) the location of the chondrosis (described in detail in Chapter 12 and Table 12.1).

Update on 130 Patients With Patellofemoral ACI

A recent update of the initial 45-patient cohort to 130 patients confirmed our initial results and improved upon them further. A total of 130 patients had treatments involving the patella or trochlea in isolation or in combination with other lesions, with a minimum follow-up of 2–9 years. These patients constitute the cohort for this study.

Baseline patient demographics are noted in Table 9.2 and outcomes as captured by validated outcomes instruments are given in Table 9.3. Osteotomy was done in this series (63 of 130 patients, 48%) in patients who had tibiofemoral malalignment, HTO, patellofemoral malalignment, TTO, or HTO-TTO (Table 9.2).

TABLE 9.2 Autologous Chondrocyte Implantation Patellofemoral Subgroup Characteristics

Subgroup	*n*	Osteotomy	Patellar Defect Location (type I–IV)	Surface Area Transplanted (cm²)	Average Age (years)
Patella	14	TTO-7	1 type II 8 type III 5 type IV	5.10	38
Trochlea	15	TTO-7	N/A	4.74	34
Patella + trochlea	5	TTO-3	3 type III 2 type IV	12.69	48
Weight-bearing condyle + patella	19	TTO-6 HTO-1 HTO+TTO-5	1 type II 7 type III 11 type IV	10.23	39
Weight-bearing condyle + trochlea	52	TTO-10 HTO-6 HTO+TTO-4	N/A	13.05	38
Weight-bearing condyle + patella + trochlea	25	TTO-7 HTO-1 HTO+TTO-6	4 type II 10 type III 11 type IV	15.84	39
Total	130	63/130 (48%)	57/63 type III + IV (90%)	11.03 cm² (average per knee)	37.5

N/A, trochlea is not applicable to patellar defect location classification.
All trochlea ($n = 98$), average surface area = 5.8 cm².
All patella ($n = 63$), average surface area = 4.72 cm².
Osteotomy was performed in this series (63/130 [48%]) of patients who had tibiofemoral malalignment (high tibial osteotomy [HTO]), patellofemoral malalignment (tibial tubercle osteotomy [TTO]), or both (HTO-TTO). Based on the patient satisfaction survey, overall satisfaction was 82%, with 11% neutral and 7% dissatisfied; 86% thought they were better, 8% the same, and 6% worse; 88% of patients said they would choose the surgery again, 4% were uncertain, and 8% said they would not. Overall, the patients rated their results as 80% good or excellent, 18% fair, and 2% poor.

TABLE 9.3 Overall Outcome Scores for Autologous Chondrocyte Implantation in the Patellofemoral Joint

Outcome Measures	Preoperative	Postoperative	*P* Value
SF-36 PCS	33.88	41.01	<.0001
SF-36 MCS	48.92	53.13	<.0001
WOMAC	38.06	21.27	<.0001
KSS–knee	51.83	79.72	<.0001
KSS–function	62.35	82.08	<.0001
Modified Cincinnati	3.58 (range 1–8)	6.03 (range 1–10)	<.0001

Large average clinical improvement was found using the Medical Outcomes Study 36-Item Short-Form Health Survey (SF-36) Physical Component Summary (PCS) and Mental Component Summary (MCS); Knee Society Score (KSS); Western Ontario MacMaster (WOMAC) osteoarthritis score; and modified Cincinnati activity score. Of these four rating measurements, only the WOMAC score is designed to decrease with patient improvement; the others increase. All of these results were statistically significant.

Results

Based on the patient satisfaction survey, overall satisfaction was 82%, with 11% neutral and 7% dissatisfied; 86% thought they were better, 8% the same, and 6% worse; 88% of the patients said they would choose the surgery again, 4% were uncertain, and 8% said they would not. Overall, the patients rated their results as 80% good or excellent, 18% fair, and 2% poor.

Table 9.3 shows the large average clinical improvement we found using the SF-36, the Knee Society Score, the WOMAC score, and the modified Cincinnati activity score. Please note that of these four rating measurements, only the WOMAC score is designed to decrease with patient improvement; the others increase. All of these results were statistically significant.

When assessing the overall size of the defects treated, there were 98 trochleas with an average surface area of 5.8 cm^2 and 63 patellas with an average surface area of 4.72 cm^2. These large areas comprised the majority of the articular surface of those joints.

There were 30 patients (23%) whose procedures failed, 14 (11%) of which were caused by failures of the weight-bearing condyle ACI graft. There were 16 failures (12%) caused by a patella or a trochlea graft failure.

Twelve patients (9%) had prosthetic reconstruction; eight patients (6%) underwent revision ACI for graft failure; five patients (4%) had no further treatment for partial graft failure; and five patients went on to develop new chondral defects (4%). Of the five patients with new defects, two had ACI, one an allograft, one an arthroscopic abrasion, and the last awaits ACI.

The failure rate of ACI in the patellofemoral joint appears to be no different than in the tibiofemoral joint in our series. Although the clinical outcomes are good (80% good or excellent, 18% fair, only 2% poor), they are less than in the tibiofemoral joint. This is common amongst different series and treatments. My preferred treatment in the patellofemoral joint remains ACI because of the high patient satisfaction and clinical outcomes.

ACI in Patients Older Than 45 Years

Background: ACI has become an accepted option for the treatment of full-thickness chondral defects of the knee in carefully selected patients. Current recommendations limit this procedure to younger patients, yet many patients older than 45 years wish to remain active and preserve their joint. The purpose of this study was to determine whether increasing patient age adversely affected clinical outcome in this patient group.[16]

Method: Patients 45 years and older treated with ACI involving the weight-bearing femoral condyles, patella, and trochlea in isolation, or in combination.

Results: Fifty-six patients 45 years and older were treated with ACI between February 1995 and February 2005. The average patient age at index surgery was 48.6 years (range 45–60 years). The minimum follow-up period was 2 years (range 2 to 11 years; mean 4.7 years). The cohort included 36 men and 20 women. The mean transplant size was 4.7 cm^2 per defect (range 1–5 cm^2) and 9.8 cm^2 per knee (range 2.5–31.6 cm^2). There were 8 failures (14%) and a need for additional surgical procedures in 24 (42%) patients. At their latest available follow-up, 72% of patients rated themselves as good or excellent, 78% felt improved, and 81% would again choose ACI as a treatment option.

Conclusion: Our results suggest that ACI can provide good clinical results even in older patients, but it is associated with a significant rate of re-operation for the arthroscopic treatment of adhesions and graft hypertrophy.

This review of prospectively collected data details the clinical and functional outcomes of ACI in 56 patients older than 45 years with a minimum follow-up of 2 years. The overall failure rate of 14% is comparable to prior reports on the results of ACI in younger patients.

Overall, patients rated their outcomes at the latest available follow-up as 72% good or excellent, 15% fair, and 13% poor; 78% felt improved by the surgery and 81% would choose to undergo ACI again. Only 8% felt their knee was worse than before the surgery and 8% would not choose to have ACI again if they were in a similar situation. When sub-categorized into simple, complex, and salvage groups, clinical improvement was seen in all three categories across all scores. Despite having the highest absolute changes in each of the functional scores, none of the improvements seen in the simple subcategory reached statistical significance because of the small number of patients ($n = 3$) in this group. For the complex and salvage subcategories, all scores showed significant improvements at the time of latest follow-up; there was no significant relationship found between complexity of defect and clinical outcome. The greatest improvement in sports activity rating was found in the most severely involved knees. Failure of treatment occurred in 8 of the 56 patients (14.3%). Surprisingly, only one failure occurred in the 16 patients treated for kissing lesions, resulting in a failure rate (6.25%) lower than the average failure rate across all patients. Of the patients treated under the Workers' Compensation Program, 6 of 15 (40%) had failed procedures, reflecting a significantly higher failure rate compared with patients having a non-work-related history. In the non-Workers' Compensation patients, 2 out of 41 failed (failure rate 5%), which is similar to the younger than 45-year-old group. Of note, five of the six patients treated in the Workers' Compensation group who had failed procedures had undergone prior marrow stimulation technique, which may have been the most significant aspect of the treatment failure in this group. Our data[17] have demonstrated that a higher failure rate with ACI will occur after prior marrow stimulation technique.

With an average transplant size of 4.7 cm^2 per defect and 9.8 cm^2 per knee, the lesions treated were substantial and generally larger than those reported in other studies of patients who, on average, were more than a decade younger. Our findings of an overall failure rate of 14% are similar to existing data in younger patient populations. We previously published our experiences with ACI in a younger patient cohort with an average age of 36 years, average transplant size of 4.3 cm^2 per defect, and overall failure rate of 13%.[12]

Most patients in this age group present to our office specifically to avoid, or postpone, prosthetic replacement; a randomized controlled study comparing cartilage repair with joint replacement was therefore not feasible. The results of a younger patient group treated at our institution by the same surgeon with identical technique and outcome instruments have shown similar results.[7] The strengths lie in the very complete and long follow-up with multiple validated outcome instruments; all patients were operated by a single surgeon with extensive experience in cartilage repair. To our knowledge, this is the first detailed report on the clinical outcome of ACI in an older age group.

Conclusion

In older patients, metabolic cell activity is assumed to be lower and defects are often large and chronic in nature, adding to concerns over the efficacy of cartilage repair procedures in these patients. Treatment of older patients with cartilage defects has therefore traditionally consisted of palliation, osteotomy, or joint replacement. With an aging population, there are an increasing number of patients who wish to remain active and are less willing to accept the limitations associated with joint replacement or who dislike the comparatively large angular corrections of isolated osteotomy. The study focuses on this group of patients who are beyond the current recommendations for cartilage repair but who are either unwilling or biologically too young to undergo joint replacement. We chose 45 years as our threshold because this age has developed as a common insurance limit for ACI, even though it is not strongly supported by data.

Our results indicate that ACI is a reliable technique for the treatment of patients 45 years and older with symptomatic, large full-thickness chondral defects of the knee. Careful indication and correction of associated malalignment is essential for a successful outcome. Patients require careful counselling with regard to the long and complex rehabilitation, the likelihood of additional surgery, and the functional gains that can be reasonably expected in order to avoid disappointment.

Prior marrow stimulation in this age group should be of concern especially in Workers' Compensation patients who may have had prolonged and problematic treatment and symptoms. In our series, the failure rate in the patients who were not under the Workers' Compensation Program was only 8% versus 40% in those patients who were, 5 of 6 of whom had prolonged symptoms and prior marrow stimulation.

Autologous Chondrocyte Implantation for Joint Preservation in Patients With Early Osteoarthritis: 2- to 11-Year Follow-Up[18]

Perhaps the most gratifying use of ACI is in the management of injured young athletes with early osteoarthritis, the young arthritics, and young people with old knees. This group of patients are outside the realm of sports medicine and too young to undergo prosthetic arthroplasty. They may still obtain successful pain relief, functional improvement, and improved quality of life after undergoing ACI.

Young patients with early osteoarthritis wishing to remain functionally active have limited treatment options. Existing studies examining the use of ACI have included patients with early degenerative changes, for whom encouraging results were reported.[7,35] No study, however, has specifically investigated the outcome of ACI in this challenging population. We hypothesize that ACI reduces pain and improves function in young, early-stage osteoarthritic patients and delays the need for joint replacement surgery.

For patient selection, we first chose all ACI patients who had completed a minimum follow-up of 2 years; however, patients whose procedure had failed within the first 2 years were also included in the study. From this group we selected those who had been categorized radiographically or clinically as having early osteoarthritic disease at the time of ACI. Radiographically, patients were eligible if they had peripheral intraarticular osteophyte formation and/or 0% to 50% joint space narrowing as defined by Ahlbäck stage 0 or 1 classification.[36] Patients were also included if they had normal radiographs but evidence of bipolar (kissing) lesions or generalized chondromalacia at the time of surgery. From the database of the 328 patients treated with ACI within the study period, 153 patients (155 knees) fulfilled the aforementioned criteria and were enrolled in the study; there were no exclusion criteria and all eligible patients were analyzed.

Autologous Chondrocyte Implantation

Patients with 2 degrees or more of malalignment were treated by realignment osteotomy and overcorrected by 2 degrees to unload and optimize the mechanical environment of the compromised compartment. We intentionally avoided more significant overcorrection by 3 to 5 degrees as recommended for isolated osteotomy because of the risk of overload and accelerated failure of the contralateral compartment. Patients with patellofemoral defects had a concurrent AMZ-TTO, lateral release, and vastus medialis obliquus advancement if there was evidence of patellar subluxation and tilt as noted by physical examination, radiographs, and/or CT scan assessment.

Outcome Measures

Our standard outcome measures were collected and we analyzed clinically important patient perceived improvements. Minimal clinically important difference (MCID) was defined as the smallest difference in score that patients perceive as beneficial.[37,38] According to previously published studies, the MCID of improvement in patients with osteoarthritis in the knee has been defined as a 17% to 22% change from baseline WOMAC subscale scores.[37,39]

Results

Patient and Defect Characteristics

The study included 153 patients with 155 treated knees. The average age of patients in this cohort was 38.3 years at the time of implantation; there were 70 women and 83 men. On average, 2.1 defects were treated per knee; the mean defect size was 4.9 cm^2 and the total area per knee was 10.4 cm^2. Fourteen percent (22 of 153) of patients were receiving workers' compensation. An average of 2.1 defects per knee were treated with an average defect size of 4.9 cm^2 and a total treated surface area of 10.4 cm^2 per knee joint.

TABLE 9.4 Functional Scores Preoperatively, at 24 Months, and at Latest Follow-up

	Preoperative (n =143)	24-Month follow-up (n = 143)	Latest follow-up (>2 years) (n = 132)	P value
Modified Cincinnati	3.6 (1–8)	6.1 (2–10)	6.7 (2–10)	<.001
KSS–knee	59.0 (24–100)	82.6 (45–100)	88.0 (50–100)	<.001
KSS–function	60.6 (15–100)	74.2 (40–100)	79.4 (40–100)	<.001
WOMAC–pain	9.6 (0–20)	5.8 (0–16)	4.7 (0–17)	<.001
WOMAC–stiffness	3.9 (0–8)	2.7 (0–7)	2.4 (0–8)	<.001
WOMAC–function	29.4 (2–62)	17.3 (0–51)	13.7 (0–49)	<.001
SF-36 PCS	37.2 (23–60)	44.0 (25–60)	45.4 (9–60)	<.001
SF-36 MCS	38.4 (9–55)	41.3 (9–53)	43.8 (9–56)	<.001

Data are given as mean (range).
KSS, Knee Society Score; modified Cincinnati, modified Cincinnati activity score; n, number of patients at the respective time point; SF-36, Medical Outcomes Study 36-Item Short-Form Health Survey; PCS, Physical Component Summary; MCS, Mental Component Summary; WOMAC, Western Ontario MacMaster osteoarthritis score.

When only considering the size of the primary, or largest, lesion in each joint, average size increased to 6.7 cm^2. Lesions were most commonly located in the following location, by order of incidence: medial femoral condyle, trochlea, patella, and lateral femoral condyle. Bipolar (kissing) lesions were present in 27% (42 of 155) of knee joints. In addition to ACI, many concurrent procedures were performed, most commonly to correct tibiofemoral malalignment in 31% (48 of 155) and patellar maltracking in 28% (44 of 155) of implanted knees.

Treatment Failures and Revision Surgery

For the purposes of this study a treatment failure was conversion to a prosthesis because avoiding prosthetic arthroplasty was the primary reason patients in this group sought treatment. Twelve knees (8%) were considered treatment failures and were revised to partial (2) or total (10) joint replacements at an average of 38 (9–118) months after ACI. The reasons for revision included complete graft failure in three patients, inadequate pain relief in one patient, and progression of osteoarthritic disease beyond the originally transplanted defect area in eight patients.

Of patients treated with ACI 8% (12 of 155) met the criteria of treatment failure because of revision with partial or total knee arthroplasty; six of these patients received payments through workers' compensation, resulting in a failure rate of 27.3% (6 of 22) in that sub-group. ACI in patients not covered by workers' compensation failed at a rate of 4.5% (6 of 133). Kaplan-Meier survival for the group is presented in Fig. 9.31.

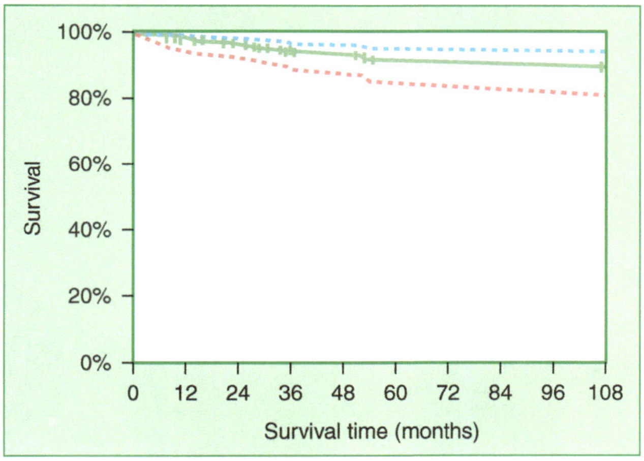

• **Fig. 9.31** Kaplan-Meier survival curve and 95% confidence interval for survival of autologous chondrocyte implantation over time.

Outcome Measures

The 92% of knees that were not considered treatment failures experienced statistically significant changes in the WOMAC pain and function scores from baseline to follow-up that exceeded the definition of MCID (Table 9.4).

Excluding patients whose treatments failed, the mean improvement in the 20-point WOMAC pain score and 68-point WOMAC function score was 4.9 points (51% improvement) and 15.7 points (53% improvement), respectively. More specifically, the proportion of patients who experienced severe or extreme pain when walking on a flat surface decreased by 73% and the percentage of patients with similar pain walking up and down stairs decreased by 76%. Similar reductions were also seen in the proportion of patients who had severe or extreme difficulty when descending stairs, ascending stairs, bending to the floor, and walking on a flat surface; the proportion of patients with this level of difficulty decreased by 78%, 75%, 73%, and 74%, respectively.

Statistically significant improvements in mean score change were also observed for the modified Cincinnati

TABLE 9.5 Functional Scores for Osteotomy Groups Preoperatively and at Latest Follow-up

	Preoperative			Latest Follow-up (>2 years)		
	HTO (n = 29)	TTO (n = 23)	P Value	HTO (n = 27)	TTO (n = 23)	P Value
Modified Cincinnati	3.4	3.3	.9	7.3	6.1	.002
KSS–knee	61.7	52.9	.03	92.0	84.1	.02
KSS–function	64.5	59.1	.2	82.6	74.3	.04
WOMAC–pain	9.5	11.5	.08	3.3	6.2	.01
WOMAC–stiffness	4.1	4.9	.1	1.9	3.2	.01
WOMAC–function	30.0	34.9	.2	10.8	19.7	.007
SF-36 PCS	36.7	35.6	.6	48.6	43.3	.03
SF-36 MCS	39.1	38.4	.7	43.7	43.7	.99

Data are given as mean.
P values compare the two groups at each time point.
HTO, high tibial osteotomy; KSS, Knee Society Score; modified Cincinnati, modified Cincinnati activity score; n, number of patients at the respective time point; SF-36, Medical Outcomes Study 36-Item Short-Form Health Survey; PCS, Physical Component Summary; MCS, Mental Component Summary; TTO, tibial tubercle osteotomy; WOMAC, Western Ontario MacMaster osteoarthritis score.

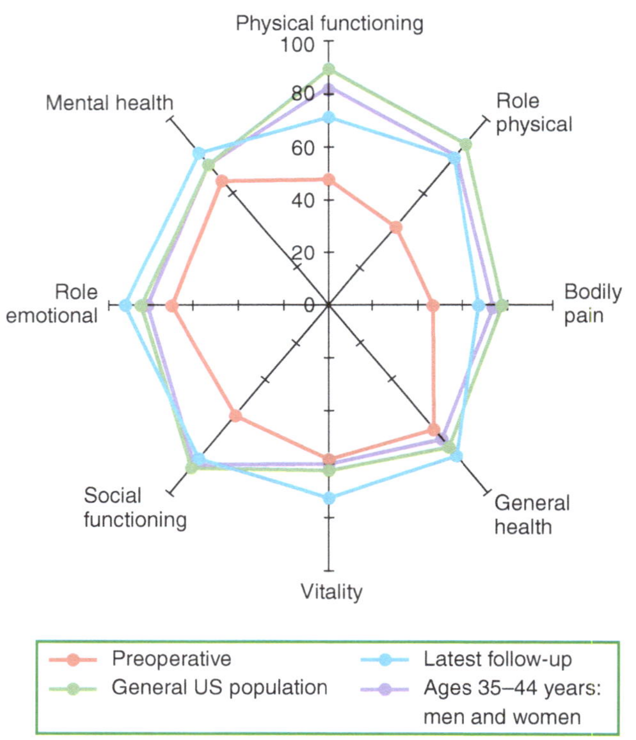

• **Fig. 9.32** Medical Outcomes Study 36-Item Short-Form Health Survey domain scores for autologous chondrocyte implantation patients preoperatively and at the time of latest follow-up. Reference values for the general US population and patients aged 35–44 years.

Knee Rating System, KSS function scale, KSS pain scale, and all eight SF-36 domain scales (Table 9.4, Fig. 9.32). Furthermore, 91.6% of patients were satisfied with the outcome after ACI treatment, 90.2% rated their knees better than before the surgery, and 91.3% would have the same procedure again.

Additional Analyses

Additional analyses were performed to test the effect of concurrent osteotomy procedures on the functional outcome of ACI. Patients with and without concurrent osteotomies experienced significant improvements in all functional scores ($P < 0.001$). There were no significant differences between patients without osteotomies and individual subgroups of patients with isolated HTO, isolated TTO, or a combination of both. Comparing patients with HTO and patients who had undergone TTO demonstrated significantly better outcomes for the HTO group at final follow-up (Table 9.5) when considering absolute levels; however, TTO patients started with worse scores.

The results from this study demonstrate that ACI results in statistically significant and clinically relevant reductions in pain and improvement in function, while delaying the need for knee arthroplasty for over 5 years in 92% of patients. Careful and thorough discussion of the invasive surgical procedure, complex rehabilitation and long recovery, and a high likelihood of repeat surgery are paramount to ensuring a reasonable level of patient expectations and satisfaction with the outcome. Given the limited treatment options for this subset of patients, ACI may be a plausible treatment for young osteoarthritic patients to delay the need for joint replacement surgery in the hope of obviating subsequent revision surgery, which is associated with much less satisfactory outcomes than primary procedures.

Our data suggest that ACI in patients with early osteoarthritis results in clinically relevant and statistically significant reductions in pain and improvement in function. A total of 92% of patients were functioning well at 5 years postoperative and were able to delay the need for joint replacement. Given the limited number of treatment options for this subset of patients, ACI may offer improved quality of life for young osteoarthritic patients

In this prospective cohort study with 2- to 11-year follow-up, we hypothesize that ACI reduces pain in young patients with early osteoarthritic changes. Our hope is to utilize ACI to delay the need for primary knee replacement until a more advanced age when the replacement might outlast the patient's lifetime, thus avoiding the need for revision surgery.

ACI in Patients After Marrow Stimulation Techniques

When I first started to perform ACI in 1995, patients who were typically sent to me had failed multiple previous treatment options and were considered to have failed the standard of care at the time, which included drilling, abrasion, and the recently introduced microfracture technique as a marrow stimulation to promote fibrocartilaginous repair in an articular defect. I noted thickened and sclerotic subchondral bone plates after debridement of the fibrocartilage repair tissue, remaining fibrous tracts within drill holes, and occasionally intralesional osteophyte formation that was very prominent and sometimes above the adjacent articular surface. My concern in taking down these intralesional osteophytes was the possibility of bleeding and mix marrow derived cells with end-differentiated chondrocytes contaminating the cell suspension, resulting in recurrent fibrocartilage repair instead of hyaline repair tissue. I initially used a bone tamp to impact the prominent bone flush with the adjacent subchondral bone to create a cavity for the recipient cells. However, I noted that several of the transplants would fill the defect and then delaminate leaving behind a very visible sclerotic subchondral bone that had been impacted. I then removed the intralesional osteophyte with a rongeur and used a high-speed bur to thin out the subchondral bone to the adjacent level of subchondral bone. I was surprised to see that bleeding was minimal given that the bone was very cortical in nature. Despite this, failures from delamination, central breakdown of the graft over the area of stiffening, and occasional deep cystic formation would occur with failure of the transplant. This did not seem to happen with articular defects that had not been previously marrow stimulated.

I had a hypothesis that the osteochondral unit had been affected by the marrow stimulation technique which lessened the success rate of integration to the subchondral bone of ACI, and a change in the subchondral bone such that its load absorbing capacity was altered and that an overlying repair tissue was subject to central overload and breakdown.

We therefore reviewed my series of ACI in a very systematic fashion to compare those that had undergone prior microfracture, abrasion, or drilling and with a control group that had not. A summary of our findings are presented.

Increased Failure Rate of ACI After Previous Treatment With Marrow Stimulation Techniques[17]

Background: Marrow stimulation techniques such as drilling or microfracture are first-line treatment options for symptomatic cartilage defects. Common knowledge holds that these treatments do not compromise subsequent cartilage repair procedures with ACI. We present our experience with ACI after prior marrow stimulation.

Hypothesis: Cartilage defects pretreated with marrow stimulation techniques will demonstrate an increased failure rate.

Study Design: Case control, Level 2 Study,

Methods: This study reviewed prospectively collected data for the first 321 consecutive patients treated at our institution with ACI for full-thickness cartilage defects that had reached more than 2 years of follow-up. Patients were grouped based on whether they had undergone prior treatment with a marrow stimulation technique. Outcomes were classified as complete failure if more than 25% of a grafted defect area had to be removed in later procedures carried out because of persistent symptoms. This includes treatment with revision ACI, allograft transplantation, partial or total knee replacement.

Results: 522 defects in 321 patients (325 joints) were treated with ACI. The average patient age was 35 years (range 13–60). There were 185 men and 136 women, with an average follow-up of 55 months (range 24–144). On average, there were 1.7 lesions per patient (range 1–5) with a transplant area of 4.9 cm^2 per lesion (range 0.5–21) and 8.2 cm^2 (range 1–30.5) per knee. Of these joints, 111 had previously undergone surgery that penetrated the subchondral bone: microfracture ($n = 25$), abrasion chondroplasty ($n = 33$), and drilling ($n = 53$). A total of 214 joints had no prior treatment that affected the subchondral bone and served as control. Within the marrow stimulation group, there were 29 (26%) failures compared with 17 (8%) failures in the control group ($P < 0.001$).

Conclusions: In our review of 321 patients, defects that had prior treatment affecting the subchondral bone failed at a rate of three times that of non-treated defects. The failure rates for drilling (28%), abrasion arthroplasty (27%), and microfracture (20%) were not significantly different ($P > 0.5$), possibly as a result of the lower number of microfracture patients in this cohort (25 of 110 marrow-stimulation procedures). Our data demonstrate that marrow stimulation techniques have a strong negative effect on subsequent cartilage repair with ACI and should therefore be used judiciously in larger cartilage defects that might require future treatment with ACI.

The marrow stimulation group of patients were very similar to the control group in all ways as noted in Table 9.6. The failure rates among the two treatment groups are noted in Table 9.7 as well as the failure rates among different categories of patients being treated.

TABLE 9.6 Patient Demographics for Control Group (no MST) and Previously Marrow-Stimulated Group (Prior MST)

Demographic Variables	No MST	Prior MST	*P* Value
No. of knees/no. of patients	214/211	111/110	–
Average age (years)	35.0 (9.2, 13–60)	35.4 (10.1, 14–55)	.7
Gender (male/female)	124/87	61/49	.6
Average follow-up time (months)	54 (27, 24–132)	56 (30, 24–144)	.4
Average no. of defects per knee	1.7 (0.9, 1–5)	1.7 (0.8, 1–4)	.9
Average defect size (cm^2)	4.6 (2.7, 0.5–21)	5.2 (3.1, 0.7–16.8)	.2
Average transplant area per knee (cm^2)	7.9 (5.0, 1.0–28.3)	8.6 (5.9, 1.5–30.5)	.3
Workers' Compensation patients	28 (13%)	24 (22%)	.1
Patients lost to follow-up after 2 years by defect category	–	–	–
Simple	3 (1%)	2 (2%)	
Complex	16 (8%)	12 (11%)	>.5
Salvage	6 (3%)	4 (4%)	

TABLE 9.7 Failure Rates for Control (no MST) and Marrow-Stimulated (MST) Groups

	No MST	Prior MST	*P* Value
Overall	214 (17, 8%)	111 (29, 26%)	<.001
Simple defects	18 (2, 11%)	9 (1, 11%)	N/A
Complex defects	97 (9, 9%)	56 (17, 30%)	<.01
Salvage defects	99 (6, 6%)	46 (11, 24%)	<.01
Subanalyses	–	–	–
Osteochondritis dissecans lesions	23 (2, 9%)	20 (6, 30%)	N/A
Workers' Compensation patients	28 (4, 14%)	24 (9, 38%)	N/A
Previous microfracture	–	25 (5, 20%)	–
Previous abrasion arthroplasty	–	33 (9, 27%)	>.5
Previous drilling	–	53 (15, 28%)	–

All values are given as overall number (no. of failures, % failure).
N/A, insufficient information to calculate.

Interestingly, even within the group of 29 knees that had failed ACI after prior treatment with MST, 14 were implanted for isolated defects and 15 for multiple defects. Among these 15 knees there were a total of 35 implanted defects, some of which had been marrow-stimulated and some of which had not: specifically, 17 had previously been marrow-stimulated (13 knees with 1 defect each and 2 knees with 2 defects each) and 18 lesions had not been treated prior to ACI. Since all knees had at least one marrow-stimulated defect and one untreated defect, we utilized the untreated defect as an internal control. Sixteen of the 17 marrow-stimulated defects failed compared with 2 of the 18 previously untreated lesions.

We have noted that marrow stimulation techniques "burn bridges" and that prior marrow stimulation techniques alter the osteochondral unit. The subchondral bone is either hypertrophic with an internal osteophyte, thickened and sclerotic, or the pick holes or drill holes developed into subchondral cysts with eventual failure of the grafts (Fig. 9.33). Accordingly, these techniques should be utilized where they have the highest chance of success and will not compromise a future reconstruction if they fail.

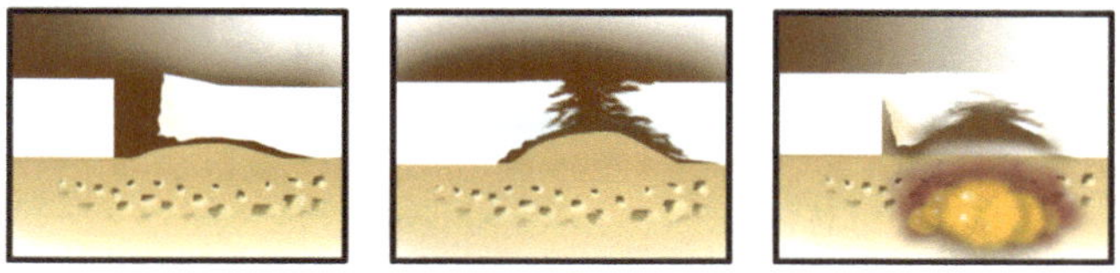

• **Fig. 9.33** Modes of failure after marrow stimulation: delamination *(left)*, intralesional osteophyte *(center)*, subchondral cyst *(right)*.

Microfracture succeeds best in patients who have defects less than 2–3 cm^2, on the weight-bearing femoral condyle, in patients younger than 40 years, in relatively acute defects less than 1 year after injury. Chronic degenerative large lesions and locations on the patella trochlea and tibia tend not to do well. A simple debridement as a first step treatment option may be adequate in these other lesions prior to recommending ACI or fresh osteoarticular allograft for these locations.

The Use of a Collagen Type I–III Membrane for ACI Compared With Periosteum

At present, the most frequently encountered postoperative adverse event with ACI is periosteal hypertrophy followed by adhesions and arthrofibrosis. A randomized prospective British study[40] comparing collagen-covered ACI (ACI-C) with periosteal-covered ACI (ACI-P) noted a dramatic decrease in periosteal hypertrophy. In this group of 68 patients with a mean age of 30 years, 33 patients were randomized to ACI-P and 35 patients to ACI-C. The mean defect size was 4.5 cm^2. All patients were followed up at 24 months. Clinical and functional assessment showed 74% of patients had good or excellent results following ACI-C compared with 67% after ACI-P at 2 years. Arthroscopy at 1 year also demonstrated similar results for both techniques. However, 34.6% of the ACI-P had periosteal graft hypertrophy required shaving for hypertrophy compared with none for the ACI-C graft at 1 year.

With a rate of hypertrophy greater than 40% in our series of multiple defects per knee, we sought to assess the use of an off-label, similar type I–III collagen membrane cover to that used in the British study.

After informed consent with the patient and IRB approval for data collection, we proceeded with the use of a collagen type I–III membrane for the use of ACI in our patients and compared it with the incidence of hypertrophy using periosteum in the previous 100 patients.

Decreased Surgical Re-Intervention Rate for Hypertrophy After ACI With Use of the BioGide Collagen Membrane

A prospective comparative study was made using a collagen type I–III membrane ACI-C to traditional ACI-P. The last 100 ACI prior to June 2007 were compared with all ACI performed after June 2007 with a minimum 1-year follow-up (54 knees). The end points were reoperation within the first year for symptomatic cover related issues and the failure rate in the first year.

The membrane used was produced by Geistlich Pharma AG (Wolhusen, Switzerland) and is of porcine origin (peritoneum), semi-permeable, type I/III collagen bilayer structure, and bio-absorbable (Fig. 9.34). Table 9.8 lists the defect size characteristics and demographics of those patients treated, which do not vary appreciably. Table 9.9 demonstrates a dramatic decrease in the incidence of periosteal hypertrophy using ACI-C.

There is no appreciable difference in the failure rate between techniques (Table 9.10) confirming prior reports from Britain demonstrating a drastic lowering of the reoperation rate for cover-related problems (6% versus 52%), with no difference in the failure rate in the first year (1% versus 1.9%).

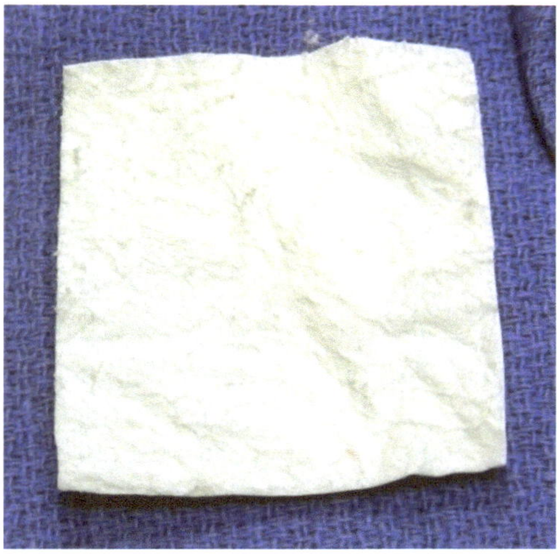

• **Fig. 9.34** Type I–III collagen bilayer membrane (porcine derived; Geistlich Pharma AG, Wolhusen, Switzerland) used as a periosteal substitute for autologous chondrocyte implantation.

TABLE 9.8 Patient Demographics Undergoing ACI-P or ACI-C

	ACI-P	ACI-C	*P* Value
No.	100	54	–
Age (years)	34.5	37.6	.06
Defect number	1.9	2.1	.25
Defect size (cm^2)	4.6	4.8	.5
Defect total surface area (cm^2)	8.8	10.2	.16

Defect size characteristics and demographics of patients treated are not appreciably different.
ACI-C, collagen-covered autologous chondrocyte implantation; ACI-P, periosteal-covered autologous chondrocyte implantation.

We have combined our results in a three-center study[19] to review our combined results with different practice patterns for a "threshold" to intervene for periosteal hypertrophy versus membrane-related problems and have found a similar marked decrease in periosteal problems with no difference in the failure rates. These demographics are summarized in Table 9.11.

The two groups were comparable for age at time of implantation with ACI and average defect size (Table 9.11). Patients treated with collagen membrane ACI had significantly more defects than those treated with periosteal ACI, resulting in a larger total area per knee implanted. The specific re-operation rate for cover-related issues, such as hypertrophy and periosteal delamination, decreased from 25.7% (77 of 300 patients) with the use of periosteum, to 4.9% (5 of 103) with the collagen membrane ($P < 0.0001$). A total of seven patients were considered as treatment failure after ACI with periosteum (2.3%), compared with four patients in the collagen membrane group (3.9%) ($P = 0.2$).

It appears that c-ACI is a reasonable substitute for periosteum. Our 2-year multicenter outcomes data will verify whether there is any decrease in outcome success as a result of this substitution. However, European studies do not show any differences and we do not anticipate any.

TABLE 9.9 ACI Membrane Hypertrophy After ACI-P and ACI-C

	ACI-P	ACI-C	P Value
Intervention for hypertrophy	52%	5.6%	1.6E-09

A dramatic decrease is seen in incidence of periosteal hypertrophy using collagen-covered autologous chondrocyte implantation (ACI-C). ACI-P, periosteal-covered autologous chondrocyte implantation.

TABLE 9.10 Failure Rate After ACI-P or ACI-C

	ACI-P	ACI-C	*P* Value
Failure rate in first year	1 (1%)	1 (1.9%)	.66

ACI-C, collagen-covered autologous chondrocyte implantation; ACI-P, periosteal-covered autologous chondrocyte implantation.

Clinical Cost-Effectiveness of ACI

ACI has proven clinically effective in restoring hyaline-like cartilage to isolated chondral defects of the knee; however, no study has quantified the quality of life or economic outcomes of this procedure. This study prospectively examined efficacy and quality of life in 44 patients undergoing ACI for full-thickness cartilage lesions and calculated the average cost per additional quality-adjusted life year.[23] The 12-month results of ACI treatment demonstrated improvement in patient function as measured by both the KSS (23% mean improvement [114.02–140.67], $P < 0.001$) and the Western Ontario and McMaster Universities Osteoarthritis Index (33% mean improvement [35.30–23.82], $P < 0.05$). Quality of life as measured by the SF-36 Physical Component Summary was dramatically enhanced from 33.32 prior to biopsy to 41.48 ($P < 0.05$) 12 months post implant. Improvement on all three scales was maintained from 12 to 24 months. Estimated cost per additional quality-adjusted life year (QALY) was $6,791. This cost-effectiveness ratio was minimally sensitive to reasonable changes in effectiveness, patient age, or procedural cost and remained very cost-effective even when assumptions were less favorable than in the base-case. Cost-effectiveness of ACI compares favorably with other interventions for chronic diseases such as intensive therapy for diabetes ($16,000/QALY) and interferon-α for hepatitis C ($4,000/QALY); it is more cost-effective than many commonly reimbursed interventions such as therapy for mild hypertension ($30,200/QALY) and lumbar discectomy for the treatment of herniated intervertebral disc ($33,900/QALY). ACI improves patient quality of life

TABLE 9.11 Demographic Data of Study Groups

	ACI-P (*n* = 300)			ACI-C (*n* = 103)			
	Mean	Min	Max	Mean	Min	Max	*P* Value
Age at ACI (years)	31.9	13.5	56.0	32.4	14.2	54.0	.762
Gender (male/female)	162/138	–	–	51/50	–	–	–
No. of defects	1.5	1.0	5.0	1.8	1.0	5.0	.001
Defect size (cm^2)	4.6	0.7	36.0	4.7	0.5	19.2	.645
Total defect area (cm^2)	6.7	1.4	36.0	8.5	0.5	29.9	.004

ACI-C, collagen-covered autologous chondrocyte implantation; ACI-P, periosteal-covered autologous chondrocyte implantation.

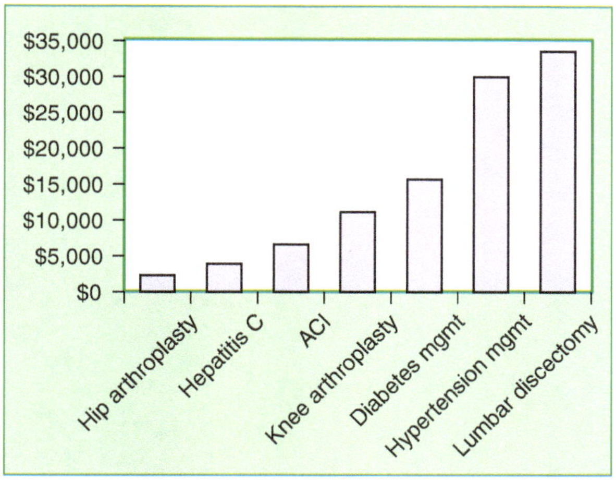

• **Fig. 9.35** Cost-effectiveness chart represented in dollars per quality-adjusted life years for procedures that are commonly performed and other disease states treated. Despite the cost of autologous chondrocyte implantation (ACI), the clinical improvement and durability of ACI in young patients are pronounced, which explains why ACI is so cost effective as a procedure when treating large focal articular cartilage defects compared with other treatment options. From Minas T. Chondrocyte implantation in the repair of chondral lesions of the knee: economics and quality of life. *Am J Orthop* 1998;27:739–744.

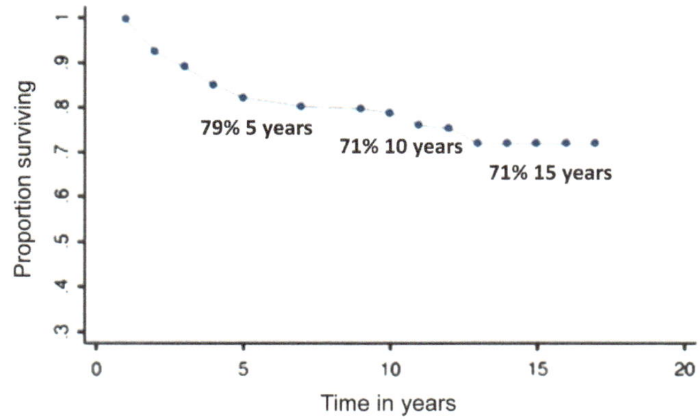

• **Fig. 9.36** Overall survival of periosteal-covered autologous chondrocyte implantation grafts. Endpoint defined as failure of graft.

and is an appropriate, cost-effective treatment for cartilage lesions of the knee.

At the time this study was performed, only 1-year follow-up data were available with clinical outcome measures (including the SF-36 standardized outcome, which was utilized to calculate the utility value for the quality adjusted life years). To date ACI grafting has been very durable,[25] the clinical outcomes improving to a maximal medical end point in the tibiofemoral joint after 2 years and in the patellofemoral joint at 3 years. As the clinical outcomes continue to improve up to 3 years, the utility calculated would also be more favorable and the procedure more cost-effective. Despite the increased cost of the procedure and cell culture process, after sensitivity analysis the conclusion does not change—ACI is very cost effective because it dramatically improves the quality of life for patients and is a durable procedure. It is very cost effective when compared with other standard surgical and medical treatments that are considered the "standard of care" for patients (Fig. 9.35).

Outcome Publication Summaries Since 2010

In 2014, My colleagues and I reported the 10-year outcomes[28] of the first 210 consecutive patients undergoing ACI-P treatment for symptomatic articular cartilage defects of the knee. There were an average 1.7 lesions per knee with a mean total surface area of 8.4 ± 5.5 cm^2. Patients provided pre- and postoperative responses to validated questionnaires, including the KSS, modified Cincinnati Rating scale, WOMAC, and the SF-36. Patients also responded to a patient satisfaction scale following surgery. All outcome scores improved statistically ($P < .0001$). Of the cohort, 78% rated their results as good-to-excellent, 16% as fair, and 6% as poor at the last follow-up visit. Survivorship analysis revealed a 79% survival rate at 5 years and 71% at 10 and 15 years of ACI-P treatment (Fig. 9.36). Fifty-three (25%) experienced one graft failure. Of the graft failures, 14 (26%) failed because of progression of disease; the original ACI graft(s) remained intact. Twelve (23%) patients experienced graft delamination and 20 (38%) failed to form durable repair tissue. Two patients (4%) failed following a traumatic event and five (9%) were classified as failed grafts because of persistent pain at the final follow-up, despite MRI evidence of an intact graft. Of the 210 patients, 19 (9%) went on to knee arthroplasty over the studied period.

Further analysis revealed risk factors for failure of ACI-P. Potential indicators included prior microfracture (MST), mechanical malalignment, defect sizes greater than 15 cm^2, and age greater than 45 years. A decline in ACI graft survival at 10 years and 15 years was particularly notable among patients with prior MST in comparison with patients without prior MST (10 years: 66% vs. 84%; 15 years: 44% vs. 79%;($P = .004$) (Fig. 9.37). Survival was also found to be higher in patients with a concomitant HTO versus no HTO ($P = .01$). When risk factors are considered, overall findings demonstrate adequate long-term survival rate of first-generation ACI.

Gomoll et al.[15] presented the findings of a large multicenter experiment reviewing 110 patients treated with ACI-P for patella and/or trochlear defects. Patients with an average defect size of 5.4 cm^2 were followed over a mean of 90 months. Collected patient reported outcome data included the SF-36, WOMAC score, modified Cincinnati activity score, KSS, and a patient satisfaction survey. A concurrent TTO was performed in 75 (69%) patients. All clinical outcome measures experienced statistical and clinically meaningful improvement at the last follow-up ($P < .0001$). Likewise, over 90% of the studied patients reported they would undergo the procedure again and 86% rated their knee good-to-excellent postoperatively. Nine patients were

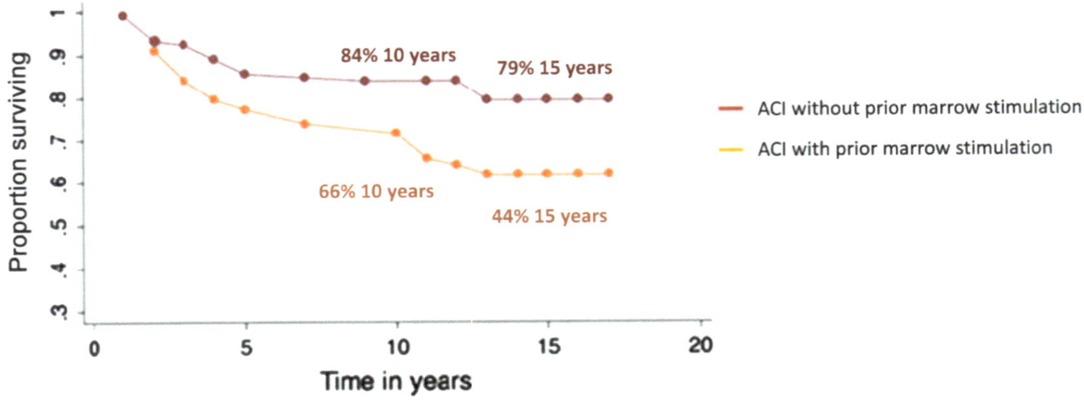

• **Fig. 9.37** Survival curves of periosteal-covered autologous chondrocyte implantation (ACI-P) grafts following marrow stimulation versus ACI-P without prior marrow stimulation. Endpoint defined as failure of graft.

classified as treatment failures. Of the nine failures, eight underwent knee replacement surgery (four total knee arthroplasty, four partial knee arthroplasty) and one patient declined further surgical treatment. The results of this study demonstrated that ACI is an excellent option for patients with isolated chondral defects of the patella or bipolar patellofemoral defects. Outcomes further suggest addressing indications of lateral patellar maltracking is critical in preserving structural integrity of the ACI graft.

In 2017, von Keudell et al.[11] reported encouraging clinical outcomes of ACI-P and ACI-C for the treatment of patella chondral lesions with correlating MRI results in a cohort of 30 consecutive patients with a mean defect size measuring 4.7 ± 2.1 cm^2. All clinical outcome measures improved significantly from baseline ($P < .001$) at 2 years postoperative with adequate repair tissue fill. A total of 25 patient (83%) reported their knee function as good-to-excellent. MOCART scoring correlated with clinical outcome findings. MRI performed at 24 months postoperatively showed complete fill of the chondral defects in 18 (75%) patients. This was the first paper to correlate graft fill and MOCART scoring to correlate with good and excellent clinical outcomes.

Four patient experienced graft hypertrophy. Three of the 16 patients who underwent ACI-P developed graft hypertrophy, whereas only 1 of the 8 patients in the ACI-C group had graft hypertrophy. Throughout the study, three ACI grafts were considered failures; all were Workers' Compensation patients. Kaplan-Meier analysis further revealed that 75% patients were able to retain their native knee up to 15 years postoperative (Fig. 9.38). Von Keudell et al. found ACI to be an effective and durable treatment option of patella chondral lesions. Further analysis went on to suggest concomitant TTO to offload the lesion improves the outcomes after ACI treatment for patella chondral lesions.

Demange et al.[41] analyzed the recurrence of osteophyte regrowth among patients with existing intralesional osteophytes removed during ACI ($n = 87$) and among patients who presented without intralesional osteophytes at the time of ACI ($n = 20$). Overall, osteophyte regrowth was observed

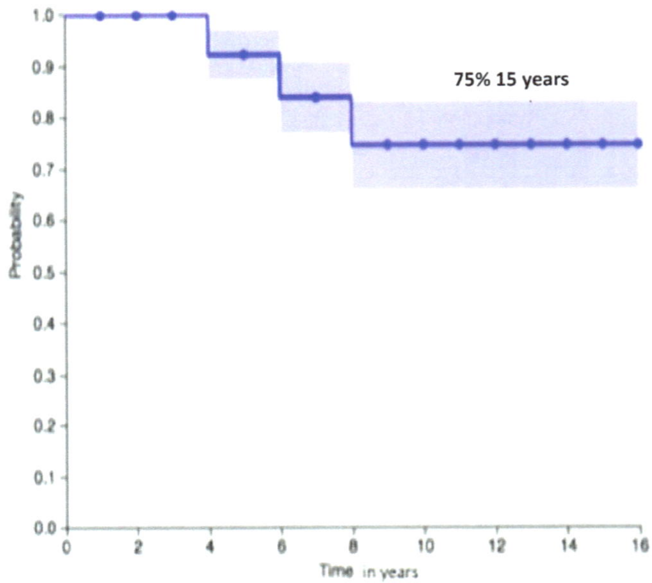

• **Fig. 9.38** Kaplan-Meier survival curve for autologous chondrocyte implantation ACI in isolated patella cartilage defects.

in 62 lesions (39.5%) or 29 patients (33.3%). Intralesional osteophyte development did not differ between the two evaluated cohorts according to MRI analysis. Sub-analysis revealed higher incidence of osteophyte regrowth in the ACI-P group compared with the collagen-covered ACI (ACI-C) ($P < 0.001$). In the ACI-P cohort, 55 lesions (45.8%) (23 patients) had osteophyte regrowth. The ACI-C group consisted of seven lesions (18.9%) (six patients) with osteophyte regrowth. The average lesion sizes were 4.2 ± 2.9 cm^2 and 4.9 ± 2.8 cm^2 for the ACI-P and ACI-C groups, respectively. Evaluation by MRI was carried out after the 1-year follow-up. Based on the findings, intralesional osteophytes do not appear to be a contraindication for ACI treatment.

In 2016, Ogura et al.[27] retrospectively evaluated the mid- to long-term clinical and radiographic outcomes of

17 patients (18 knees) who underwent concurrent ACI and meniscal allograft transplantation (MAT) over a mean 7.9-year follow-up. The mean total defect surface area was 7.6 ± 5.3 cm^2. Six knees were classified as failures with total knee arthroplasty being performed in four of them. Of the 12 successful knees, 7 underwent subsequent surgical procedures (SSP). Despite the elevated SSP rate, clinical outcome scores in relation to radiographic outcomes revealed significant improvement over the study period. Patient-reported outcome scores obtained from the modified Cincinnati Knee Rating Scale, WOMAC, VAS, and SF-36 all improved significantly, and 10 patients (11 knees; 92%) reported a high level of satisfaction. Radiographic results resembled these findings. No significant osteoarthritis progress was observed radiographically based on K–L grading in the successfully operated knees. Results suggest ACI treatment with concurrent MAT is an adequate joint-preserving procedure. Preoperative discussion with the patient regarding the possibility of a subsequent surgical procedure is advised.

In 2017, Ogura et al.[12] evaluated the long-term clinical outcomes and graft survival of 23 adolescents (24 knees) under the age of 18 years (mean 15.9 years) undergoing ACI treatment for symptomatic, grade III/IV chondral defects. The mean number of defects treated per knee was 1.5. The mean total defect surface area measured 6.2 cm^2 (range, 2.0–23.4 cm^2). Ten knees were treated with ACI-P and 13 knees were treated with ACI-C. Clinical outcome evaluation consisted of completion of the modified Cincinnati Knee Rating Scale, WOMAC, VAS, and SF-36, which all improved statistically from baseline ($P < .001$). Analysis showed an 89% graft survival at 5 and 10 years postoperatively (Fig. 9.39). Three patients had graft delamination with one patient refusing realignment surgery to correct genu varum. SSPs were performed on 20 knees, primarily because of graft hypertrophy. Despite the high SSP rate, 90% of patients were satisfied following surgery, rating knee-specific outcomes as good or excellent. At final follow-up, 96% of patients rated their knee as improved and all patients stated they would undergo the procedure again.

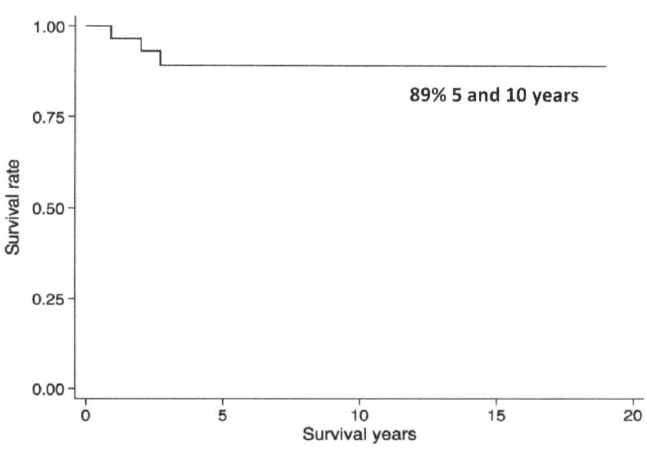

• **Fig. 9.39** Kaplan-Meier survival curve for adolescent autologous chondrocyte implantation patients. Endpoint defined as failure of graft.

The study demonstrates excellent outcomes in adolescent patients treated with ACI.

In 2017, Pike et al.[26] presented mid- to long-term results (mean follow-up, 95 months) of combined ACI with ACL reconstruction in 26 patients with large chondral defects (mean total defect surface area 8.4 ± 4.3 cm^2). Thirteen patients underwent primary ACL reconstruction and 13 underwent revision ACL repair. The mean defect total surface area was significantly greater in the ACL revision group, measuring 10.27 ± 4.22 cm^2 compared with 6.57 ± 3.99 cm^2 in the primary ACL group. Of the 26 patients, 8 were defined as clinical failures. There was no correlation between failures and primary versus revision ACL reconstruction. Clinical outcome scores, including modified Cincinnati Rating scale, VAS for pain, and WOMAC, significantly improved from baseline ($P < .001$). Patients undergoing revision ACL repair with ACI greater defect surface areas were clinically worse off at baseline with lower modified Cincinnati score. However, the ACL revision group saw greater improvements over the studied period compared with the primary reconstruction group, resulting in equivalent functional outcomes at final follow-up.

Ogura et al.[22] assessed the 20-year long-term outcomes of 23 patients (24 knees) with a mean defect surface area of 11.8 cm^2 (range, 2.4–30.5 cm^2) undergoing ACI-P treatment for grade III/IV chondral lesions. The survival rate was 63% at 10 and 20 years. Nine knees were considered failed treatments. Of the clinical failures, five knees underwent revision ACI. One revision ACI failed because of a traumatic injury. This knee eventually went on to arthroplasty. The remaining four knees with revision ACI did well throughout the study. A total of 80% of the patients maintained their original knee. Four knees were converted to arthroplasty at a mean of 5.9 years primarily as a result of disease progression. All 15 knees with retained grafts had significant improvement in measured clinical score at 20 years postoperatively, apart from the WOMAC stiffness subscore and the SF-36 mental component summary. Greatest clinical improvements were evident within the first 2 years. Of the 15 patients with retained grafts, 14 patients reported improved knee function, rating their knee as good or excellent 2 years after treatment. Eleven patients rated their knee as good or excellent 20 years postoperatively. Despite the technical challenges of ACI-P, the outcomes of this studied cohort support first-generation ACI as a reliable, long-term treatment.

Minas et al.[42] compared the clinical outcomes and graft survival in patients undergoing the ACI sandwich technique with autologous bone grafting (ABG) ($n = 24$) to a historical, matched patient cohort who underwent ABG treatment alone ($n = 13$). The average defect size measured 6.9 ± 3. 5 cm^2 and 7.1 ± 3. 5 cm^2 for the respective groups. The mean depth measured 1.2 ± 0.4 cm for the ABG group and 1.1 ± 0.3 cm for the ACI full sandwich group. Over the course of the study, the ACI full sandwich cohort consistently experienced greater improvement in clinical outcome and satisfaction scores. Radiographic studies and survival analysis

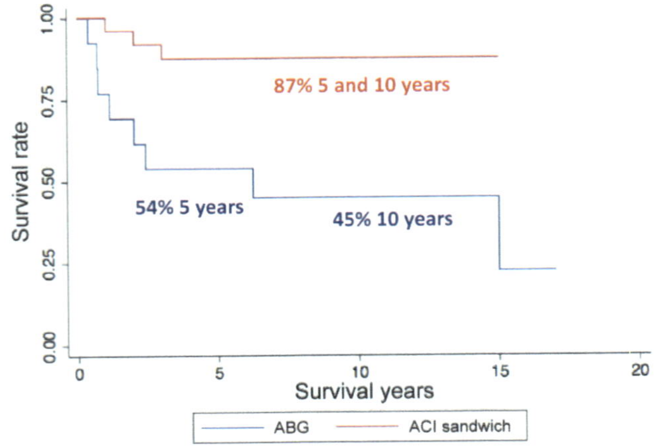

• **Fig. 9.40** Kaplan-Meier survival curves of autologous bone graft versus autologous chondrocyte implantation sandwich. Endpoint defined as failure of graft.

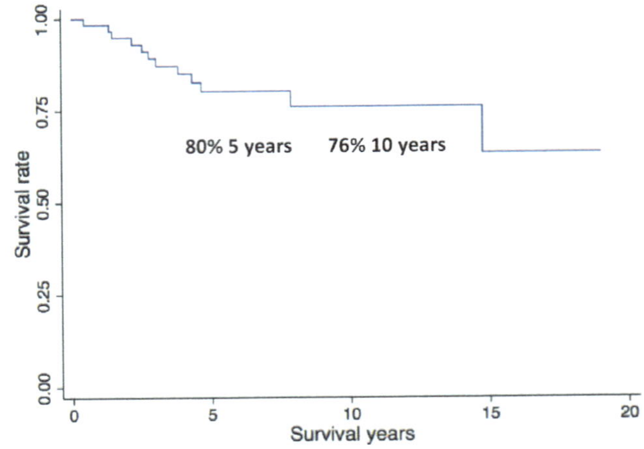

• **Fig. 9.41** Overall Kaplan-Meier survival curves with endpoint defined as graft failure.

results correlated with the reported clinical outcomes. As demonstrated in Fig. 9.40, the ACI full sandwich group had a significantly higher survival rate of 87% at 5 and 10 years postoperatively compared with the ABG group (54% at 5 years and 45% at 10 years postoperative). In total,11 patients were considered clinical failures: 8 patients in the ABG group and 3 patients in the ACI full sandwich group. The three ACI full sandwich failures underwent subsequent arthroscopic chondroplasty, which resolved their symptoms. Of the eight ABG failures, five proceeded with ACI revision surgery. One patient had a re-revision ACI treatment, eventually followed by a unicompartmental knee arthroplasty at 6.2 years postoperative. The other patient was converted to a TKA 15 years after ACI index surgery and one patient had revision with bone allograft followed by ABG and then ACI revision treatment at 8.3 post-index surgery. Clinical results and survival analysis demonstrated superior outcomes in the ACI full sandwich technique group in comparison with the ABG group.

Ogura and colleagues[20] carried out a case-series analysis of 57 patients (58 knees) undergoing either ACI-P ($n = 23$) or ACI-C ($n = 35$) for the treatment of tibiofemoral bipolar lesions, which demonstrated excellent survival rates of 80% at 5 years and 76% at 10 years postoperative (Fig. 9.41). Subanalysis showed significantly better survival in those treated with ACI-C versus ACI-P at 5 years postoperative (97% vs. 64%, Fig. 9.42) ($P = .0014$). The average defect sizes were: medial femoral condyle 8.3 ± 3.8 cm^2, medial tibial plateau 3.4 ± 1.8 cm^2, lateral femoral condyle 9 ± 3.4 cm^2, lateral tibial plateau 3.4 ± 1.5 cm^2. Fifteen patients had an HTO and six patients had a distal femoral osteotomy (DFO) at the time of index surgery.

Over the study period, 84% maintained their biological knees, avoiding joint arthroplasty. Clinical failures included 12 patients; 9 were converted to arthroplasty at a mean of 4.4 ± 4.0 years, 2 had revision ACI at 5 and 17 months postoperatively, and one patient did not require revision

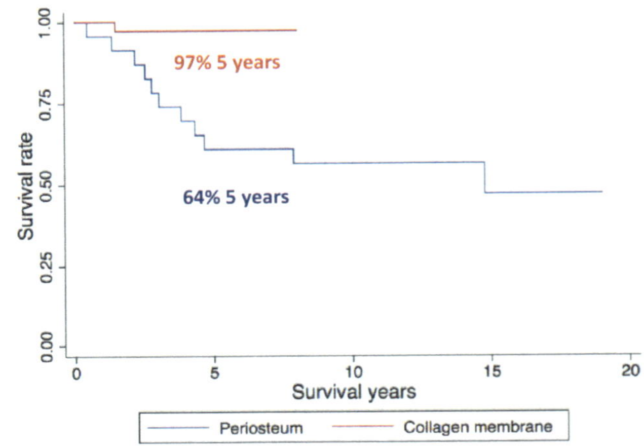

• **Fig. 9.42** Kaplan-Meier survival curves for periosteal-covered autologous chondrocyte implantation versus collagen-covered autologous chondrocyte implantation. Endpoint defined as failure of the graft.

surgery. Concomitant HTO surgery increased survival of medial compartment ACI grafts. No correction was seen between ACI with DFO and without DFO in the lateral compartment. Patient-reported outcome measures increased significantly with clinically meaningful improvement in all patients with retained grafts. Over 90% of the patients were satisfied with the outcome of their surgery at the final postoperative visit (mean 8.3 years). Findings support the use of ACI for the treatment of bipolar lesion in the tibiofemoral compartment with high rates of survival and patient satisfaction.

In 2018, Merkely et al.[43] conducted a case-control study to evaluate the outcomes and safety of anterior meniscal takedown, a technique commonly used to access and treat chondral defects on the tibial plateau and posterior femoral condyle with ACI. The meniscal takedown with refixation group, consisting of 62 patients, was compared with a matched cohort of patients who did not undergo meniscal

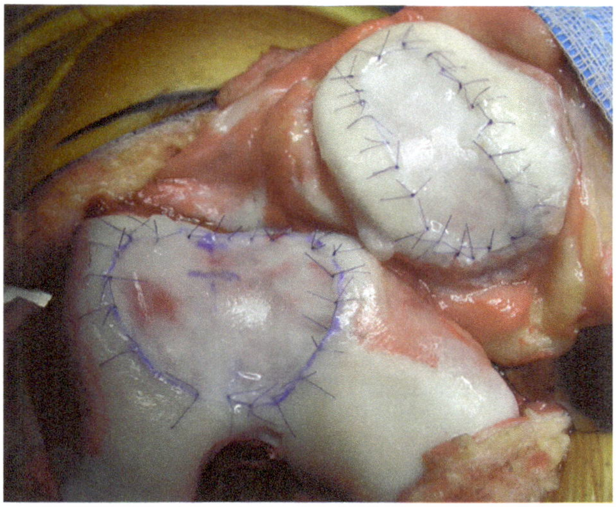

• **Fig. 9.43** Bipolar patellofemoral autologous chondrocyte implantation (ACI) using second generation collagen ACI.

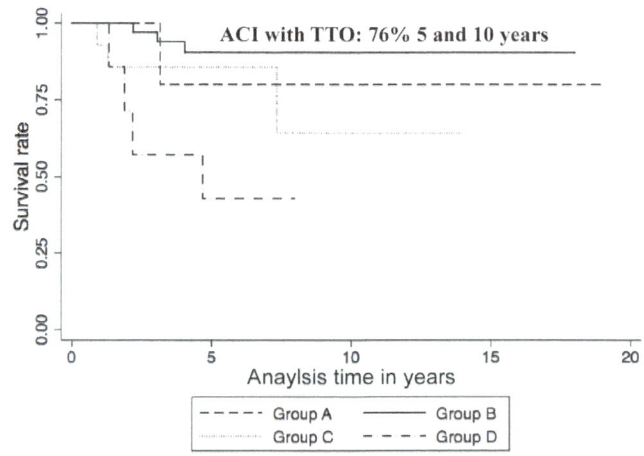

• **Fig. 9.44** Kaplan-Meier survival curve per subgroup. Overall 10-year survival 79%. Subanalysis: group A, ACI alone 80% ($n = 5$); group B, ACI with TTO 91% ($n = 34$); group C, failed TTO with subsequent ACI ± TTO 64% ($n = 14$); group D, failed MST ± TTO with subsequent ACI ± TTO 43% ($n = 7$). Endpoint defined as failure of graft. *ACI*, autologous chondrocyte implantation; *MST*, marrow stimulated technique; *TTO*, tibial tubercle osteotomy.

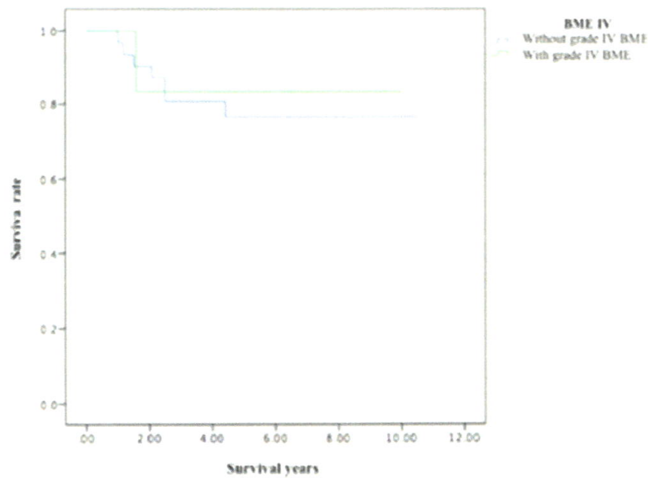

• **Fig. 9.45** Kaplan-Meier survival curves (control group has no microfracture) with and without bone marrow edema (BME) before autologous chondrocyte implantation in patients. Endpoint defined as failure of graft.

takedown, serving as the control group. Matching criteria included age, BMI, defect size, and affected compartment. It was not feasible to use specific defect location as a matching criterion. MRI evaluation indicated no significant difference in absolute meniscus extrusion (preoperative 1.6 ± 2.5 mm vs. postoperative 1.3 ± 1.5 mm; $P = .265$) or relative percentage of extrusion (RPE) (preoperative 14 ± 21 mm vs. postoperative 21 ± 24 mm; $P = .265$) among the patients who underwent meniscal takedown and refixation. Likewise, neither meniscal extrusion nor RPM differed significantly between the investigational arm ($P = .108$) and control group ($P = .306$). In conclusion, the study identified meniscal takedown and refixation as a safe and effective technique to expose the tibial plateau and posterior femoral condyle for ACI treatment.

In 2019, Ogura et al.[21] presented the clinical outcomes and survival rates of 58 patients with 60 knees treated with ACI for bipolar chondral defects in the patellofemoral compartment over a mean of 8.8 ± 4.2 years. The lesions were large: patella defects 5.6 cm^2 (82% Fulkerson type IVB) and trochlear defects 4.2 cm^2 (Fig. 9.43).

Patients responded to baseline and postoperative functional outcome assessments, including the modified Cincinnati Knee Rating Scale, WOMAC, and the SF-36, and a patient satisfaction survey. Radiographic assessment using Iwano classification and Kaplan-Meier analysis were performed to assess progression in patellofemoral osteoarthritis and overall survival. Kaplan-Meier analysis showed an overall survival of 83% and 79% at 5 and 10 years postoperatively. Highest survival rates were seen in patients who underwent a concomitant TTO at the index procedure without a prior failed microfracture or TTO, measuring 91% at 5 and 10 years postoperatively (Fig. 9.44). In total, 11 patients (19%) failed at a mean of 2.9 ± 1.9 years. Five of these patients were treated with ACI-C and six patients underwent ACI-P. Prior marrow stimulation appeared to be an indicator of an inferior outcome, consisting of 57% of the failures (Fig. 9.45). Revision surgeries included six ACI treatments and two arthroplasties and one patient required no further surgery. Of the retained grafts, all functional outcome measures improved significantly with a satisfaction rate of 88% recorded at the last postoperative visit. Radiographic evaluation of 28 knees with intact grafts demonstrated no increase of the Iwano classification in 26 of the 28 knees. Findings substantiate the durability and effectiveness of ACI treatment of bipolar patellofemoral lesions, highlighting the importance of resolving patellar maltracking with a concurrent TTO.

In 2019, Merkely et al.[44] compared the functional and radiographic outcomes of patients undergoing arthroscopic or open lateral MAT with transosseous suture refixation using a bone bridge-in-slot technique ($n = 20$). MRI scans at 1 year after the index procedure revealed no statistically significant difference in absolute meniscal extrusion between techniques. However, a significant difference was observed in mean RPE. The arthroscopic MAT group had a significantly greater RPE than the open MAT group (31 ± 27 mm vs. 10 ± 29 mm; 95% CI, −0.4 to −0.02 mm; (P <.03). Meniscal extrusion of more than 3 mm was evident in five patients (50%) following arthroscopic MAT. Meanwhile, no patients experienced meniscal extrusion of 3 mm in the open MAT cohort (P < .01).

In 2019, Ogura et al.[45] (2019) evaluated the efficacy of the ACI segmental-sandwich technique for the repair of deep osteochondral defects in 15 consecutive patients with a mean defect size of 6.0 ± 3. 5 cm^2 (range 1.5–13.5 cm^2) and a mean depth of 1.0 cm using ABG. Patients completed the modified Cincinnati Knee Rating System, VAS pain score, WOMAC, and the SF-36 preoperatively and at a mean follow-up of 7.8 years. All patient-reported outcome scores exhibited statistical and clinically meaningful improvement (P <.05), with 13 patients (87%) reporting good to excellent outcomes. Radiographic measures reflected the clinical and functional findings. K–L grades revealed no significant osteoarthritic progression in nine of the ten evaluated patients and 83% had complete or near-complete filling and integration to adjacent cartilage at 3 years postoperative (mean MOCART score, 64.2 ± 19.9 cm^2). There were no treatment failures, and Kaplan-Meier survival analysis demonstrated a survival rate of 100% over the course of the study. Findings suggest the ACI segmental-sandwich technique is a viable and durable treatment choice for large osteochondral lesions, with favorable functional outcomes and excellent survival rates.

In 2019, Ogura et al.[46] analyzed survival of revision ACI treatment. The study enrolled 53 patients (62 cartilage lesions) who failed initial ACI treatment and subsequently underwent revision ACI. Forty-nine of these patients underwent initial ACI-P treatment and the other four had ACI-C. For revision ACI, periosteum was used to treat 36 patients and collage type I/III membrane was used in 17 patients. An additional 31 cartilage lesions resulted from progression of disease and were treated at the time of revision ACI. ACI graft survival rates following revision were 71% at 5 years and 53% at 10 years postoperative. A greater survival rate was observed among the patients without previous cartilage repair before the initial ACI than in those with previous cartilage repair surgeries prior to the index ACI surgery (81% vs. 62% at 5 years; 64% vs. 42% at 10 years) (Fig. 9.46). The type of membrane cover, ACI-P or ACI-C, did not impact survival. Failed revision ACI cases consisted of 26 patients: 15 were converted to arthroplasty at a mean of 4.6 years and 11 underwent revision cartilage repair at a mean of 5.4 years. Functional scores improved significantly and standard radiographic assessment showed no progression of osteoarthritis among the patients with retained grafts ($n = 27$). Results suggest revision ACI is effective; however, a cartilage repair procedure prior to the initial ACI treatment appears to impact graft survival adversely.

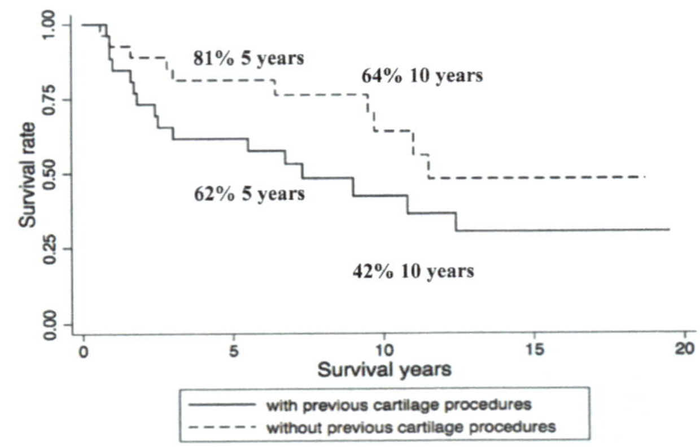

• **Fig. 9.46** Kaplan-Meier survival curves with and without previous cartilage procedure before initial autologous chondrocyte implantation. Endpoint defined as failure of graft.

Matrix/Membrane Autologous Chondrocyte Implantation

The **SUMMIT** trial, **Su**periority of **M**ACI implant versus **Mi**crofracture **T**reatment, was instrumental in demonstrating clearly that the clinical responsiveness and durability of membrane autologous chondrocyte implantation (MACI) was superior to microfracture in obtaining US FDA approval for MACI in December 2017 and available for US surgeons in January 2018.

This was a prospective randomized clinical trial of 144 patients in 14 different clinical centers randomized to MACI versus microfracture. In both the 2-year[47] and 5-year[48] follow-up, the clinical outcomes were significantly superior with the use of MACI.

MACI consists of a porcine collagen bilayered ACI with a uniform cell density of 1 million cells/cm^2. The technique involves the same biopsy and cell culturing process as ACI but cells are then precultured uniformly throughout the collagen membrane for 48–72 hours prior to delivery for implantation. The MACI procedure involves the same radical debridement of articular cartilage as ACI and then uses fibrin glue to attach the membrane with the cell layer facing the subchondral bone without the use of sutures (Fig. 9.47)

Patients suffering posttraumatic articular cartilage injuries or chronic articular injuries and patients having undergone marrow stimulation technique frequently exhibit sclerotic subchondral bone, intralesional osteophytes, or shallow subchondral cysts. This abnormal subchondral bone increases the likelihood of poor integration and failure of the MACI graft.[17] A technique that has been developed without the use of bone graft and used for deeper lesions is a very shallow MACI sandwich technique as illustrated in Figs. 9.48 and 9.49.

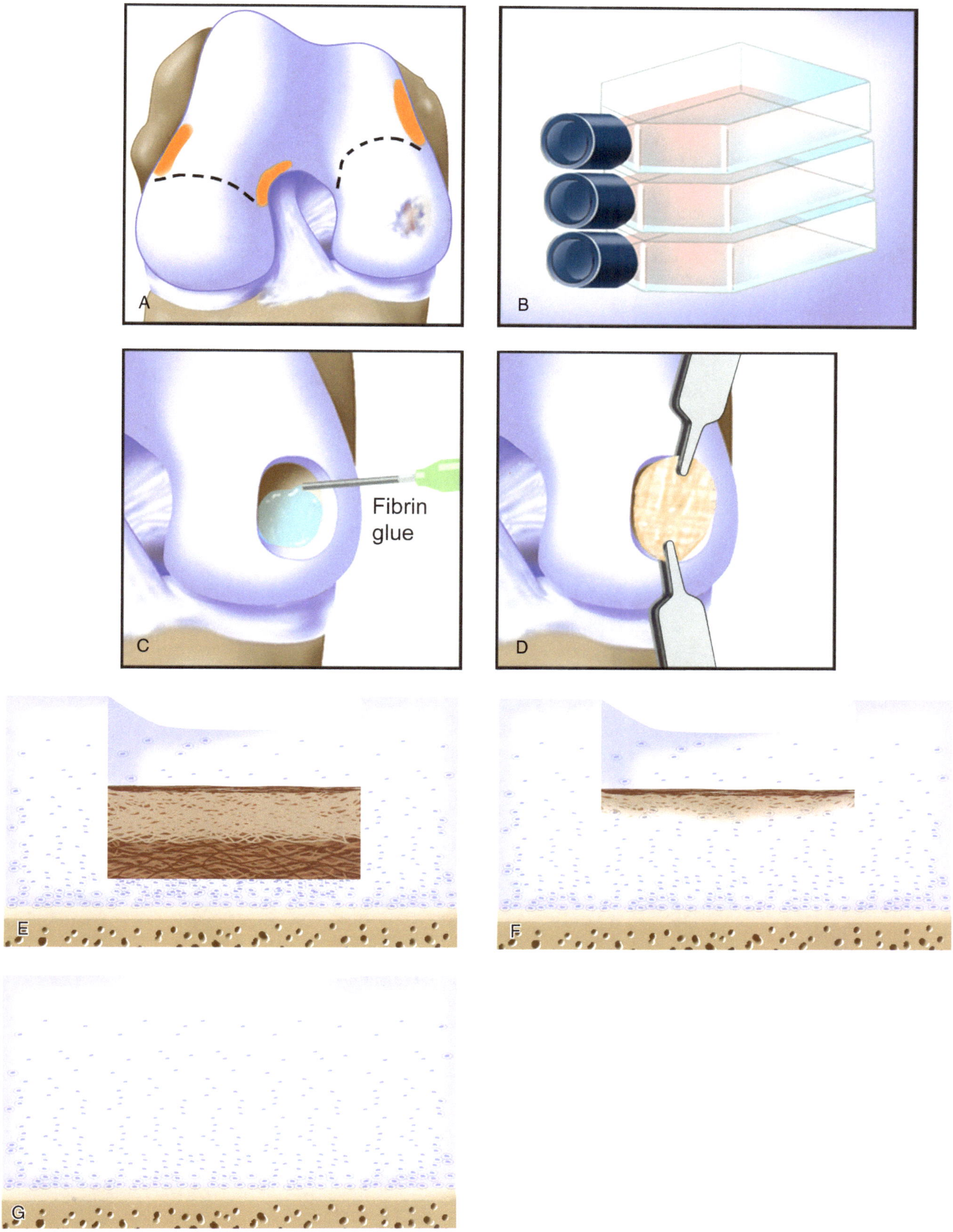

• **Fig. 9.47** (A) Well-contained focal articular defect suitable for membrane autologous chondrocyte implantation (MACI). (B) MACI is pre-cultured in a bilayered collagen membrane and transported to the operating room in its transport culture media. (C) As per ACI, a radical debridement is performed to the subchondral bone removing the calcified layer of cartilage. Fibrin glue is then applied to the base of the defect. (D) The MACI membrane is then applied with the cell layer facing downward to the subchondral bone and gently held in place with a neural patty or the surgeon's gloved thumb until the glue sets. (E,F) Defect with cells filling it from below over time, until (G) completion.

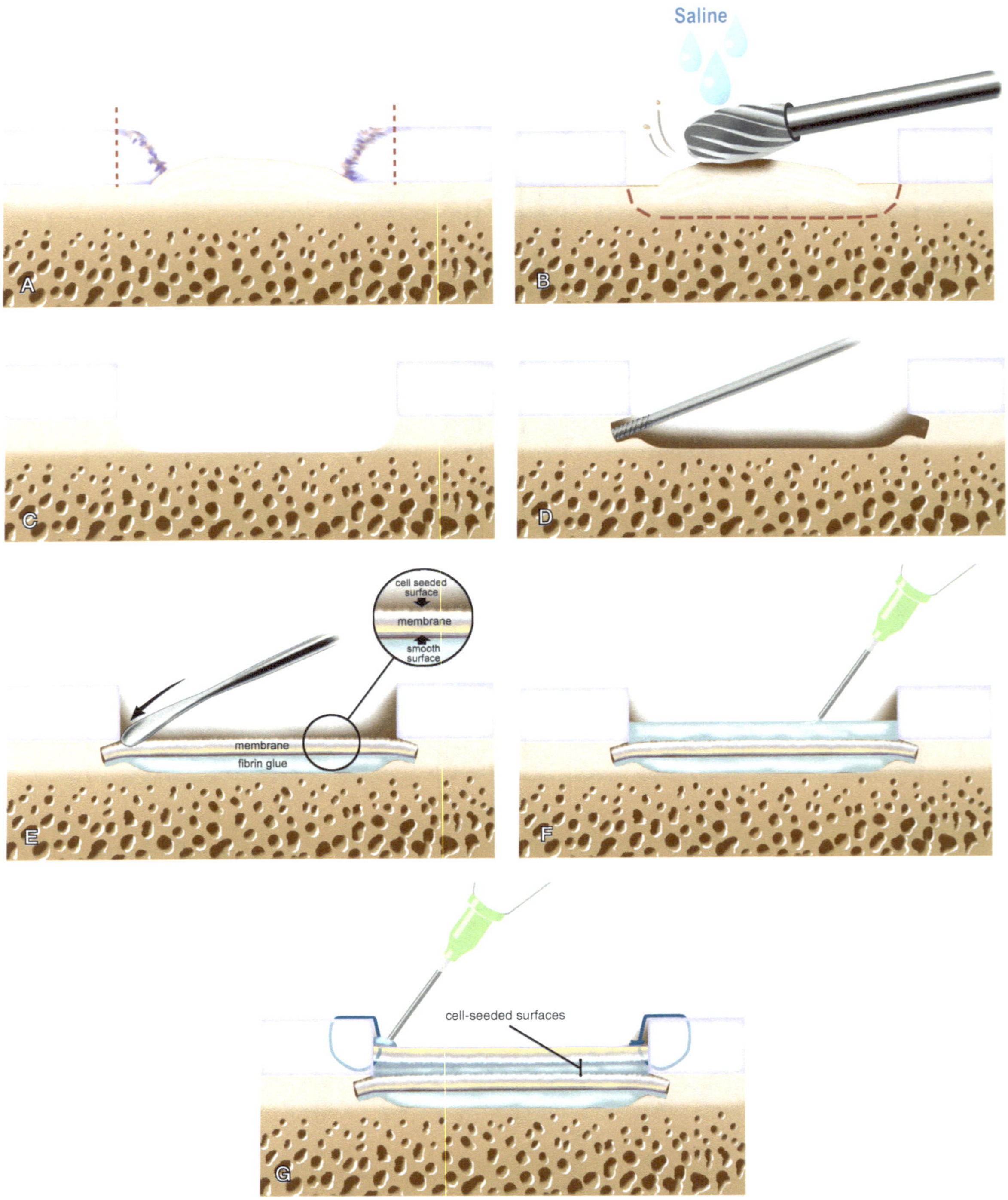

• **Fig. 9.48** (A) A defect suitable for cartilage repair with membrane autologous chondrocyte implantation (MACI) sandwich technique without the use of bone graft. This image shows an articular defect with thickened chronic-appearing subchondral bone similar to an intralesional osteophyte after marrow stimulation technique or a chronic lesion. (B) The defect must be radically debrided back to healthy subchondral bone with vertical articular margins. The abnormal thickened and sclerotic subchondral bone is then pared down with a high-speed egg-shaped 4–6 mm bur back to healthy-appearing subchondral bone under continuous saline irrigation. (C) The abnormal bone has been removed back to healthy-appearing subchondral bone not entering the cancellous marrow space if possible. Subchondral bone removal should not be any deeper than 2 mm. (D) A high-speed pencil-tip bur is utilized around the articular cartilage to release it slightly (1–2 mm) so that the MACI membrane may be placed under its surface with fibrin glue. This allows separation of the marrow elements from the surface with release of the tourniquet. The MACI membrane is orientated with the cell seeded surface to face outward. (E) Fibrin glue is applied to the base of the defect, a Freer is utilized to help place the MACI membrane circumferentially under the margins of the defect with the cell-seeded surface facing outward. A neural patty is then gently applied to the defect and the tourniquet is let down to seal it from any marrow derived elements. (F) A second thin layer of fibrin glue is applied to the cell-seeded surface. (G) The second MACI membrane is then applied to the defect with its cell-seeded surface facing downward toward the first layer thereby sandwiching the cells between the two membranes. A thin seal of fibrin glue is then applied circumferentially around the margins to help secure the membrane and if the defect is very large, several circumferential tacking sutures with 6-0 Vicryl absorbable sutures can be added. The procedure is now complete.

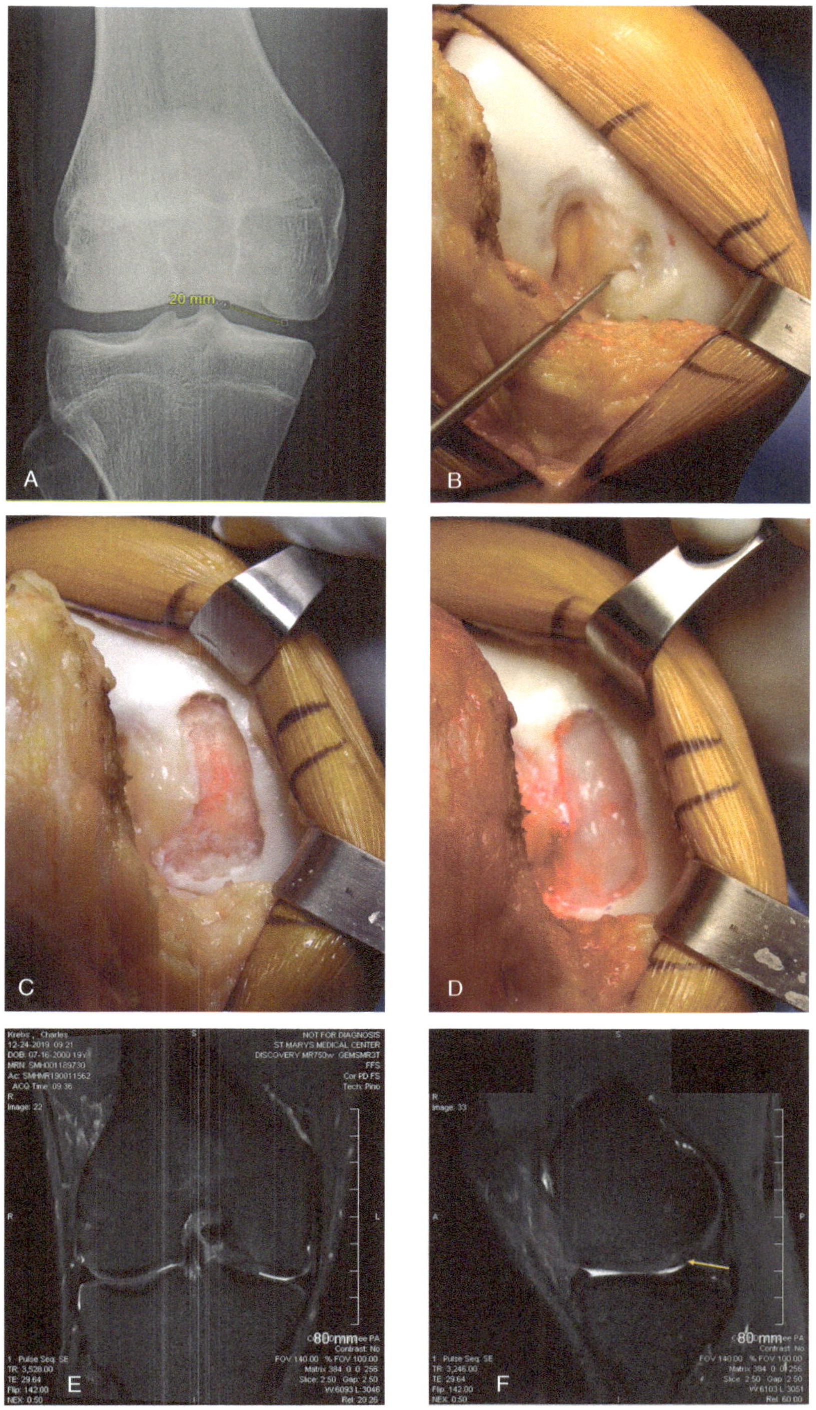

• **Fig. 9.49** (A) Standing AP x-ray image of a 19-year-old hockey player who injured his knee while playing as a goaltender. Atypical osteochondritis dissecans (OCD) on the lateral aspect of the medial femoral condyle is evident. The fragment is probably unstable because the patient is having mechanical symptoms of catching and locking of the knee. (B) Open arthrotomy for membrane autologous chondrocyte implantation (MACI). Arthroscopy and cartilage biopsy for MACI has been performed as well as removal of the unstable fragment more anterior in the OCD lesion. The biopsy site is evident at the lateral intercondylar notch at the time of open arthrotomy. The remainder of the fragment is intact but clinically evident and unstable. (C) The radically debrided chondral defect showed very sclerotic subchondral bone, which was pared down with a high-speed bur and a ring curet back to healthy subchondral bone in preparation for a sandwich technique without bone graft. (D) Appearance of the sandwich technique MACI performed for this sclerotic OCD lesion. The first membrane cell-seeded surface facing outward was sealed to the subchondral bone using fibrin glue with its edges under the surrounding cartilage margins. A neural patty was applied to the surface gently and the tourniquet was let down ensuring that there was no leakage into the articular surface of the marrow elements. The second MACI was glued with its cell-seeded surface face down toward the first. The margins were then sealed with fibrin glue below the level of the articular surface. Sutures were not required because the membranes were stable through a range of motion. (E) Fat-suppressed MRI scan at 18 months postoperative shows absence of bone marrow edema and complete fill of the articular injury to the medial femoral condyle. (F) Sagittal MRI image shows a complete repair tissue fill of the articular surface with no subchondral edema at 18 months postoperative. Clinically the patient is doing very well with no pain discomfort and is able to play sports once more.

Summary

It has been known for over 200 years that articular cartilage does not heal after injury.[49] ACI provides a durable hyaline repair tissue when patients are carefully chosen, background factors responsible for the chondral injury are addressed surgically at the time of ACI, and a careful surgical technique and rehabilitation are performed.

ACI clearly has outstanding clinical results in the juvenile athlete and high-level soccer player when the injury is treated within the first year of injury. Delays in treatment or multiple treatments result in less successful clinical outcomes probably as a result of the athlete's leg becoming less fit.

ACI in the patellofemoral joint has been successful for a difficult treatment management problem when careful attention is paid to patellar tracking. ACI has been successful in pan-patellar injuries (Fulkerson type IV patella) and medial patellar facet injuries (Fulkerson type III patella). It is effective in managing defects of the trochlea, which has been a problem area until the advent of ACI. ACI has a complementary role in managing patellofemoral chondral defects in those maltracking knees where realignment osteotomy alone is not successful. Even when lesions are large and bipolar the clinical results are excellent at 10 years: 91% survival with good and excellent outcomes in the 85% range when it is performed as the primary treatment with TTO to realign and unload the patellofemoral joint.[21] At the moment, ACI gives outstanding clinical results for injury of the patellofemoral joint including bipolar lesions and demonstrates excellent durability. It is probably the preferred treatment for any articular injury in the patellofemoral joint.

Patients older than 45 years continue to do favorably. We have found that if the patient is physiologically young and active with a localized chondral defect, the success rate after treatment remains 95%. However, if the patient has been previously microfractured and is covered by Workers' Compensation, the success rate drops to 60%. This finding is more likely secondary to microfracture in the Workers' Compensation group; however, separating the two factors is difficult.

Young arthritic patients pose a particular management dilemma because these patients are frequently too young to be considered for prosthetic arthroplasty and traditional sports medicine techniques are not effective in alleviating pain by repairing articular cartilage. This group of patients is generally older (39 years old) and requires large areas of surface repair (average 11 cm^2). The clinical outcomes in this group have been very positive with a patient satisfaction rate of 87% overall. Of this group 7% went onto prosthetic replacement over the course of this study.

Marrow stimulation techniques appear to alter the osteochondral unit. If a surface treatment such as ACI is then performed, the success rate drops from 92% for a native chondral defect to 74% in a chondral defect previously treated by MST that has failed. When all other factors are controlled, it appears that MST, irrespective of the type (abrasion, drilling, or microfracture) jeopardizes the success of ACI. It is therefore recommended that microfracture be utilized for those lesions that are smaller than 2–3 cm^2 and are confined to the femoral condyles in patients younger than 40 years with acute lesions that are known to do the best with this technique. Failed MST remains a treatment dilemma. Alterations in the management of the subchondral bone such as thinning of the bone prior to ACI or replacing the osteochondral unit with a sandwich technique ACI or osteoarticular allograft may be more suitable.

Updated research has shown that MRI is a useful tool to predict the outcome of ACI after MST. ACI failure rate is low in our series (overall approximately 8%). However, when there is Grade IV BME (bone marrow edema) prior to ACI the failure rate is 21.4%. If there is grade IV BME after MST prior to ACI, the failure rate skyrockets to 83.7% by 5 years. This suggests the best treatment is to repair the entire osteochondral unit with ACI sandwich technique with autologous bone graft or a fresh osteochondral allograft when grade IV BME is present after MST.

A bioabsorbable collagen type I–III membrane replacing periosteum in ACI appears not to diminish the clinical outcomes but improves the problem of periosteal hypertrophy. This has been demonstrated in a randomized controlled trial comparing the two membrane covers.[40] We have confirmed with a prospectively matched comparison that our hypertrophy rate is dramatically diminished and nearly abolished when using collage instead of periosteum.[19]

The clinical outcomes of patella ACI[15] and the treatment of bipolar injuries in the patellofemoral[21] and tibiofemoral[20] joints demonstrate excellent patient-reported clinical outcomes all approximately 85% good-to-excellent and with 10-year durability above 90% when they are treated primarily with ACI and osteotomy when indicated as the primary treatment, but not after MST.

With the arrival of MACI, the ACI procedure becomes less invasive with the delivery of a collagen carrier that is bioabsorbable with a uniform seeded density of chondrocytes to the defects, which is easier to perform. MACI remains an open procedure, although it has been performed arthroscopically for small defects. Attention to the background factors remains critical to maintain successful clinical outcomes. Careful rehabilitation will result in a good clinical outcome. Newer generation ACI techniques that involve cell-seeded transport media or membranes that are arthroscopically delivered will improve upon the ease of recovery for patients and easier surgery. These new techniques are addressed in Chapter 16 and represent exciting advancements.

References

1. Brittberg M, Lindahl A, Nilsson A, Ohlsson C, Isaksson O, Peterson L. Treatment of deep cartilage defects in the knee with autologous chondrocyte transplantation. *N Engl J Med.* 1994;331(14):889–895.
2. Minas T, Marchie A, Bryant T. *SF-36 as a predictor of clinical outcome after autologous chondrocyte implantation in the knee.* Toronto Ontario Canada: International Cartilage Repair Society;; 2001. [poster].

3. Mithofer K, Minas T, Yeon H, Micheli LJ. Functional outcome of knee articular cartilage repair in adolescent athletes. *Am J Sports Med.* 2005;33(8):1147–1153.
4. Peterson L, Minas T, Brittberg M, Lindahl A. Treatment of osteochondritis dissecans of the knee with autologous chondrocyte transplantation: results at two to ten years. *J Bone Joint Surg Am.* 2003;Suppl 2(85-A):17–24.
5. Curl WW, Krome J, Gordon ES, Rushing J, Smith BP, Poehling GG. Cartilage injuries: a review of 31, 516 knee arthroscopies. *Arthroscopy.* 1997;13(4):456–460.
6. Minas T, Neher S. Current concepts in the treatment of articular cartilage defects. *Orthopedics.* 1997;20(6):525–538.
7. Minas T. Autologous chondrocyte implantation for focal chondral defects of the knee. *Clin Orthop Relat Res.* 2001;391 Suppl:S349–S361.
8. Peterson L, Karrlson J, Brittberg M, et al. Patellar Instability with recurrent dislocation due to Patellofemoral Dysplasia results after surgical treatment. 48. *Bulletin of the Hospital for Joint Disease Orthopaedic Institute.* 1988:130–139.
9. O'Driscoll SW, Salter RB. The induction of neochondrogenesis in free intra-articular periosteal autografts under the influence of continuous passive motion. An experimental investigation in the rabbit. *J Bone Joint Surg Am.* 1984;66(8):1248–1257.
10. Rodrigo J, Steadman R, Fulstone H. Improvement of full-thickness chondral defect healing in the human knee after debridement and microfracture using continuous passive motion. *Am J Knee Surg.* 1994;7:109–116.
11. von Keudell A, Han R, Bryant T, Minas T. Autologous chondrocyte implantation to isolated patella cartilage defects. *Cartilage.* 2017;8(2):146–154.
12. Ogura T, Bryant T, Minas T. Long-term outcomes of autologous chondrocyte implantation in adolescent patients. *Am J Sports Med.* 2017;45(5):1066–1074.
13. Mithöfer K, Peterson L, Mandelbaum BR, Minas T. Articular cartilage repair in soccer players with autologous chondrocyte transplantation: functional outcome and return to competition. *Am J Sports Med.* 2005;33(11):1639–1646.
14. Minas T, Bryant T. The role of autologous chondrocyte implantation in the patellofemoral joint. *Clin Orthop Relat Res.* 2005;436:30–39.
15. Gomoll AH, Gillogly SD, Cole BJ, et al. Autologous chondrocyte implantation in the patella: a multicenter experience. *Am J Sports Med.* 2014;42(5):1074–1081.
16. Rosenberger RE, Gomoll AH, Bryant T, Minas T. Repair of large chondral defects of the knee with autologous chondrocyte implantation in patients 45 years or older. *Am J Sports Med.* 2008;36(12):2336–2344.
17. Minas T, Gomoll AH, Rosenberger R, Royce RO, Bryant T. Increased failure rate of autologous chondrocyte implantation after previous treatment with marrow stimulation techniques. *Am J Sports Med.* 2009;37(5):902–908.
18. Minas T, Gomoll AH, Solhpour S, Probst C, Byrant T. Autologous Chondrocyte Implantation for Joint Preservation in Patients with Early Osteoarthritis - 2 to 11 year follow-up. *Clinical Orthopaedics and Related Research.* 2009
19. Gomoll AH, Probst C, Farr J, Cole BJ, Minas T, et al. The use of a Type I/III bi-layer collagen membrane to decrease re-operation rates for symptomatic hypertrophy after autologous chondrocyte implantation. *Am J Sports Med.* 2009;37(1):20S–23S.
20. Ogura T, Bryant T, Mosier BA, Minas T. Autologous chondrocyte implantation for bipolar chondral lesions in the tibiofemoral compartment. *Am J Sports Med.* 2018;46(6):1371–1381.
21. Ogura T, Bryant T, Merkely G, Minas T. Autologous chondrocyte implantation for bipolar chondral lesions in the patellofemoral compartment: clinical outcomes at a mean 9 years' follow-up. *Am J Sports Med.* 2019;47(4):837–846.
22. Ogura T, Mosier BA, Bryant T, Minas T, et al. A 20-year follow-up after first-generation autologous chondrocyte implantation. *Am J Sports Med.* 2017;45(12):2751–2761.
23. Minas T. Chondrocyte implantation in the repair of chondral lesions of the knee: economics and quality of life. *Am J Orthop.* 1998;27(11):739–744.
24. Lindahl A, Brittberg M, Peterson L. Health economics benefits following autologous chondrocyte transplantation for patients with focal chondral lesions of the knee. *Knee Surg Sports Traumatol Arthrosc.* 2001;9(6):358–363.
25. Peterson L, Brittberg M, Kiviranta I, Akerlund EL, Lindahl A. Autologous chondrocyte transplantation. Biomechanics and long-term durability. *Am J Sports Med.* 2002;30(1):2–12.
26. Pike AN, Bryant T, Ogura T, Minas T. Intermediate- to long-term results of combined anterior cruciate ligament reconstruction and autologous chondrocyte implantation. *Orthop J Sports Med.* 2017;5(2):2325967117693591.
27. Ogura T, Bryant T, Minas T. Biological knee reconstruction with concomitant autologous chondrocyte implantation and meniscal allograft transplantation: mid- to long-term outcomes. *Orthop J Sports Med.* 2016;4(10):2325967116668490.
28. Minas T, Von Keudell A, Bryant T, Gomoll AH. The John Insall Award: a minimum 10-year outcome study of autologous chondrocyte implantation. *Clin Orthop Relat Res.* 2014;472(1):41–51.
29. Ware Jr. JE, Sherbourne CD. The MOS 36-item short-form health survey (SF-36). I. Conceptual framework and item selection. *Med Care.* 1992;30(6):473–483.
30. Insall JN, Dorr LD, Scott RD, Scott WN. Rationale of the knee society clinical rating system. *Clin Orthop Relat Res.* 1989;248:13–14.
31. Bellamy N, Buchanan WW, Goldsmith CH, Campbell J, Stitt LW. Validation study of WOMAC: a health status instrument for measuring clinically important patient relevant outcomes to antirheumatic drug therapy in patients with osteoarthritis of the hip or knee. *J Rheumatol.* 1988;15(12):1833–1840.
32. Noyes FR, Barber SD, Mooar LA. A rationale for assessing sports activity levels and limitations in knee disorders. *Clin Orthop Relat Res.* 1989;246:238–249.
33. Peterson L, Minas T, Brittberg M, Nilsson A, Sjogren-Jansson E, Lindahl A. Two- to 9-year outcome after autologous chondrocyte transplantation of the knee. *Clin Orthop Relat Res.* 2000;374:212–234.
34. Pidoriano AJ, Weinstein RN, Buuck DA, Fulkerson JP. Correlation of patellar articular lesions with results from anteromedial tibial tubercle transfer. *Am J Sports Med.* 1997;25(4):533–537.
35. Minas T. Autologous chondrocyte implantation in the arthritic knee. *Orthopedics.* 2003;26(9):945–947.
36. Ahlback S, Aeschlimann A, Michel BA, Stucki G. Osteoarthrosis of the knee: a radiographic investigation. *Acta Radiologica.* 1968; Suppl 277:7–72.
37. Angst F, Aeschlimann A, Michel BA, Stucki G. Minimal clinically important rehabilitation effects in patients with osteoarthritis of the lower extremities. *J Rheumatol.* 2002;19:131–138.
38. Jaeschke J, Singer J, Guyatt G. Measurement of health status. Ascertaining the minimal clinically important difference. *Controlled Clinical Trials.* 1989;10:407–415.

39. Goldsmith CH, Boers M, Bombardier C, Tugwell P. Criteria for clinically important changes in outcomes: development, scoring and evaluation of rheumatoid arthritis patient and trial profiles. OMERACT committee. *J Rheumatol.* 1993;20(3):561–565.
40. Gooding CR, Bartlett W, Bentley G, Skinner JA, Carrington R. A prospective, randomised study comparing two techniques of autologous chondrocyte implantation for osteochondral defects in the knee: periosteum covered versus type I/III collagen covered. *Knee.* 2006;13(3):203–210.
41. Demange MK, Minas T, Von Keudell A, Sodha S, Bryant T, Gomoll AH. Intralesional osteophyte regrowth following autologous chondrocyte implantation after previous treatment with marrow stimulation technique. *Cartilage.* 2017;8(2): 131–138.
42. Minas T, Ogura T, Headrick J, Bryant T. Autologous chondrocyte implantation "sandwich" technique compared with autologous bone grafting for deep osteochondral lesions in the knee. *Am J Sports Med.* 2017;363546517738000.
43. Merkely G, Minas T, Ogura T, Ackermann J, Barbieri Mestriner A, Gomoll AH. Safety, feasibility, and radiographic outcomes of the anterior meniscal takedown technique to approach chondral defects on the tibia and posterior femoral condyle: a matched control study. *Cartilage.* 2018;12(1):62–69.
44. Merkely G, Ogura T, Ackermann J, Mestriner AB, Minas T, Gomoll AH. Open meniscal allograft transplantation with transosseous suture fixation of the meniscal body significantly decreases meniscal extrusion rate compared with arthroscopic technique. *Arthroscopy.* 2019;35(6):1658–1666.
45. Ogura T, Merkely G, Bryant T, Winalski CS, Minas T. Autologous chondrocyte implantation "segmental-sandwich" technique for deep osteochondral defects in the knee: clinical outcomes and correlation with magnetic resonance imaging findings. *Orthop J Sports Med.* 2019;7(5):2325967119847173.
46. Ogura T, Bryant T, Merkely G, Mosier BA, Minas T. Survival analysis of revision autologous chondrocyte implantation for failed ACI. *Am J Sports Med.* 2019;47(13):3212–3220.
47. Saris D, Price A, Widuchowski W, et al. Matrix-applied characterized autologous cultured chondrocytes versus microfracture: two-year follow-up of a prospective randomized trial. *Am J Sports Med.* 2014;42(6):1384–1394.
48. Brittberg M, Recker D, Ilgenfritz J, Saris DBF, Group SES. Matrix-applied characterized autologous cultured chondrocytes versus microfracture: five-year follow-up of a prospective randomized trial. *Am J Sports Med.* 2018;46(6):1343–1351.
49. Hunter W. On the structure and diseases of articulating cartilages. *Clin Orthop Relat Res.* 1995;(372):3–6.

10 Tibial Osteotomy

TOM MINAS, MD, MS

CHAPTER OUTLINE

Arthritis and Malalignment

The premise of knee osteotomy surgery is to correct malalignment at the site of the deformity and relieve pressure on the overloaded or arthritic compartment. In general, medial compartment osteoarthritis of the knee coexists with a varus knee secondary to deformity in the metaphysis of the tibia. The joint line is generally horizontal to the floor. Femoral varus is unusual but may occur secondary to metabolic bone disease such as rickets or trauma but are usually excluded with long alignment x-ray images. Hence tibial osteotomy is usually performed for varus leg alignment with medial compartment overload or osteoarthritis.

Similarly, valgus malalignment of the knee with lateral compartment osteoarthritis usually coexists with deformity in the distal femur, which consists of dysplasia or hypoplasia of the lateral column of the distal femur. There is usually a superior and lateral directed joint line. Osteotomy through the distal femur thereby corrects the deformity at its location and produces a horizontal joint line. If a varus proximal tibial osteotomy was performed in this situation, further superior lateral joint line obliquity would result with the risk of subluxation of the tibia on the femur. Although Coventry described the use of proximal tibial varus osteotomy for valgus osteoarthritis of the knee, he recommended that this be performed for a deformity of less than 10 degrees and noted the risk of subluxation.[1]

Why Osteotomy?

In 1994, the Centers for Disease Control and Prevention reported[2] that by the year 2020 osteoarthritis will have the largest increase in numbers of new patients of any disease in the United States. Approximately 60 million Americans referred to as Baby Boomers are at risk, which is 20% of the population of the United States. Total knee arthroplasty has become one of the most commonly performed procedures with reproducibly good results in the United States. This is in part largely a result of generically designed anatomic implants with universal knee instrumentation. Prior to its development, high tibial osteotomy was commonly performed. However, in 2008, 220,000 total knee replacements were performed in patients under the age of 55 and a total of 450,000 total knee replacements were performed overall. As good as total knee replacement surgery is, patient satisfaction only remains approximately 80%. Reasons for dissatisfaction include persistent pain, stiffness, and prosthetic arthroplasty failure. Failures typically result from polyethylene osteolysis, mechanical loosening, joint infection, or problematic revision surgery secondary to ligamentous laxity or bone deficiency. The re-evaluation of joint preservation techniques have led to a resurgence of osteotomy and cartilage repair surgeries as well as more bone-sparing partial prosthetic arthroplasties.

Tibial osteotomy had been a procedure routinely performed in patients with tibial varus malalignment and medial unicompartmental disease over the age of 50 years. The average age for tibial osteotomy in the Coventry series[1] was 63 years. Today, it would be difficult for a surgeon to do a tibial osteotomy at this age because of the reproducible long-term results with total knee arthroplasty surgery in this age category.

However, unicompartmental arthrosis is becoming prevalent among patients in their 20s, 30s, and 40s. As Baby Boomers age and activity levels remain high because of interest in sports, injuries to the anterior cruciate ligament, meniscus, and articular cartilage predispose to unicompartmental disease in patients much younger than those treated in the past. The average age of high tibial osteotomy patients for bone-on-bone medial compartment disease in my practice was 44 years old when reviewed (Harvard hip and knee course, Korbyl, Minas, 2003.). Unicompartmental and total knee arthroplasty cannot offer these patients a long-term, high functional level of activity.

Sharma et al.[3] have demonstrated that the risk of progression of unicompartmental osteoarthritis with malalignment is four times more common in a varus knee than a neutrally aligned knee and five times more common in a valgus than a neutrally aligned knee, over an 18-month period with evidence of progression on standing radiographs. Osteoarthritis in the malaligned limb with unicompartmental disease remains a problem in young athletes and adults. Tibial osteotomy remains the procedure of choice in limbs with unicompartmental osteoarthritis with malalignment.

A long-term Swedish study[4] evaluating the natural course of arthrosis of the knee over 20 years noted that patients with Ahlbäck stage 1 osteoarthrosis (50% joint space narrowing) would have progression of disease in 61% of the cases with 39% remaining stable without further reduction in the joint space. In patients with Ahlbäck stage 0 arthrosis, defined by osteophytes or subchondral bone sclerosis with normal joint space, 57% would not progress over time. In more advanced cases with Ahlbäck stages 2, 3, 4, and 5, the condition would progress over time.

If we are to use tibial osteotomy in our treatment algorithm to help these young patients, it is important to avoid both technique-related problems and patient-related issues that have led to the disfavor of tibial osteotomy in the past.

Technique-Related Issues Against High Tibial Osteotomy

Arthroplasty surgeons have conceptual difficulty with osteotomies because of the potential to make the arthroplasty more challenging and to compromise the results of a primary arthroplasty. Issues that have led to these problems include placement of skin incisions, patella baja, infrapatellar tendon contracture, contracture of the lateral ligament and posterolateral corner with release of the proximal tibial fibular joint, obliquity of the joint line, and distortion of the upper anatomy of the tibia (see Fig. 10.1). Excessive valgus correction has also resulted in difficult arthroplasty balancing of the flexion/extension gap and obtaining adequate alignment and increases the risk of peroneal nerve palsy. The total joint literature is abundant with reports of inferior outcomes following tibial osteotomy to primary total joint replacement; others report that results are equivalent but that experienced surgeons with modified surgical techniques are needed to obtain results equal to total knee replacement as a primary procedure. If we are to pursue osteotomy surgery as a treatment for our young patients undergoing cartilage repair, treatment for instability or unicompartmental arthritis, we must not compromise or make more difficult the eventuality of total knee replacement.

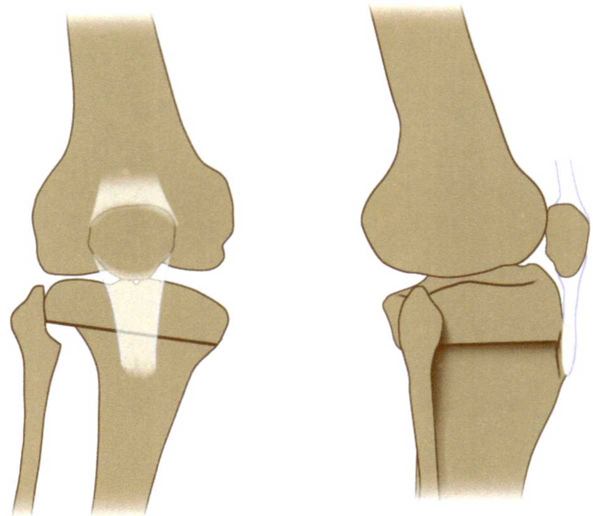

• **Fig. 10.1** This illustration demonstrates common sequelae of the classic closing wedge Coventry osteotomy with cast immobilization postoperatively. There is metaphyseal-diaphyseal mismatch, proximalization of the fibula with lateral collateral laxity, patella infera, and marked overcorrection into valgus. These aspects of the osteotomy made it unfavorable to patients because of cosmetic alignment and functional issues, as well as a deterrent to surgeons because of the difficulties when performing total knee replacement in the future.

Patient-Related Issues

Closing wedge osteotomy with staple fixation and postoperative casting in full extension often lead to patient dissatisfaction arising predominantly from overcorrection into valgus with cosmetic disfigurement (see Fig. 10.2). Release of the proximal tibiofibular joint leads to lateral laxity, which results in the sensation of a sloppy knee secondary to posterior-lateral ligament instability. Cast immobilization leads to various problems for the patient and the surgeon. Patients have difficulty ambulating and challenges returning to work. The treating surgeon is faced with managing patella infera, lateral contracture, and decreased joint

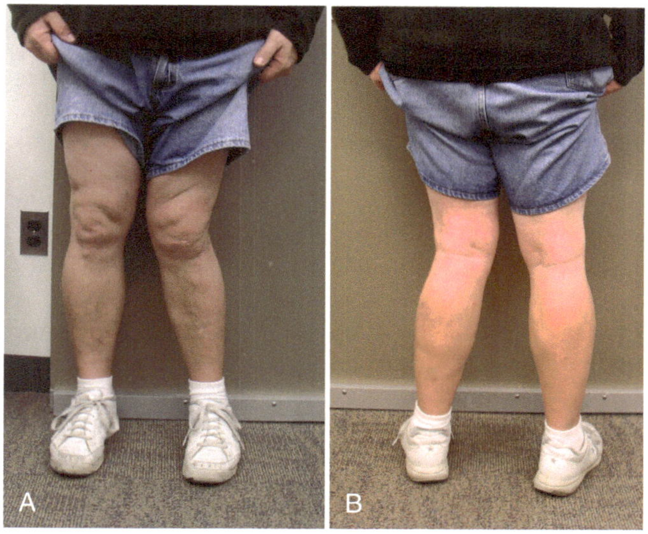

• **Fig. 10.2** Frontal and rear view of the patient standing after tibial osteotomy. This patient had left knee medially-based pain with a neutrally aligned lower extremity. He underwent a closing wedge valgus tibial osteotomy and was very dissatisfied with the procedure because of his altered gait pattern resulting from overcorrection into too much valgus. His medially-based pain did not resolve.

motion, as previously discussed. These problems can be avoided or eliminated by appropriate procedural osteotomy technique selection, patient selection, and careful pre- and postoperative planning and care. Renewed interest in joint preservation and cartilage repair has led to innovative new osteotomy techniques that are more precise and improved technical ease with reproducible results.

Procedural Planning

In a multi-variate analysis of predictors of good outcome, Coventry's findings[1] were that the long-term outcome was determined by the mechanical correction to 8 degrees or more of tibiofemoral valgus, and ideal body weight of the patient was less than 1.32 times normal. Rinonapoli[5] noted that the longevity was also proportional to the stage of disease at the time of osteotomy. Updated reports with experimental cadaveric loading have demonstrated similar findings.[6] The authors found that when tibiofemoral alignment was shifted from varus to valgus alignment, a decrease in medial contact pressure and medial contact area occurred. For defect chondral sizes of 10 to 20 mm, all contact pressures within the medial compartment were shifted to the lateral compartment at between 6 and 10 degrees of tibiofemoral valgus. Contact pressures were found to concentrate around the defect rims for all defect sizes. It was recommended that 6 to 10 degrees of tibiofemoral valgus be the optimal axial alignment to favor cartilage repair.

My experience is similar; if the patient is relatively slim, i.e., ideal body weight less than 1.32 times normal, a nonsmoker, highly motivated, and has unicompartmental medial disease with varus deformity, they are a good candidate for osteotomy surgery. An arc of range of motion of 90 degrees or better is desired. Patellofemoral symptoms can be accepted if they can be dealt with by a concomitant tibial tubercle osteotomy. Attention to clinical varus thrust and baseline leg length discrepancy is also important.

Preoperative x-ray examinations (see Fig. 10.3) include long axial alignment x-rays on 54" cassettes to include the hip, knee, and talus as a standing film in extension. Rosenberg 45-degree bent PA films, standing AP, lateral, and skyline films, and radiograph measurement of leg length are important.

The mechanical axis is measured from the center of the femoral head to the center of the talus. If this falls through the medial joint compartment with evidence of peripheral osteophyte formation, flattening of the articulation, subchondral bone sclerosis, and/or joint space narrowing, the patient is a candidate for osteotomy surgery if they do not have subluxation of the tibiofemoral joint or lateral symptoms. Lateral symptoms must be assessed to disprove lateral compartment degenerative changes or meniscal tear. A high-resolution MRI scan is the most sensitive method of assessing the lateral and patellofemoral compartments if in doubt. I use MRI routinely to rule out pathology in the other two compartments prior to osteotomy.

Preoperative Planning for Angular Correction of Tibial Osteotomy

Consider the normal tibiofemoral alignment of the knee; a neutral mechanical access requires that a line passes from the center of the femoral head through the center of the knee into the center of the ankle (see Fig. 10.4). This assumes that the neck shaft angle at the hip joint is within normal limits, 130 to 135 degrees, and that the tibiofemoral axis at the knee is 5 to 7 degrees of valgus.

My desired angular correction for medial OA (Fig. 10.5) is to place the mechanical axis through the center of the lateral intercondylar spine or just to the downslope of this. This is 2 degrees overcorrected from a neutral mechanical axis. This is different from the classic teaching that the mechanical axis is recommended to pass through the Kurosaka point at 62% across the width of the tibia. I feel that this is overcorrected to a level that is cosmetically unacceptable to patients and alters the kinematics of the patient's athletic endeavors so that they are difficult to perform. If the osteotomy is performed for a cartilage repair procedure with an intact joint space, the mechanical axis should pass through the center of the knee joint and not be overcorrected. In addition to the mechanical axis, consider the tibiofemoral axis. From previous basic science research, a 6- to 10-degree tibiofemoral valgus angle is sufficient to unload a medial compartment.[6] If there is varus in the proximal femur, the knee alignment may be markedly overcorrected by looking only at the mechanical varus of the overall leg alignment.

Assuming that the proximal femur has a normal neck shaft angle, my preferred technique to calculate the angular correction is as follows (Fig. 10.6). A simple angular correction as measured on the long axial standing films is performed as follows. Pass a line from the center of the femoral head to the desired axis at the knee joint, e.g., the lateral intercondylar spine. A second line from the center of the talus then intersects this same point. The acute angle between the two is the angular correction desired. Ligamentous instability of the medial complex and anterior cruciate ligament (ACL) should be assessed so that if there is laxity it can be accounted for at the time of osteotomy to ensure that marked overcorrection does not ensue.

Cartilage Repair, Osteoarthritis, Instability

There is a renewed interest in the use of tibial osteotomy. Patients are maintaining a higher level of fitness and aerobic activity as they age and generally wish to preserve their joints as long as possible. Newer techniques of both opening and closing wedge tibial osteotomies give predictable angular corrections with reliability. The increased technical accuracy and reduced risk of complications make it more appealing for both surgeon and patients to pursue joint preservation. Three broad categories for the indications for osteotomy surgery presently exist. It is generally agreed that cartilage repair in the presence of malalignment usually results in failure as the source of the cartilage breakdown in the first place is generally malalignment in addition to other traumatic factors such as meniscal deficiency, ACL injury, or articular cartilage injury. Osteotomy has therefore become an adjuvant procedure that has been deemed to be necessary when articular cartilage injury being repaired is greater than 2 degrees of malalignment if the lesion is considered to be greater than 2 cm^2 with a cell-based treatment such as microfracture or autologous chondrocyte implantation (ACI).

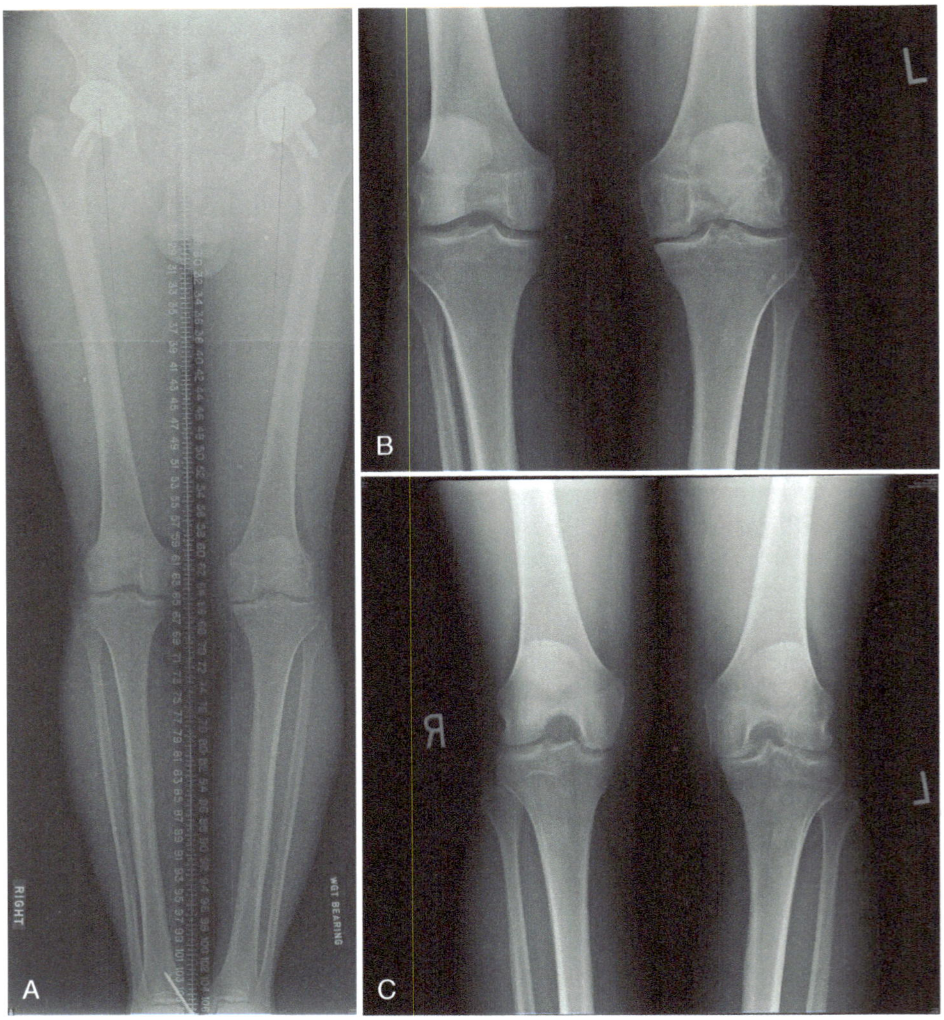

• **Fig. 10.3** Standard series of x-ray images used to evaluate a patient for tibial valgus osteotomy. This 54-year-old police officer who had undergone hip resurfacing procedures wishes to remain physically very active and avoid total knee replacement. (A) Long axial alignment x-ray images demonstrate that the left knee is in mechanical varus with the mechanical axis falling into the medial compartment with medial compartment joint space narrowing. (B) Standing AP evidence of previous anterior cruciate ligament (ACL) reconstruction is noted with tibial and femoral tunnels present. (C) Standing PA Rosenberg views demonstrate loss of posterior cartilage space on the medial joint compartment typical for a chronic ACL-deficient knee as normal where pattern for the medial compartment is anterior and medial noted on the standing AP x-ray image.

Continued

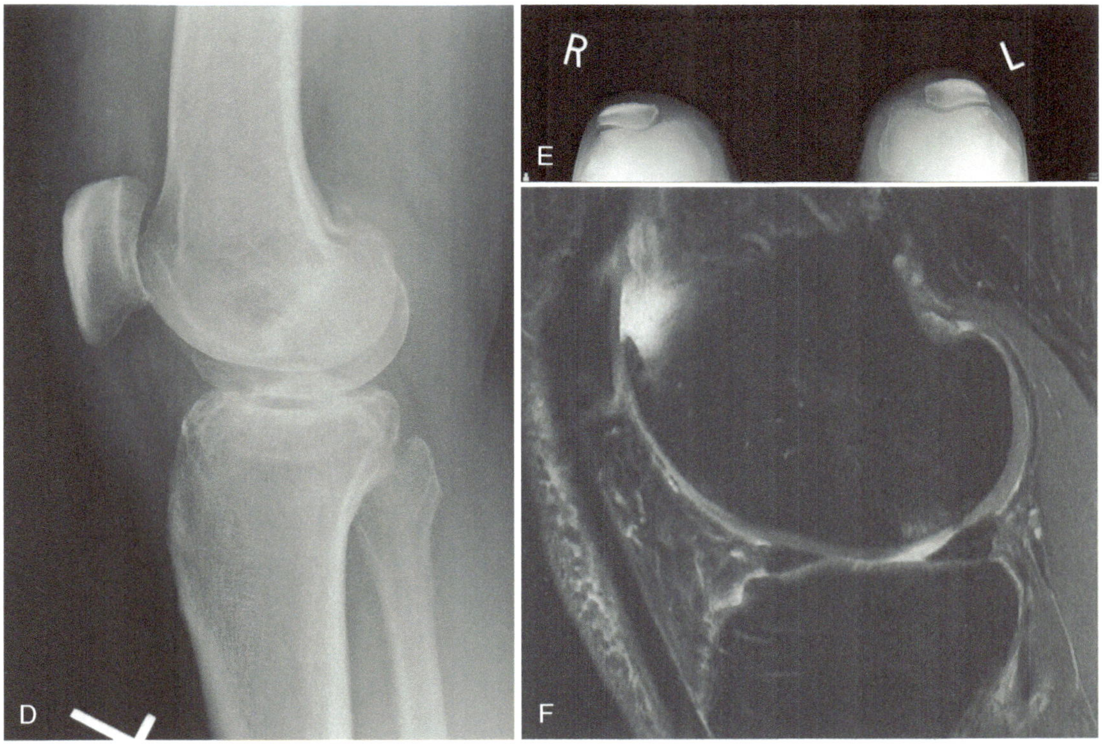

• **Fig. 10.3 Cont'd** (D) The lateral x-ray image further demonstrates central posterior erosion of the tibiofemoral joint on the medial compartment and the formation of a cupola (cupping of the joint). Loss of the intercondylar notch is also noted with chronic ACL-deficient knees. (E) A high-resolution MRI scan performed on a 1.5 Tesla magnet demonstrates a full-thickness articular cartilage loss in the center of the lateral femoral condyles with underlying bone marrow edema; the cartilage defect measures approximately 2 cm in length by 1 cm wide. This defect corresponds with laterally based discomfort in the patient. (F) As tibial valgus-producing osteotomy loads the lateral tibiofemoral compartment, the MRI scan here is very useful as it demonstrates that the osteotomy is contraindicated in this patient.

The goal of realignment osteotomy with cartilage repair without evidence of joint space narrowing is to restore normal mechanical alignment and mechanics to the knee joint prior to bringing the mechanical axis to the midline or restoring at least 6 degrees of tibiofemoral valgus.[6] When bone-on-bone changes are present on x-ray examination and joint preservation with cartilage repair is not indicated, osteotomy remains effective as a pain-relieving procedure, which still allows improved levels of activity. However, overcorrection is recommended in this situation with 2 degrees of overcorrection to the lateral tibial spine being our preferred amount. Anterior-posterior instability may also be improved upon by altering the tibial slope when performing osteotomy surgery for recurvatum or hyperextension deformity secondary to neuromuscular disorder or anatomical joint line deformity by performing flexion osteotomies. ACL-deficient knees or knees with fixed flexion deformities may be improved upon by extension osteotomies either in isolation or in combination with tibial valgus osteotomies.

Technique Selection for High Tibial Osteotomy

The factors to consider when performing proximal tibial valgus osteotomy include leg length discrepancy, medial joint laxity, ACL laxity, the presence or absence of an osteochondral defect on the medial femoral condyle, joint-line obliquity, a patient who is a prior smoker or who currently smokes, opiate requirements at baseline, ethanol use, and a cooperative and compliant patient. Recent basic science work evaluating the effect of open versus closing wedge osteotomy on the changes in load distribution across the knee[7] have demonstrated that with a less than 5-degree osteotomy correction, the closing wedge provided superior results in load transfer from medial to lateral compartments than that seen with an opening osteotomy. However, at 10-degree osteotomy correction there was no significant difference in load transfer in the knee compartments between the two surgery modes, opening versus closing wedge osteotomy.

With regard to the patient-related factors, I exclude patients who have addictive behavior patterns (smoking or baseline opiates) from osteotomy surgery. Postoperative pain management is very difficult for both surgeon and patient because of the possibility of delayed or nonunion of the tibia with smoking and persistent pain. If the patient has unrealistic expectations about the recovery after surgery, return to work, or the inability to use crutches, they should also not be considered for osteotomy surgery.

The technique of open wedge tibial valgus osteotomy has become my preferred technique. It addresses the deformity where it occurs on the medial aspect of the metaphyseal-diaphyseal junction of the proximal tibia. It does not distort the anatomy of the upper tibia so that total knee

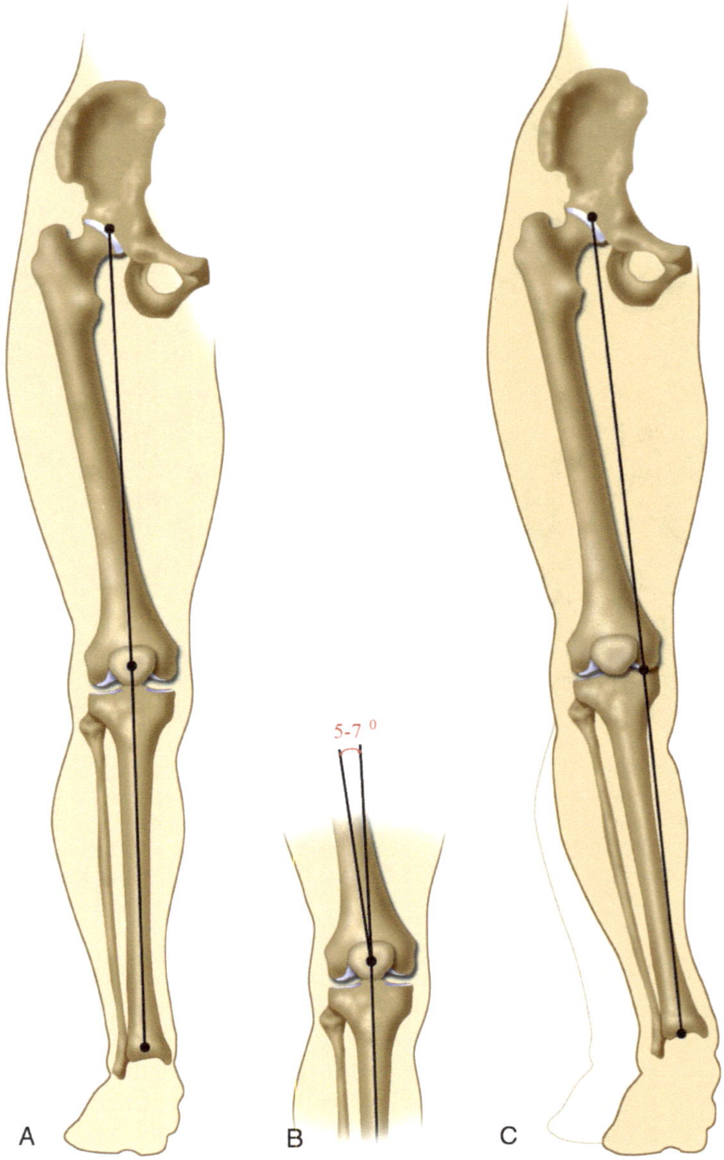

• **Fig. 10.4** (A) Normal mechanical axis. A line drawn through the center of the femoral head to the center of the talus should fall to the center of the knee. This assumes a normal hip neck shaft angle of 130 degrees and (B) a tibiofemoral valgus anatomical axis angle of 5 to 7 degrees. (C) Demonstrates varus mechanical axis.

replacement is more easily performed than after traditional closing wedge Coventry osteotomy. When performed for early osteoarthritis, medial joint laxity can be corrected easily and secondary laxity of the ACL can be lessened by decreasing the sagittal slope of the tibia by placing the osteotomy fixation device more posteriorly. However, it requires special care to ensure that the hamstring insertions are not overly tightened by lengthening the medial column of the tibia or by increasing the patellofemoral contact forces with large opening corrections. Additionally it requires the use of bone graft at the osteotomy site, which increases the time to union of the osteotomy. Opening wedge osteotomy can increase leg length and this is advantageous if the leg is short at baseline but can be problematic otherwise. The average time to union of a tibial opening wedge osteotomy is 10–12 weeks and a closing wedge osteotomy is 6 to 8 weeks. This may play a factor in someone who has to return to work in a physical capacity earlier with regard to procedure selection. These technical details will be discussed further.

Closing wedge osteotomies are currently performed for corrections less than 10 degrees, specifically for conditions of osteochondritis dissecans, large osseous bone cysts, or avascular necrosis of the medial femoral condyle. The autologous bone graft that is harvested with the osteotomy is used as the restorative bone graft for the osteochondral defect on the medial femoral condyle. In this way, malalignment is corrected and the osseous defect is repaired in a single setting (see Chapter 13 on osteochondral defects). Other indications for a closing wedge osteotomy include patients who are previous smokers or laborers who require a quick

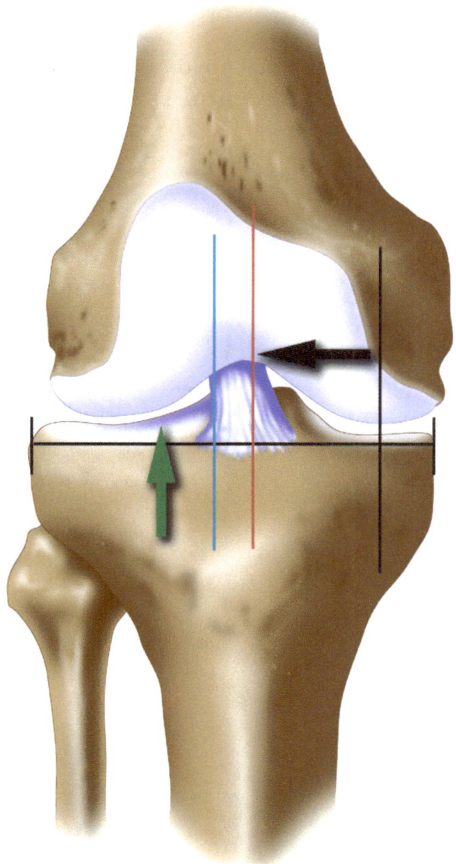

• **Fig. 10.5** Mechanical axis correction. Classic mechanical axis correction for tibial valgus-producing osteotomy is recommended by several authors to pass through the Kurosaka point at 62% across the width of the tibia (*broad green arrow*). This results in a tibiofemoral valgus angle of approximately 10 to 12 degrees. My preference is to correct the mechanical axis to the midline (*red line*) when correcting the varus with cartilage repair for a focal medial defect and to overcorrect by only 2 degrees to the lateral tibial spine if the patient has a very large medial femoral condyle chondral defect, "kissing" medial chondral defects, or established osteoarthritis with greater than 50% loss of the joint space on weight-bearing x-ray images.

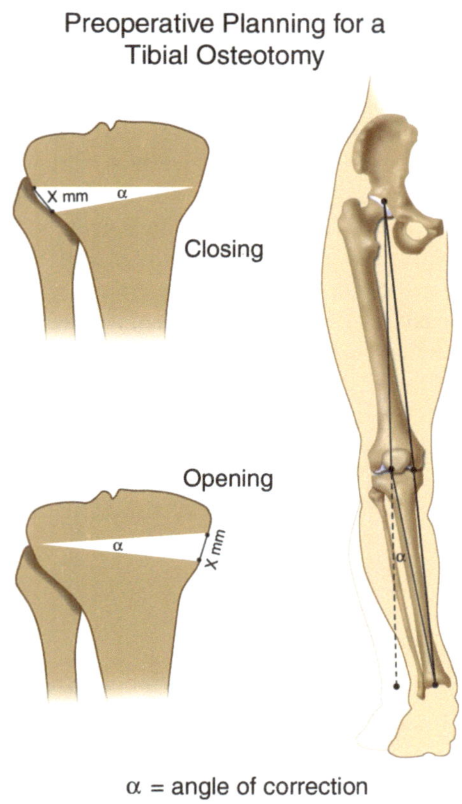

• **Fig. 10.6** Osteotomy planning is a straightforward procedure when the varus is in the proximal tibial metaphysis as is the most common situation. A line is drawn from the center of the femoral head to the desired point of correction (see Fig. 10.5), in this case from the lateral tibial spine, to the proposed position of the foot at the center of the ankle. The angle between the center of the talus and the proposed position is the angle of correction, α. Using calibrated digital x-ray images and software that is readily available (General Electric, Centricity, web-based software), the actual opening in millimeters, *x*, may be calculated for an opening wedge osteotomy. Similarly, the exact number of millimeters for angle α for a closing wedge osteotomy may be calculated or the angle may be taken directly off the osteotomy closing wedge calibrated angular system, which is typical. Intraoperative check with clinical appearance of the limb after osteotomy as well as using intraoperative checks with long alignment wires or rods under fluoroscopic control confirm accurate angular corrections.

return to work because cancellous bone to cancellous bone healing usually occurs within 6 to 8 weeks.

A reverse dome osteotomy, as popularized by Paley,[8] is very powerful for large corrections, i.e., 15 to 30 degrees. It has the advantage of maintaining the anatomy of the upper tibia and correcting large deformities. It is technically demanding and requires a freehand technique with a concomitant fibular osteotomy and a fixed angle device for fixation or external fixator, and usually is longer in its healing, i.e., 3 to 4 months.

Surgical Setup, Hospital Course, and Postoperative Care

Osteotomies are performed on a radiolucent table which allows visualization of the hip, knee, and ankle accompanied by image intensification. General anesthesia is used, a pericapsular infiltration (my mixture is prepared by our pharmacy and available for every major surgery: clonidine 80 µg, epinephrine 0.5 mg, ketorolac 30 mg, ropivacaine 0.5% 49.25 mL QS with normal saline to final volume of 100 mL) with inclusion of a saphenous nerve block at the end of surgery providing excellent pain relief for 24–36 hours on average. Tranexamic acid (TXA) 1 gram IV at the onset of surgery and 1 gram at the end of surgery markedly decreases bleeding. Drains are left under the muscle compartments overnight until only 30 cc or less over 8 hours and then they are removed to prevent a muscle compartment syndrome. Patients are placed on DVT prophylaxis during the surgery with foot pump compression (to avoid calf muscle compression), light graduated compression stockings with a light gauze dressing only at the end of surgery, and are started on aspirin 81 mg bid for 3 weeks postoperatively starting the day of surgery. Postoperative pain management is important. A continuous ice water closed compression system is applied in the OR and sent home with the patient. Intravenous ketorolac 30 mg IV every 6 hours for 3 doses and oral acetaminophen 1 gram every 6–8 hours for the first several weeks and intermittent oxycodone 5–10 mg every 8–12 hours for the first 1–2 weeks is all that is needed. Patients are generally discharged on the day after surgery or the same day in a removable hinge knee brace, a continuous passive motion (CPM) machine, and two crutches touch weight-bearing, foot flat to the ground with weight of leg supported. Ice cryotherapy is generally very helpful for swelling and discomfort. It is recommended that patients take vitamin D 3000 IU and 1000 mg of calcium daily for bone healing and avoid nonsteroidal antiinflammatory drugs, which may delay osteotomy healing. As noted earlier, we do not perform osteotomies on patients who are cigarette smokers because of the known risk of nonunion.

Anatomical Considerations

When performing high tibial osteotomy, avoidance of neurovascular injuries and compartment syndrome is critical. Understanding the course of the femoral artery and its normal and abnormal anatomy as well as the course of the peroneal nerve is important to avoid injury from an oscillating saw blade during performance of the procedure. Upon performing a closing wedge osteotomy, the author inadvertently cut through a small artery located directly on the back of the tibia, a vascular consult was obtained, the tourniquet was let down, and Doppler pulses of the foot noted a good distal circulation. The small vessels were then tied off and fortunately no further sequelae occurred. Upon further investigation, it was discovered that this was an aberrant anterior tibial artery (see Fig. 10.7). Upon reviewing

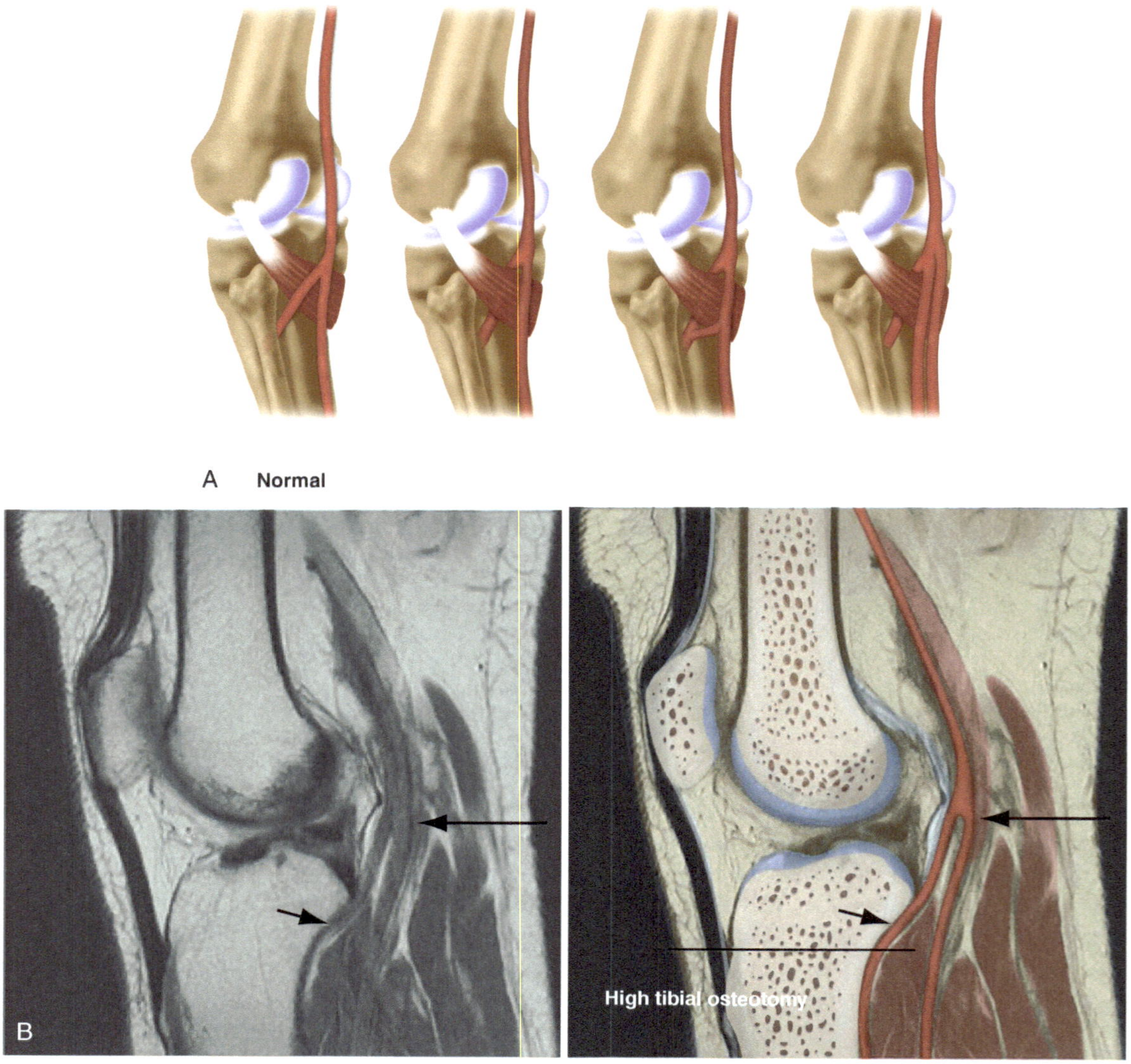

• **Fig. 10.7** (A) Variations of an aberrant tibialis anterior artery are depicted. A division of the popliteal artery into the tibialis anterior artery and the peroneal artery trunk may have aberrancies with the tibialis anterior artery going deep to the popliteus muscle and lie directly on the posterior tibial cortex as noted. This vessel may then be inadvertently transected during procedures on the upper end of the tibial metaphysis. It is especially at risk during tibial osteotomy. An aberrant tibialis anterior artery occurs in approximately 2.1% of knees.[9] (B) The MRI and corresponding diagram illustrate the aberrant anterior tibial artery deep to the popliteus muscle lies directly on the posterior cortex of the tibia at risk at the usual position of high tibial osteotomy.

Continued

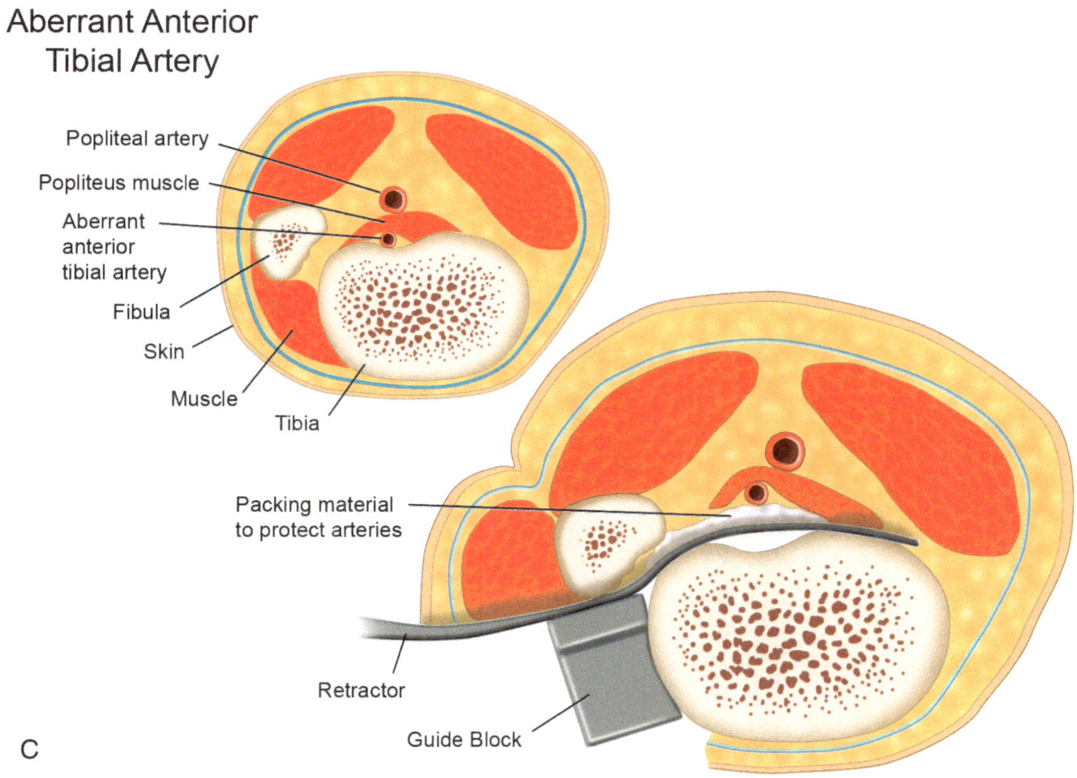

• **Fig. 10.7 Cont'd** (C) Careful posterior subperiosteal dissection of the tibia protects an aberrant anterior tibial artery from injury. The incidence of this variation is 2.1%[9] and can be visualized on preoperative MRI scan if this is performed.

the malpractice cases against osteotomies in the Boston area, it was discovered that there were two cases of arterial injury, one resulting in a compartment syndrome of the anterior musculature with necrosis requiring excision of the anterior muscle compartment and tendon transfer to the foot. The second resulted in avascularity to the foot resulting in amputation. I collaborated with my radiology colleagues to investigate the incidence and significance of the aberrant anterior tibial artery.[9] The angiographic literature has reported a prevalence of high division of the popliteal artery from 3% to 8% and in our MRI surveillance of 1116 knees there was an incidence of 23/1116 or 2.1% of an aberrant anterior tibial artery lying directly on the posterior cortex of the tibia deep to the popliteus muscle. The vessel is an embryological remnant of the deep popliteal artery having undergone developmental arrest.

Another recent study[10] using Duplex ultrasonography on 100 knees in 50 patients visualized the popliteal artery at the level of total knee arthroplasty, 1–1.5 cm distal to the articular surface, moved only 1.4 mm further posterior at 90 degrees of flexion in 76% of knees but closer to the posterior cortex in 24% with flexion. At the level of tibial osteotomy, 1.5–2 cm distal to the articular surface, 85% of the arteries moved further away posterior at 90 degrees of flexion by only 1.7 mm; however, 15% moved closer to the tibia at 90 degrees of flexion. Hence as it is technically more difficult to perform an osteotomy at 90 degrees of flexion and there is no guarantee the vessels may not be brought closer to the tibia and at greater risk of injury, I prefer to do the osteotomy in full extension after having dissected out the back on the knee protecting the neurovascular structures with sponges and retractors. I then perform an accurate and safe osteotomy, fixing the osteotomy in full extension to ensure that a fixed flexion deformity does not arise (which may occur if fixation is performed with the knee flexed), which is a big mistake when performing osteotomy surgery.

Closing Wedge Osteotomy

There are several companies that use calibrated osteotomy jigs in 1- and 2-degree increments allowing very accurate reproducible Coventry wedge, closing osteotomy corrections. A closing wedge osteotomy can generally be performed without elevation of the tibial tubercle of up to 10 degrees of angular correction. Removal of the medial portion of the fibular articular surface, leaving intact the proximal tibiofibular joint capsule is preferred with corrections of 8 degrees or less (see Fig. 10.8). Corrections of 10 degrees or greater are difficult without going to a mid-shaft fibular osteotomy to allow an easy closing osteotomy, otherwise the proximal tibiofibular joint would be completely released, rendering the lateral ligamentous complex lax and the fibula migrating proximally above the lateral tibiofemoral joint line. For osteotomies between 10 and 14 degrees,

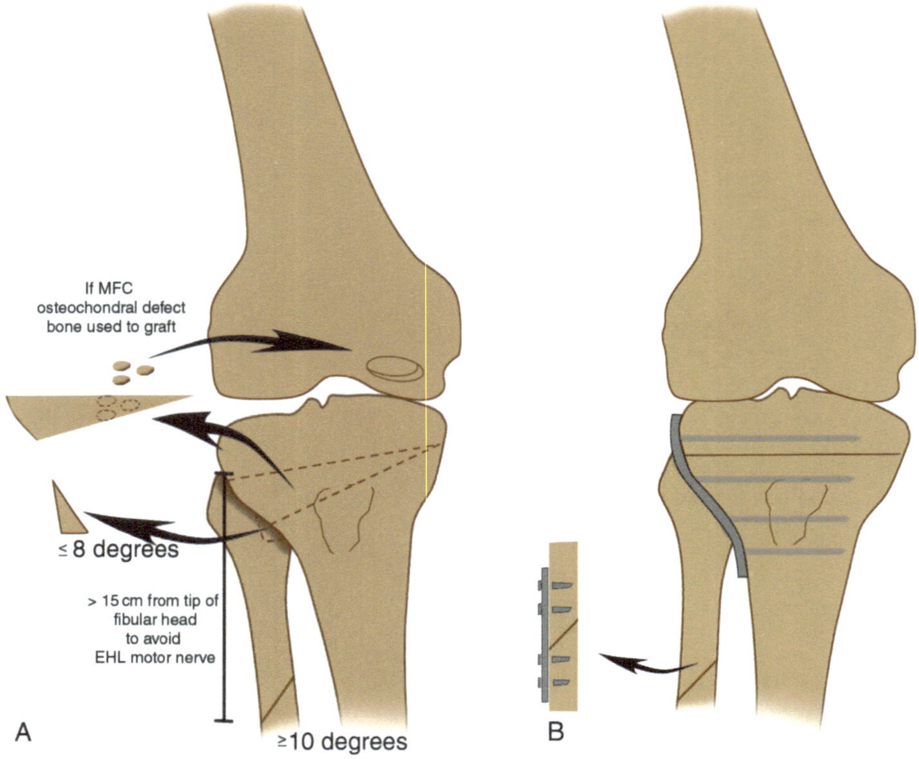

• **Fig. 10.8** (A) The present primary indication for a closing wedge tibial valgus osteotomy is to provide bone for a medial femoral condyle bone grafting of an osteochondral defect and restore the alignment of the leg to neutral mechanical alignment. If the angular correction is 8 degrees or less, then the medial aspect of the fibular articular surface is removed. If the correction is greater than 10 degrees, a mid-shaft fibular osteotomy is performed and then fixated (B). *EHL*, Extensor hallucis longus; *MFC*, medial femoral condyle.

the tubercle is generally elevated and a retrotubercular osteotomy is performed. This allows the osteotomy to be performed lower down on the tibial surface so as not to produce a metaphyseal-diaphyseal mismatch and not to remove as much bone. However, there is risk of the medial cortex fracturing because it is in diaphyseal bone and displacement of the osteotomy. A medial plate or fixation staple would be required if this were to happen. This is performed with a concomitant mid-shaft fibular osteotomy. Fixation of both osteotomies is performed.

A skin incision is made just off the midline (see Fig. 10.9, a stepwise surgical approach, and Fig. 10.10, postoperative x-ray images) slightly laterally from the superior pole of the patella to the inferior aspect of the tibial tubercle. Full thickness medial and lateral flaps are made to the posterior medial and posterior lateral corner of the knee joint. The lateral patella tendon margin is dissected sharply to the anterior tibial crest and along the anterior compartment muscle fascia. A second deep incision is made transversely from the anterior aspect of the proximal tibiofibular joint, transversely to the patella tendon below Gerdy's tubercle. The anterior lateral muscle compartment is then subperiosteally dissected from distal to proximal with an elevator being used distally and sharp knife dissection on the metaphysis. The anterior and inferior aspects of the fibular head are then subperiosteally dissected leaving intact the joint capsule of the proximal tibiofibular joint. The posterior aspect of the tibia is dissected subperiosteally and extracapsularly to the back of the knee joint and is packed full of saline-soaked sponges to protect the neurovascular structures. The patella tendon is skeletonized to its insertion on the tubercle. The iliotibial band (ITB) is then reflected proximally off Gerdy's tubercle to the coronary ligament of the lateral meniscus. Stay sutures are used to hold the soft tissues (ITB) proximally.

If the angular correction is 8 degrees or less, the calibrated jig is applied to the proximal tibial joint margins and the transverse cut is made to the medial cortex but not through. The angled cut is then made to the medial cortex in extension because the posterior structures are packed with sponges.

If the correction is greater than or equal to 10 degrees, a separate 3–5 cm incision is made between the superficial posterior muscle compartment and the lateral compartment at the level of the mid-shaft fibula, through the skin and the fascia only. Blunt finger dissection is made to the posterior lateral corner of the fibula where the periosteum is sharply incised with a knife and a circumferential subperiosteal dissection is then performed. Retractors are applied to the fibula. An oblique osteotomy is then made with a sagittal saw and the osteotomy is allowed to slide on itself once the proximal tibial osteotomy is closed. This is then fixated with a 1/3 semi-tubular 4-hole plate after the proximal osteotomy

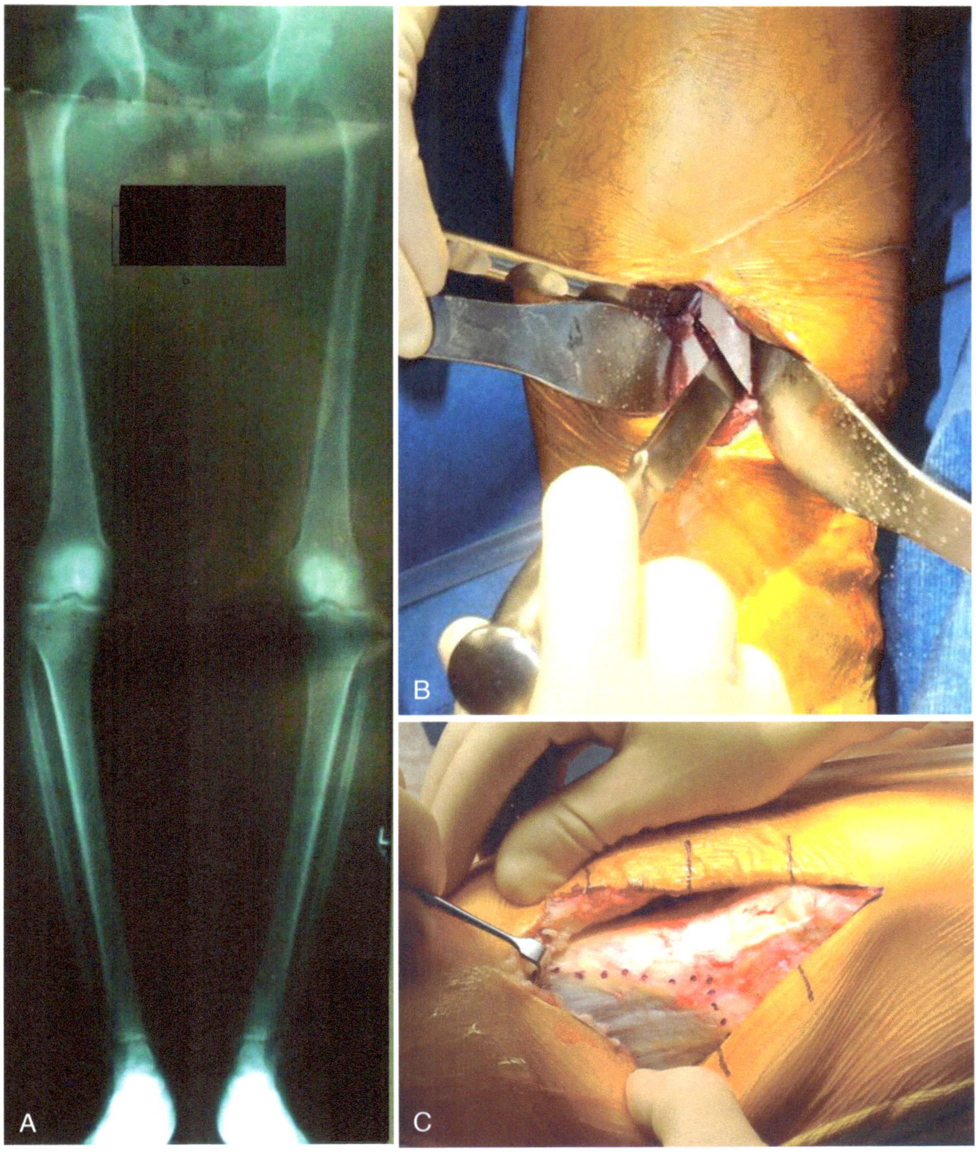

• **Fig. 10.9** (A) 54-inch long alignment x-ray image demonstrating marked varus malalignment of both knees in a 30-year-old male. The left knee has medially-based pain. A 10-degree angular correction places the mechanical axis to the lateral tibial spine unloading the medial compartment, which has early joint space narrowing. (B) A 3-cm skin incision is made at the level of the mid-shaft of the fibula at least 15 cm distal to the fibular head to avoid injury to the motor nerve of the extensor hallucis longus muscle. This is made at the junction of the lateral and posterior muscle compartments. A blunt finger dissection is all that is required to get to the posterior lateral corner of the fibula, which has the fascial attachments. These are then sharply incised longitudinally and a subperiosteal dissection to the deep and superficial aspect of the fibula reveals the bone clearly as seen in the photograph. A small sagittal saw creates an oblique osteotomy to the deep cortex, which is then opened with an osteotome to allow easy motion of one segment relative to the other. (C) A longitudinal incision is made at the level of the superior lateral pole of the patella to the inferior aspect of the tibial tubercle. Full-thickness flaps at the level of the fascia are then performed around the tibia to the posterior medial aspect of the upper tibia and to the posterolateral aspect. The proposed takedown of the anterolateral muscle compartment is then identified as indicated by the sterile marking pen dots on the photograph. (D) The anterolateral muscle compartment is then sharply taken down subperiosteally to the posterior lateral corner of the tibia and the proximal tibiofibular joint. The iliotibial band attachment to Gerdes tubercle is also subperiosteally dissected sharply with a knife as a single flap to the level of the coronary ligament of the lateral meniscus and then sutured onto the capsule to keep it out of the way. The infrapatellar fat pad is then released from the anterior tibia to identify the pretibial bursa and protecting the patellar tendon. (E) A small elevator is placed along the posterior proximal tibiofibular joint capsule. The anterior aspect of the fibular head is then carefully subperiosteally dissected. The inferior half of the joint capsule of the proximal tibiofibular joint is then released anteriorly and posteriorly through the anterior approach. This allows the proximal portion of the fibula to mobilize minimally when the fibular osteotomy is later fixated with a one-third semi-tubular plate. If this was a correction less than or equal to 8 degrees, a fibular osteotomy would not be required and the osteotomy correction would be entirely through excision of the medial one-third of the proximal fibular articular surface leaving only the proximal capsule attached to the tibia. This allows the osteotomy of the tibia to close without proximal migration of the fibula and resultant laxity of the fibular collateral ligament and popliteus tendon attachments. In addition, the posterior muscle compartment is sharply subperiosteally dissected from the back of the tibia to protect the neural-vascular structures. A small wet sponge is placed in a distal to proximal direction directly on the bone and extracapsularly on the posterior joint line.

Continued

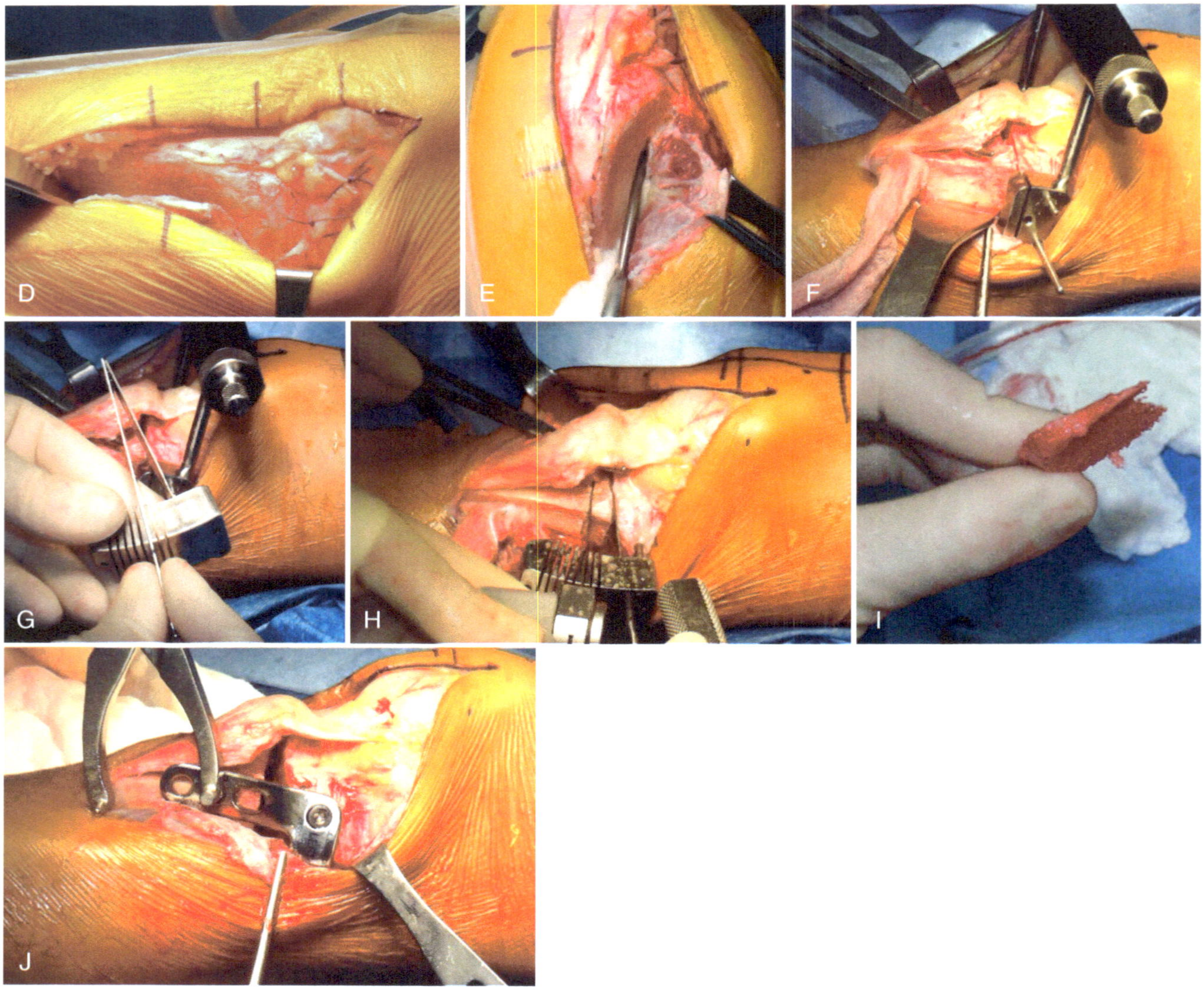

• **Fig. 10.9 Cont'd** (F) A transverse tibial tubercle osteotomy is first performed 1 cm posterior to the anterior cortex with the distal hinge remaining intact. This allows the transverse component of the osteotomy to be performed further distally on the metaphysis thereby removing less bone with the same angular correction. In addition, the tibial tubercle may either be elevated using the bone that has been extracted from the tibial closing wedge osteotomy or just medialized to improve patellar tracking. A radiolucent calibrated jig is then placed across the medial and lateral aspects of the tibia parallel to the joint line and confirmed on image intensification. The transverse osteotomy is now performed to the medial cortex through both the anterior and posterior cortices protecting the posterior neurovascular structures with sponges that had been packed on the posterior cortex after it has been carefully subperiosteally dissected. In this way if there is an aberrant tibialis anterior vessel on the posterior cortex it is avoided. (G) Most closing wedge osteotomy jigs are calibrated in varying increments. This jig is calibrated from 6 degrees to 20 degrees at 2-degree increments. The sawblade as shown, when placed through the jig, will need to go to the opposite tip at which the transverse osteotomy rests, in this case the medial proximal cortex of the tibia. (H) With the second calibrated jig now being applied to the proximal cut, a second bony cut is made at 10 degrees to the first to the opposite medial cortex through both anterior and posterior cortices. This is checked under image intensification as it is being performed to ensure that the medial cortex has not been violated. (I) Using a 0.25-inch osteotome at the level of the proximal and distal closing wedge osteotomy cuts, the bony fragment is then easily removed. Note that as this 10-degree fragment has been removed from the metaphysis at a more distal location its size is quite small. This makes the metaphyseal-diaphyseal mismatch very little and the distortion of the upper end of the tibia is therefore minimized. If a total knee replacement were required in the future, an offset tibial stem would probably not be required and the procedure would be facilitated by the utilitarian midline incision that was used for the osteotomy instead of a classic hockey-stick type of incision. (J) The osteotomy is now slowly closed after the medial cortex has been multiply drilled with a 3.2-mm drill bit to ensure that a controlled closure occurs. A compression clamp is attached to the off-set L-plate that is used with the system and after the proximal two 6.5-mm screws have been placed in the plate. The mid-shaft fibular osteotomy is carefully palpated and through its separate incision to insure that it moves easily to allow closure of the tibial osteotomy. When the osteotomy is completely closed, the distal two screw holes are utilized. If there is a crack of the medial cortex, either a staple is placed at that site to prevent translation of the tibial shaft laterally or the medial cortex from opening. The other option is to use an oblique lag screw through the oblong hole within the plate, which was performed in this case for added stability and to prevent breakage of the medial side.

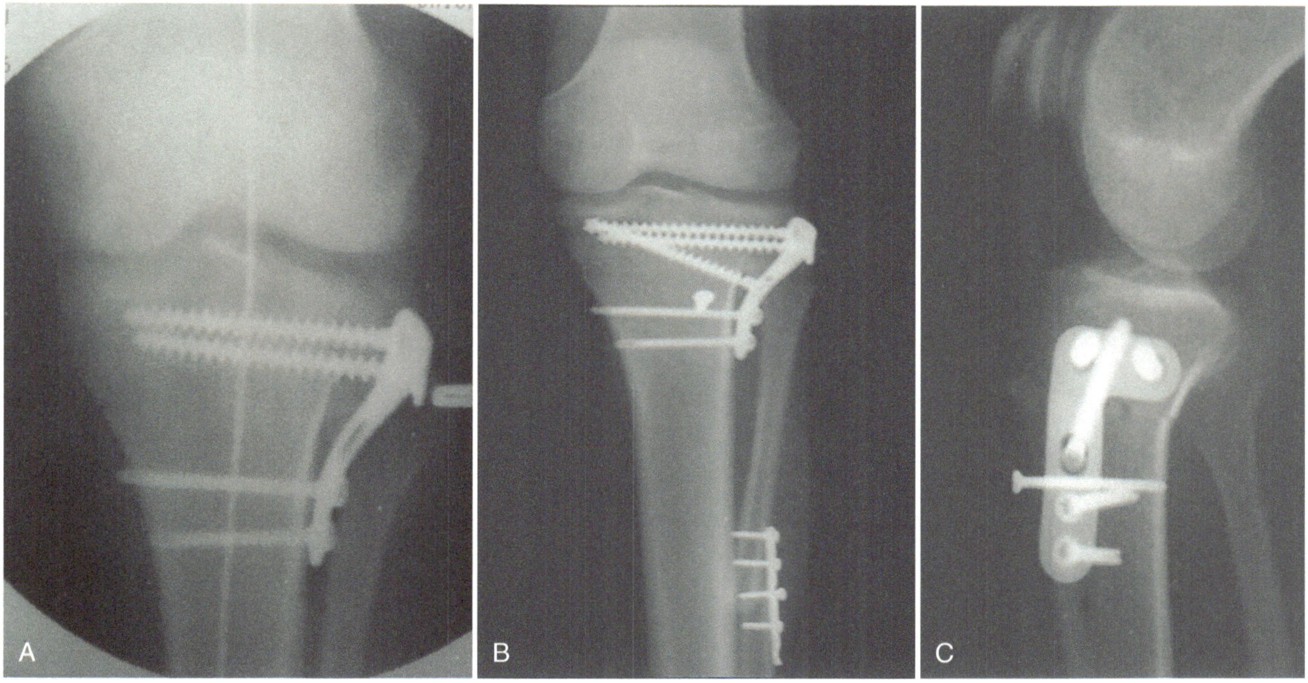

• **Fig. 10.10** (A) An intraoperative check is performed using a Bovie cord on the radiolucent table from the center of the femoral head to the center of the talus at the ankle joint to ensure that the proposed angular correction is to the lateral tibial spine as planned preoperatively. (B) The tibial tubercle is slightly medialized to ensure central patellar tracking and fixated with a single anterior-to-posterior lag screw to the posterior cortex of the tibia. The fibula is separately plated with a small one-third semi-tubular plate. X-ray examination demonstrates the final radiographic appearance. Note the minimal deformity of the upper end of the tibia, also that the proximal fibula is at its native position insuring that the posterior lateral ligamentous complex has not been made lax. (C) Final radiographic appearance on the lateral x-ray image. Note that the tibial tubercle osteotomy performed in this case was to facilitate a lower osteotomy position and not to unload the patellofemoral joint. In corrections that are less than 10 degrees, a tibial tubercle osteotomy is generally not utilized unless the position of the patellar tendon attachment is very proximal and near the joint line. A tibial tubercle osteotomy in that situation would be useful to protect the patellar tendon from injury.

has been fixated. This allows ease of comfort postoperatively and rapid union of the fibula.

If the osteotomy of 10 degrees or greater intersects the patellar tendon, the tibial tubercle is osteotomized, leaving it intact distally and elevating it. The closing wedge osteotomy is then performed. The osteotomy closure is performed slowly with a compression device through an L plate so as not to fracture and make unstable the medial cortex (the cortex is usually pre-drilled). The tubercle is finally re-fixated with one or two 3.5-mm screws in a compression mode through the posterior cortex. Usually, if there is some lateral patella facet disease along with this, a full thickness lateral release will be performed and the closing wedge bone graft is placed under the tibial tubercle in order to elevate it.

The sponges are now removed and the tourniquet is let down and electrocautery is used for any bleeders. Hemovac drains (two arms) are placed in the wounds. One arm is placed posterior to the tibia, loosely re-approximating the iliotibial band to the superior aspect of the anterior lateral muscle compartment. The anterior aspect of the muscle fascia is left completely opened. Closure of the subcutaneous tissues and the skin follows. The drains are left in overnight and taken out in the morning. The muscle compartments are clinically inspected every 4–6 hours to monitor for anterior muscle compartment syndrome as needed. Foot compression pumps are used immediately after surgery to diminish swelling and DVT risk. They are the preferred mechanical compression device as they improve venous return without pressure on the muscle compartments.

Opening Wedge Osteotomy

Opening wedge osteotomy is the preferred osteotomy because of its technical ease, very accurate dial-in correction, and lack of deformity to the proximal tibia, which presumably will result in an easier conversion to total knee replacement in the future. It is especially useful if there is leg length shortening on the affected side, joint line obliquity inferior-medially with a varus thrust because it restores leg length and produces a horizontal joint line. If there is medial laxity, it is corrected by adding to the medial column deep to the medial collateral ligament and if there is ACL laxity or posterior cruciate ligament (PCL) laxity, it can be improved by extension or flexion of the tibial sagittal slope respectively. The osteotomy is performed at the deformity of the tibia vara, which is usually at the metaphyseal-diaphyseal junction. When performing an osteotomy, it is important to direct the cut to the proximal tibiofibular joint and not

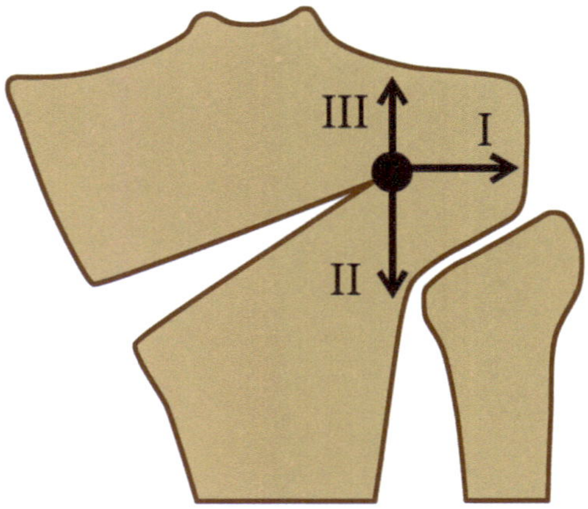

• **Fig. 10.11** Takeuchi classification of lateral hinge fracture[11] with open wedge high tibial valgus osteotomy (an avoidable complication). Type I continues into the lateral metaphysis and may cause translation of the fragments and delayed union. Type II is below the tibiofibular joint into the lateral cortex with instability of the tibia, and Type III extends into the lateral tibial plateau articular surface.

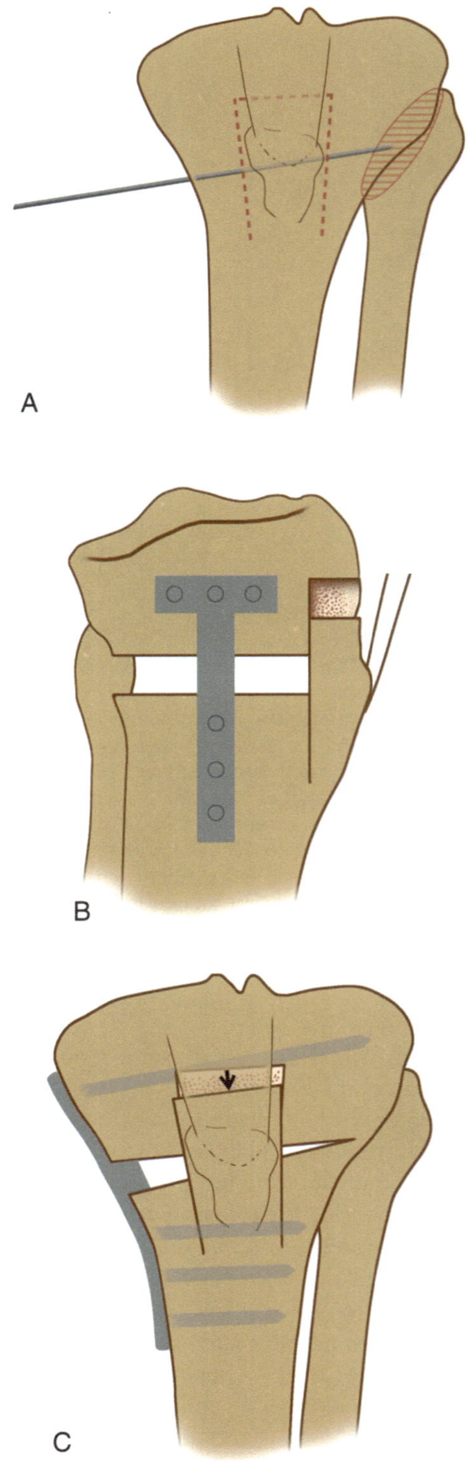

• **Fig. 10.12** (A) The guidewire is placed obliquely across from the medial metaphyseal-diaphyseal junction to the tibiofibular joint. It is directed behind the tibial tubercle which is cut leaving it attached to the lower osteotomy fragment. (B) The osteotomy cut is made behind the tubercle towards the tibiofibular joint. It is then opened. The tubercle is cut 1 cm posterior to the anterior cortex. The tubercle remains attached distally. (C) The final appearance of the open wedge high tibial valgus osteotomy. Note that the tibial tubercle has migrated distally but rests on the proximal fragment adding stability to the construct.

the upper lateral metaphysis because upon opening a lateral hinge fracture (LHF) may occur as described by Takeuchi[11] (Fig. 10.11). The osteotomy is often at the level of the patellar tendon attachment but usually retro-tubercular. This is performed proximal to the pes anserinus insertion obliquely directed toward the proximal tibiofibular joint to within 5 mm of the lateral cortex. I find this is at the strongest attachment of tibiofibular joint capsule, which resists displacement at opening and avoids LHF as has been shown by others as well.[12] Opening wedge osteotomies may be performed up to approximately 20 degrees. I always release the pes anserinus tendons from the medial subcutaneous border of the tibia to allow the medial column to lengthen and not develop a flexion deformity from soft tissue tightness. They are reattached to the superficial medial collateral ligament (MCL) over the plate at the end of the surgery. Similarly, performing the osteotomy behind the tibial tubercle prevents the extensor mechanism from tightening with increasing opening wedge osteotomy (see Fig. 10.12).

A longitudinal incision is made from the superior medial pole of the patella to the inferior aspect of the tibial tubercle. Fig. 10.13 shows a stepwise surgical technique for an opening wedge tibial valgus osteotomy. A full thickness medial subcutaneous flap is then made and pes anserinus tendons are identified on the subcutaneous border of the tibia medially. The superior aspect of these tendons are then incised and the tendons are released subperiosteally from anterior to posterior and are repaired at the end. A transverse incision is made through the periosteum in the deep portion of the MCL from the posterior aspect of the tibia to the anterior aspect of the tibia, proximal to the pes insertion. The MCL is then subperiosteally dissected to within 1 cm of the joint line to the coronary ligament of the medial meniscus. The MCL is then tagged with a suture and tacked to the capsule proximally to be out of the way and reattached to the pes

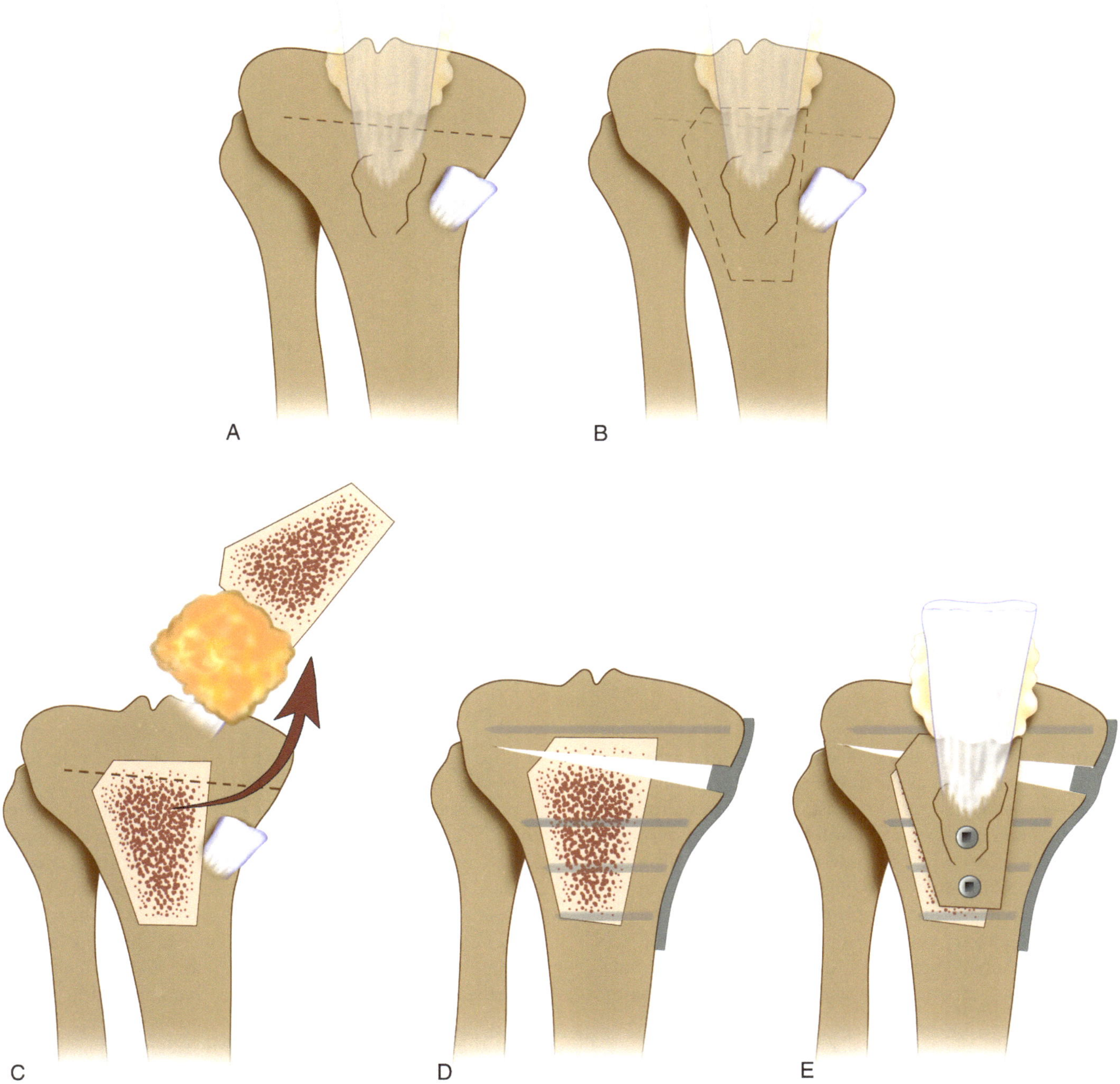

• **Fig. 10.13** (A) Step 1: the *dotted line* represents the proposed level of the tibial opening wedge valgus-producing osteotomy from the metaphyseal-diaphyseal junction of the proximal tibia to the proximal tibiofibular joint. (B) Step 2: outline of the proposed level of the tibial tubercle anteromedialization osteotomy (Fulkerson osteotomy) with a transverse proximal counter cut and an oblique distal counter cut, followed by the medial to posterolateral osteotomy typical of the Fulkerson osteotomy. The steepness will vary based on the amount of anteriorization versus medialization required for extensor mechanism unloading and proper tracking. The posterior lateral cortex of the tibia must always remain intact. (C) Step 3: the tibial tubercle osteotomy is now performed, Hoffa's fat pad is released off the anterior tibial interval anterior to the intrameniscal ligament, and the origins of the anterior horns of the medial and lateral menisci. A lateral sub-vastus arthrotomy is performed to visualize the joint and unload the patella and a medial sub-vastus arthrotomy is performed to the level of the insertion of the vastus medialis obliquus on the joint capsule. (D) Step 4: the opening wedge tibial valgus-producing osteotomy is now performed and fixated. (E) Step 5: the tibial tubercle is now replaced at the level of its original proximal transverse counter cut and positioned in the anterior and medial directions necessary to centralize and unload the tibial tubercle. Pointed reduction forceps or a K-wire holds the tubercle in position while two anterior to posterior lag screws are used to fixate the tibial tubercle. Note that the distal cut of the tibial tubercle is not a straight anterior to posterior transverse cut, but slopes distally and anteriorly to avoid a stress riser and potential postoperative stress fracture at this position. There is usually a gap at this position, which is then bone grafted with a combination of demineralized bone matrix and cancellous allogeneic bone chips.

Continued

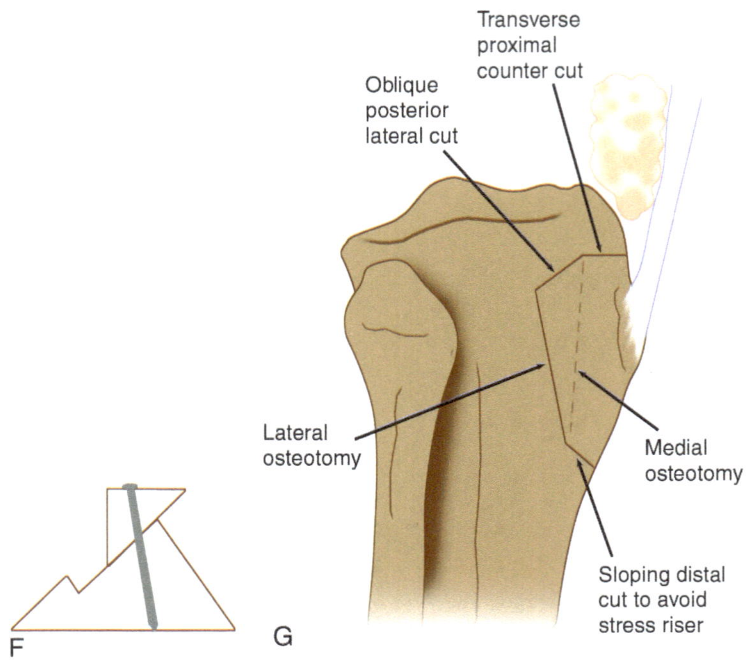

• **Fig. 10.13 Cont'd** (F) This diagram illustrates the cross-sectional appearance of the tibia at the level of the tibial tubercle after it is mobilized and fixated. The deficient lateral bone stock is replaced with demineralized bone matrix as is the overhanging medial tibial tubercle supplemented underneath its overhang. The medial periosteal sleeve, which includes the past anserinus tendons, is cold over the bone graft substitute and reattached to the patellar tendon on the tibial tubercle to have a smooth medial subcutaneous border with no bony prominences (see technique of tibial tubercle osteotomy [TTO] in Chapter 12). (G) View of the TTO from the lateral side. The distal aspect of the TTO is sloped anteriorly to lessen the stress riser and possibility of postoperative fracture. The proximal counter cut is transverse to allow the osteotomy to "lock in" when finally positioned and reduce the chance of proximal migration postoperative aiding in stability of the osteotomy.

tendons over the plate at the closure leaving intact the deep and superficial aspects of the medial collateral ligament. The patella tendon is skeletonized on its insertion, distally. With the knee then flexed in a figure-of-4 position, the posterior aspect of the tibia is dissected and extracapsularly dissected. The gastrocnemius-soleus origin on the exposed posterior aspect of the knee is then sharply released off the back of the tibia allowing a very careful subperiosteal dissection across the tibia from medial to lateral to the proximal tibiofibular joint. Small wet sponges are packed behind the knee to the level of the lateral tibiofibular joint and proximally to the level of the joint and this is easily palpated.

Under image intensification, a guidewire is placed obliquely at the level of the metaphyseal-diaphyseal junction, proximal to the patella tendon insertion if possible, to the level of the proximal tibiofibular joint. If the patellar tendon insertion is very proximal, a retrotubercular osteotomy is performed (which is my usual and preferred technique). This is done by making an axial sawcut at the level of the patellar tendon insertion followed by a medial to lateral saw cut for 1 to 2 cm distal to this at a level of 1 cm posterior to the anterior tibial tubercle cortex. In this way the tibial tubercle is still attached to the distal fragment. A saw cut is then made on top of the guidewire with the knee in full extension visualized under image intensification guidance to the lateral cortex of the tibia, to the tibiofibular joint, but not through it. Opening wedge tines are then used to open the medial aspect of the tibia. If the correction is large (>10 mm) or there is a fracture through the lateral cortex at the tibiofibular joint, I use a lateral staple across the osteotomy to ensure stability and non-displacement (see Fig. 10.14). The correct amount of angular correction is documented with an intraoperative guidewire/guide rod assessment placing a Bovie cord wire from the center of the femoral head to the center of the talus falling through the lateral intercondylar spine. This will coincide with the desired degree of angular correction. Puddu plates are then placed, 6.5-mm cancellous screws are used proximally through the plate, and 4.5-mm screws are placed distally. I have found that the first generation stainless steel T Puddu plate utilized for the femur is more robust because it has three proximal screws and four distal screws about the osteotomy site. I have used it for several years on the tibia without failure of the plate or loss of correction. It is also a low-profile implant and is not usually felt by the patient. I have used cancellous autograft dowels in the past but I currently use allograft freeze-dried cancellous chips. The autografts were taken from the distal femoral metaphyses above the MCL origin. The tourniquet is then let down and an excellent marrow "blush" of marrow elements permeates the allograft bone. No irrigation is used so that none of these bone-forming cells and elements are lost. I have found that healing is similar to autograft bone and I have not used iliac crest bone since 2001.

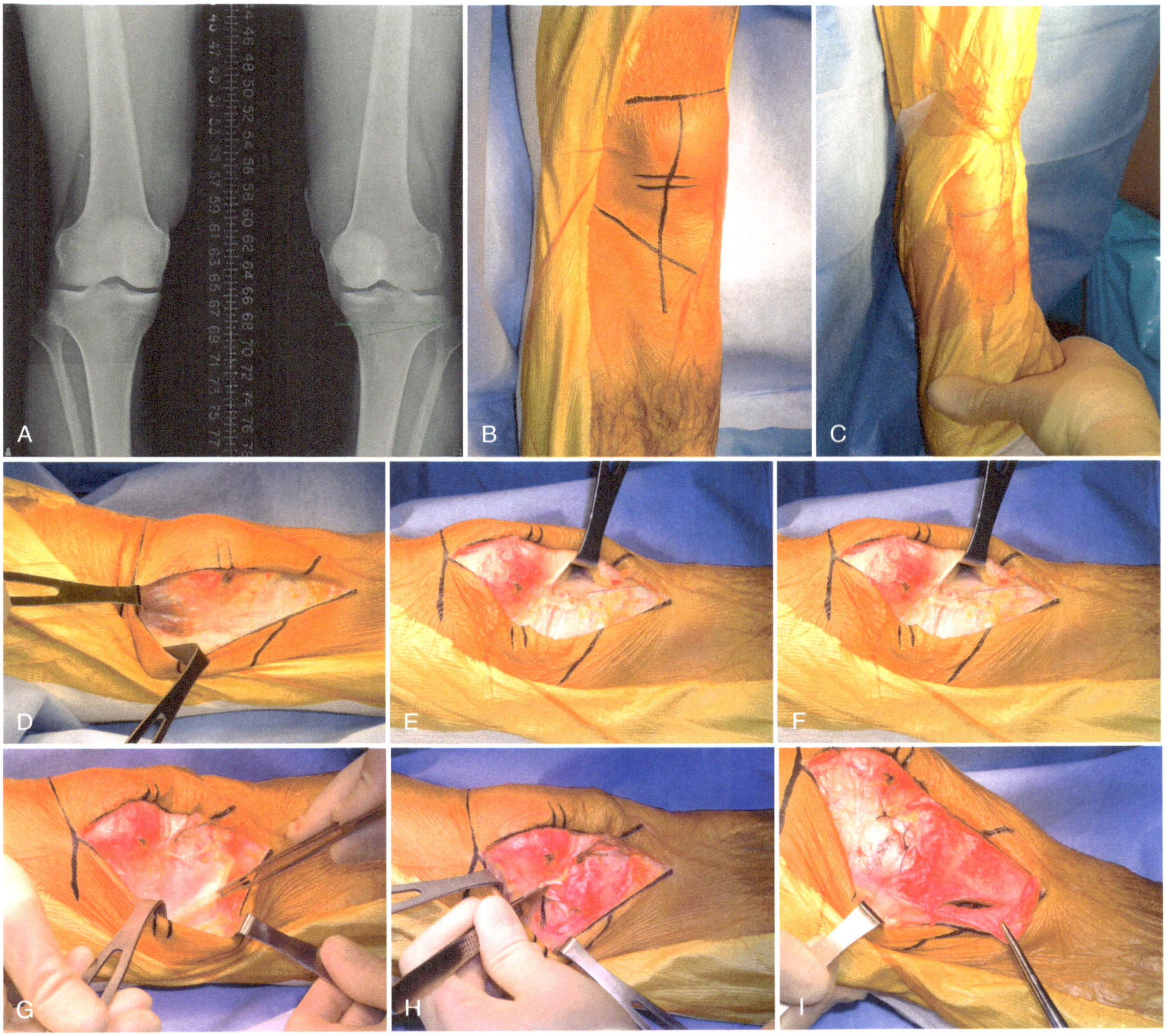

• **Fig. 10.14** (A) Digital long x-ray images demonstrating varus alignment used to calculate the opening wedge correction to place the mechanical axis through lateral tibial spine of the knee. Digital templating of this standing AP x-ray image demonstrates that an 11-degree correction places the mechanical axis through the center of the knee corresponding to a 12.5-mm opening wedge tibial valgus-producing osteotomy. (B) Intraoperative skin incision to demonstrate the extent of the incision and the oblique marking indicates the pes anserinus tendon insertions on the subcutaneous border of the tibia. If the joint needs to be opened or there is a need for autograft bone for the high tibial valgus osteotomy, the skin incision is brought proximal to the double hash lines. Otherwise, the incision is shorter, just distal to the double hash lines. (C) I am holding the foot and the center of the ankle is separately marked and confirmed on fluoroscopy. (D) A medial sub-vastus exposure to the distal femur is prepared for harvesting of autologous bone graft for the tibial valgus osteotomy. The soft tissue flaps are directly down to fascia and remaining full-thickness fasciocutaneous flaps that are well vascularized. (E) A periosteal dissection is made just above the femoral origin of the medial collateral ligament in preparation for cancellous bone graft harvesting with a dowel harvester. (F) In preparation for the tibial osteotomy, the medial border of the patellar tendon is dissected into the infrapatellar bursa to the tendinous insertion on the tibial tubercle. (G) The proximal border of the pes anserinus tendons is localized. (H) A sharp subperiosteal dissection release is the pes anserinus tendons off their insertion distally and posteriorly to the tibia. The superficial medial collateral ligament is transected and subperiosteally dissected in a proximal direction to within 1 cm of the joint line, which is marked with a sterile marking pen. They are then held out of the way of the osteotomy with stay sutures. The knee is now placed in a figure-of-four position so that the posterior soft tissue envelope may be sharply subperiosteally dissected from the posterior tibial cortex in a lateral direction to the proximal tibiofibular joint. (I) The past tendons are held with a Kocher and the origin of the soleus muscle is sharply incised from the back of the tibia and the posterior structures are dissected sharply off the back of the tibia.

Continued

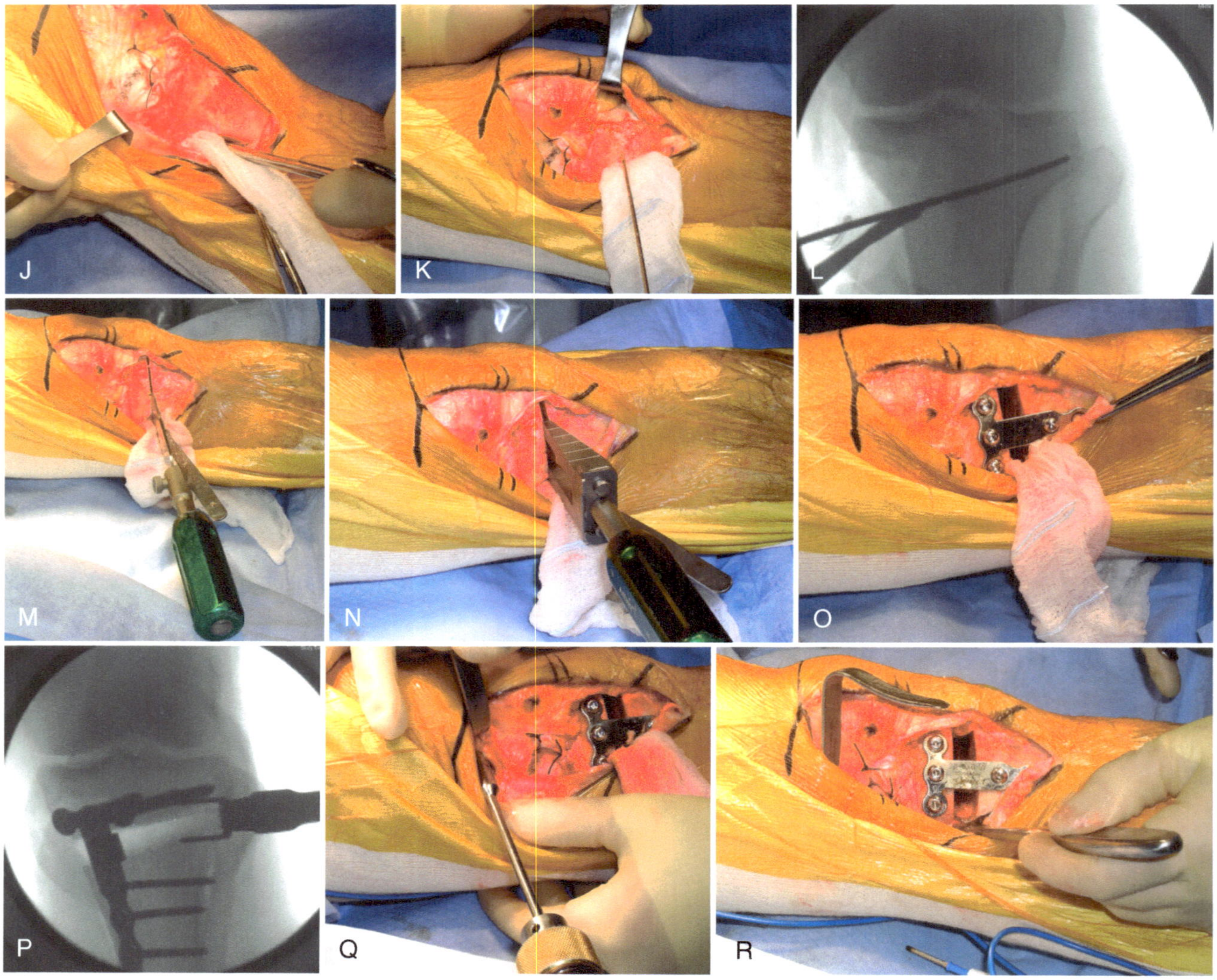

• **Fig. 10.14 Cont'd** (J) A small saline-soaked sponge is packed directly against the posterior aspect of the tibia protecting the neurovascular structures before osteotomy. (K) In preparation for the tibial osteotomy, a guidewire is directed to the midportion of the proximal tibiofibular joint and confirmed under image intensification while the knee is in full extension for good oscillating saw control. The pin is then broken away short of the cortex, the leg is stabilized, the guidewire is used to stabilize the sawblade as first the anterior cortex and then the posterior cortex are cut two-thirds of the way to the opposite cortex. A large osteotome is then utilized for the final one-third so that the lateral cortex is not broached but left intact so that the osteotomy may hinge on the intact cortex and proximal tibiofibular joint capsular tissues. (L) The breakaway pin is well positioned in the metaphyseal bone of the proximal tibia at the level of the tibiofibular joint. There is at least 2.5 cm to the lateral tibial joint line to ensure that there is not an insufficiency fracture into the articular surface. The proposed osteotomy goes to the soft spongy lateral cortex of the metaphysis and not the diaphysis where it is more likely to crack and displace. (M) A broad osteotome is used to complete the osteotomy to the lateral cortex but not through it. This is confirmed on image intensification. Note that the medial cortical osteotomy opens up symmetrically anteriorly and posteriorly. If this were not the case, there would be concern that the osteotomy was not completed either anteriorly or posteriorly, which would make for a difficult angular correction. (N) With counterpressure at the level of the proposed osteotomy and a slight valgus force at the level of the ankle, the opening wedge tines are gently impacted in the direction of the lateral cortex ensuring that full extension of the knee is always obtained. A bolster under the ankle is utilized to confirm this full extended knee position. (O) I prefer a femoral T Puddu plate on the tibia because of its improved fixation and low profile when the desired correction is obtained. (P) When large opening corrections are required, a prophylactic lateral staple is applied through the same midline anterior incision. This is also utilized in the event of a lateral cortical fracture or displacement. If this were to occur, the osteotomy position would be closed laterally and the staple applied. (Q) An 11-mm diameter harvester is then utilized through a single cortical entry to harvest several 20-mm autologous cancellous bone dowels from the distal metaphysis of the femur. (R) The autologous bone graft dowels are positioned both anteriorly and posteriorly at the cortical margins to enhance cortical bony union and prevent any movement of allograft cancellous bone chips into the soft tissue envelope.

Continued

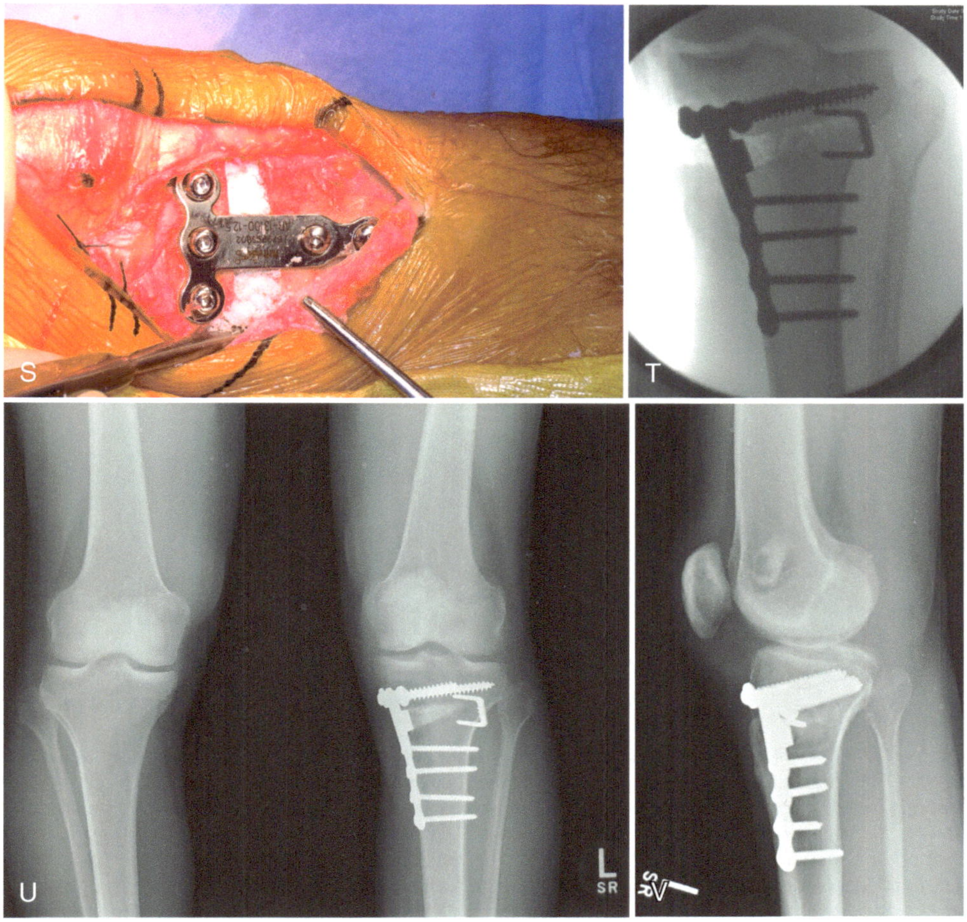

• **Fig. 10.14 Cont'd** (S) Final appearance after cancellous allogeneic bone chips are used to fill the central void of the osteotomy and the donor bone graft site. Drains are now positioned posterior to the tibia and in the subcutaneous envelope. The past tendons are loosely reattached to the superficial medial collateral ligament and medial retinacular sleeve with interrupted suture. The tourniquet is then let down and the marrow elements permeate the entire bone graft site with marrow stem cells enhancing the union of the construct. No irrigation is utilized on this area. Small bleeders are then cauterized and a light dressing with a compression sock is supplied from toes to groin. A cryotherapy sleeve is applied over the knee and then a knee immobilizer accompanied by a Venodyne pump for DVT prophylaxis. Continuous passive motion is started the following day. (T) The immediate postoperative appearance of the osteotomy. (U, V) Radiographic appearance of osteotomy 1 year after surgery, (U) AP view and (V) lateral view.

Opening Wedge High Tibial Valgus Osteotomy Accompanied by Anteromedialization Tibial Tubercle Osteotomy

Combined osteotomies are performed when either large corrections are required, i.e., 10 to 20 mm opening wedge, or there is specific patellofemoral maltracking or lateral facet cartilage wear. If the tibial tubercle is left attached to the tibia with a large opening wedge osteotomy being performed above the patellar tendon insertion, the patella will be effectively distalized, increasing contact forces across the patellofemoral joint, which will result in pain and articular cartilage wear. In this situation a retrotubercular osteotomy may be performed, leaving the tubercle attached to the proximal fragment, or the entire tubercle may be removed and placed back at its most proximal insertion, correcting for patellar alignment (diagrammatically demonstrated in Fig. 10.13).

Reverse Dome Tibial Valgus Osteotomy

For corrections greater than or equal to 15 degrees I prefer a reverse dome osteotomy below the tibial tubercle with a mid-shaft fibular osteotomy. This is a very powerful osteotomy[8] because it does not distort the upper anatomy of the proximal tibia such that future reconstruction is not compromised. It is technically the most difficult to perform of the three types of tibial osteotomies described here and has a longer time to osseous union (3–4 months). This usually requires a fixed angle device such as a blade plate fixation to allow the correction to be stable (Figs. 10.14 and 10.15).

The exposure is similar as per closing wedge valgus osteotomy. Fig. 10.16 shows stepwise surgery for a reverse dome tibial valgus osteotomy. However, depending on the location of the proposed arc of the osteotomy on the proximal medial tibia, the pes anserinus tendons may have to

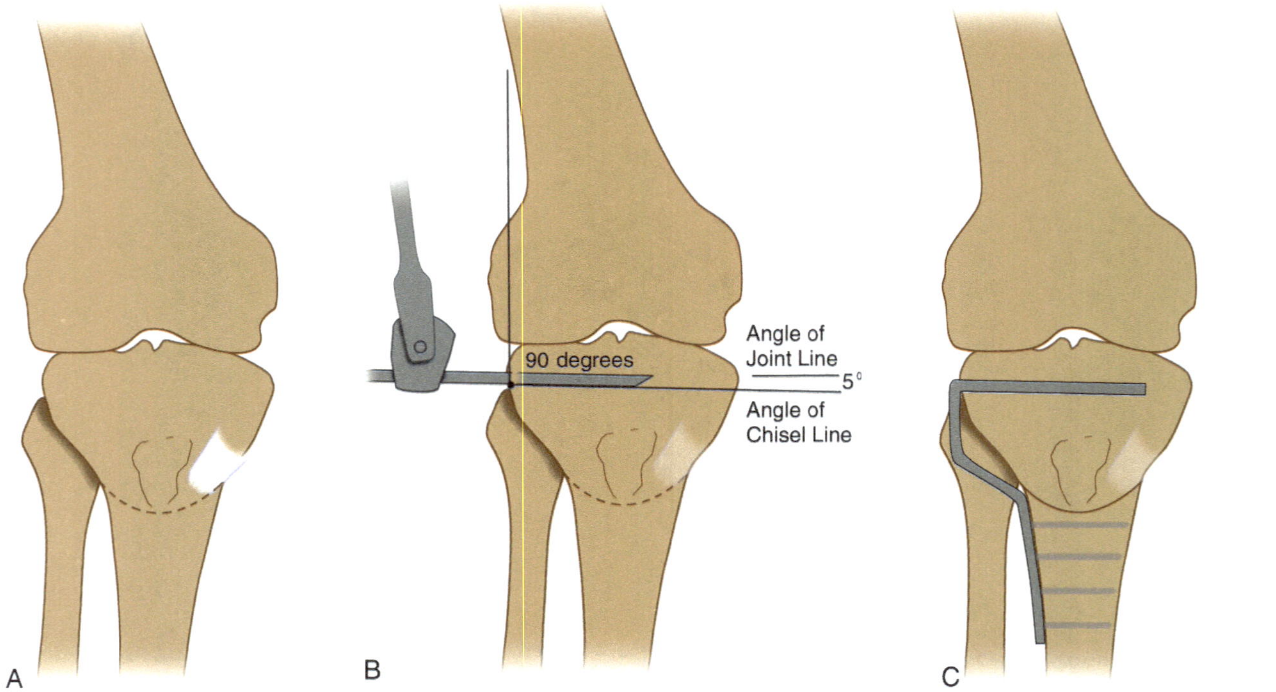

• **Fig. 10.15** Reverse dome osteotomy. If a corrective osteotomy requires greater than or equal to 15 degrees, a reverse dome osteotomy[8] is performed below the level of the tibial tubercle allowing a very large angular correction of up to 30 degrees without distorting the proximal tibial geometry for eventual total knee arthroplasty. A mid-shaft fibular osteotomy is also required and a fixed angled device such as a 90-degree offset blade plate is used for fixation. (A) Step 1: the upper end of the tibia is exposed, the arc of rotation to the metaphysis of the medial and lateral tibial plateau below the tibial tubercle is outlined and marked on the tibia with a marking pen. (B) Step 2: under image intensification guidance, a guidewire is placed parallel to the tibial articular surface and up to 5 degrees divergent from the surface to produce a tibiofemoral angle of zero to 5 degrees of valgus. A seating chisel for blade plate placement is then seated to the depth desired. (C) Step 3: A 90-degree offset blade plate is then placed, fixated, and a reticulated compression device used to compress the osteotomy, the desired angular correction will be obtained. The fibula is then fixated with a one-third semi-tubular plate.

be subperiosteally released in a posterior medial direction as per the opening wedge tibial valgus osteotomy in order for them to slide proximally and not be injured during the reverse dome osteotomy portion of the procedure. Prior to osteotomy, however, the chisel for the 90-degree blade is placed at the desired obliquity to the tibiofemoral joint usually with a 15–20 mm offset to the tibia. The correction is determined by the angle of entry into the tibia relative to the tibial plateau surface. Usually a 5–7 degree tibial femoral axis is desired, which requires entry 5–7 degrees parallel to the tibial plateau surface. The shaft of the tibia is then brought to the proximal fragment after the osteotomy and the desired correction is obtained. After chisel placement, reverse dome osteotomy is made usually with a series of drill holes through a pre-made drill guide from anterior to posterior. The drill holes are connected with small 1/8" osteotomes, first the anterior cortex followed by the posterior cortex, and then the mid-shaft fibular osteotomy. The blade plate is then placed and the angular correction is made under manual valgus force, distracting and re-approximating the tibial osteotomy. An articulated compression device is then used through the blade plate to provide compression to the osteotomy to obtain the angle of correction desired. Postoperative wound care and analgesic is the same as for the other tibial osteotomies described.

Postoperative Care

Patients generally stay in hospital for 3–4 days after high tibial osteotomy. Deep muscle compartment drains are left in for 3 days postoperatively with 48 hours of epidural. If the drains fall out, the epidural is immediately discontinued and careful monitoring of the compartment status with clinical examination is performed. Continuous passive motion begins the second day after surgery to help restore motion. The patient is generally sent home with a continuous passive motion machine for 3 weeks postoperatively unless intra-articular work is added, in which case CPM is used for 6 weeks to prevent adhesions and enhance cartilage repair or health. Non-steroidal antiinflammatory medications are not used after surgery because they may interfere with bone healing. Patients remain touch weight-bearing until there is radiographic evidence of bony healing prior to allowing a graduated weight-bearing program.

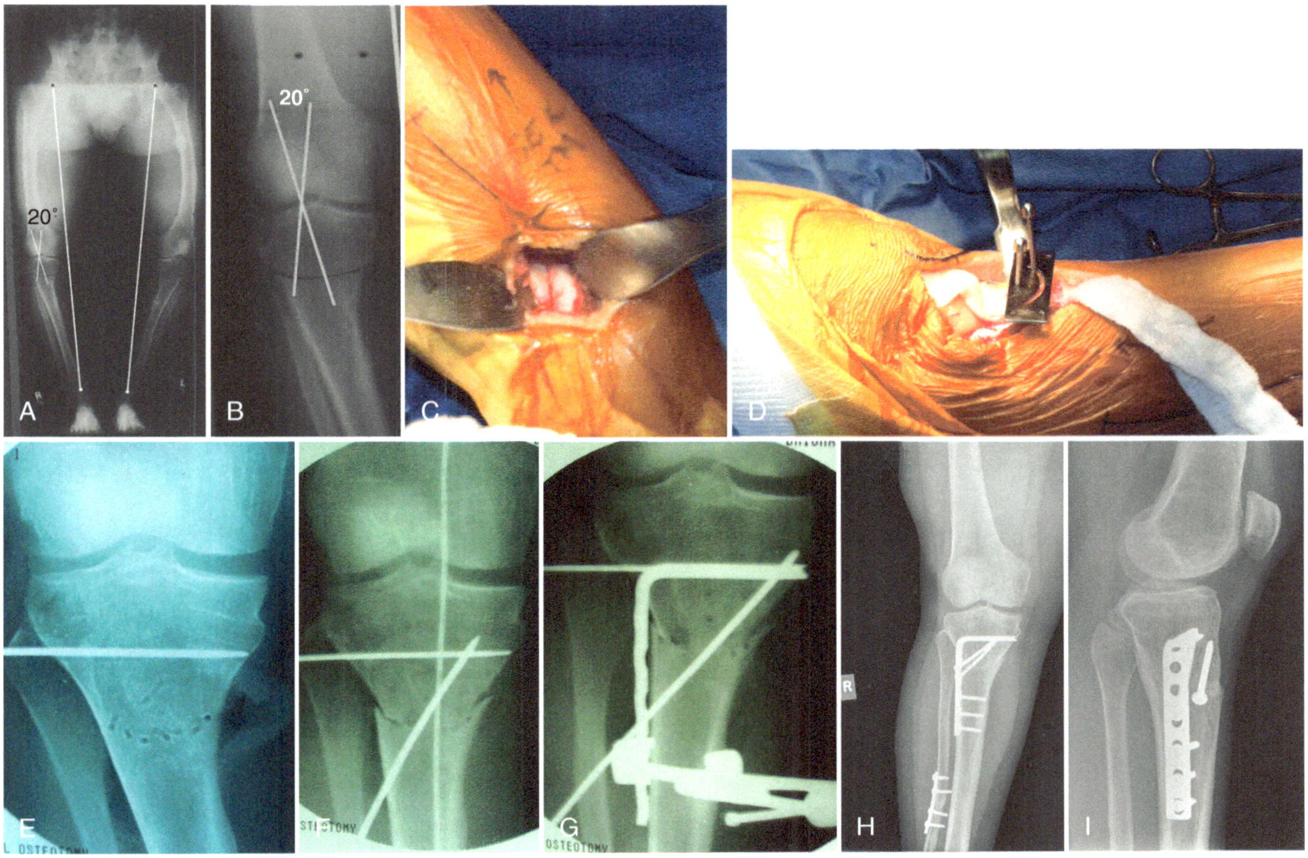

• **Fig. 10.16** (A) Long alignment films of a 31-year-old female with familial vitamin D-resistant rickets. X-ray images demonstrate severe varus malalignment with mechanical axis falling outside the medial aspect of the knee joints. The right knee is very symptomatic with medially-based pain. There is mild deformity in the femur with varus bow malalignment but there is more in the proximal tibia. (B) A 20-degree angular correction is required to place the mechanical axis through the lateral tibial spine unloading the medial compartment. This can be performed partly through the femur and the tibia; however, it was decided that because the femoral contribution to the deformity was not severe (unlike the left knee), the correction would be performed entirely through the tibia with a reverse dome tibial valgus osteotomy. The outline of the proposed dome osteotomy is demonstrated in the metaphysis of the proximal tibia. This will be performed below the level of the tibial tubercle around a center of arc of rotation at the center of the knee. (C) A mid-shaft fibular osteotomy is first performed at the junction between the superficial posterior muscle compartment and the lateral muscle compartment in an oblique fashion. (D) Several different crescentic jigs are available that match the width of the proximal metaphyseal curve. An appropriate jig is chosen and centrally several small drill holes are made through the tibia from anterior to posterior to be used to connect the dots with a thin sharp 0.25-inch osteotome. (E) Fluoroscopic x-ray image taken after the dome drill holes have been made through the tibia. As this patient is very small in stature, a pediatric blade plate guidewire is placed parallel to the joint line to produce a 90-degree cannulated blade plate. Sponges are placed behind the tibia after a dissection is made to take down the anterolateral muscle compartment and to release the superficial medial collateral ligament and the pes anserinus tendon attachments to the medial aspect of the tibia. The osteotomy is then performed from anterior to posterior with an osteotome. The distal fragment is then gently distracted, hinged around the dome osteotome, and placed on the lateral side to produce the desired correction. (F) Fluoroscopic x-ray image after the fragment has been fixated with a temporary K wire at the proposed level of correction. A Bovie cord has been placed from the center of the femoral head to the center of the talus at the ankle demonstrating that the mechanical axis to fall to the medial tibial spine. This is felt to be an adequate correction for this severe deformity. (G) A 90-degree cannulated pediatric blade plate (no offset available) is applied to the proximal fragment and an articulated compression device is placed distally to compress the two fragments together before screws are placed. (H) The final appearance of the tibia 1 year after osteotomy surgery. Note that there is minimal deformity in the upper end at the tibia despite such a large angular correction. This does not jeopardize any potential future reconstructive needs for the patient. (I) Lateral x-ray image after reverse dome tibial valgus-producing osteotomy.

Osteotomy for Instability: the Sagittal Correction

Tibial osteotomy is also very powerful in the sagittal plane. Opening and closing wedge osteotomies may be performed to correct hyperextension of the knee and reduce PCL insufficiency with a flexion osteotomy (Fig. 10.16) or decrease a flexion deformity of the knee and reduce ACL insufficiency with extension osteotomy (Fig. 10.17). If there is ACL insufficiency, the more posterior slope that is present the more likely the tendency for the tibia to translate forward. Lessening this tibial slope with an extension osteotomy reduces the tendency for anterior translation of the tibia. Similarly, if there is minimal posterior slope with a PCL-insufficient knee with femoral rollback, the tibia tends to slide posteriorly. Increasing tibial slope with a flexion osteotomy lessens the likelihood of posterior tibial translation. These principles can also be used for hyperextension

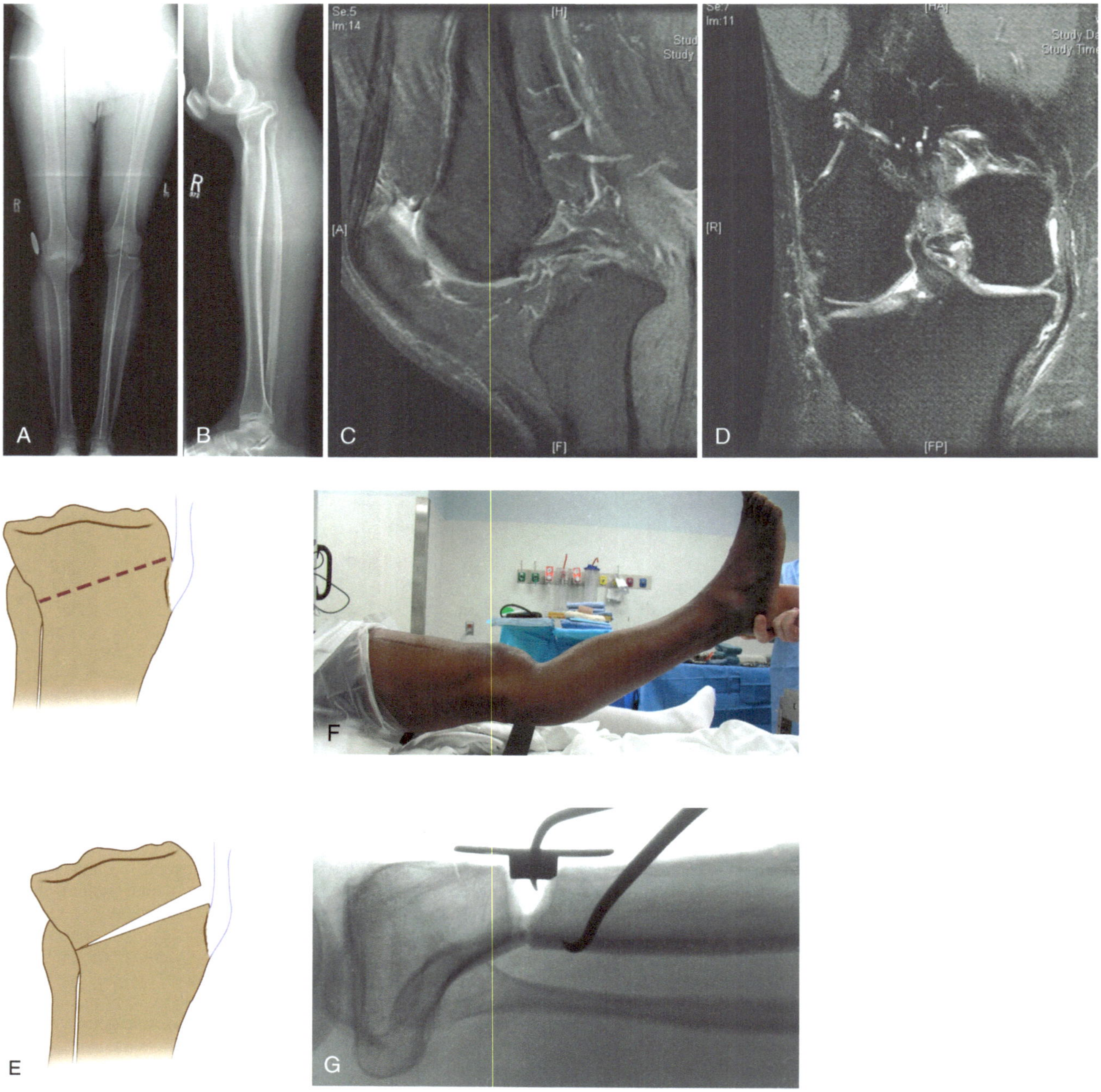

• **Fig. 10.17** (A) Recurvatum/posterior cruciate ligament insufficiency. Long axial alignment x-ray images in a 50-year-old male who has had difficulty with weight-bearing over the last 6 months prior to x-ray examination. He has experienced hyperextension instability of his knee. He has had a previous femoral fracture as a boy treated by a skeletal traction with a tibial traction pin. The tibial traction pin was applied through the proximal tibia presumably injuring his anterior epiphyseal plate resulting in growth arrest anteriorly and a deviated sagittal tibial slope. His joint line is not visible on standing AP or long alignment AP x-ray examination. (B) Weight-bearing x-ray images in the lateral plane demonstrate posterior translation of the tibia with a tibial upslope in the sagittal plane secondary to anterior tibial growth plate arrest following pediatric use of a tibial skeletal traction pin. (C) MRI in the sagittal plane demonstrates that the posterior cruciate ligament is intact and the articular surfaces of the patellofemoral joint are intact. (D) Coronal MRI demonstrating intact collateral ligaments and anterior cruciate ligament with loss of articular cartilage on the medial femoral condyle. (E) This case demonstrates the need for corrective osteotomy by increasing the posterior sagittal slope. This particular patient had a reversed sagittal slope with an upslope in the posterior direction secondary to an anterior tibial epiphyseal arrest from a traction bow. The principles for correction require restoration of a posterior sagittal slope with an anterior to posterior osteotomy leaving the posterior hinge intact until the recurvatum disappears which is noted immediately intraoperatively (see Fig. 10.16G). The same technique can be performed to prevent posterior translation of a tibia when there is symptomatic posterior cruciate instability accompanied by medial compartment osteoarthritis. A tibial valgus-performing osteotomy is performed with the osteotomy opened more anteriorly than posteriorly and in this manner the tibial slope is increased and the posterior cruciate ligament instability is lessened in addition to unloading the damaged medial compartment. (F) Clinical evaluation of the knee during the operative correction with approximately 30 degrees of hyperextension deformity. (G) Anterior flexion osteotomy is performed after removing the tibial tubercle to obtain exposure at the level of the deformity at the metaphyseal-diaphyseal junction. The osteotomy is opened anteriorly until full extension without hyperextension is obtained. A spacer plate of the appropriate anterior opening is applied to temporarily confirm the osteotomy position as noted.

Continued

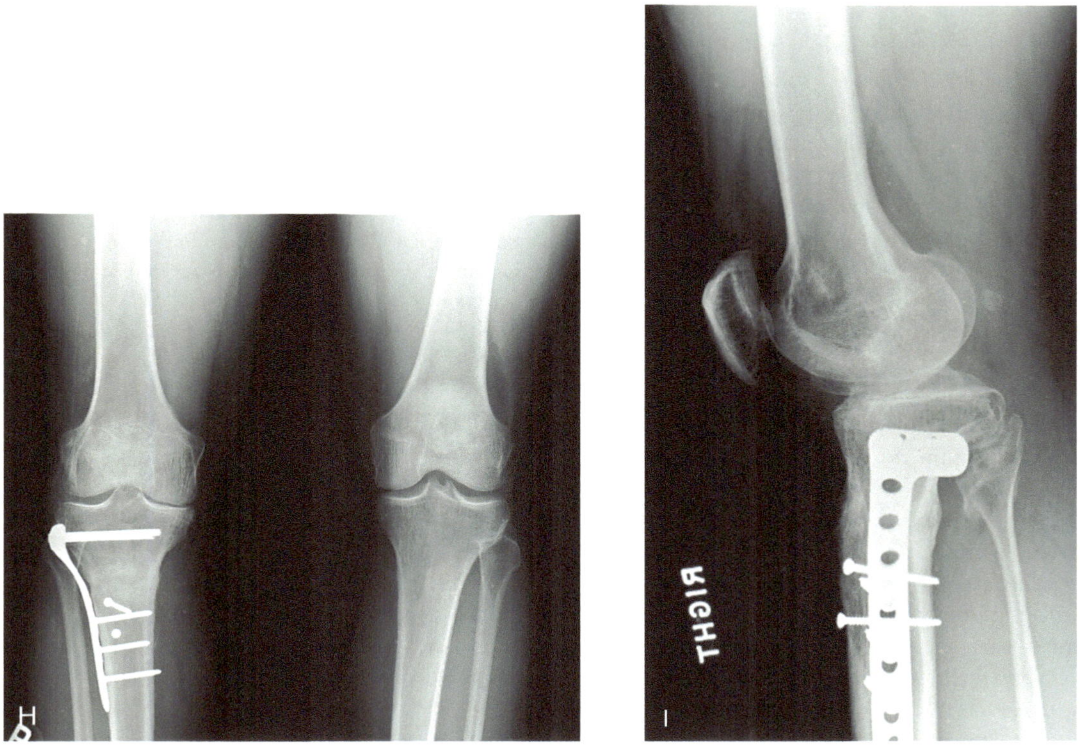

• **Fig. 10.17 Cont'd** (H) Postoperative (AP views) appearance 1 year after surgery when the osteotomy is solidly united demonstrating tangential articular joint views. A locking plate was used for the fixation. (I) A lateral x-ray image demonstrates a 0-degree tibial slope without hyperextension deformity and a femur that is centrally located on the tibia and is not subluxed anteriorly. The patient remains asymptomatic many years later.

deformities of the knee as well as fixed flexion deformities around the knee. They can also be combined with valgus-producing tibial osteotomies although this increases the complexity of the osteotomy.

ACL Laxity with Varus

The ACL-injured knee frequently has varus alignment and often an increased tibial sagittal slope. This puts ACL reconstruction at increased risk of failure. Articular injury at the time of ACL disruption is often on the medial compartment of the joint; reconstruction will therefore require attention to all background factors for successful clinical outcome. Restoring neutral alignment in the frontal plane will optimize the chance of success for cartilage repair in the medial compartment or osteoarthritic degenerative change in the medial compartment. Improving and restoring to normal amounts (3–5 degrees) the sagittal slope, by decreasing the sagittal slope will decrease the tendency towards anterior translation of the tibia. In this situation, an opening wedge valgus-producing tibial osteotomy in combination with an extension osteotomy may be performed by placing the opening wedge plate more posteriorly, thereby decreasing the sagittal slope of the tibia. An anterior staple may help prevent anterior opening. Using a small sagittal saw to make a rectangular space for a rectangular spacer block plate posteriorly by taking some extra bone from the distal fragment insures that the slope is lessened. Intraoperative x-ray examination or fluoroscopy to assess the lateral view of the tibia and the sagittal slope is necessary for confirmation (Fig. 10.18).

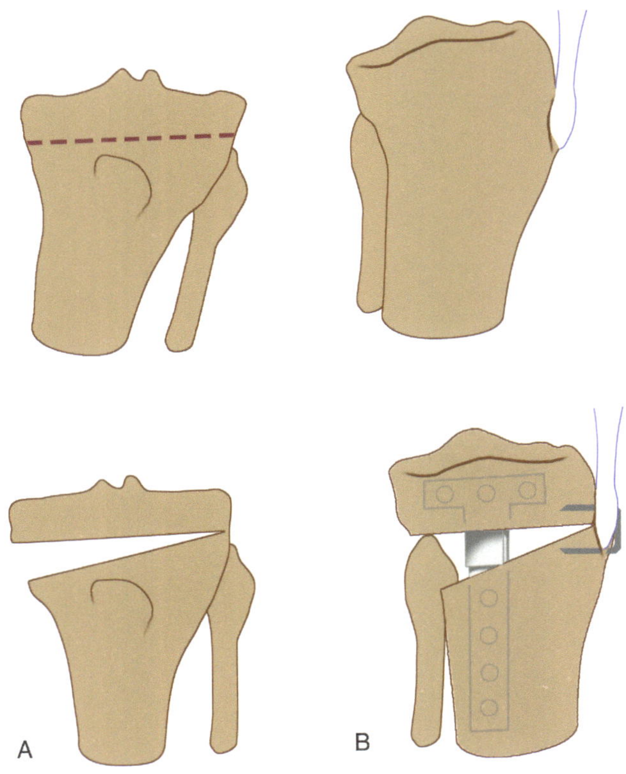

• **Fig. 10.18** Anterior cruciate ligament (ACL) insufficiency is frequently associated with increased posterior tibial sagittal slope. (A) Frontal view: a valgus-producing osteotomy in an ACL-deficient knee decreases the posterior sagittal slope. (B) Lateral view: a tibial valgus extension osteotomy will assist in stabilizing the tendency towards anterior translation of the tibia by preferentially opening the osteotomy posteriorly as shown.

Conclusion

Using the techniques described, I have found that high tibial osteotomy is a procedure that is safe, reproducible, and does not jeopardize future prosthetic reconstruction of the knee joint. Its original indications were for unloading medial compartment osteoarthritis with varus deformity. This remains true to date; however, improved techniques of osteotomy provide accurate corrections with minimal cosmetic disfigurement or change in the shape of the proximal tibia. In addition, the indications now include optimizing the success of cartilage repair for medial lesions in the varus knee with mechanical correction to normalize the mechanical environment of the joint and place the mechanical axis to neutral alignment. Exciting improvements in osteotomy have resulted from understanding the effect of altering the sagittal slope of the tibia to improve stability in the anterior-posterior plane of the knee joint.

When performed accurately, high tibial osteotomy is a reproducible and satisfying procedure for patients that may optimize the outcome of cartilage repair, joint instability, or alleviate the pain of osteoarthritis and allow improved levels of activity with joint preservation.

References

1. Coventry MB, Ilstrup DM, Wallrichs SL. Proximal tibial osteotomy. A critical long-term study of eighty-seven cases. *J Bone Joint Surg Am.* 1993;75(2):196–201.
2. Centers for Disease Control and Prevention. Arthritis prevalence and activity limitations–United States, 1990. *JAMA.* 1994;272(5):346–347.
3. Sharma L, Song J, Felson DT, et al. The role of knee alignment in disease progression and functional decline in knee osteoarthritis. *JAMA.* 2001;286(2):188–195.
4. Sahlstrom A, Johnell O, Redlund-Johnell I. The natural course of arthrosis of the knee. *Clin Orthop Relat Res.* 1997;340:152–157.
5. Rinonapoli E, Mancini GB, Corvaglia A, Musiello S, et al. Tibial osteotomy for varus gonarthrosis. A 10- to 21-year followup study. *Clin Orthop Relat Res.* 1998;353:185–193.
6. Mina CM, Garrett WE Jr., Pietrobon R, Glisson R, Higgins L. High tibial osteotomy for unloading osteochondral defects in the medial compartment of the knee. *Am J Sports Med.* 2008;Volume 36(number 5):949–955.
7. Ogden S, Mukherjee DP, Keating ME, Ogden AL, Albright JA, McCall RE. Changes in load distribution in the knee after opening wedge or closing wedge high tibial osteotomy. *J Arthroplasty.* 2009;24(1):101–109.
8. Paley D. *Principles of Deformity Correction.* Berlin: Springer-Verlag; 2002.
9. Klecker RJ, Winalski CS, Aliabadi P, Minas T. The aberrant anterior tibial artery, magnetic resonance appearance, prevalence, and surgical implications. *Am J Sports Med.* 2008;Vol. 36(No.4):720–727.
10. Shetty AA, Tindall AJ, Qureshi F, Divekar M, Fernando KWK. The effect of knee flexion on the popliteal artery and its surgical significance. *J Bone Joint Surg -British.* 2003;85-B(2):218–222.
11. Takeuchi R, Ishikawa H, Yamaguchi Y, et al. Fractures around the lateral cortical hinge after a medial opening-wedge high tibial osteotomy: a new classification of lateral hinge fracture. *Arthroscopy.* 2012;28(1):85–94.
12. Nakamura R, Komatsu N, Fujita K, et al. Appropriate hinge position for prevention of unstable lateral hinge fracture in open wedge high tibial osteotomy. *Bone Joint J.* 2017;99-B(10):1313–1318.

11

Femoral Varus Osteotomy

TOM MINAS, MD, MS

CHAPTER OUTLINE

Introduction

The valgus knee (see Fig. 11.1) is usually associated with hypoplasia of the lateral femoral condyle and a superior lateral directed joint line. The ankle joint is frequently obliquely orientated to the floor parallel to the knee joint in this situation. Corrective osteotomy performed at the level of the femoral deformity to restore the joint line parallel to the floor will also make the ankle parallel to the floor. For this reason, correction of valgus malalignment is performed through the femur. As in tibial corrective osteotomies, osteotomies may be closing wedge, opening wedge, or reverse dome osteotomies. Each has its own advantages and disadvantages. The clinical outcomes following femoral osteotomies parallel those of tibial osteotomies; however, they are much less common as is the literature[1,2] on them. Valgus knees are less frequent than varus knees and the disease pattern frequently involves the patellofemoral joint when the knee is in valgus. Correction of both lateral and patellofemoral arthritic conditions is technically more demanding and less predictable.

Indications

Femoral varus-producing osteotomy is indicated for unloading a laterally based articular cartilage defect, pain secondary to lateral compartment overload, or lateral compartment osteoarthritis with intact medial and patellofemoral articulations. Unlike tibial osteotomy, which is very effective for addressing instability such as anterior cruciate ligament (ACL) or posterior cruciate ligament (PCL) secondary to sagittal slope correction, changing the flexion or extension of the distal femur has no influence on instability. Overall, femoral osteotomies are technically more challenging to perform because of the larger soft tissue envelope, the longer lever arm, which can displace the osteotomy as it is being performed, and its proximity to the articular surface of the trochlea and the femoral artery. My choice of which type of femoral osteotomy to utilize is dependent upon the degree of correction, the leg length discrepancy, and the need for bone grafting of an osteochondral defect. Like opening wedge tibial osteotomies, an opening wedge femoral osteotomy is technically easier to perform than the closing wedge or reverse dome osteotomies because it allows a "dial-in" accurate correction. It has the disadvantage of requiring the use of bone graft; however, I have found that allograft materials (specifically a combination of cancellous allograft bone chips with demineralized bone matrix) heal in the same amount of time as autograft bone.

I use opening wedge femoral osteotomies for corrections up to 15 degrees because I find that for greater corrections there is a tendency for the distal fragment to flex because it remains hinged on the medial side at the level of the adductor tubercle, which is in a relatively posterior axis. The medial hinge on the femur, however, is not supported by an additional structure such as the fibula when performing high tibial valgus osteotomy (HTO) and is more prone to fracturing and displacing. In addition, the iliotibial band starts to become very tight when corrections greater than 15 degrees are attempted. A shortened leg length on the affected side is

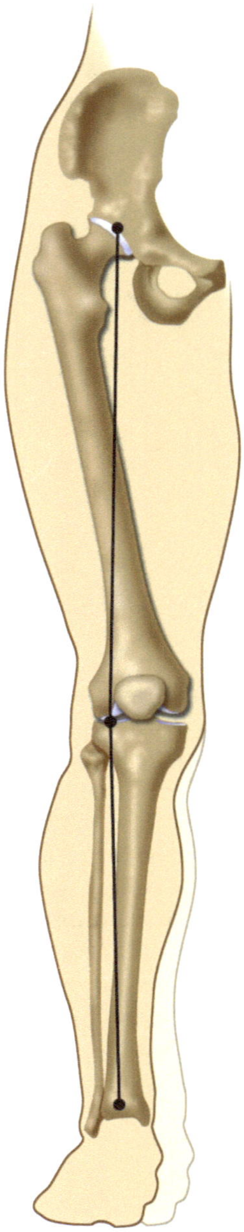

• **Fig. 11.1** Valgus mechanical alignment is associated with hypoplasia of the lateral femoral condyle and a superior lateral directed joint line.

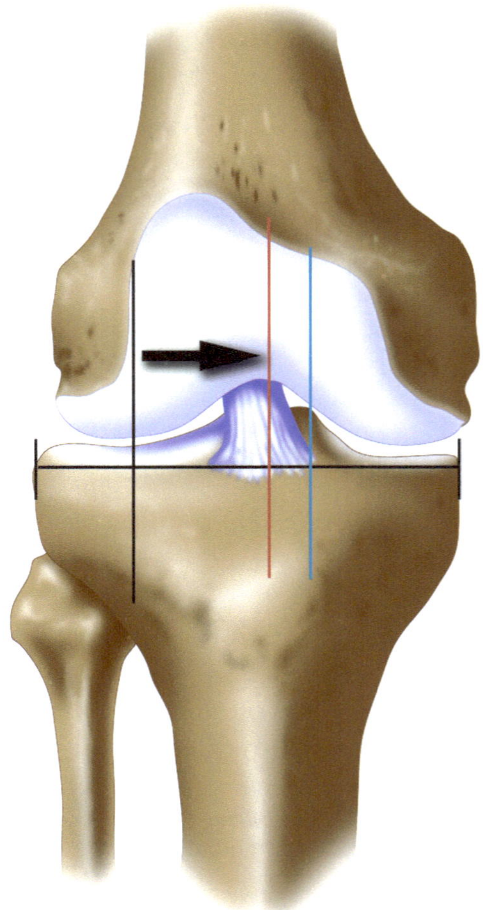

• **Fig. 11.2** The desired mechanical axis correction is to the midline of the knee *(red line)* in a situation of cartilage repair when there is no joint space narrowing of the lateral compartment, or a 2-degree overcorrection to the medial tibial spine *(blue line)* when there is osteoarthritis or joint space narrowing present.

another relative indication to use an opening wedge varus-producing osteotomy, which tends to equalize leg lengths.

The supracondylar reverse dome osteotomy[3] remains a very powerful osteotomy for large angular corrections and is my choice for corrections greater than 15 degrees. It traditionally required the use of an angled blade plate to obtain stable fixation; however, locking plates or retrograde intramedullary nails have made fixation much easier.

Closing wedge varus-producing femoral osteotomies heal more rapidly than the other two and provide a source of autogenous bone graft in the event there is an osteochondral defect of the lateral femoral condyle that requires osseous bone grafting. If the affected leg is longer, a closing wedge osteotomy is preferred to equalize leg lengths. Fixation has always been described using a 90-degree angled blade plate[4]; however, medial locking buttress plates now make the procedure technically much easier to perform with more precise corrections.

Planning

The goal of femoral osteotomy correction is similar to that of tibial valgus-producing osteotomy. If weight-bearing x-ray images demonstrate intact joint spaces and valgus malalignment is present with mechanical axis forces through the lateral compartment, correction of the mechanical axis is to the midline if an articular cartilage defect is being unloaded (see Fig. 11.2). This normalizes forces across the joint. If there is joint space narrowing or a large articular cartilage defect that is undergoing repair, the aim is to unload the lateral compartment by only 2 degrees, which corresponds to the top of the medial tibial spine. In this way, a premature wear of the medial compartment is less likely.

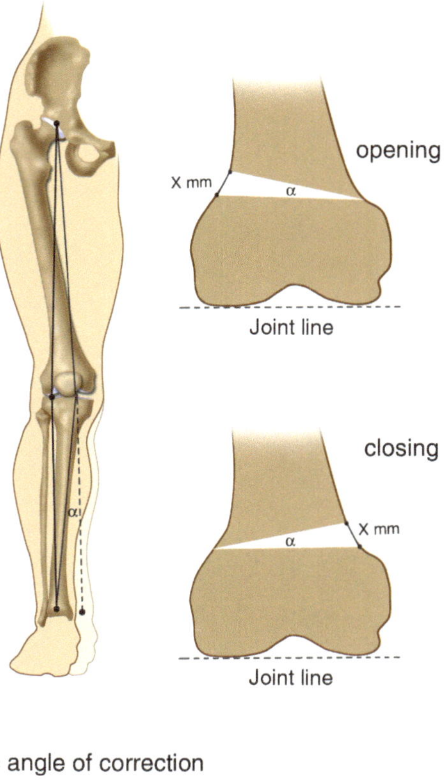

• **Fig. 11.3** The angle of correction for a varus-producing femoral osteotomy is measured on a long alignment x-ray image. The angle from the existing center of the ankle to the proposed mechanical axis at the knee (Fig. 11.2) and back to the new position of the ankle represents the angular correction. This angle is applied to the level of the opening or closing wedge osteotomy on the distal femoral metaphyseal–diaphyseal junction. The measurement in millimeters, *x*, is the correct opening or closing osteotomy. Opening wedge systems generally have spacer plates in millimeters that correspond to the preoperative planning. Closing wedge systems usually have angular increments on the osteotomy jigs that accurately measure in degrees the angular correction. Digitized x-ray systems with built-in software, calibrated for magnification error, make the planning very straightforward (General Electric web-based Centricity software [GE Healthcare, Waukesha, WI, USA]).

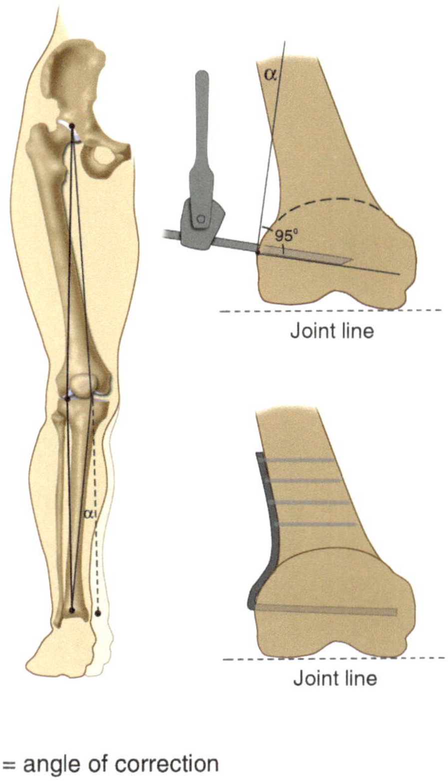

• **Fig. 11.4** The angular correction is calculated identical to Fig. 11.3. A 95-degree blade plate is used for fixation of a supracondylar reverse dome varus femoral osteotomy, although other fixed angle devices may be used such as a locking plate. The corrective angle alpha is measured from the lateral cortex of the femur to the intersection of the proposed position of the 95-degree angled blade plate. Generally, angled metallic triangles that have the angle alpha are placed along the plate portion of the angled blade plate. This allows a guidewire to be placed along the plane of the entry blade. The seating chisel then passes along the guidewire prior to the supracondylar femoral dome osteotomy. Once the osteotomy is completed, the 95-degree blade plate is placed along the tract of the seating chisel, the alignment of the leg corrected with a varus force until the plate portion fits flush to the lateral femoral cortex. An articulated compression device is then applied, the osteotomy site compressed, and screw fixation completes the stabilization of the osteotomy.

Long alignment x-ray images in a double stance AP phase are required for calculating angular correction (see Figs. 11.3 and 11.4). A line from the center of the femoral head is projected to the desired mechanical axis of either the center of the knee or the medial tibial spine to the proposed position of the foot. An angular correction then goes from the existing center of the ankle to the proposed mechanical axis point at the knee and then to the new ankle position. This acute angle is the angular correction. This angular correction is then converted to opening or closing millimeters using digital x-ray templates to plan for an opening wedge osteotomy on the lateral side of the distal femur or a closing wedge osteotomy on the medial side of the femur above the adductor tubercle and trochlea. This angle also allows the placement of a chisel to be planned for the use of an angled blade plate relative to the tibial femoral joint line (Fig. 11.4).

Opening Wedge Varus Femoral Osteotomy

Technique and Aftercare

An opening wedge femoral varus-producing osteotomy is performed through a midline incision. (Fig. 11.5 demonstrates an appropriate case example and Fig. 11.6 outlines the surgery in a stepwise fashion.) The deep exposure may be performed through a lateral sub vastus approach to approach the lateral distal femur for an extra-articular surgery. The lateral sub vastus approach may be combined with a tibial tubercle osteotomy to expose the entire distal femur and joint without a muscle split. I usually use a lateral parapatellar arthrotomy to expose the distal lateral femur and the patellofemoral articulation.

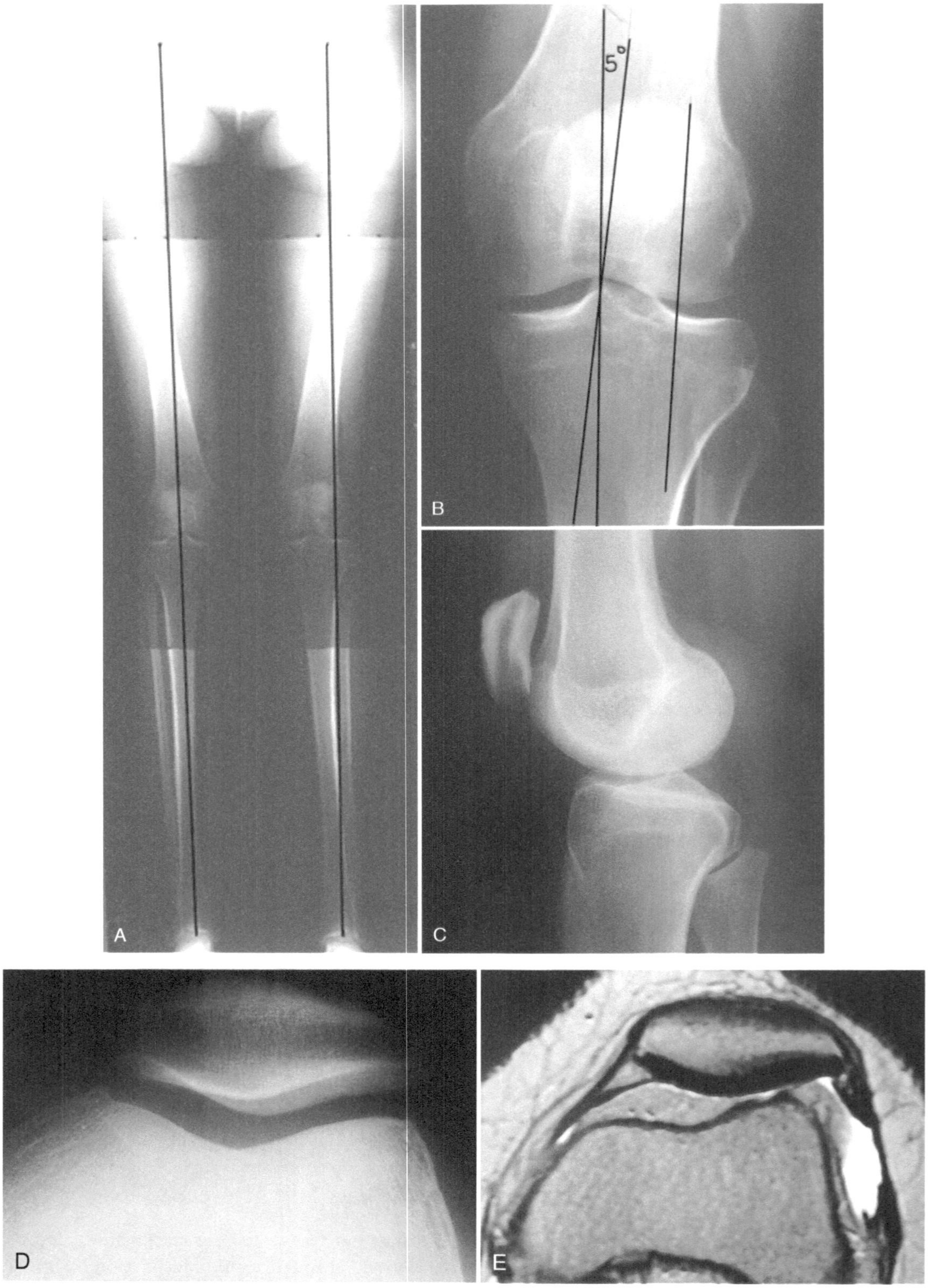

• **Fig. 11.5** (A) Long alignment x-ray images taken from a 23-year-old woman, 6 feet 1 inch tall, who has suffered disabling anterior and lateral knee pain for 9 months. Her clinical appearance demonstrates that she has valgus malalignment to her left leg with equal leg lengths, she has patellofemoral lateral maltracking with subluxation and tilt of the patella, in addition to a positive J-sign as she flexes her knee from a fully extended position. She has a positive patellar compression test, mild crepitus, lateral joint line tenderness, and a stable knee to collateral and anterior-posterior testing. (B) Mechanical axis to the left knee falls through the center of the lateral tibiofemoral compartment. A 5-degree angular correction is required to place her mechanical axis to the medial tibial spine. (C, D) Lateral and skyline x-ray images demonstrate mild patella alta with a well-centered patella on a 45-degree tangential skyline x-ray image with intact joint spaces. (E) The corresponding axial MRI scan demonstrates intact articular surfaces to the patella and the trochlea with lateral patella subluxation. A plan for a combined varus femoral osteotomy in addition to an anteromedialization of the tibial tubercle (Fig. 11.6) is planned to unload and normalize her joint forces and thereby alleviate her symptoms.

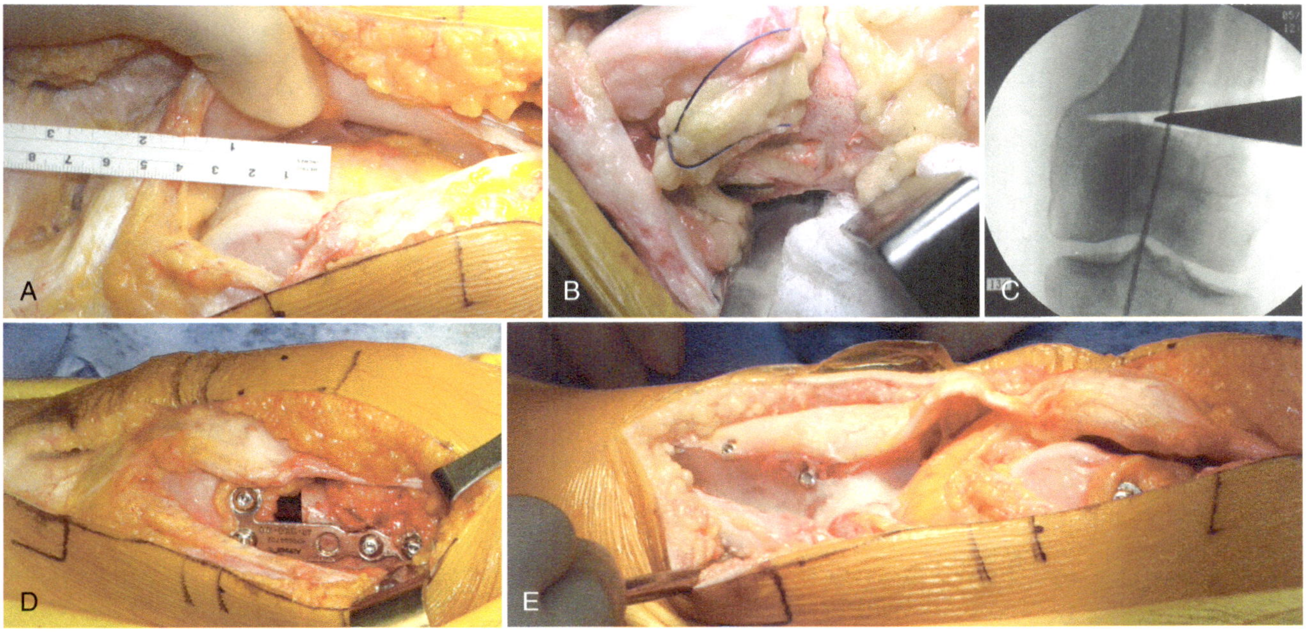

• **Fig. 11.6** (A) A midline surgical approach was performed to the knee. (The foot is to the left of the image and the head on the right.) A lateral parapatellar arthrotomy demonstrates the lateral wear of the trochlea and exposes the distal lateral femur. (B) In preparation for a distal femoral varus osteotomy, the intermuscular septum is dissected sharply off the linea aspera on the lateral side for an opening wedge osteotomy (and the distal medial femur to the adductor tubercle on the medial side when performing a closing wedge osteotomy). With the knee flexed and the intermuscular septum having been released off the sharp posterior lateral distal corner of the femur, it is very easy to sweep off digitally the fatty area and any tissue and the neurovascular structures off the back of the femur all the way to the adductor tubercle on the opposite side. Small wet sponges and a retractor are then easily placed directly on the back of the femur to protect the neurovascular structures prior to the use of an oscillating saw for the distal femoral osteotomy. The osteotomy is performed with the knee in full extension, easily stabilized by an assistant, with minimal risk to the neurovascular structures posteriorly, and with good saw control anteriorly to avoid the trochlea. (C) Opening wedge tines are gently impacted to the desired level of opening that is preoperatively planned. The assistant provides counterpressure on the medial side of the knee to avoid breaking through the metaphyseal medial hinge. An intraoperative check using a Bovie guidewire from the center of the femoral head to the center of the ankle passes to the desired level at the medial tibial spine. In addition, the clinical appearance of the leg appears to be neutral to minimal varus. At this time, the osteotomy can be fixated in its desired position and bone grafted. (D) Once the femoral osteotomy is stabilized with internal fixation, the tracking of the patella is assessed after the valgus alignment is corrected with a full-thickness lateral release being left open. In this case, the patella continues to track laterally, there is thinning of the articular surface of the trochlea laterally, and it is felt that an unloading tibial tubercle osteotomy is necessary to centralize and unload the lateral patellofemoral facet. Autologous bone graft from the left iliac crest was used to bone graft the femoral osteotomy in this patient, who was treated in 2003. Since then, combined allograft cancellous bone chips and demineralized bone matrix have been used as an allograft mixture. The allograft mixture is placed in the defect at the completion of the osteotomy and prior to releasing the tourniquet. When the tourniquet is released, marrow-derived elements permeate the allograft mixture completely with bone-forming cells and growth factors. I have found this to heal as quickly as autologous bone graft and have used this mixture in the place of autologous bone graft, which has lessened the morbidity of the procedure. (E) A Fulkerson osteotomy (anteromedial tibial tubercle osteotomy, see Chapter 10) with the distal hinge intact is then performed. Three 3.5-mm cortical screws are used to lag the osteotomy in place. Stable fixation is obtained and continuous passive motion starts the next day.

A key part of the exposure is to protect the posterior neurovascular structures. This may be performed by releasing the vastus lateralis attachment to the lateral intermuscular septum and the linea aspera distally for 3 cm off the back of the femur sharply. With the knee flexed, the posterior structures on the back of the femur are then very easily dissected with a finger bluntly. Small wet sponges are then packed behind the femur with a Hohmann retractor to protect the femoral artery and the other neural vascular structures. A breakaway notched guidewire is then placed across the femur from the supracondylar lateral position of the proposed osteotomy just proximal to the trochlea across to the adductor tubercle on the medial side. The supracondylar synovium is then split and subperiosteally dissected leaving a cuff attached distally to the trochlea. Methylene blue is used in a longitudinal fashion at the level of the osteotomy to make a mark to correct rotation. The guidewire is then broken at one of its notches near to the lateral femoral cortex and the leg is kept in full extension with the posterior neurovascular structures being protected with a Hohmann retractor and sponges. I usually place a padded bump just proximal to the knee joint underneath the femur so that at the time of the osteotomy there is no flexion of the distal femoral fragment. An oscillating saw is used to cut obliquely across the femur along the path of the guidewire under direct visualization and image intensification on a radiolucent operating room table. The last 1 cm is cut using an osteotome to the medial cortex but not through it at the level of the metaphyseal bone to allow a "greenstick type" opening without fracture and displacement of the two fragments. Opening wedge tines or laminar spreaders are utilized to open the lateral cortex gently to the desired amount as per the preoperative plan. When the desired opening is attained, a secondary check is made with intraoperative assessment by clinical appearance and image intensification assessment using a solid rod or a Bovie cord that extends from the femoral head to the talus at the ankle to assess the desired mechanical axis. (An opening of 15 mm is generally the maximum that can be performed based on tightness of the lateral structures of the knee, especially the iliotibial band. More than this the possibility of a reverse dome osteotomy should be considered.) A femoral Puddu plate with the desired opening spacer block is then applied to the distal femur and fixated with distal cancellous screws and proximal cortical screws or a locking plate. Bone graft supplement is utilized to fill the defect. My preference is a combination of cancellous allogenic bone chips combined with demineralized bone matrix. I have stopped using autograft bone since 2003 and have found that union is predictable and as fast as autograft, without the associated patient morbidity. The supracondylar synovium is then sutured overtop of the bone graft to remain outside the joint space. The tourniquet is then let down and the bone marrow elements permeate the bone graft enhancing its biological capacity to heal. Anti adhesion membrane (Seprafilm, Genzyme Biosurgery, Cambridge MA, USA) is placed directly on top of the synovium to prevent postoperative adhesions. Suction drains are placed in the soft tissue envelope subcutaneously. I generally do not close all of the lateral retinaculum adjacent to the patella to avoid increased mechanical pressures across the patellofemoral joint. A tight subcutaneous closure is then performed. A light dressing and a hinged knee brace combined with cryotherapy is utilized postoperatively. DVT prophylaxis in the form of baby aspirin 81 mg twice a day orally is prescribed for 3 weeks postoperatively. Continuous passive motion is utilized for 3 weeks postoperative and touch weight-bearing. A check x-ray examination is made postoperatively as a baseline, followed by x-rays at 3, 8, and 12 weeks. Generally opening wedge femoral osteotomy heals between 10 and 14 weeks solidly. Fig. 11.7 shows 6-month follow up x-ray image. Partial weight-bearing is allowed starting at 6 weeks based on the appearance of radiographic union; full weight-bearing is not permitted until solid healing has been confirmed by x-ray examination.

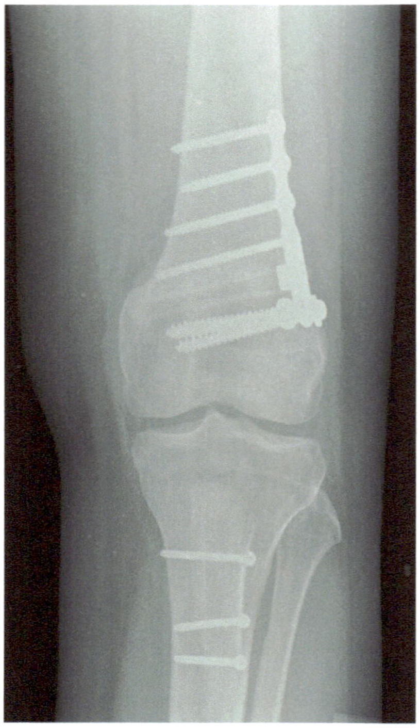

• **Fig. 11.7** Final radiographic appearance following femoral varus osteotomy and tibial tubercle osteotomy 6 months after the procedure. The patient has become pain-free and continues to function well at latest follow-up 6 years later.

Reverse Dome Femoral Varus Osteotomy

The reverse dome distal femoral varus-producing osteotomy as described by Paley[3] is my preferred osteotomy for correction of greater than 15 degrees. The osteotomy is based on the center of rotation arc (CORA) around a central point at the center of the knee. By creating a circular osteotomy about this center, which captures the width of the medial and lateral distal femoral metaphyseal flares, the lower leg can be rotated about this pivot point without appreciable distortion of the femoral anatomy. The soft tissue structures remain balanced and are not overly tightened. Future reconstruction with total knee arthroplasty is not compromised. The surgical technique is described in the diagrammatic representations in Fig. 11.8 and followed by a clinical example in Fig. 11.9.

Closing Wedge Varus Femoral Osteotomy: Classical Technique

A diagrammatic representation of a classic femoral closing wedge osteotomy is illustrated in Fig. 11.10. The surgical stepwise technique is shown in Fig. 11.11 and performed as shown in Fig. 11.12. An anterior incision is made to the knee with a medial sub vastus arthrotomy performed. This allows exposure to the distal femur and to the joint. The distal aspect of the medial intermuscular septum at its insertion on the adductor tubercle and supracondylar femur is released off the posterior aspect of the femur. With the knee flexed a blunt finger dissection sweeps away the neurovascular structures off the back of the femoral cortex where they can be protected with small wet sponges and a retractor, as well as one to retract the anterior quadriceps such that good circumferential visualization is adequate. A guidewire is placed parallel to the tibial femoral joint for the placement of a 90-degree offset blade plate chisel. The entry site is started with three 4.5-mm drill bits at least 2.5 cm above the joint line and above the intercondylar notch to avoid penetrating the intercondylar anterior and posterior

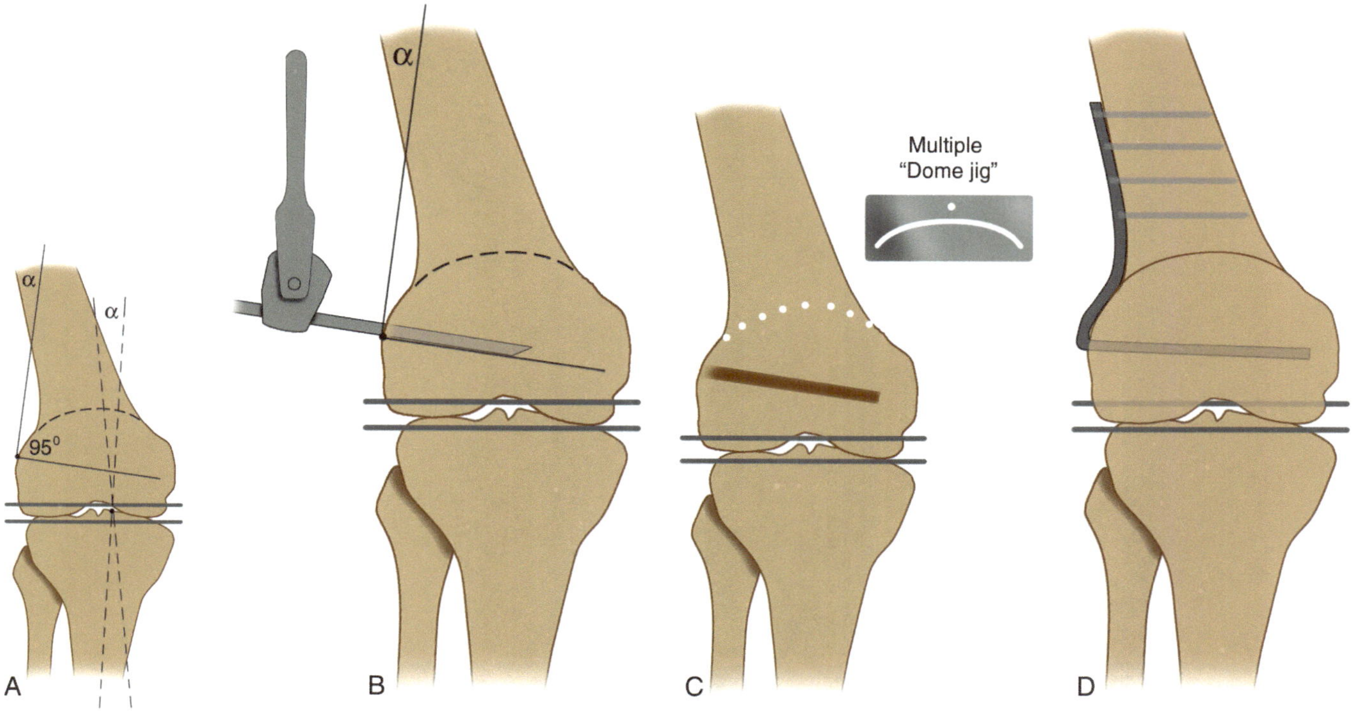

• **Fig. 11.8** (A) Step 1: the desired angular correction for the femoral osteotomy, angle alpha, is calculated as per Fig. 11.3. I prefer to use a 95-degree angled blade plate for accurate fixation for a reverse dome osteotomy. The seating chisel entry to the distal femoral metaphysis is key for the correction of the osteotomy. Using a 95-degree angled blade plate, a guidewire may be placed along the path of the blade entry noting that the correction angle alpha is the angle between the plate and the lateral femoral cortex, which can usually be referenced with a metallic angled triangle used for osteotomies. (B) Step 2: the seating chisel for the blade plate is then introduced along the path of the guidewire in the usual fashion of drilling the outer cortices and seating the chisel inward and outward under fluoroscopic guidance to ensure the path is along the guidewire. (C) Step 3: several crescentic domes are then applied to the distal femoral metaphysis until an appropriate arc that matches the metaphyseal width is chosen. This is pinned to the anterior femur. Multiple 2-mm drill holes are penetrated from anterior to posterior cortex in this semicircular fashion. The posterior aspect of the knee neurovascular structures are protected with radiolucent retractors and small wet sponges. The dots are connected with 0.25-inch narrow osteotomes and the distal fragment is mobilized through the osteotomy. (D) Step 4: with the osteotomy being mobilized with osteotomes, the leg is gently manipulated with traction and a varus force until the leg is straight. The blade plate is applied through the previous chisel tract, the plate portion is then applied against the lateral femoral cortex, an articulated compression device may be used to apply further compression if necessary, and the screw fixation stabilizes the osteotomy.

cruciate ligaments. The chisel tract is then performed to at least 50 to 60 mm deep.

The femoral osteotomy is performed at least 2.5 cm above the proposed blade plate chisel entry site so that there is an adequate bone bridge during compression of the osteotomy preventing the blade chisel from breaking through into the osteotomy site. The lateral cortex is left intact. A small wedge of bone is then taken from the proximal fragment of approximately 5 mm in width.

The 90-degree offset blade plate is then inserted and compressed axially such that the proximal fragment impales the distal fragment until the plate portion fits to the proximal cortical fragment. Screws are now utilized to fix the plate to the proximal fragment. This produces a tibiofemoral axis of zero degrees, with the femur collinear to the tibia. The mechanical access will depend on the varus at the hip and its offset. It may actually be through the center of the medial compartment or outside of the medial compartment depending on the proximal femoral anatomy. A closing wedge osteotomy with the technique as described by Gross[4] will produce a tibiofemoral angle of 0 degrees. This is because the 90-degree blade plate is positioned parallel to the articular surfaces and the fragment is closed down until the plate portion fits the femoral cortex, always producing a tibiofemoral axis of 0 degrees. It is a simple and reproducible technique that provides excellent fixation stability. However, it does not take into account the neck shaft angle of the hip joint and deformity in the proximal femur and may therefore result in an overcorrection into varus, which may lead to premature wear of the medial compartment. This may present a larger problem for a younger patient undergoing cartilage repair surgery where a more accurate angular correction to neutral or at the medial tibial spine may be required. This technique does not allow such a precise correction. A calibrated osteotomy correction device may be required for a closing wedge osteotomy fixed with a tension band plate for precise corrections as will be described.

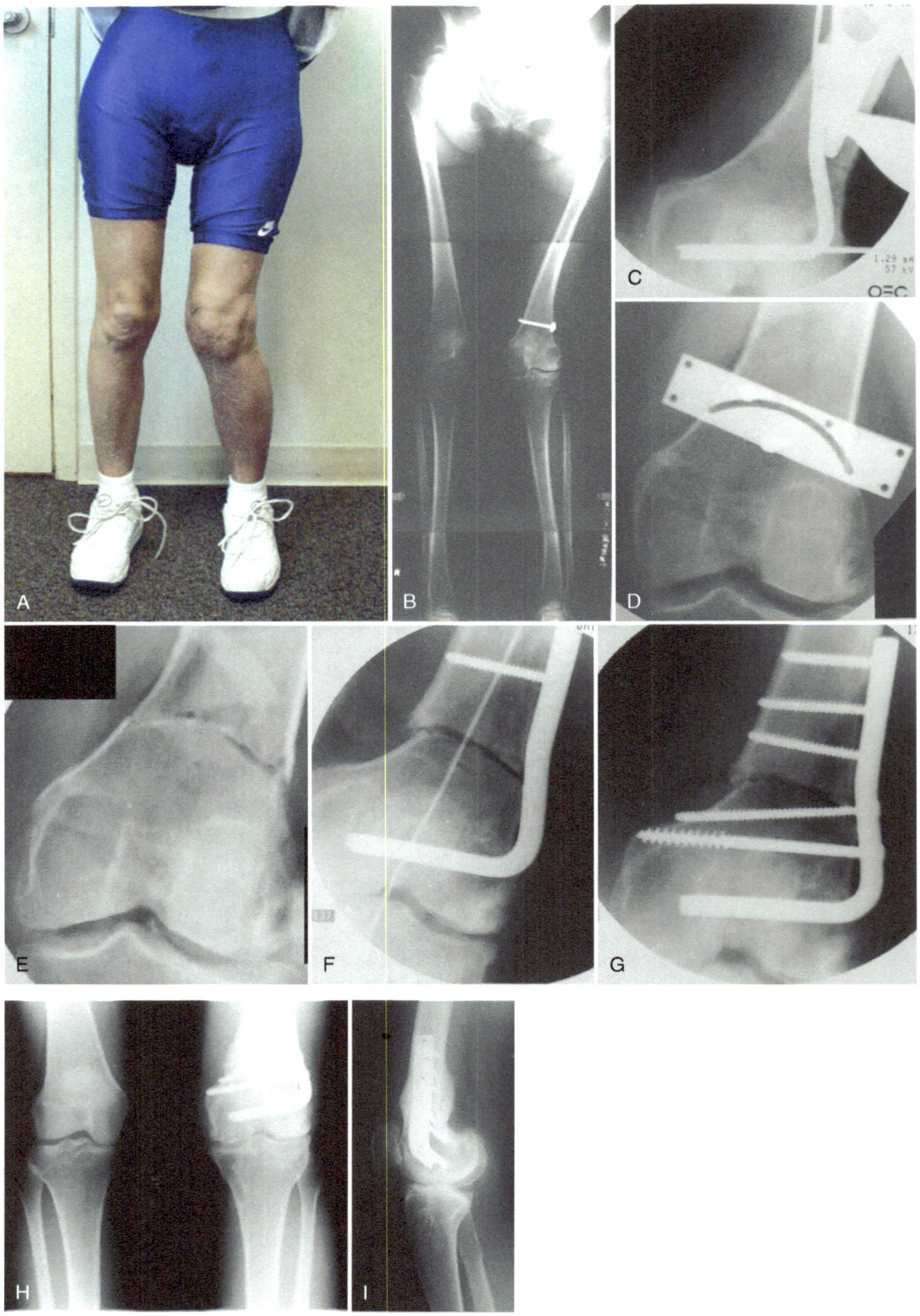

• **Fig. 11.9** (A) A 36-year-old woman who has had a left knee anterior cruciate ligament (ACL) reconstruction for instability. She has a mild form of congenital insensitivity to pain with arthritis of her right hip and her left knee with valgus malalignment. She experiences mild discomfort and persistent instability in her knee. A varus femoral osteotomy will be performed for a 20-degree angular correction with a supracondylar reverse dome femoral osteotomy and blade plate fixation. (B) Long alignment x-ray images of the patient in Fig. 11.9A. (C) A guidewire is placed in the proposed path of the blade portion of the 95-degree angled blade plate with a 20-degree angled triangle parallel to the lateral cortex, which delineates the angle of correction for this osteotomy. A blade plate seating chisel is used to enter the distal femur along the plane of the guidewire to provide an appropriate angle correction for the osteotomy. (D) Intraoperatively, a jig of an appropriate arc of radius is applied to the distal femur with two pins for fixation in preparation for the osteotomy. Once this is done, the supracondylar osteotomy is performed with 2-mm drill bit perforations from anterior to posterior, and the back of the knee is protected with retractors and small wet sponges. (E) A ¼-inch osteotome is utilized to connect the dots from anterior to posterior until the distal femoral fragment is mobilized. The distal fragment is mobilized with osteotomes through the osteotomy site with gentle traction on the foot and a varus force on the distal fragment until the limb is almost straight. The blade plate is applied to the distal fragment from the previous chisel tract until the plate portion lies flush to the femoral cortex and then the osteotomy site is compressed and reduced accurately to ensure that there is no flexion or extension of the distal fragment and screw fixation is performed for stabilization. (F) Intraoperative confirmation of correction of the mechanical axis using a Bovie cord from the center of the femoral head to the center of the talus falls through the center of the knee. (G) The final intraoperative appearance of the osteotomy when the fixation is complete. (H, I) Radiographic appearance of the healed osteotomy 1 year after surgery in the frontal and lateral projections. Robust callus formation is noted around the osteotomy site. The anatomy of the distal femur is not distorted to avoid jeopardizing potential future reconstruction with total knee arthroplasty. This is a key advantage to reverse dome osteotomy about the knee.

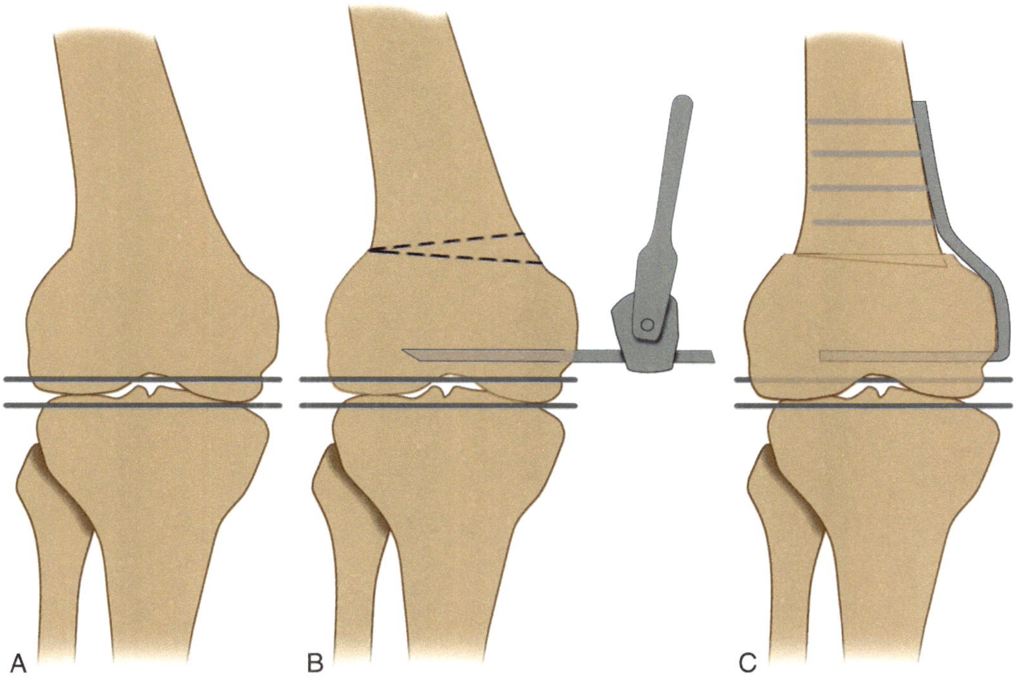

• **Fig. 11.10** (A) Step 1: with a medial sub vastus arthrotomy having been performed to expose the joint line and the proximal distal medial aspect of the femur, a guidewire is placed along the joint line and one parallel to this into the bone above the intercondylar notch as a guide for the direction of the blade plate chisel. (B) Because of the trapezoidal shape of the distal femur with the anterior aspect being narrow and the posterior aspect being broad, it is important to ensure that the seating chisel is placed parallel to the shaft of the femur (the anterior one-third of the distal condyles), and as the seating chisel is then inserted parallel to the guidewire (Fig. 11.10A), it should not pass more than two-thirds across the width as confirmed on image intensification so that it does not break through the opposite lateral cortex on the more narrow anterior aspect of the femur. Once the seating chisel has exited the distal femur, a transverse osteotomy above the trochlea to the lateral cortex is performed, and a 5-mm wedge medially based is then removed after a proximal cut is performed to the opposite apex leaving the lateral cortex intact. (C) The 90-degree offset blade plate is then seated completely to the distal fragment. Axial compression on the lower leg will allow the proximal shaft of the femur to impale itself within the softer cancellous bone of the distal fragment until the plate portion of the fixed angle device rests against the medial cortex of the proximal fragment of the distal femur. An articulated compression device is not utilized on the medial aspect of the femur because this puts the femoral artery at risk as it exits Hunter's canal at the distal one-third of the femur. Screws are placed to complete the fixation of the osteotomy. It is not uncommon for the lateral cortex to break during the compression and stabilization of the blade plate device. With newer medially based precontoured locking plates available, the classic technique is generally not recommended because the mechanical access correction is less precise. The osteotomy may be closed and fixated with a precontoured medially based locking plate for a precise and accurate correction.

Distal Femoral Varus Closing Wedge Osteotomy for Valgus Malalignment with Osteochondral Repair

At this time, I rarely use a 90-degree blade plate fixation with closing wedge osteotomy. Although a blade plate offers excellent fixation stability, if there is any malplacement of the chisel portion of the device, the plate may not sit flush on the femoral cortex medially or the angular correction of the osteotomy may change and the lateral cortex may break in so doing. Also, impaling the proximal cortex into the distal metaphysis is not as simple as it sounds. With present generation locking plate devices, blade plates are no longer necessary. Fixation is secure and stable.

For these reasons, I currently use a calibrated jig that allows a precise angular correction as planned preoperatively. This is performed from the medial side of the distal femur as described through a medial sub vastus arthrotomy or a medial parapatellar arthrotomy. The fixation device can then be a contoured locking plate (Synthes Tomofix Medial Locking Plate [Synthes, Solothurn, Switzerland]), which is a lateral tibial locking buttress plate flipped upside down that fits the distal medial femur perfectly, or a non-locking tension band L-plate (as in Fig. 11.13).

In addition, the indication for a closing wedge distal femoral varus-producing osteotomy is usually for a leg aligned in valgus with a lateral osteochondral defect. This is performed to obtain the desired varus correction to unload the defect and autologous bone graft for the osseous defect through the same incision without the need for supplemental autologous bone graft source. The distal femoral metaphyseal bone is of excellent quality and a good source of autologous bone graft. The example in Fig. 11.13 illustrates such a case.

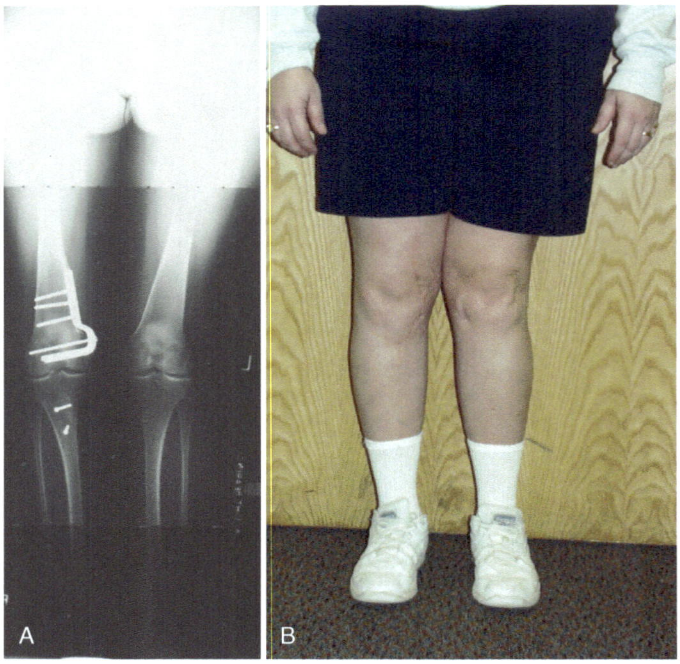

• **Fig. 11.11** (A) Long alignment frontal x-ray images of a 44-year-old woman who had undergone a closing wedge femoral osteotomy with tibial tubercle osteotomy on the right knee for lateral tibiofemoral osteoarthritis and lateral patellar facet osteoarthritis. She now presents with valgus alignment and lateral and anterior debased pain in the left knee. (B) Clinical appearance of her lower extremities 4 years later, now symptomatic on the left side. She was pleased from the pain relief that the osteotomy offered and her clinical appearance and wished to pursue osteotomy for the same problem in the opposite left knee at the age of 48 years. A classic closing wedge femoral osteotomy with 90-degree angled offset blade plate is performed as per the technique described by Alan Gross.[2,4]

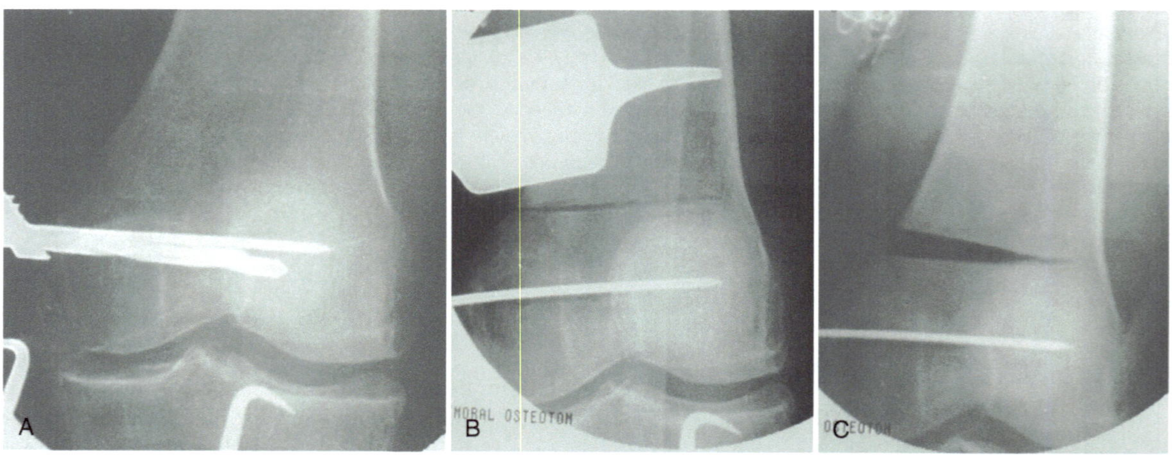

• **Fig. 11.12** (A) A triple drill guide is utilized collinear with the guidewire, which is parallel to the joint line from a medial sub vastus approach to the distal femur. This prepares a cortical pathway for the seating chisel to enter the distal femur and be guided by the guidewire. (B) The seating chisel is introduced with a slap hammer back and forth along the distal femur to prevent it from becoming jammed within the dense cancellous bone. It is then removed and the proximal closing wedge osteotomy is performed. A transverse osteotomy is performed under direct visualization of the anterior cortex to the lateral cortex leaving this intact. The anterior dissection involves a transverse incision from medial to lateral across the supracondylar synovium, then subperiosteally dissecting it distally towards the trochlea, and proximally for 1 cm to allow reapproximation of the synovium over the osteotomy once it is closed and completed. The posterior neurovascular structures are protected with small wet sponges. (C) A 5-mm medially based osteotomy is performed by freehand technique to meet the opposite lateral osteotomy site. The bone wedge is then removed. (D) The 90-degree offset blade plate is then chosen by the offset that is measured from the medial aspect of the femur to the cortical shaft when a trial closing reduction is performed and directly measured. The blade plate was then seated and axial compression applied once more until the plate portion rested upon the medial cortex of the proximal fragment. Bone-holding clamps may be required and cortical fixation is then performed with 4.5-mm screws. In this case the lateral cortex fractures, which is common because of the compression required to close the osteotomy and implode the proximal shaft into the distal fragment. This is of no consequence as the fixation is stable and the device is rigid and not a tension band device. The mechanical axis is checked intraoperatively on the radiolucent table using a Bovie cord from the center of the femoral head to the center of the ankle, which in this case falls into the center of the medial joint compartment. This is more than usually recommended with this technique

(*Continued*)

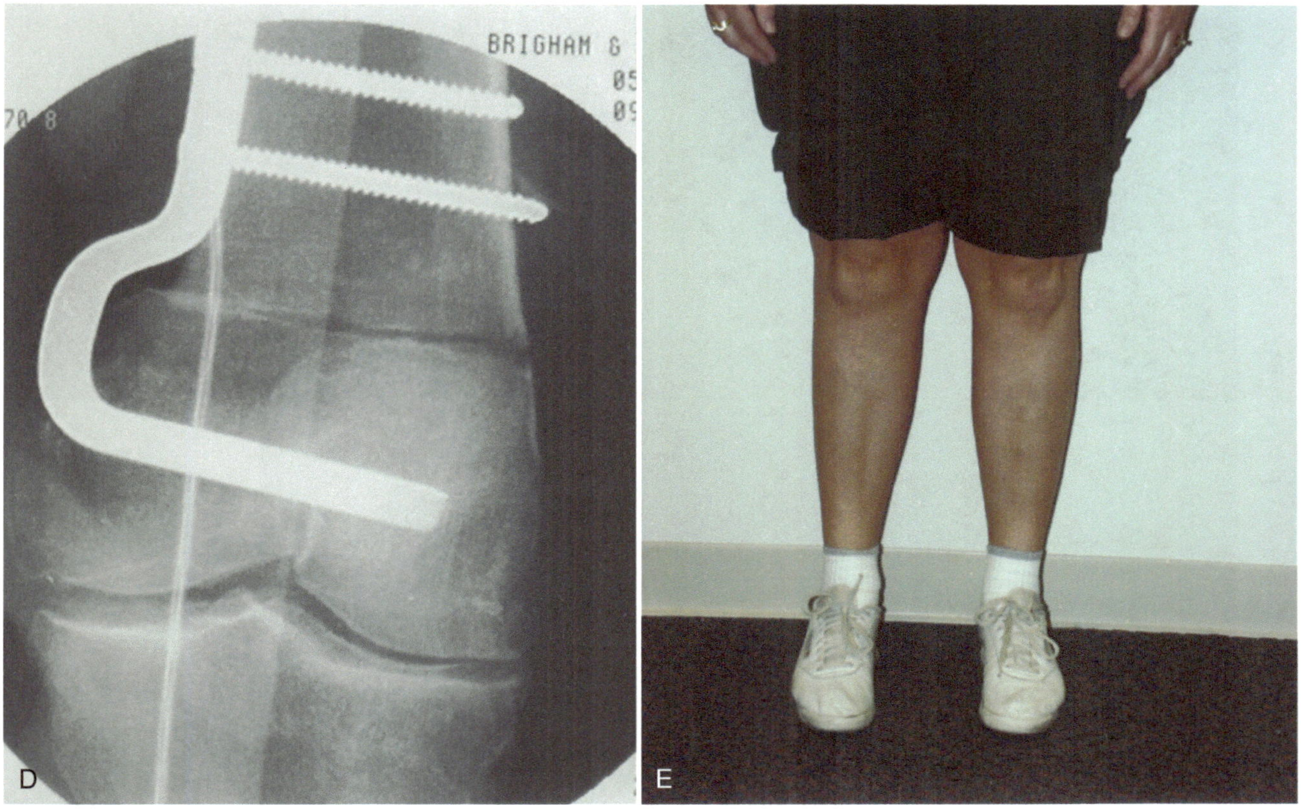

• **Fig. 11.12 Cont'd** but common using the classic closing wedge technique with a 90-degree blade plate. (E) Final clinical appearance after correction with osteotomy on both knees. There is only slight varus, equal leg lengths, and good pain relief.

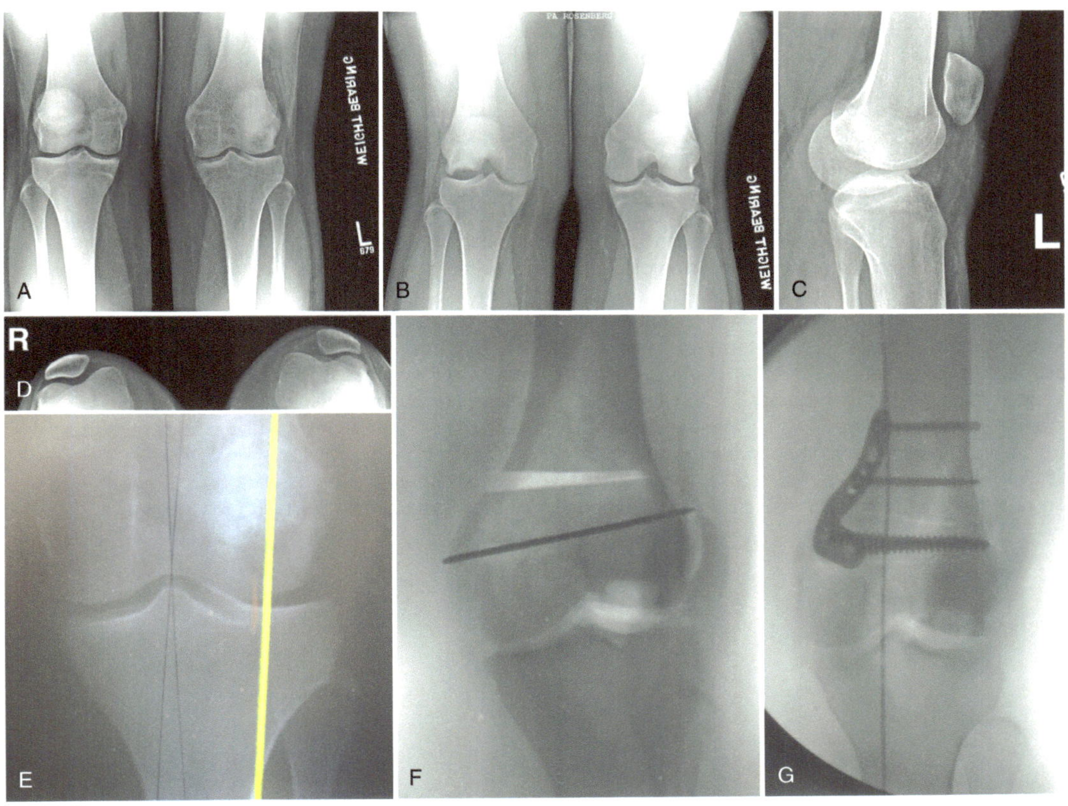

• **Fig. 11.13** Closing wedge distal femoral osteotomy with fixation using lateral tibial locking buttress plate. The lateral tibial locking buttress plate flipped upside down fits the distal medial femur perfectly. Standing AP (A), and PA (B) x-ray images of a 17-year-old woman with osteochondritis

(*Continued*)

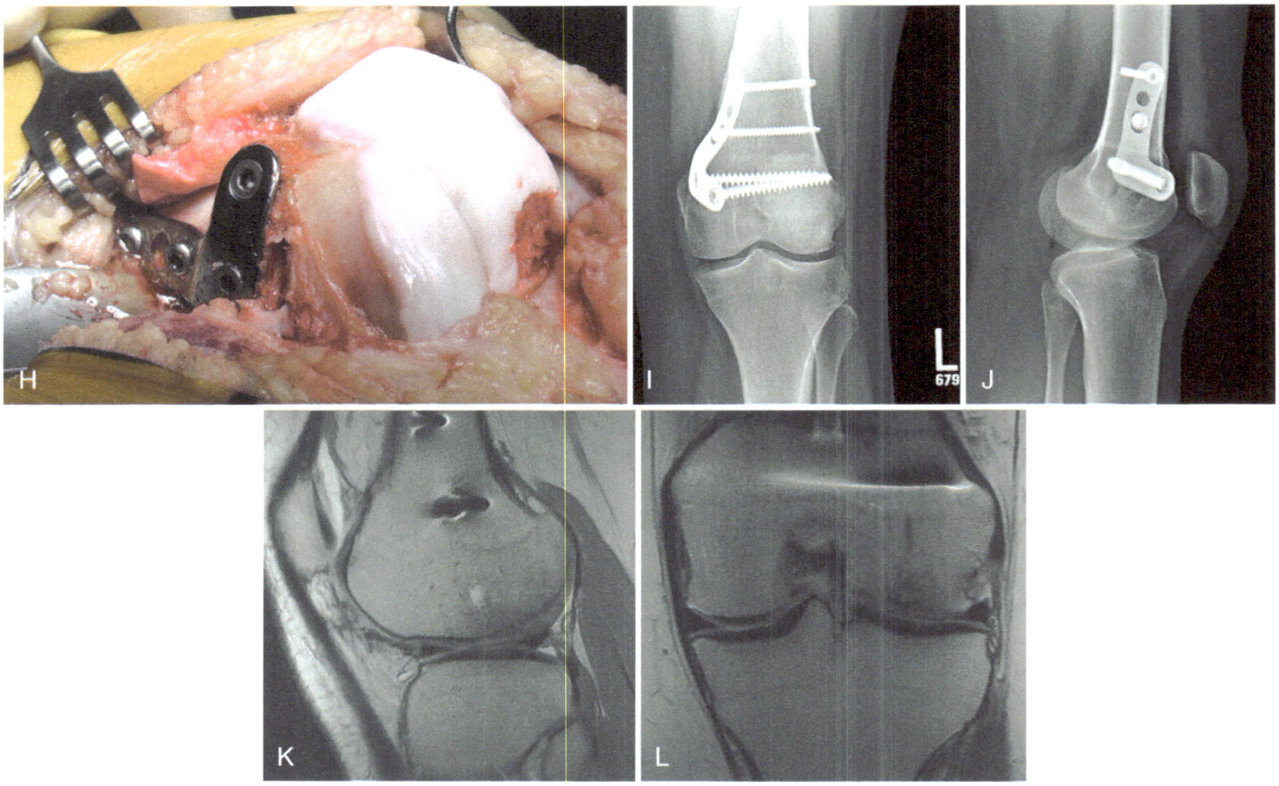

• **Fig. 11.13 Cont'd** dissecans of the posterior lateral femoral condyle. There has been fragmentation of the osteochondritis dissecans fragment and it has been removed arthroscopically. This leaves a osseous and cartilaginous defect to the lateral femoral condyle. Lateral (C) and skyline (D) x-ray images of the left knee demonstrate the posteriorly located osteochondritis dissecans lesion on the lateral femoral condyle and the evidence of patellar tilt of the left knee. (E) Close-up view taken from a long-leg alignment x-ray image of the left knee demonstrates the mechanical axis (*yellow line*) to fall through the center of the lateral femoral condyle. Any type of cartilage repair to the osteochondritis dissecans lesion would be at risk of premature failure without mechanical axis correction to the medial tibial spine (the defect is large and there is early joint space narrowing noted on Rosenberg PA views); an 8-degree angular correction is necessary. (F) A supracondylar 8-degree closing wedge varus-producing osteotomy has been performed. The lateral cortex remains intact. (G) The osteotomy is closed with a tension band L-plate used for proximal tibial osteotomies contoured to the proximal femur noting that the intraoperative mechanical axis is successful in placing the axis to the medial tibial spine as preoperatively planned. (I would use a medially based locking contoured plate today because it is now available, fits more precisely, and is more rigid.) The bone taken from the osteotomy is then utilized as an osseous repair for the lateral femoral condyles osteochondritis dissecans lesion. (H) Intraoperative appearance through a medial peripatellar arthrotomy of the L-plate used as a tension band plate placed on the medial side of the joint in combination with autologous bone grafting to the lateral femoral condyle osteochondritis dissecans. Today I would perform a lateral matrix-induced autologous chondrocyte implantation sandwich technique using this autologous bone graft to restore the osteochondral unit. (I, J) Final AP and lateral radiographs following osseous union of the osteotomy site and the lateral femoral condyle osteochondritis dissecans lesion. (K, L) No further cartilage repair was required for the osteochondritis dissecans lesion in this patient. The patient's own bone marrow cells under the influence of a cartilage rehabilitation with continuous passive motion and protected weight-bearing gave the patient a fibrocartilaginous surface and the patient became asymptomatic. This was followed with high-resolution MRI scanning to ensure that there was a repair surface and not an empty bony defect (sagittal and coronal proton-density fast-spin echo images). The patient remains asymptomatic and has returned to sporting activities. A biopsy for cultured articular chondrocytes was taken at the time of the open reconstruction for the possibility of failure of the fibrocartilaginous surface repair and the need for second stage autologous chondrocyte implantation (ACI). However, 4 years later the patient continues to remain asymptomatic. She is followed with annual clinical examinations to assess for crepitus, swelling, and other symptoms and by annual x-ray examinations with standing AP and flexed PA views to assess for the potential of joint space narrowing. If symptoms were to develop or clinical findings, high-resolution MRI scan would be repeated after the first 2 years with the possibility of arthroscopy for confirmation and cartilage repair with ACI or fresh osteoarticular allograft as deemed necessary.

Summary

Distal femoral varus osteotomy can be performed for either valgus deformity with lateral osteoarthritis or valgus deformity with cartilage or osteochondral repair to the lateral joint compartment. Long alignment x-ray images confirm that the deformity is in the distal femoral metaphysis with a superior and lateral directed joint line. The angle of the tibiotalar joint is also usually obliquely aligned indicating that osteotomy through the femur will make both the knee and ankle joint parallel to the floor.

Deformity correction of the mechanical axis is to the midline for cartilage repair with an intact lateral joint line or to the medial tibial spine when there is joint space loss or a large chondral defect in the lateral tibiofemoral compartment. Overcorrection is not desired.

Opening wedge femoral osteotomy is generally utilized for corrections up to 15 degrees for cartilage or arthritic lateral disease with valgus malalignment and possibly a short leg. Closing wedge femoral osteotomy is generally used when there is a need for autologous bone grafting to the lateral tibiofemoral compartment or there is a long leg on the affected side. Closing wedge femoral osteotomy provides more rapid healing that is predictable especially in prior smokers or perimenopausal women. A supracondylar reverse dome osteotomy is generally utilized for corrections of 15 to 30 degrees with a lateral 95-degree blade plate fixation for distal femoral lateral locking plate or retrograde intramedullary femoral locking rod. This is a very powerful osteotomy that does not distort the anatomy of the distal femur. The technique should always be considered so that future reconstruction such as total knee arthroplasty is not jeopardized. Femoral osteotomy is technically more difficult to perform than tibial osteotomy but provides very reproducible outcomes when chosen and performed as described in the techniques in this chapter.

References

1. Healy WL, Anglen JO, Wasilewski SA, Krackow KA. Distal femoral varus osteotomy. *J Bone Joint Surg Am*. 1988;70(1):102–109.
2. McDermott AG, Finkelstein JA, Farine I, Boynton EL, MacIntosh DL, Gross A. Distal femoral varus osteotomy for valgus deformity of the knee. *J Bone Joint Surg Am*. 1988;70(1):110–116.
3. Paley D. *Principles of Deformity Correction*. Berlin: Springer-Verlag; 2002.
4. Gross AE, Hutchinson CR. Realignment osteotomy of the knee–part 1: distal femoral varus osteotomy for osteoarthritis of the valgus knee. *Oper Tech Sports Med*. 2000;8(2):122–126.

12

Patellofemoral Malalignment, Tibial Tubercle Osteotomy, and Trochleoplasty

TOM MINAS MD, MS

CHAPTER OUTLINE

Introduction

This chapter is meant to offer the practicing orthopedist a practical management approach to dealing with patellofemoral disease. The key to successful treatment relies on an accurate diagnosis of the underlying pathomechanics responsible for the pain.

Chronic patellofemoral pain is a common and problematic management issue. The term "chondromalacia" has often been applied to anterior knee pain. Chondromalacia (soft cartilage), a pathologic term, may not even be present. Pain is a multifactorial perception. It is important to ensure that the pain is local and not referred, that it is not caused by a local soft tissue inflammatory or neurogenic process, and that it arises from the patellofemoral joint. This is usually determined by a careful history and physical examination. The emotional well-being of the patient may modify the subjective response of pain. Even with obvious patellofemoral pathomechanics, if physical therapy has not been performed adequately to address these problems, a repeated course of carefully directed physical therapy is worthwhile.

Many factors have been implicated as a source of abnormal forces across the patellofemoral joint. These include patella alta, trochlea dysplasia, an abnormally increased quadriceps or Q-angle, with secondary soft tissue problems, weakened or hypoplastic vastus medialis oblique (VMO) quadriceps muscle with a contracted lateral retinaculum. These pathomechanics lead to abnormal forces across the patella resulting in secondary degenerative changes or injury to the articular surfaces with cartilage defects of the patellofemoral joint acutely or chronically.

The prevalence of patellofemoral cartilage defects is controversial because it is unknown what percentage of lesions become symptomatic enough to prompt evaluation. Several studies have reported the presence of high-grade focal chondral defects in 11%–20% of knee arthroscopies. Among these defects, 11%–23% were located in the patella and 6%–15% in the trochlea.[1–3] A group investigating asymptomatic NBA basketball players with knee magnetic resonance imaging (MRI) found articular cartilage lesions in 47%, patellar lesions in 35%, and trochlear lesions in 25% of players; however, only approximately half of these defects were characterized as high-grade lesions.[4] These reports emphasize the importance of a thorough history and physical evaluation of the entire kinetic chain from pelvis to foot, a gait analysis, and assessment of all knee structures (tendons, ligaments, and soft tissues) before attributing a patient's symptoms solely to the presence of a chondral defect.

History

Patellofemoral articular defects frequently present as anterior knee pain; patients often report their pain to be located retropatellar, peripatellar, occasionally radiating down the shin bone, or in the instance of trochlear defects, the pain at times is located posteriorly in the popliteal area. Secondary pain may be from synovial or capsular irritation from joint distension secondary to an effusion or caused by exposed subchondral bone overload from a chondral defect. Thus, in light of this secondary nature of pain, other factors may also contribute, making it difficult to assign a percentage of pain to the cartilage pathology. Large defects can cause clicking or popping, giving way, and activity-related swelling. Distension of the joint often causes an aching sensation with a loss of motion and function but not necessarily complaints of pain. Standard patellofemoral symptoms are often reported such as increased pain with prolonged flexed knee position and stair climbing as maximal patellofemoral forces are in the flexed knee position when patellar engagement in the trochlea occurs greater than 30 degrees (Fig. 12.1A,B). Patients are approximately evenly split in reporting a traumatic versus a more gradual onset of symptoms; sports participation was the most common inciting event associated with the diagnosis of chondral lesions. Patellar dislocation is associated with damage to the articular surface, with chondral defects of the patella seen in up to 95% of patients[5] (Fig. 12.2A,B). It is the author's opinion that patellar dislocations usually occur because of baseline mechanical abnormalities with increased quadriceps angles (Q-angles) and/or dysplasia of the trochlea; despite the history of trauma, it is usually a minor twist during participation in sports. Patients often report extended courses of physical therapy, bracing and taping, or prior knee surgery.

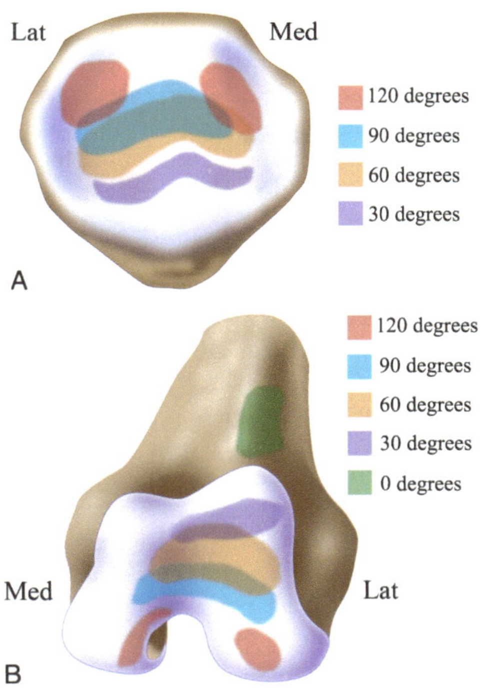

• **Fig. 12.1** (A) Portions of the patella that are engaging at different angular degrees of flexion. (B) Corresponding portions of the trochlea that are engaging with the patella at different angular degrees of flexion. (Modified from Aglietti P, Insall JN, Walker PS, Trent P. A new patella prosthesis. Design and application. *Clin Orthop Relat Res*. 1975;107:175–187.)

Physical Examination

Gait abnormalities, such as intoeing or hip abductor weakness, and an increase in femoral anteversion and valgus malalignment of the lower extremity are frequently seen in this patient population, especially adolescents. Adaptations in gait are also seen such as hip and knee external rotation and contractures of the hip abductors and iliotibial band. Traditionally, the Q-angle (Fig. 12.3) has been used in the evaluation of patellofemoral symptoms. Many different methods of measuring this angle have been reported and the high interobserver variability makes its usefulness questionable.[6,7] As described, the Q-angle should be evaluated in both full extension and approximately 30 degrees of flexion, because in some cases a laterally subluxated patella in full extension can falsely decrease the Q-angle (the patella should be repositioned in the central sulcus before measuring the Q-angle). My preference is to examine and measure the Q angle is full extension with the patella manually reduced in the trochlea with medially directed force on the patella (I call it the Thumb Reduction Test). Ask the patient to contract the quadriceps and you can see and feel the patella sublux laterally. Q-angles in asymptomatic patients are 14 degrees in males and 17 degrees in females.[8] Quadriceps wasting, especially of the vastus medialis, is common in long-standing patellofemoral symptoms. Recently, more emphasis has been placed on core muscle weakness, especially of the hip abductors, hip extensors, and pelvic stabilizers. Weakness in this group can be demonstrated by asking the patient to single-leg stand on the affected limb, resulting in a pelvic drop on the contralateral side. In addition to poor pelvic support, dynamic internal rotation of the femur and dynamic valgus positioning of the limb can be observed. Activity-related swelling and, in particular, a joint effusion indicate more advanced disease. Palpation of the medial and lateral retinaculum can elicit pain; the lateral structures are often contracted (tested by attempting to reverse patellar tilt) and the medial soft tissues can be attenuated (such as chronic patholaxity of the medial patellofemoral ligament [MPFL]). Patellar mobility, tilt, and subluxation should be assessed and quantified medially and laterally. Normally the patella should be able to "glide" 30% of its width medially and laterally without the patient experiencing apprehension of a subluxation or dislocation. Catching with mobilization of the patella against the trochlea is suggestive of larger defects. Knee range of motion is usually preserved but may be inhibited by pain or large effusions in acute cases. The J-sign (the patient slowly extends the knee from full flexion, the patella subluxes laterally once it leaves the constraints of the trochlear groove near full extension) may occur in normal patients but is exaggerated in patients with patellar maltracking and often implies incompetence of the medial restraining structures, including the MPFL.

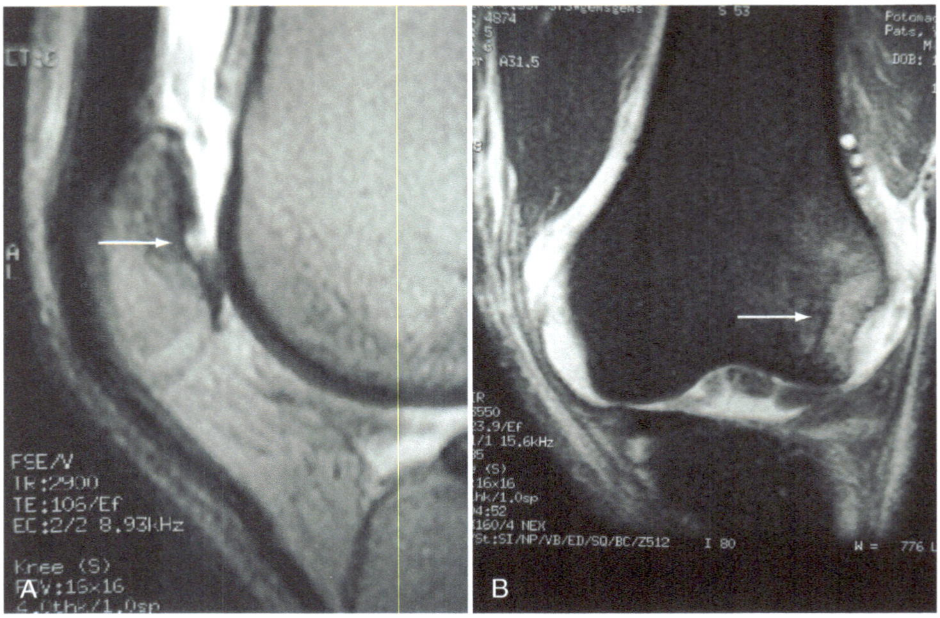

• **Fig. 12.2** (A) Sagittal MRI scan demonstrating central full-thickness articular cartilage loss (*arrow*) after patellar dislocation. (B) Coronal MRI scan with fat suppression, demonstrating intense bone marrow edema at the location of the patellar dislocation at the distal lateral trochlea (*arrow*). This is a classic MRI appearance of the articular injury patterns following patellar dislocation.

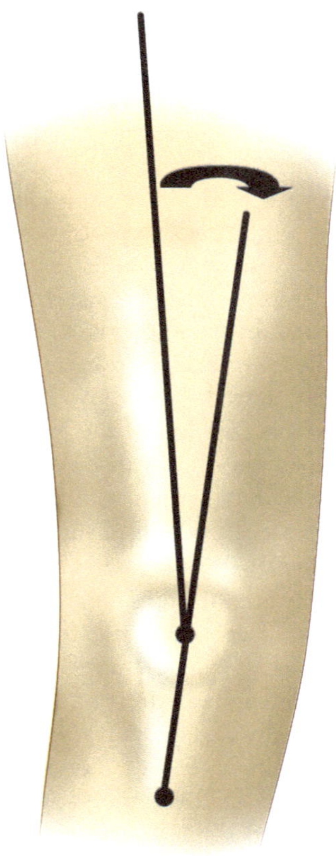

• **Fig. 12.3** Diagrammatic representation of the quadriceps or Q-angle. A line drawn from the anterior-superior iliac spine to the central pole of the patella (with the patella reduced in the trochlea in full extension) follows an angle with a line drawn from the central patella pole to the patellar tendon insertion at the tibial tubercle. This angle averages 14 degrees in men and 17 degrees in women. (From Aglietti P, Insall JN, Cerulli G. Patellar pain and incongruence. I: measurements of incongruence. *Clin Orthop Relat Res*. 1983;176:217–224.)

Physical Therapy

The goal of physical therapy is to restore soft-tissue balance in the patellofemoral joint, including muscular and capsuloligamentous balance often remote from the joint. Rehabilitative exercises should include a stretching regimen to restore flexibility of the quadriceps, hamstrings, and iliotibial band, as well as patellar mobilizations as needed to optimize capsular structure balance (e.g., reverse tilt) of the quadriceps and patellar tendon. After flexibility has been restored, a strengthening program should be instituted, emphasizing the core proximal musculature, including the hip abductors and external rotators, because most patients have previously received too much emphasis on isolated quadriceps strengthening. When quadriceps strengthening is emphasized it should be performed with closed-chain activities such as elliptical trainer, leg presses, and squats with the knee less than 30 degrees of flexion from full extension to prevent maximal patellofemoral contact forces. Open-chain resisted quadriceps extensions should be avoided so that patellofemoral pain or cartilage damage are not aggravated. Short-arc open-chain quadriceps extensions are performed when the patella is not engaged in the trochlea in the first zero to 20 degrees of flexion of the knee. Gait training should focus on avoidance of an intoeing gait, which results in functional femoral anteversion. Throughout rehabilitation, it is important to protect the patellofemoral articulation by using isometric and short-arc closed-chain concentric and eccentric muscle strengthening, which is individually designed to avoid specific arcs of pain or loading of cartilage defects. A trial of patellar McConnell taping or patellar bracing to centralize a maltracking patella is worthwhile, especially when symptoms are limited to certain activities, such as athletic endeavors. The patient should understand the comprehensive McConnell approach, which uses taping to allow pain-free rehabilitation, i.e., the taping is not an end in itself. Patients should understand that they have mechanical reasons for their imbalance and resultant pain in their extensor mechanism. Therefore it is important that they maintain their stretching and strengthening regimen to stay within their envelope of function, their own personal equilibrium. If they are able to experience benefit with physical therapy but have recurrent relapses of discomfort, they should rest, elevate, and ice the extremity along with taking nonsteroidal anti inflammatory medications until they are able to resume their quadriceps rehabilitation regimen. Only when they fail therapy should they then seek definitive surgical intervention for resolution of symptoms and restoration of function.

Imaging Studies

Useful tests to assist in determining the diagnosis include standard radiographs to include standing AP, 45-degree PA (Rosenberg views), lateral and skyline (Merchant views), and standard 54" axial alignment x-ray examinations. X-ray images are useful with any patellofemoral joint to determine joint space narrowing or osteoarthritis on a standard Merchant view. Merchant view is taken at 45 degrees of flexion during which the patella is normally well engaged in the trochlea distally. It is not an effective view for assessing maltracking. When maltracking occurs, it is usually in the first 0–30 degrees of flexion from extension. The dislocated or subluxed patella in full extension travels medially as it travels distally capturing the trochlea as it reduces. This is the clinical finding of a J-sign. Dejour et al.[9] have shown the advantages of a true lateral radiograph in assessing trochlear dysplasia and patellar tilt not appreciated on the Merchant view.

Assessment of articular cartilage injury is receiving more attention with high-resolution 3.0 Tesla MRI magnets and thin 1-mm slice acquisitions orthogonal to the axis of the joint surface, improved upon with cortical enhancement magnets. Although intravenous gadolinium as an indirect arthrogram with MRI scan was popular in early 2006, reports of complications related to injury to the kidneys have discontinued its use in our practice. The high-resolution MRI images that are presently available rarely require an arthrogram to enhance the effect of the imaging. If so, direct injection of gadolinium is necessary prior to the MRI scan. Although the gold standard for assessing articular injury remains arthroscopy, sensitivity and specificity > 90% can be obtained with high-resolution MRI scan using even a standard 1.5 Tesla magnet with appropriate orthogonal gantry tilting to surfaces of the trochlea and appropriate sequences.[10,11] This is our preferred method of assessing articular cartilage injury to localize the site and size of articular injury in the patellofemoral articulation.

To assess patella subluxation accurately, spiral computed tomography (CT) of the patellofemoral joint is performed with the leg in full extension, once with the quadriceps relaxed and again with the muscle maximally contracted (Fig. 12.4). It is especially helpful in determining dysplasia of the bony patellofemoral joint (Figs. 12.5 and 12.6). Computed tomography also allows a more precise evaluation of patellar and trochlear anatomy than the Merchant view (Fig. 12.7). Accurate documentation of subluxation can be determined with a CT scan when clinical findings are difficult, especially in obese patients.

The addition of intra-articular contrast gadolinium helps to reveal any articular cartilage defects on the patella or the trochlea or both and the exact location and size. I have found that my preferred test for patellofemoral maltracking, location of the articular cartilage defect, and assessment of dysplasia of the trochlea, is a CT arthrogram performed with the quadriceps first relaxed and then contracted in the fully extended position of the knee (Fig. 12.8).

Furthermore, superposition of two CT images, one through the patellofemoral articulation, the other through the tibial tubercle, allows calculation of the tibial tubercle to trochlear groove (TT-TG) distance: the center of the trochlear groove and the center of the tibial tubercle are marked, and the medial-to-lateral distance between the two is measured (Fig. 12.9). A TT-TG distance of >15 mm is considered normal; values >20 mm are abnormal and these cases should be considered for a tibial tubercle osteotomy.[12] It is also possible to use MRI images obtained during routine knee evaluation to measure the TT-TG distance (Schoettle et al.[13] demonstrated the equivalency of CT and MRI TT-TG measurements) and the Caton-Deschamps measurement of patellar height[14] (alta, infera, normal), thus providing additional information without added cost.

Despite the enthusiasm over the use of the TT-TG distance, I am reluctant to use solely that measured reference to determine patellar maltracking. In a small person's knee, 15 mm is a large distance and would often result in severe subluxation of the patella in comparison with a very large person. I am more inclined to use clinical examination and CT arthrogram with the knee in the extended position both

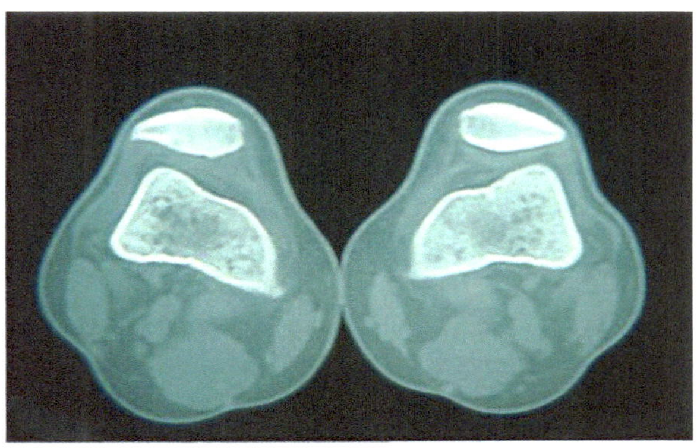

• **Fig. 12.4** CT scan of bilateral subluxed patellas with quadriceps contracted with the knees in full extension.

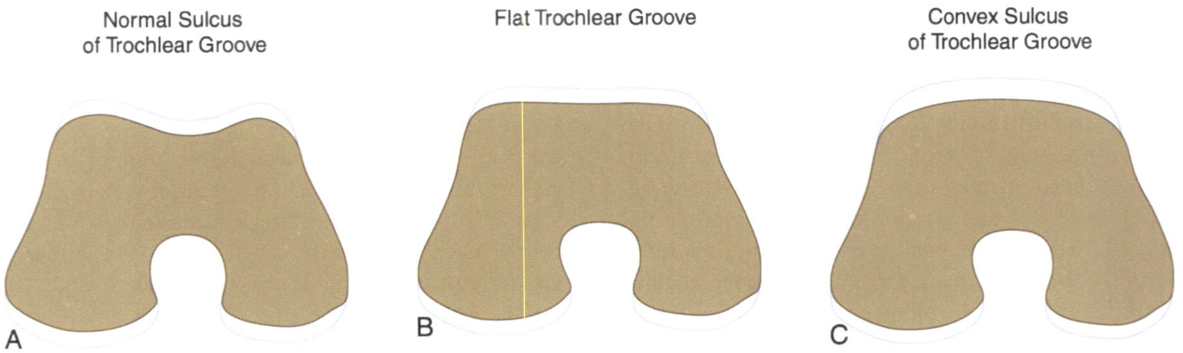

• **Fig. 12.5** (A) Coronal view of a normal trochlea with a central concave groove. Variations of trochlea dysplasia may cause flattening of the groove (B) or a convex groove (C). When this occurs developmentally, the sesamoid patella articulation is congruent to the dysplastic trochlea and is also abnormally shaped.

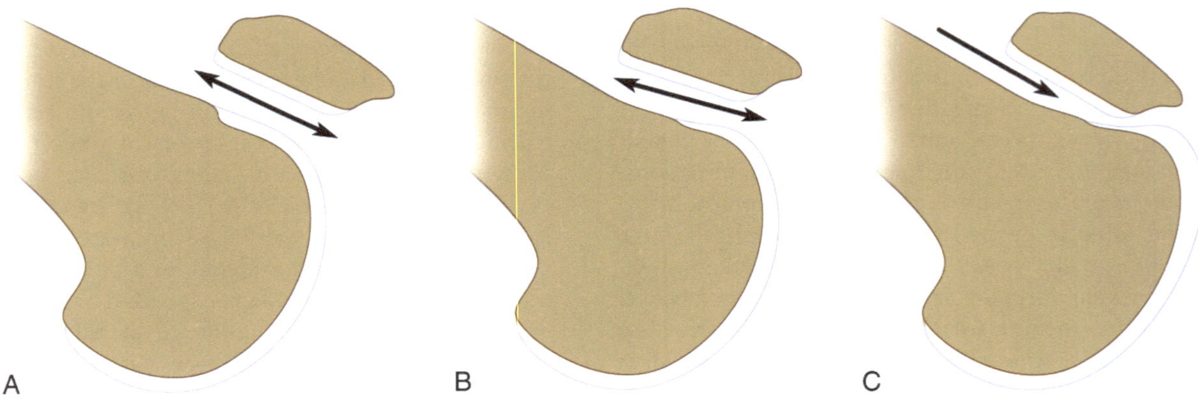

• **Fig. 12.6** Trochlea dysplasia in the sagittal view may exhibit (A) a smooth entry sulcus or (B) a prominence that drives the patella inferior pole into a "speed bump." Severe changes (C) or a trochlea "spur" as noted by Dejour if there is a commonly associated patella alta, predisposing to abnormal forces to subluxation and premature articular cartilage wear. (From Dejour H, Walch G, Neyret P, Adeleine P. Dysplasia of the femoral trochlea [French]. *Rev Chir Orthop Reparatrice Appar Mot*. 1990;76(1):45–54.)

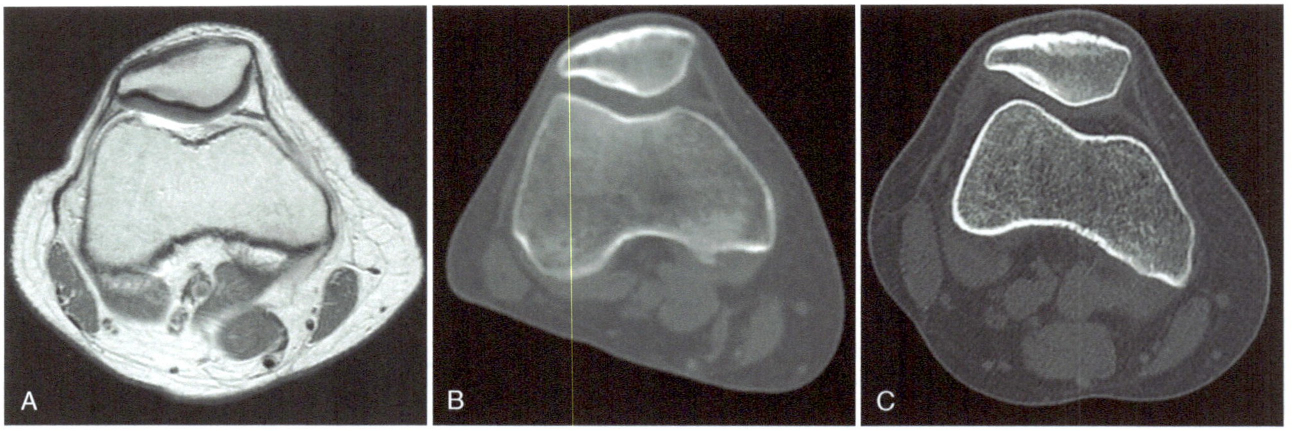

• **Fig. 12.7** (A) A high-resolution MRI scan with intravenous gadolinium utilized as an indirect arthrogram effect. Notice the intact full-thickness nature of the lateral patellar articular cartilage. This 32-year-old woman has had a history of chondromalacia since the age of 12 years. She has undergone multiple courses of physical therapy, taping, and bracing. She has been offered a patellar lateral arthroscopic release and has sought another opinion. (B) This is a CT scan of the patella in a well reduced position. Notice the thickening of the subchondral bone to the lateral patellar facet. This is indicative of chronic lateral maltracking, overload with remodeling of the subchondral bone. (C) The patient's quadriceps is contracted with the leg in extension. Notice the lateral subluxation of the patella. The patient requires isolated medial translation of the tibial tubercle accompanied by a patellar lateral retinacular release. The articular cartilage shown in (A) was normal, therefore there was no need for anterior translation of the tubercle.

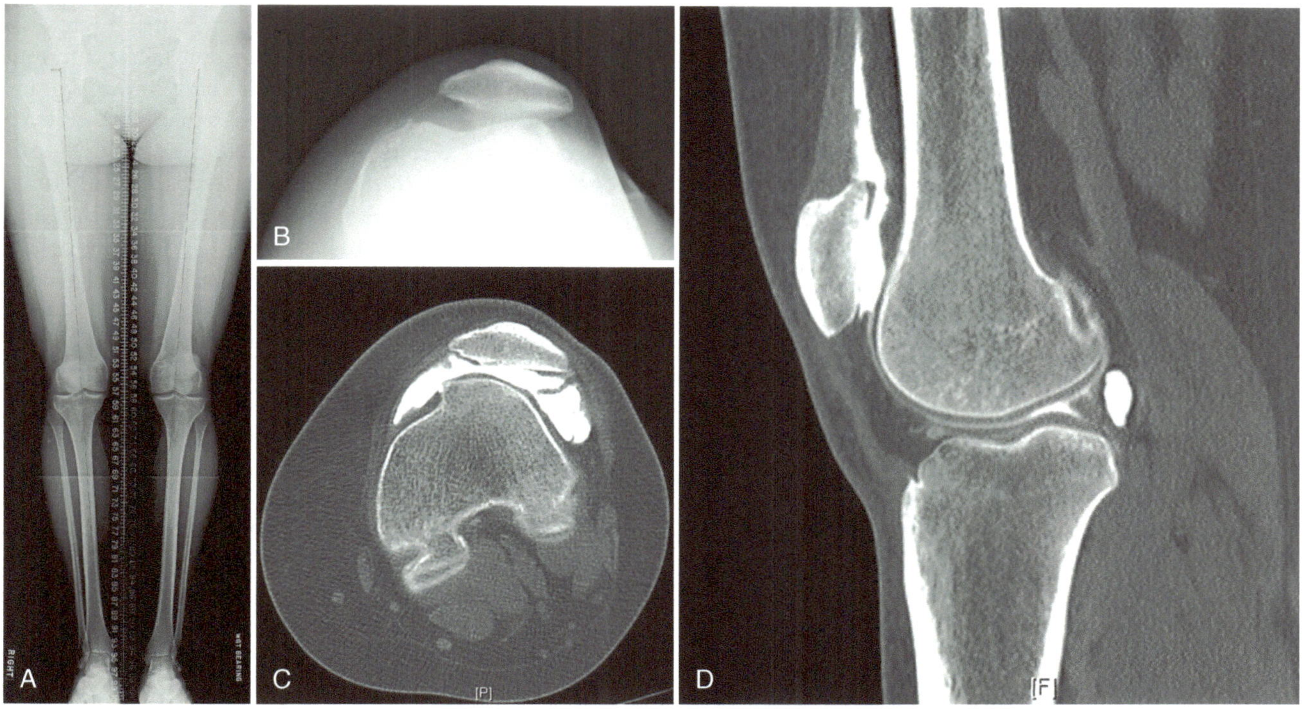

• **Fig. 12.8** (A) Long alignment x-ray image in a young woman with patellofemoral pain demonstrating a neutral mechanical axis. (B) A Merchant or skyline x-ray examination demonstrates patellar subluxation with intact articular surfaces. (C) A coronal CT arthrogram with the quadriceps contracted demonstrating subluxation of the patella as it is perched on the superior lateral dysplastic trochlea. A full-thickness articular cartilage loss is noted on the patella centrally and laterally. A spiral CT arthrogram as a single test is the preferred study for patellofemoral disease. The dye clearly outlines the localization of the cartilaginous loss. Dysplasia of the trochlea is clearly visualized and the test can be performed rapidly and can assess the position of the patella with the quadriceps in the contracted and relaxed positions. This is especially helpful in obese patients where clinical examination is less reliable. (D) The sagittal CT scan arthrogram demonstrates complete loss of cartilage on the patella lateral facet except for a small rim proximally.

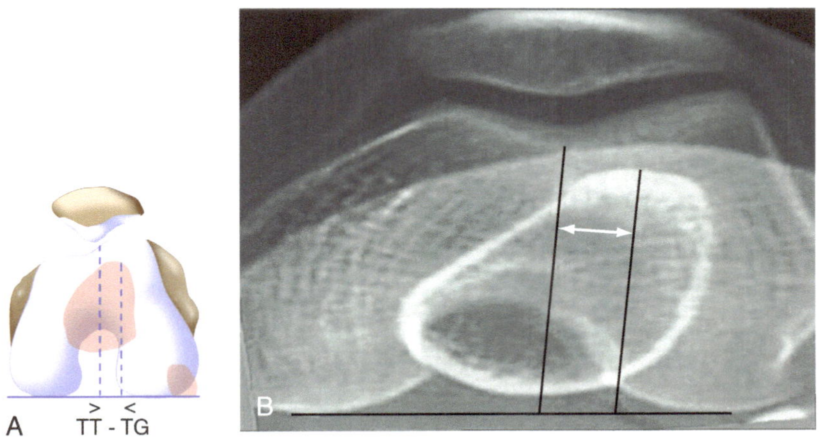

• **Fig. 12.9** (A) Diagrammatic representation of the tibial groove–tibial tubercle (TG-TT) distance. Anything greater than 20 mm is clearly considered abnormal. This does not take into account the size of the patient. It is an absolute number that assists in determining patellofemoral maltracking. (B) The TT-TG distance can be measured directly from a CT scan from the axial cuts that are overlapped at the level of the tibial groove and the level of the tibial tubercle.

relaxed and contracted to determine patellar subluxation rather than the use of the TT-TG distance.

When the pain pattern is suggestive of arising from the patellofemoral articulation, a bone scan may be useful in difficult cases of evaluation when other studies are negative to determine increased activity in that part of the joint, but is rarely necessary.

Identify the Pathomechanics: Successful Surgery

In a patient with persistent patellofemoral pain and functional disability, there are certain factors that need to be determined prior to appropriate treatment of the patient with patellofemoral disease. These factors are determined after the history, physical examination, x-ray examination, MRI scan, and CT scan. The factors include long leg alignment, patellar tilt, patellar subluxation, location on the patella articular chondrosis, location on the trochlea articular chondrosis, the quadriceps angle, and secondary factors: VMO quadriceps hypoplasia or atrophy, patella alta, and dysplasia of the trochlea. Once these factors are accurately determined, an appropriate surgical treatment plan can be recommended.

The primary factors that I have found to guide my treatment algorithm include patellar tilt, subluxation, and localization of the chondrosis (Table 12.1).

Patellofemoral disease represents a spectrum with differing severities of long leg alignment, patellar subluxation, chondrosis, or arthrosis. This algorithm addresses the different stages of disease in a stepwise fashion of increasing severity dependent on the findings.

I will assume that the long leg alignment is in neutral mechanical axis and the factors at the present time are those related to patellofemoral tracking in a neutrally aligned leg. However, the valgus knee with patellofemoral dysplasia and lateral maltracking is a difficult variant to address. Such an example is shown in Fig. 12.10.

Isolated Patellar Tilt: Lateral Release

The procedure of arthroscopic lateral release is an overly utilized procedure. It is effective for isolated patellar tilt without subluxation of the patella when the lateral retinacular structures of the patella are contracted and mobility of the patella is limited. There may be early grade II Outerbridge chondromalacia associated with a chronically contracted and non-subluxated patella. The procedure should be performed either arthroscopically or open from the superior lateral pole of the patella to the inferior lateral aspect of the patellar tendon. The superior-lateral and inferior-lateral geniculate arteries are cut with this procedure and must be isolated, coagulated, or tied. It is important not to release the tendinous portion of the vastus lateralis muscle from the superior lateral patella because of the ensuing weakness that will develop. Any loose partial thickness chondrosis flaps should be removed at the time of the lateral release to limit any pain resulting from mechanical causes.

If subluxation is associated with patellar tilt, arthroscopic lateral release should not be performed. Persistent subluxation, mechanical overload with subsequent progressive chondral wear and pain will persist, resulting in failure of the procedure and unnecessary surgery for the patient (Figs. 12.11 and 12.12). The importance of an accurate diagnosis in differentiating tilt and subluxation can be seen in the case presented in Fig. 12.7 because an isolated lateral release would not have been effective. Instead, an isolated medialization of the tibial tubercle with lateral release is indicated and was performed.

TABLE 12.1 Treatment Algorithm for the Surgical Management of Patellofemoral Disease

Clinical algorithm useful for the management of patellofemoral disease. The role of patellar tilt, patellar subluxation, Fulkerson classification of patellar chondrosis, and obliteration of a radiographic skyline joint space determine the treatment pathway.

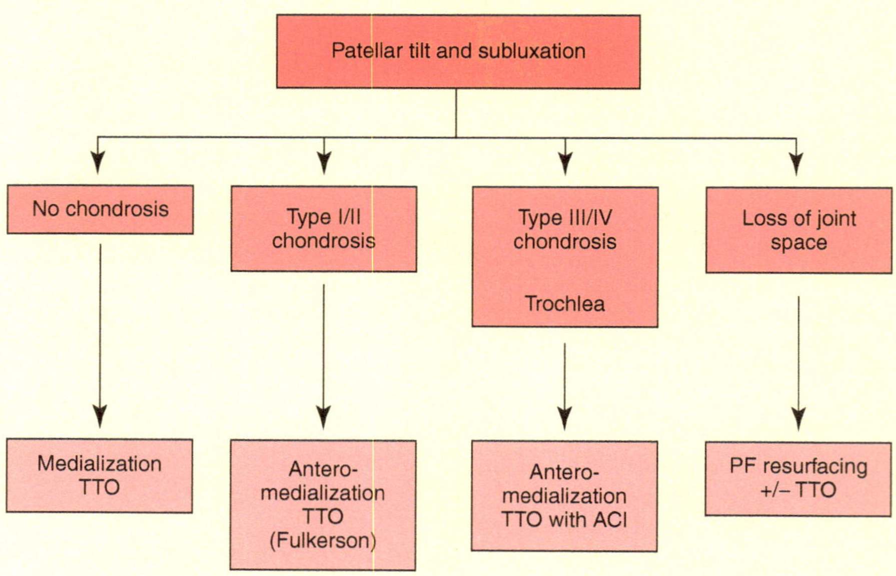

ACI, autologous chondrocyte implantation; *TTO*, tibial tubercle osteotomy.

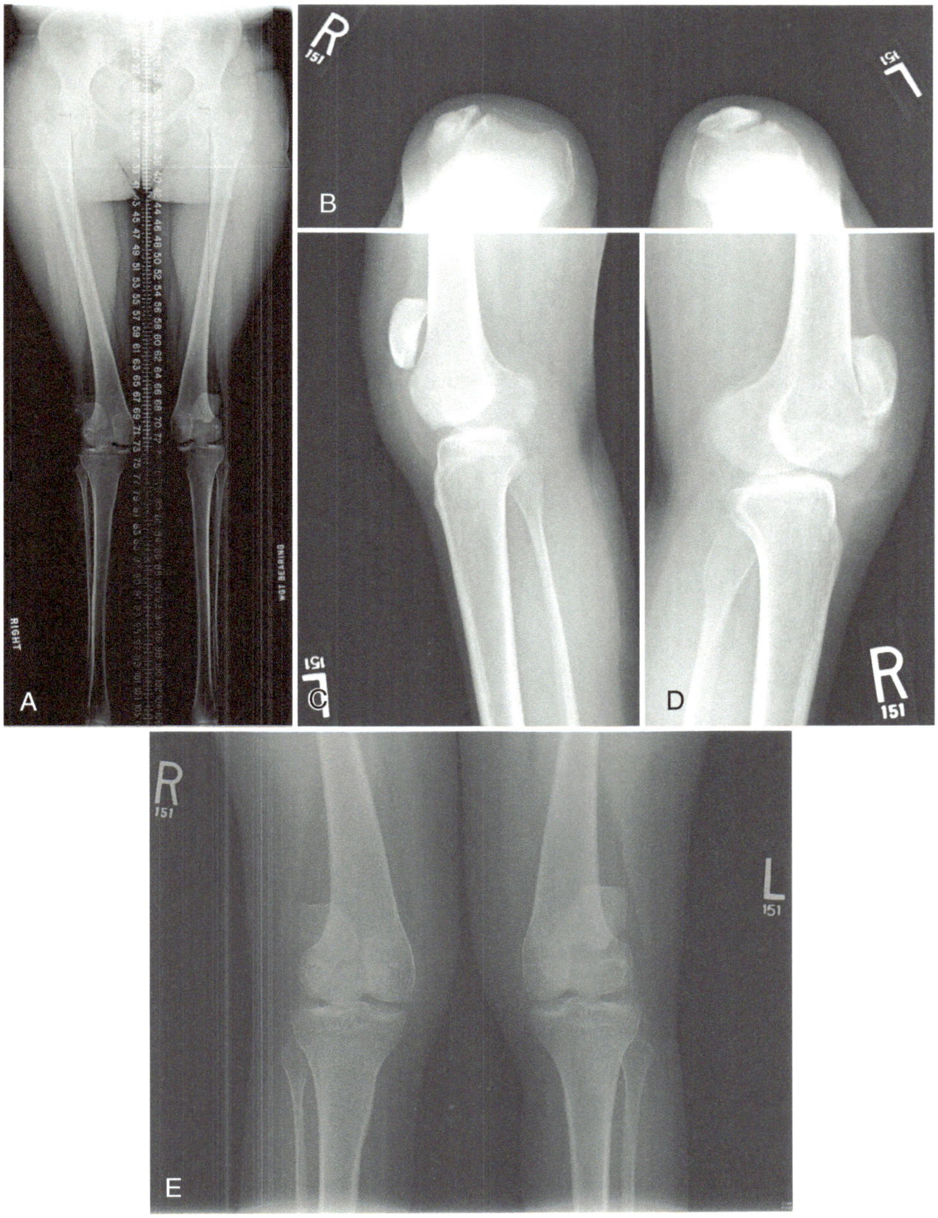

• **Fig. 12.10** (A) The long alignment x-ray images of a 19-year-old woman who has valgus mechanical alignment. She has suffered from anterior knee instability and pain since early adolescence. Valgus malalignment is occasionally associated with trochlea dysplasia, a hypoplastic lateral femoral condyle, and patellar instability as in this case. This is an uncommon variant of trochlea dysplasia that is very difficult to manage because of the combined deformities, which promote patellar instability. (B) Bilateral skyline x-ray images demonstrate dislocation of the patella on the right and medial subluxation of the patella on the left. (C, D) Lateral x-ray images of both knees demonstrating patella alta. (E) Bilateral AP x-ray images demonstrate laterally positioned patellas and intact tibiofemoral joint spaces.

Patellar Tilt and Subluxation With or Without Chondrosis

Fulkerson Types I and II Chondrosis: Anteromedialization Tibial Tubercle Osteotomy

When there is a combination of patellar subluxation and tilt, the usual causes include a lateralized tibial tubercle patellar tendon insertion, with an abnormally increased Q-angle, accompanying soft tissue medial attenuation and lateral retinacular contracture. Chondrosis may have developed and dysplasia of the trochlea may be present.

The surgical correction of the abnormal quadriceps vectors resulting from a lateralized tibial tubercle and lateral retinacular contracture need to be addressed. There have been various forms of tibial tubercle osteotomy (TTO) with lateral retinacular release performed over the years. The Fulkerson anteromedialization (AMZ) TTO[15] has gained popularity in the United States (Fig. 12.13) as a modification of the Elmslie-Trillat[16] procedure in that it

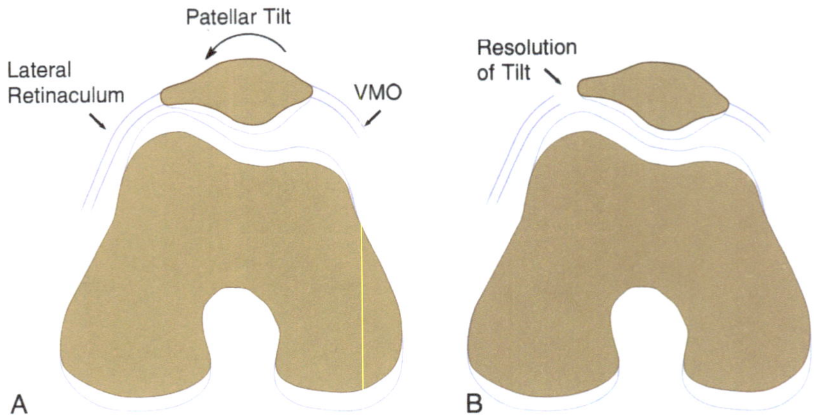

• **Fig. 12.11** (A) Isolated patellar tilt without subluxation is uncommon and due to a tight lateral retinaculum, (B) isolated lateral release from the superior pole of the patella distally will keep the insertion of the vastus lateralis muscle attached to the superior pole of the patella and unload the lateral patellar facet. This is an effective but rarely required and overly performed procedure. *VMO*, vastus medialis oblique.

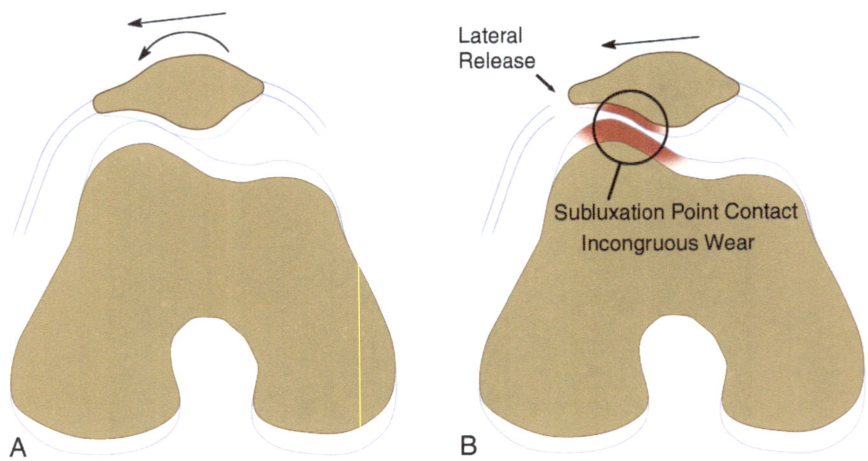

• **Fig. 12.12** The more common situation clinically is a patella that has both lateral patellar tilt and subluxation (A). However, a lateral release performed in this situation (B) resolves tilt but not subluxation and pain often persists. Lateral release in this situation is contraindicated.

allows a more aggressive anterior translation than that provided by the latter. The soft tissue balancing required in order to centralize the patella in the trochlea may also be concomitantly performed (Fig. 12.14). This procedure off-loads the lateral and inferior poles of the patella by the anterior and medial translation of the tibial tubercle. It therefore loads the proximal and medial poles of the patella. Successful clinical outcomes have been achieved when the chondrosis involved with maltracking has been localized to the lateral patella facet or inferior patella pole. Conversely, it has demonstrated poor clinical outcomes in the presence of articular damage to the proximal or medial patella surfaces, or central trochlea involvement.[17] This has led to a classification of articular chondral injury to the patella locations corresponding to: type 1, chondral injury to the inferior patella pole; type 2, chondral injury to the lateral patella facet; type 3, chondral injury to the medial patella facet; type 4, chondral injury to the proximal pole or panpatellar surface (Fig. 12.15A–D).

Patellar Tilt and Subluxation With or Without Chondrosis

Types III and IV Chondrosis: AMZ TTO+ACI

After reviewing the clinical outcomes of the first 45 patients to have been treated by ACI with full-thickness chondral lesions involving the patellofemoral joint, patients reported 70% good and excellent results with type III and type IV articular injuries of the patella.[18] As our experience grew, our clinical results treating type III and type IV patellar lesions also improved. Including the first cohort of 45 patients, our recent experience of 130 patients involving the patella, trochlea, or both articulations, noted 80% good and excellent results as reported by patients with 18% of patients noting improved clinical outcomes (fair), and only three patients reporting being the same as or worse than they were before the surgery (see Chapter 9 on ACI). At the moment, ACI is our preferred treatment option for articular lesions

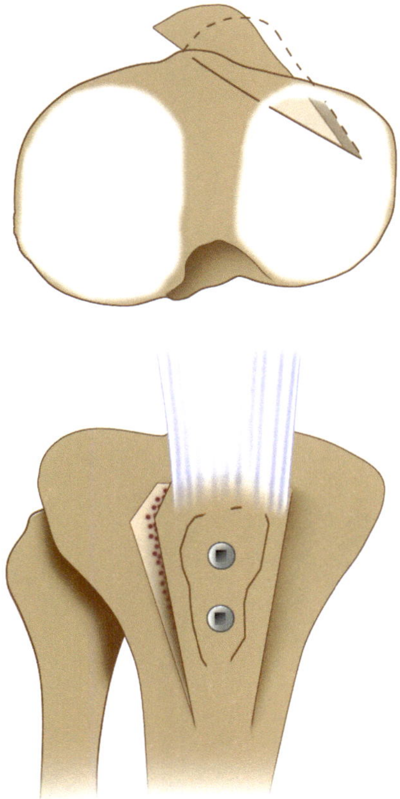

• **Fig. 12.13** Fulkerson osteotomy is a modification of the Elmslie-Trillat operation. It allows anterior translation of the tibial tubercle along with medial translation dependent on the obliquity of the osteotomy from anterior medial to posterior lateral. This is demonstrated in the diagram.

in the patellofemoral joint when osteotomy alone (types III and IV patellar chondral injury with maltracking) is not indicated, and joint preservation is desired.

Modified Surgical Technique of AMZ TTO (Fulkerson)[15]

TTO is a well described treatment for a variety of patellar related problems including recurrent instability, maltracking, unloading chondral defects, and arthrosis.[16,19–22] The most common types of osteotomy involve some degree of medialization and/or some degree of anterior displacement of the tubercle, while leaving the distal cortical hinge intact. The amount of anterior and medial displacement can be adjusted based on the steepness of the osteotomy. This is determined by the nature of the pathology. Typically, in cases of instability, the osteotomy is flatter and the translation is more medial than anterior. When treating chondral defects or arthrosis, the purpose of the osteotomy is to decompress and unload the patellofemoral joint. Therefore, a steeper osteotomy is performed, whereby the tubercle is translated more anterior than medial.

When performed for the proper indications, the results of TTO are good. However, there are a number of possible complications[23] associated with the procedure. In the past, I have found that patients often complained of a prominent bony ridge along the medial border of the osteotomy. This was seen more commonly after a steeper osteotomy had been performed. Typically, patients complained of tenderness over the area, especially with kneeling. Female patients often complained of difficulty shaving their legs. Some patients were also unhappy about the "knobby" appearance of their knee after an osteotomy. In an attempt to reduce these problems, I have developed a simple and reproducible technique for diminishing the bony prominence along the anteromedial border of the tuberosity after performing a TTO. This has significantly reduced the number of postoperative complaints associated with the procedure.

Surgical Technique

The patient is placed in the standard supine position. I utilize a lateral post at the level of the greater trochanter to prevent external rotation of the leg, as well as a post at the mid-calf in order to maintain the knee in full extension and allow approximately 90 degrees of flexion during the procedure if necessary. A longitudinal incision is made slightly lateral to midline so that the incision is not directly over the tubercle and the hardware used for fixation is not prominent. If wound breakdown were to occur, it would be over muscle and not bone (Fig. 12.16).

Evaluation of the articular pathology to determine the degree of anteriorization versus medialization is performed first, typically a full subvastus lateral release in combination with a TTO. Full-thickness medial and lateral flaps are made first. The lateral border of the patellar tendon is identified and a full-thickness release is made through capsule and synovium into the joint along the lateral border of the patella. The iliotibial band attachment from the iliotibial tract to the lateral superior pole of the patella is released and the posterior border of the vastus lateralis muscle is identified and released from the synovium and the lateral intramuscular septum. This allows complete mobility to the patella and direct inspection of the trochlea and patella while leaving the medial sleeve intact. The areas of chondrosis can then be localized and the amount of medialization and anteriorization of the tibial tubercle can be determined to unload the damaged segment. The tibial tubercle is exposed in its entirety utilizing full-thickness medial and lateral subcutaneous flaps (Fig. 12.17). An elevator is used from distal to proximal to lift the anterior muscle compartment off the tibia and expose the posterolateral border of the proximal tibia. A small Hohmann or Bennett retractor is then placed behind the tibia to protect the neurovascular structures during the osteotomy.

Medially, an elevator is also used to create a large, full-thickness subperiosteal flap. Dissection is carried nearly to

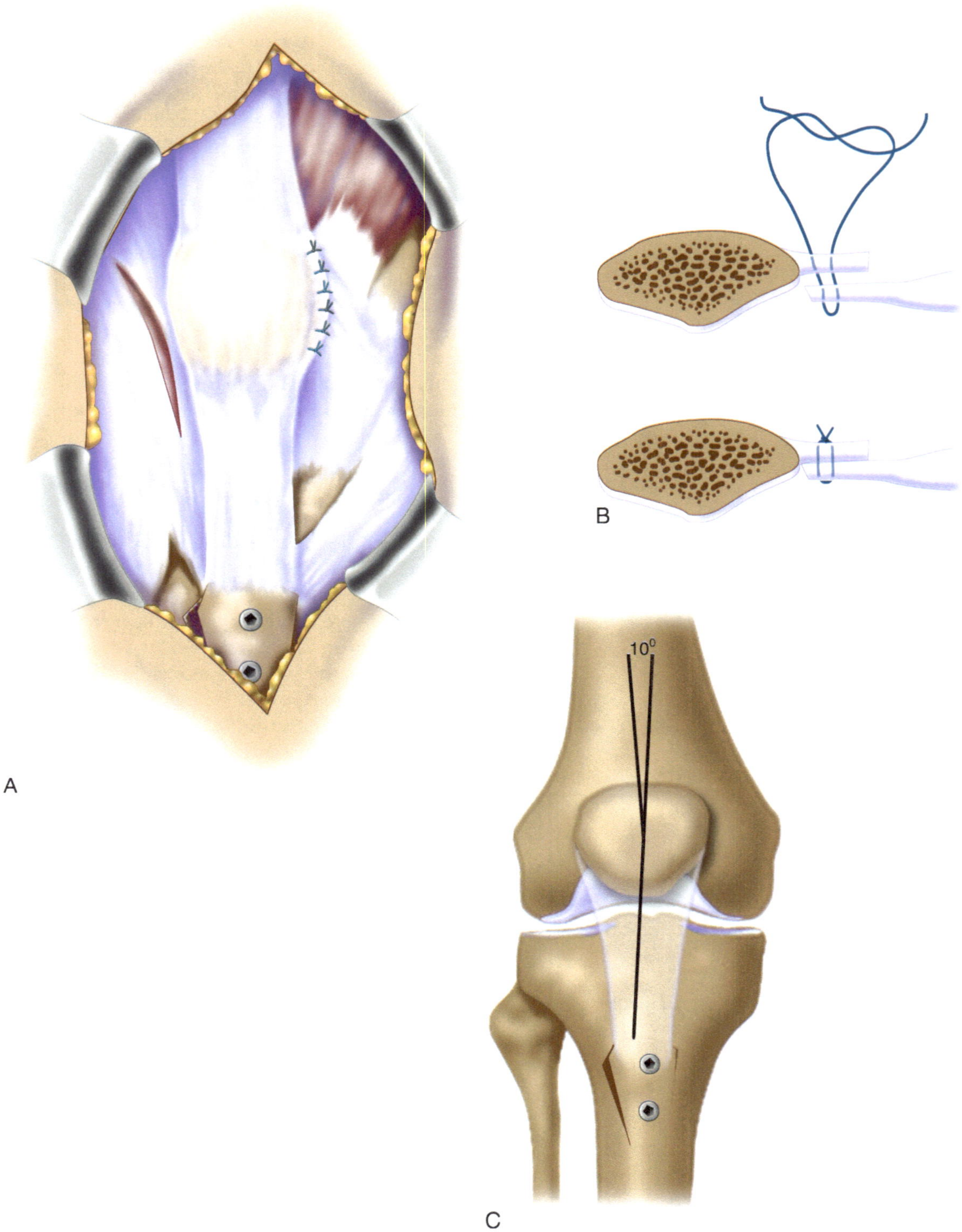

• **Fig. 12.14** In order to translate the patella in response to the direction of translation of the tubercle, a soft tissue balancing must be performed. (A) Laterally, the lateral capsule and the iliotibial band attachment to the superior pole of the patella are released to the posterior lateral intramuscular septum performing a lateral sub vastus approach to the joint. This preserves the integrity of the quadriceps and especially the vastus lateralis attachment to the superior pole of the patella. Alternatively, a lateral lengthening can be performed by releasing the ileopatellar attachment of the IT band from the lateral border of the patella, then releasing the synovium posteriorly off its attachment to the femur. At the end of the procedure, the lateral joint can be effectively closed by reattaching the posterior aspect of the synovium, which is still attached to the patella, to the anterior aspect of the ileopatellar attachment of the IT band at 90 degrees of flexion when it would be maximally out to length. This is presently my preferred technique. (B) On the medial side, I prefer a medial parapatellar arthrotomy, identification of the MPFL (medial patella-femoral ligament) attachment of the synovial capsular condensation to the abductor tubercle and a vest-under-pants advancement of the MPFL and capsule under the patellar retinaculum to anteriorize the patella further away from the trochlea unloading the articular surfaces as shown. (C) After the procedure is completed, the tubercle is usually co-linear to the tibial spines resulting in a postoperative Q-angle of 0–10 degrees.

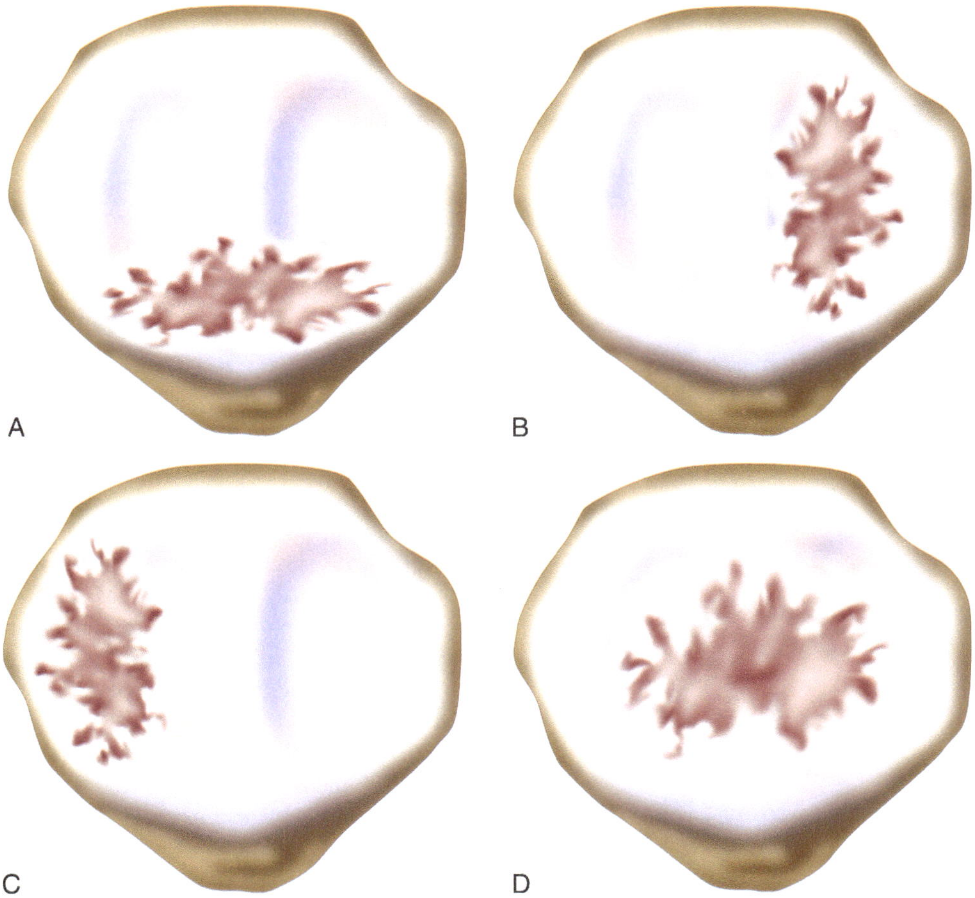

• **Fig. 12.15** Fulkerson Classification of chondral defects to the patella. (A) type I: inferior patella pole. (B) type II: lateral patella facet. (C) type III: medial patella facet (often associated with a trochlea injury). (D) type IV: central panpatellar injury.

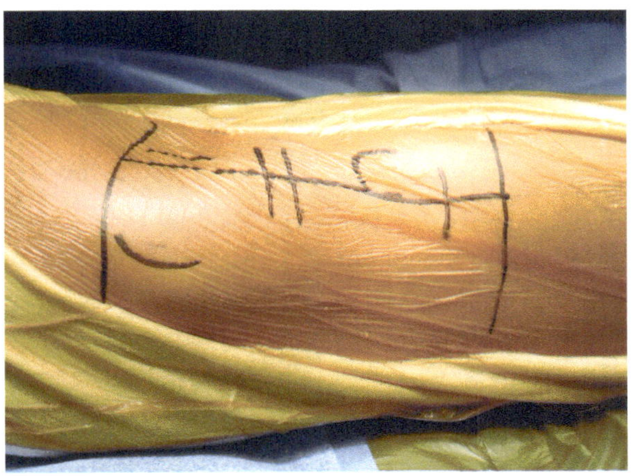

• **Fig. 12.16** Skin incision from superior pole of patella to inferior border of tibial tubercle. Note the incision is slightly lateral to the patella. This preserves the saphenous nerve skin sensory innervation of the anterior skin medial to the incision.

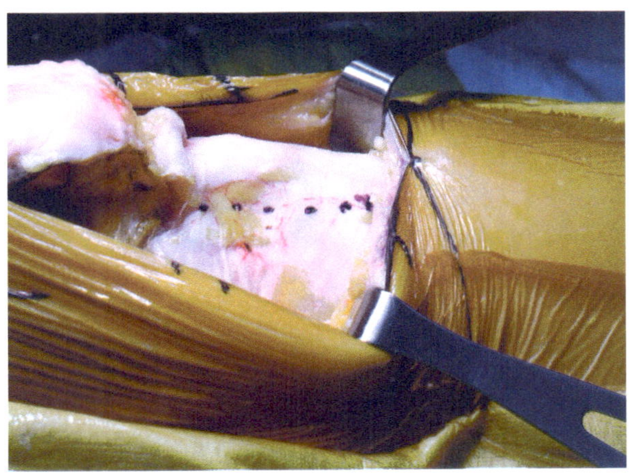

• **Fig. 12.17** Complete exposure of tibial tubercle after creation of full-thickness medial and lateral skin-subcutaneous flaps.

the superficial MCL (Figs. 12.18 and 12.19). This step is key for later repair to the osteotomized segment.

Lastly, the retropatellar bursa is incised and an army-navy retractor is placed under the patellar tendon exposing the proximal aspect of the tuberosity.

Next are the bony cuts. Initially, a counter cut is made just proximal to the tuberosity, taking care to protect the patellar tendon. This is done with a small sagittal saw from the medial to lateral border of the patellar tendon insertion. An oblique cut is then made laterally to prevent propagation

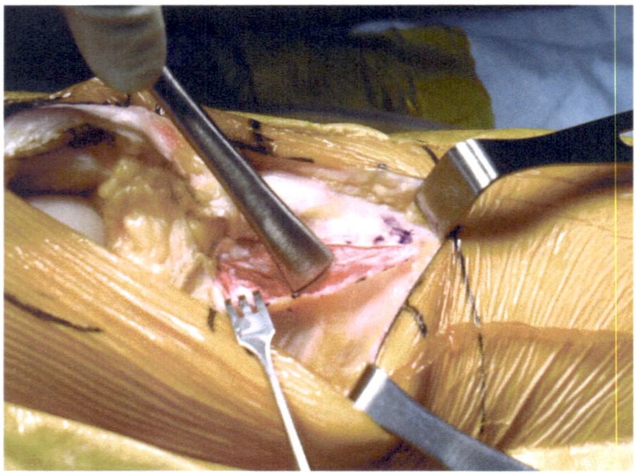

• **Fig. 12.18** Creation of medial subperiosteal flap nearly all the way to the posteromedial border of the tibia including the pes tendon insertions and the superficial medial collateral ligament.

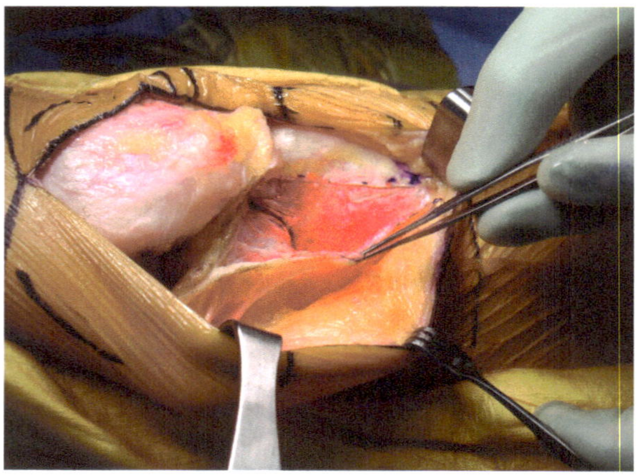

• **Fig. 12.19** Creation of medial subperiosteal flap nearly all the way to the posteromedial border of the tibia including the pes tendon insertions and the superficial medial collateral ligament.

of the osteotomy toward the lateral cortex or the joint. The location of the osteotomy on the medial cortex is determined by the desired steepness of the osteotomy. Steeper osteotomies begin more anteriorly, just adjacent to the tuberosity. Flatter osteotomies begin more posteriorly down the medial face of the proximal tibia. Osteotomy angles vary from 30 degrees for an average steepness to 60 degrees of obliquity to the posterior lateral corner of the tibia for a steep anterior translation of the tubercle. The line of the osteotomy can be marked on the medial cortex with a marking pen or electrocautery. As the osteotomy proceeds distally, the direction of the cut should become flatter, so that the distal cortical hinge is maintained. If intra-articular work is required such as ACI, the distal hinge is cut obliquely and more steeply to elevate the entire tubercle proximally (see Chapter 9, ACI.)

Initially, a saw is used to perforate the medial cortex along the entire extent of the osteotomy. Next, the exit point on the lateral cortex is determined and marked. This can be done with the use of a jig (AMZ Tracker, Depuy, Warsaw, IN) or free-hand, which is my preference. Again, the level of the cut should become more anterior as the osteotomy proceeds distally. Once the lateral cortex is marked, the cortex is perforated using a small sagittal saw. Finally, the osteotomy is completed by connecting the medial and lateral cortical perforations using a sagittal saw. The osteotomy should be deep enough so that it traverses entirely cancellous bone except the distal hinge. Copious irrigation is required to avoid thermal necrosis to the bone. This will lead to rapid healing. However, care must be taken that the osteotomy is not too deep and perforates the posterior cortex, which can lead to iatrogenic fracture.[23,24] When the osteotomy has been completed, an osteotome can be used at all the corners to ensure that the tuberosity is mobile. This should not involve a great deal of force.

Once mobile, the tuberosity can be translated into the desired position. I place the tuberosity so that the patellar tendon is directly co-linear and anterior to the tibial spines. I then temporarily stabilize the tuberosity with large pointed reduction forceps while I make sure that I have not over-medialized the tubercle resulting in medial subluxation. At 90 degrees with neutral foot rotation the tubercle–sulcus angle should be collinear or 0 degrees. The tuberosity is stabilized with large pointed reduction forceps and fixed with two bicortical 3.5-mm fully threaded cortical screws placed using a lag technique orthogonal to the osteotomy site. I have not had loss of fixation with the smaller cortical screws and not had prominent hardware and have a tight pitch capture to the posterior cortex with excellent lag effect and compression.

At this point, there is often a large, sharp edge of bone overhanging medially (Fig. 12.20). This is trimmed vertically flush with the medial cortex of the tibia using a small sagittal saw. It can then be divided and used laterally as bone graft.

Finally, Optium DBM (demineralized bone matrix; LifeNet Health, Virginia Beach, VA) is packed tightly along the medial border of the osteotomy site (Fig. 12.21). The medial subperiosteal sleeve is closed over the graft and repaired back to the periosteum on the anterior aspect of

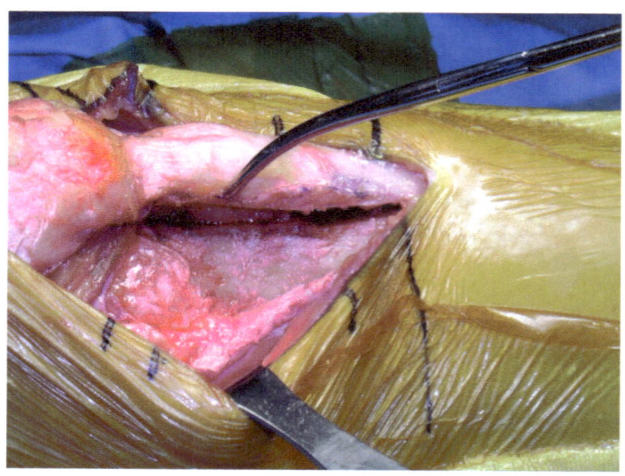

• **Fig. 12.20** Medially overhanging bone after fixation of the osteotomy.

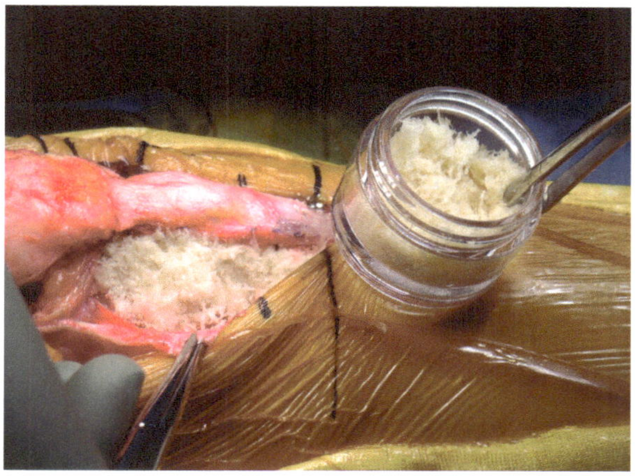

• **Fig. 12.21** Packing of demineralized bone graft under medial periosteal flap.

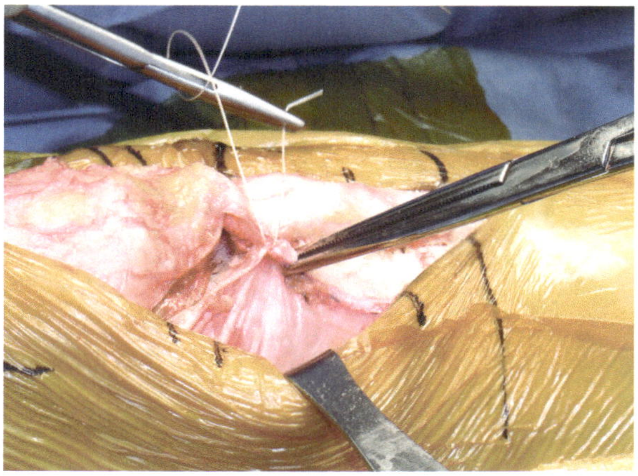

• **Fig. 12.22** Closure of medial periosteal flap to the medial border of the patellar tendon insertion on the mobilized tibial tubercle after fixation over demineralized bone graft without undue tension.

the tuberosity (Figs. 12.22 and 12.23). This can usually be done with minimal tension if an adequate flap has been raised initially. The envelope contains the superficial MCL pes anserinus insertion with periosteal sleeve to the posterior medial corner of the tibia. I routinely perform a lateral release (Fig. 12.24) as part of my initial exposure.

A medial advancement of the MPFL to the mid patellar pole bringing it under the medial patellar retinaculum with a horizontal mattress suture both stabilizes the patella and advances it (Fig. 12.25). Normally, the MPFL inserts at approximately the mid-pole of the patella.[25] It is always easy to find by grasping the medial synovium and capsule anterior to the abductor tubercle attachment of the MPFL with a Kocher and identifying a very stable check rein that includes the ligament. This is then advanced to the mid-pole of the patella. It is nearly always present and an MPFL reconstruction is rarely required using autologous tissue or allograft tissue. I use a vest–under-pants technique for performing a medial advancement with the MPFL capsular sleeve coming under the patellar retinaculum (Fig. 12.26). This advances the VMO as needed while using the MPFL capsular sleeve as a soft tissue interposition[26] to elevate the patella further and not compress posteriorly the medial patella facet as is typically performed with a "reefing."

Routine closure and postoperative care is then performed (Fig. 12.27). Patients are allowed 50% weight-bearing in extension with a hinge knee brace locked in extension immediately. Crutches are utilized. Progression to full body weight occurs by 4–6 weeks. Passive range of motion is also begun on the day of surgery. Isometric straight leg raises are performed in the brace locked in extension until there is evidence of bony healing by 4–6 weeks. Stationary bicycling out of the brace is begun at 3 weeks after surgery. Patellar mobilizations are begun immediately after surgery and are critical to prevent Hoffa's fat pad fibrosis and maintain normal patellar mobility. I have found that these osteotomies generally heal rapidly by 6–8 weeks and have not seen any complications directly related to this modification in technique.

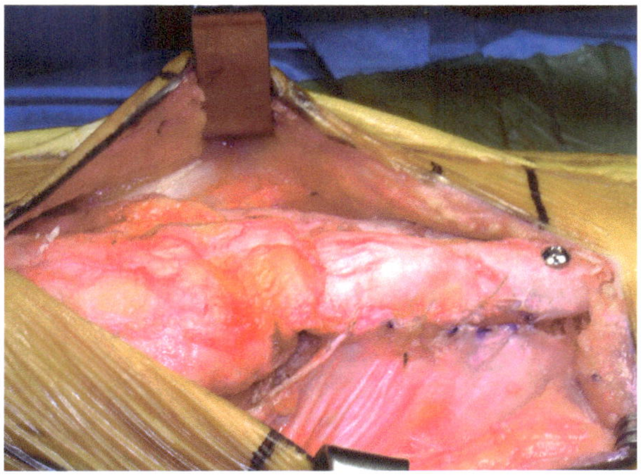

• **Fig. 12.23** Closure of medial periosteal flap to the medial border of the patellar tendon insertion on the mobilized tibial tubercle after fixation over demineralized bone graft without undue tension.

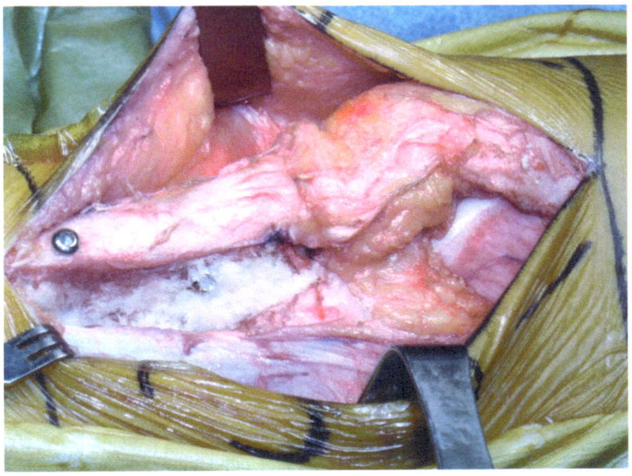

• **Fig. 12.24** Completed osteotomy viewed laterally. Demineralized bone graft has also been added to the cancellous bed of the mobilized tibial tubercle which lessens bleeding and enhances bone union. Note that a full-thickness lateral subvastus release has been performed.

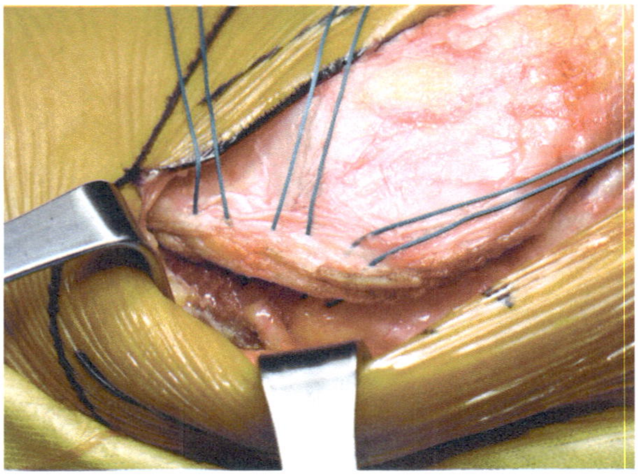

• **Fig. 12.25** Pants-under-vest technique for medial advancement of the medial patellofemoral ligament (MPFL). The MPFL insertion is advanced to the mid-pole of the patella and taken under the patellar retinacular sleeve to enhance anterior translation of the patella. Advancing the MPFL to this position also provides a stable check rein to lateral translation of the patella. I prefer to have approximately 30% glide medial and lateral of the patella in full extension so that the patellofemoral joint is not overly compressed. Horizontal mattress sutures are used to the mid patellar pole and tied. Distal sutures are not used so as not to overtighten the soft tissue envelope of Hoffa's fat pad.

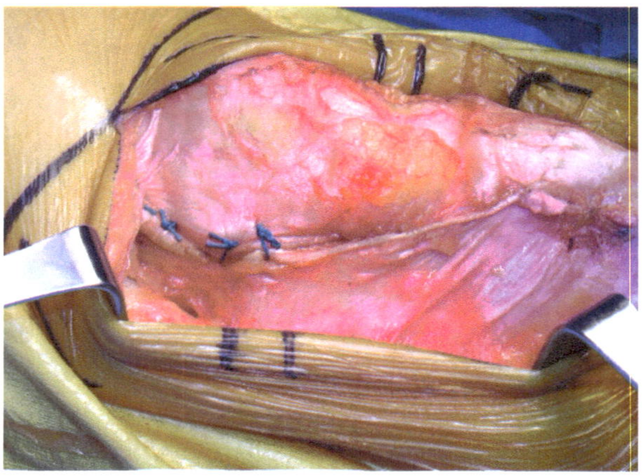

• **Fig. 12.26** Pants-under-vest technique for medial advancement of the medial patellofemoral ligament (MPFL). The MPFL insertion is advanced to the mid-pole of the patella and taken under the patellar retinacular sleeve to enhance anterior translation of the patella. Advancing the MPFL to this position also provides a stable check rein to lateral translation of the patella. I prefer to have approximately 30% glide medial and lateral of the patella in full extension so that the patellofemoral joint is not overly compressed. Horizontal mattress sutures are used to the mid patellar pole and tied. Distal sutures are not used to avoid overtightening the soft tissue envelope of Hoffa's fat pad.

TTO is a relatively common procedure with predictable results. This technique differs only slightly from standard descriptions. The careful dissection of the full-thickness medial periosteal sleeve to the posteromedial border of the tibia is the key step in the procedure. Most techniques describe only a limited medial subperiosteal dissection. When only a limited flap is raised, it is difficult to repair

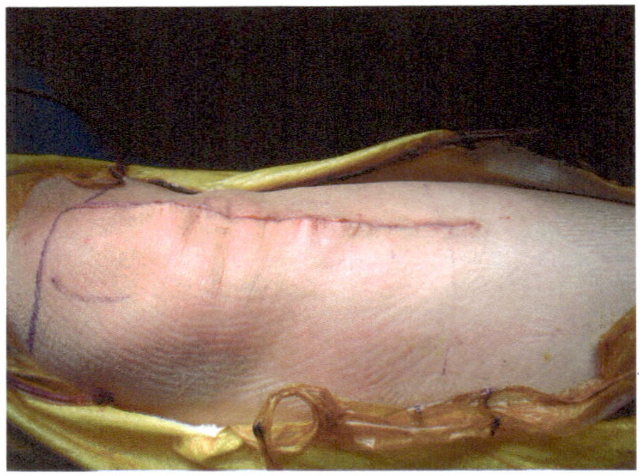

• **Fig. 12.27** Skin closure. Note there is no large prominence of the tuberosity as the medial contour has been restored.

at the end of the procedure. Often, a prominent edge of bone remains medially. The subcutaneous tissues are generally very thin in this region and this prominent edge of bone can be seen and felt by the patient. By excising the prominent bone and repairing the periosteum over demineralized allograft bone matrix, a more normal contour can be restored to the proximal tibia. Although this may not affect patient outcomes with regard to restoration of stability or reduction of patellofemoral pain, overall patient satisfaction with the procedure is very high.

Trochlea Dysplasia

Accurate assessment of patellofemoral maltracking should always include an assessment for trochlea dysplasia in order to have a successful surgical outcome. My assessment for trochlea dysplasia is part of any routine evaluation of patellar instability. However, my treatment for trochlea dysplasia with surgical trochleoplasty is the last part of a decision to stabilize the patella and I use the technique sparingly. Lateral maltracking secondary to an increased quadriceps angle is the most usual situation that I encounter. The typical surgical algorithm first involves a lateral subvastus arthrotomy to release the tight lateral structures. This allows visualization of articular injury to the patella, trochlea, and dysplasia of the trochlea. A tibial tubercle osteotomy is then performed to centralize and possibly unload damaged articular surfaces as assessed intraoperatively. ACI to the patella or trochlea is my preferred method of cartilage repair in the patellofemoral joint because of its excellent clinical outcomes. The need for this has already been determined prior to the procedure. A VMO advancement is then performed as needed to stabilize the patella. However, at this stage, if the trochlea is dysplastic, ongoing instability issues may be encountered. Slight over-tensioning of the VMO may lead to medial subluxation and under-tensioning to lateral subluxation if trochlea dysplasia is present. At this point, the last part of the stabilization procedure is a trochleoplasty.

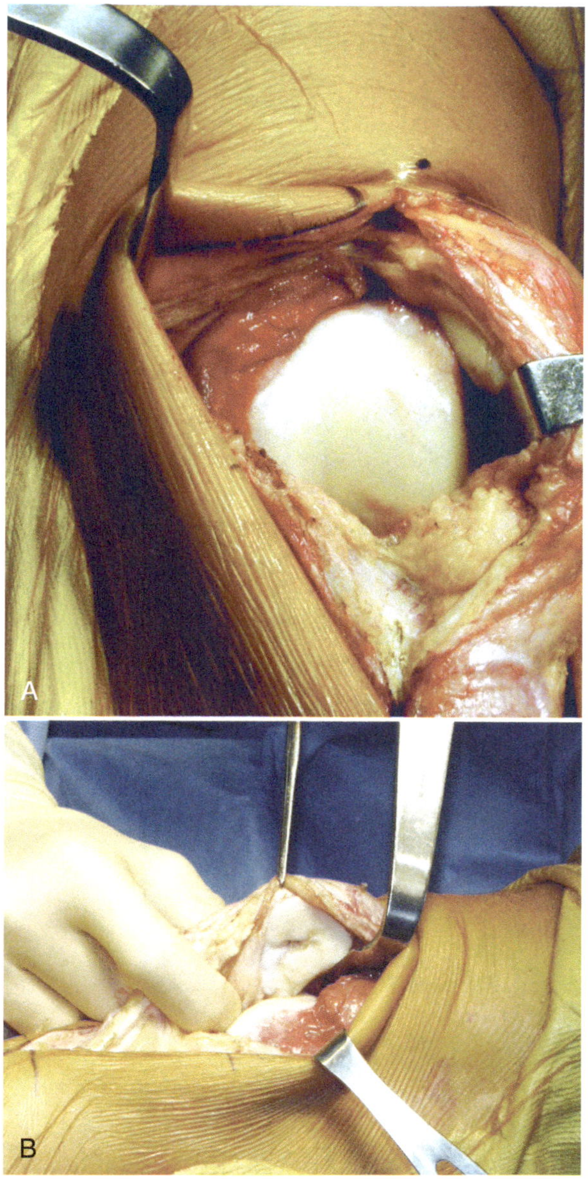

• **Fig. 12.28** (A) Moderate dysplasia of the trochlea as viewed from below with a superior lateral boss. (B) Severe patellar damage to the central and inferior pole of the patella secondary to chronic instability and maltracking.

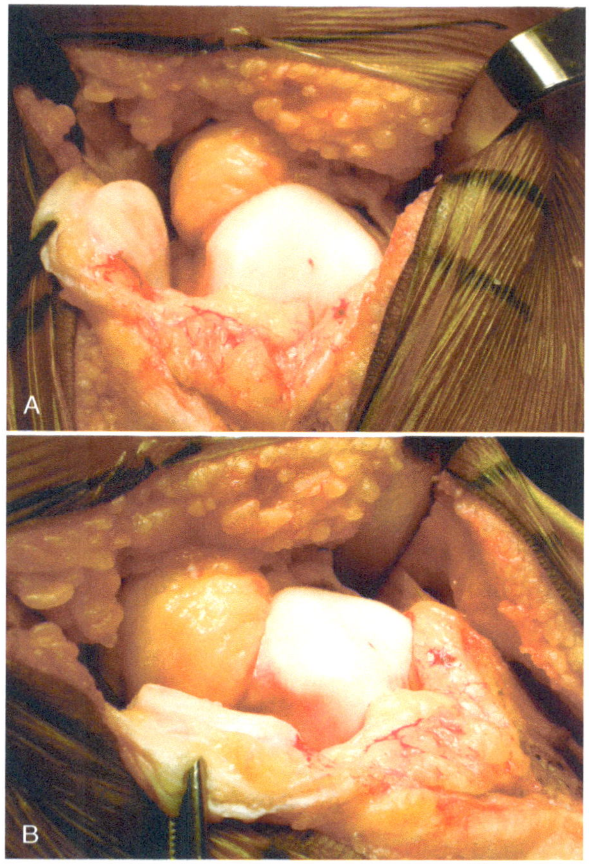

• **Fig. 12.29** (A) Another case of trochlea dysplasia in a more severe form. Note the prominent bulbous proximal entry site to the trochlea ("trochlea spur" as described by Dejour) that is poorly formed, viewed from below. (B) The same patient as in (A) viewed from lateral noting the prominent anterior spur of the trochlea relative to the anterior femoral cortex. If associated patella alta is present, then severe instability results, as the inferior pole of the patella is not engaged in the trochlea sulcus. If early engagement is present, instability is less severe.

Dysplasia of the trochlea of the distal femur is an uncommon developmental abnormality leading to patellar instability and premature degeneration of the patellofemoral joint. It is occasionally associated with dysplasia of the lateral femoral condyle leading to a valgus deformity accompanied by patellofemoral instability (Fig. 12.10). The degree of dysplasia is variable from subtle flattening of the proximal entry site (Fig. 12.28) to the trochlea to a bulbous convex entry site leading to severe instability (Fig. 12.29). Because the patella is a sesamoid bone that develops secondary to its congruity with the trochlea, it is frequently flattened or concave on its large lateral facet to match the shape of the trochlea. Like congenital dislocation of the hip (CDH) leading to premature osteoarthritis in the fifth decade of life, dysplasia of the trochlea also usually presents with instability, anterior knee pain, a diagnosis of chondromalacia, and end-stage isolated patellofemoral arthritis more commonly in women in the fifth decade of life.

The diagnosis requires attention to the possibility of recurrent patellar instability secondary to dysplasia of the trochlea. If a patient has recurrent instability, a lateral x-ray examination frequently demonstrates a prominent proximal barrel-shaped trochlea as noted by Dejour[9] with a "crossing sign" and a trochlea spur. His proposed description and classification of dysplasia has been published[27] and is noted in Table 12.2. Fig. 12.30A–D demonstrates the morphological phenotypes that he has described, which relate to the radiological findings in Table 12.2. A CT scan gives the most accurate diagnosis, but MRI scan is also useful.

Patients have frequently had multiple prior failed surgeries, which include proximal soft tissue balancing of the patella along with distal tubercle transfer and a failed clinical outcome with further instability episodes (see Fig. 12.31). Once the diagnosis has been established as

TABLE 12.2 Henri Dejour's Grades of Dysplasia of the Trochlea, Radiographic, and CT Appearance

Grade	Conventional Radiography	Computed Tomography
A	Crossing sign	Trochlear morphology preserved
B	Crossing sign supratrochlear spur	Flat or convex trochlea
C	Crossing sign	Asymmetry of trochlear facets
D	Crossing sign supratrochlear spur	Asymmetry of trochlear facets

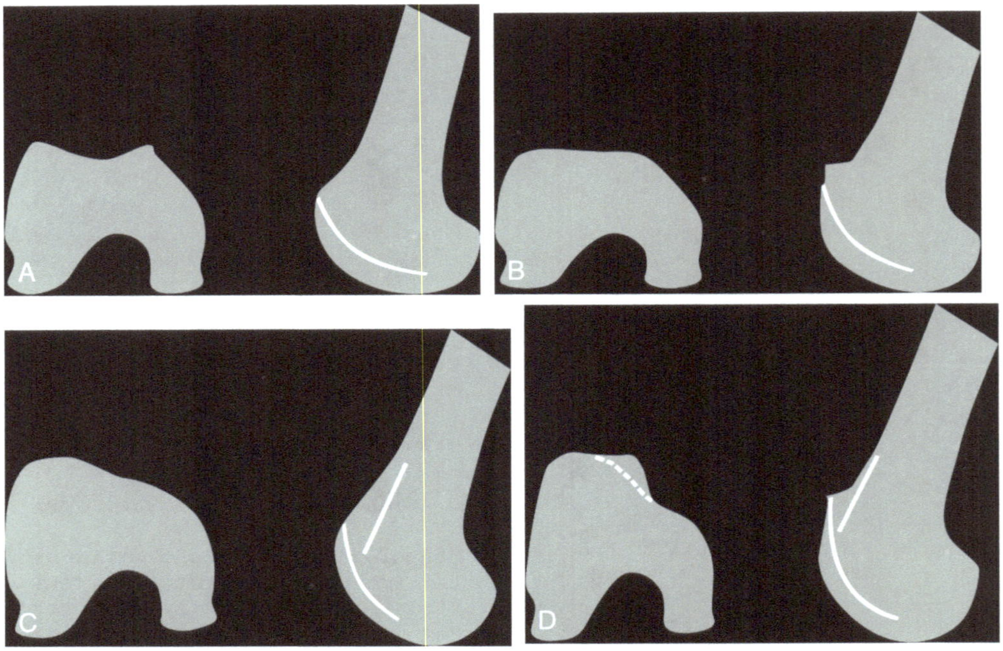

• **Fig. 12.30** Classification by Henri Dejour (see Table 12.2) of morphologic variations in trochlea dysplasia. (A) Grade A: dysplasia of the trochlea. (B) Grade B: dysplasia of the trochlea. (C) Grade C: dysplasia of the trochlea. (D) Grade D: dysplasia of the trochlea.

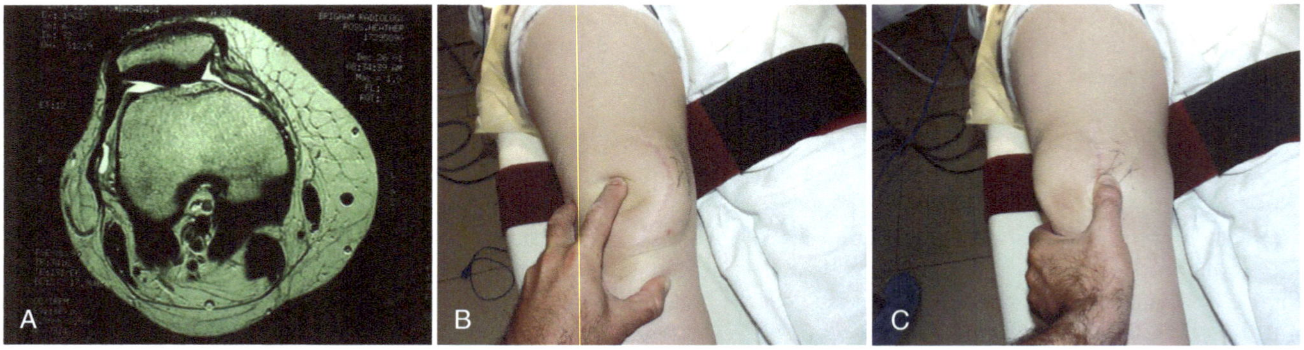

• **Fig. 12.31** (A) Axial image of a CT scan in a young woman who has had previous proximal and distal realignment surgery that has been unsuccessful with continued recurrent patellar instability. The MRI scan notes a flattened proximal trochlea sulcus. (B, C) The same patient as in (A). Note the marked medial and lateral instability of the patella with previous skin incision.

instability secondary to trochlea dysplasia, surgical reconstruction is necessary. With trochlea dysplasia in addition to an abnormal shape to the trochlea with flattening or convexity, there is often too much cartilage present proximally and centrally. This acts as a type of speed bump over which the patella is guided away from the central sulcus in flexion. Removing and contouring the proximal entry point to the patella capture is the goal of a synovial interposition trochleoplasty (Fig. 12.32). This allows the patellofemoral joint to remain congruent because it does not

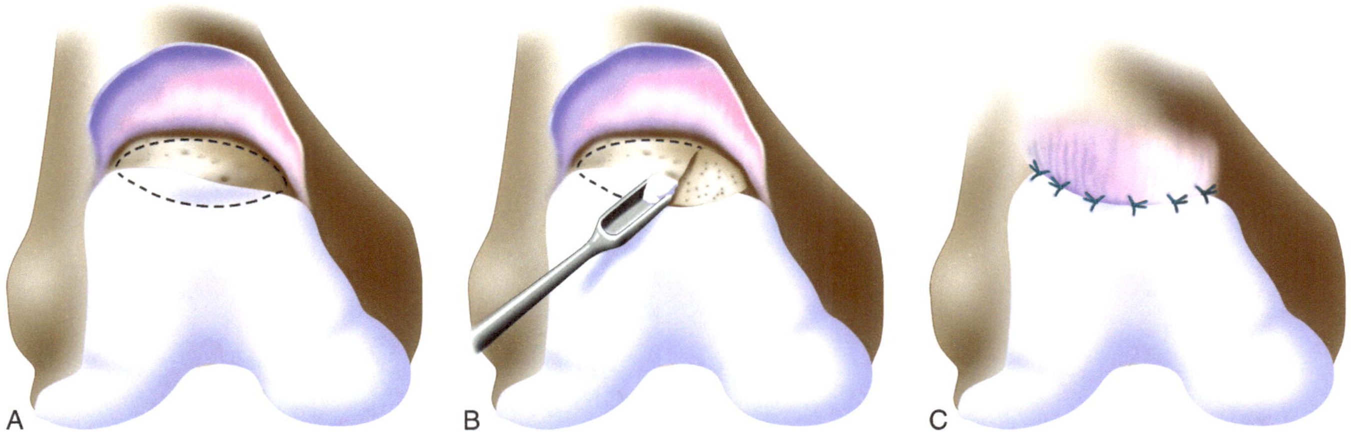

• **Fig. 12.32** (A) Diagram of a Peterson synovial interposition trochleoplasty (as described in Peterson L, Karrlson J, Brittberg M. Patellar instability with recurrent dislocation due to patellofemoral dysplasia. Results after surgical treatment. *Bull Hosp Jt Dis Orthop Inst*. 1988;48:130-139.) The synovium is reflected proximally from the trochlea attachment. The central proximal 1–1.5 cm of cartilage and bone at the level of the lower patellar pole in engagement to the trochlea is removed in line with the intercondylar notch to allow capture of the lower patellar pole into the trochlea. It is recessed toward the anterior femoral cortex. (B) Diagram of removal of cartilage and bone centrally at the most proximal aspect of the trochlea where the initial instability of the patella occurs when it does not find a central leading sulcus. (C) Diagram of the synovium advanced and sewn through the articular surface to allow a congruence and smooth the entry site for the patella to engage into the trochlea.

distort the shape of either articulation. The surgical correction by interposition soft tissue synovial trochleoplasty can be performed with good success.[28] Fig. 12.33 shows the technique used for the case in Fig. 12.32. Another example of interposition trochleoplasty as developed and described by Peterson[28] is given in Chapter 15, case studies.

Bony reconstruction of the trochlea was first described by Albee in 1915.[29] This involved the lateral trochlea osteotomy and elevation with a bone block autograft taken from the proximal tibia and fixated with a bony nail. It was performed through a direct lateral approach, it was successful in stabilizing the patella; however, because of the increased contact forces on the lateral patella facet, it was prone to develop osteoarthrosis.

Dejour has described a bony contouring of the trochlea,[9,30] which has also been successfully performed by others.[31–34] The technique (see Fig. 12.34) involves an open arthrotomy, recession of the synovium from the attachment of the proximal trochlea to expose the distal femur at the entry site of the trochlea. A bur that has a measured resection from the articular surface then excavates bone deep to the proximal articular surface of the trochlea. The central sulcus is then cut with a knife, the medial and lateral trochlea facets are impacted with a bone tamp to form a central sulcus, the osteochondral facets of the trochlea are stabilized with a staple, absorbable screw, or screw that has a countersunk head. The potential complications include delayed or nonunion of the trochlea, chondrolysis, arthrofibrosis, persistent pain because of patellar articular changes, or progression to patellar articular chondrosis secondary to incongruency of the joint.

It is the incongruency of the joint that concerns me specifically and for this reason I have utilized the technique as described by Lars Peterson[28] with synovial interposition advancement.

Awareness of the importance of the shape of the femoral sulcus as a component of patellar instability has gained more acceptance over the last decade. Consequently, surgical deepening of the sulcus has been introduced. The indications, techniques, and rehabilitation as well as evaluation of results are therefore still being systematically sought and clarified. However, recurrent patellar instability after surgical treatment should always raise suspicion of dysplasia of the trochlea.

Patellar Tilt and Subluxation: Radiographic Loss of Joint Space, Patellofemoral Replacement With or Without TTO, Patellofemoral Prosthetic Arthroplasty

When collapse of the joint space radiographically has occurred, as viewed by the Merchant or skyline x-ray image, cartilage repair by ACI is no longer possible. Isolated osteotomy is not possible if paned patellar cartilage loss is present. The procedure relies on intact full-thickness cartilage margins to maintain the joint space so that the growing cartilage repair tissue may fill the defect. If medial or proximal cartilage is absent, a tibial tubercle osteotomy with anterior and medial translation is not effective. In this situation, I have found that for middle-aged patients too young for a total knee replacement, a patellofemoral prosthesis offers pain relief and improved functionality and preserves bone stock. Initially,

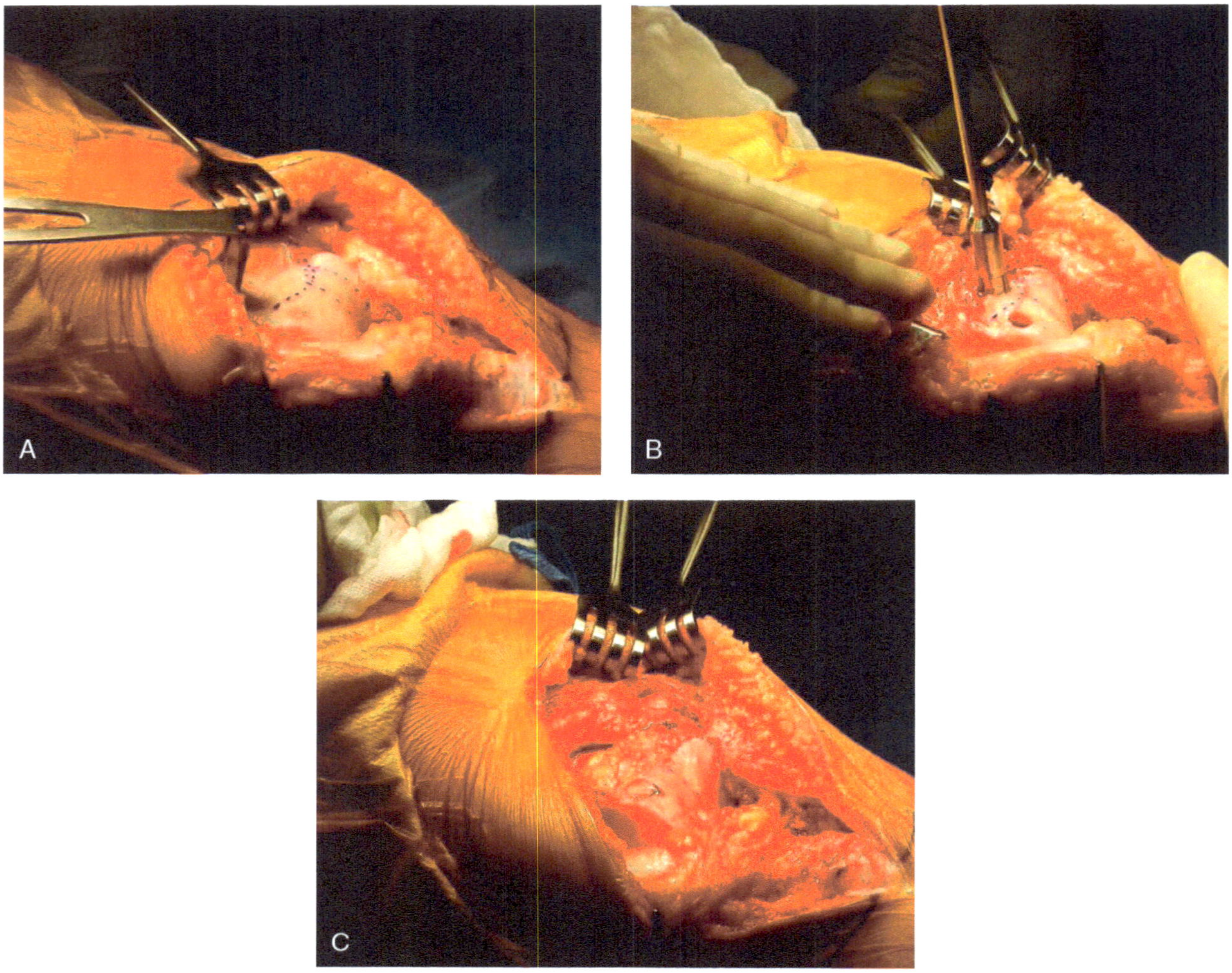

• **Fig. 12.33** (A) Clinical example of a Peterson Interposition Trochleoplasty: open appearance with central markings toward the intercondylar notch demonstrating the central tracking path of the patella. The transverse curvilinear proximal markings represent the cartilage and bone to be removed centering on the distal tracking pathway. (B) A donor osteochondral plug is being harvested from the proposed area of discarded cartilage and bone. The donor osteochondral plug is oversized by 1 mm and measured to the same recipient depth to ensure a good press fit into the recipient site, noted empty on the lateral trochlea. (C) The final appearance of the joint after the synovium has been advanced to the remaining proximal cartilage and bone. The knee joint is closed with a medial advancement of the vastus medialis oblique. One year postoperatively the patient is asymptomatic with no recurrent instability of the patella and an absence of anterior knee pain. The opposite knee has failed open proximal and distal realignment procedures and will also undergo open trochleoplasty to ensure stability. Bilateral disease is common in this condition.

a custom trochlea inset metal prosthesis with a standard polyethylene patella button has been used. A standard medial parapatellar arthrotomy is performed with a standard patellar resurfacing. The trochlea prosthesis is only 3 mm thick and removes little cartilage and bone (Fig. 12.35). It is easily converted to a total knee replacement if the tibiofemoral cartilage degenerates. It does not jeopardize future reconstructions, yet it allows adequate pain relief and functionality for activities of daily living.

Several companies currently offer off-the-shelf implants.

Summary

Patellofemoral disease is one of the most problematic management issues for the orthopedist dealing with knee reconstructive surgery. Once nonoperative management has failed in alleviating pain and improving functionality, a careful assessment to determine the underlying pathomechanics causing the instability and/or degenerative process is necessary for successful management. These factors include limb alignment and patellar pathomechanics, patella alta, an increased quadriceps angle, dysplasia of the trochlea, secondary soft tissue imbalance, and localized chondrosis to the patella and the trochlea.

The management algorithm presented attempts to deal with these identified factors and the secondary degenerative processes. Although MPFL reconstruction has been recently popularized using autograft tendon or allograft tendon, I have found that the native MPFL is nearly always present and attached to the adductor tubercle and may be advanced when necessary. Reconstruction of the MPFL without identifying the other background factors for instability will usually result in persistent instability and pain. When identified carefully, the options of patellar lateral release, anteromedial

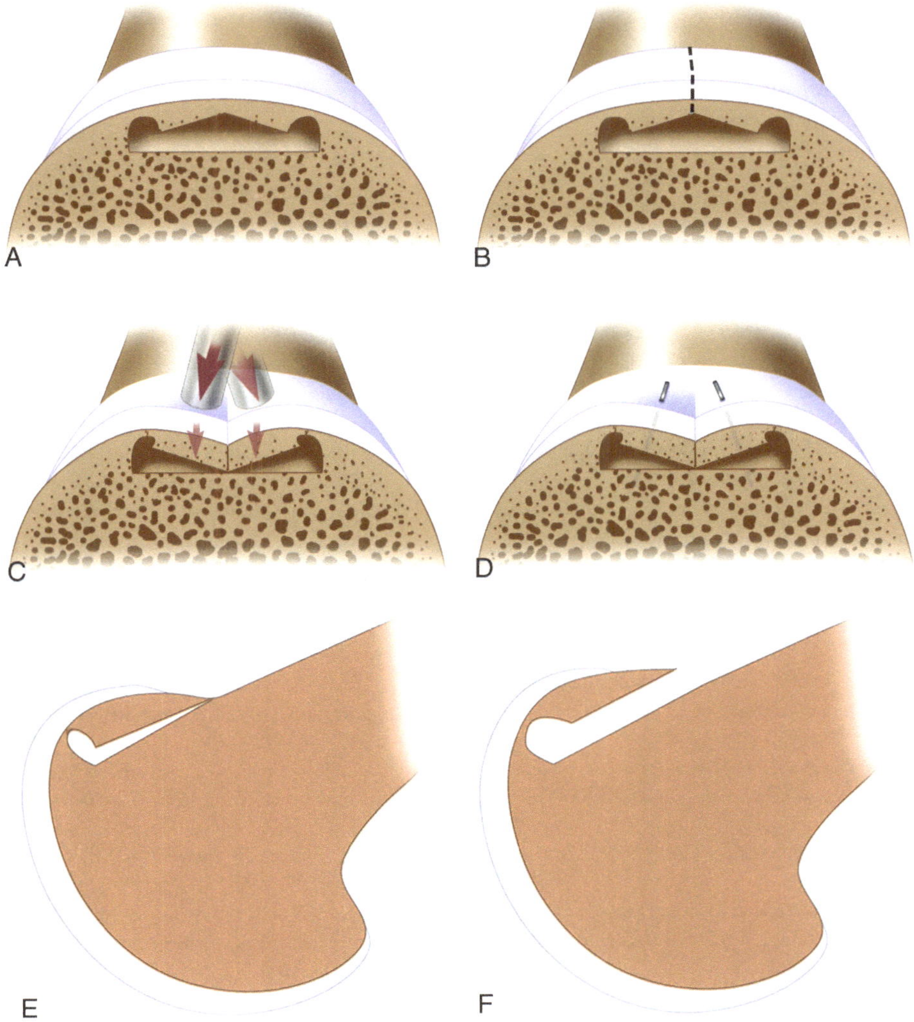

• **Fig. 12.34** The steps in performing a Dejour trochleoplasty. (A) The anterior femoral cortex is exposed proximal to the trochlea by elevating and moving proximal the synovium and leaving it intact. Using a measured distance micro-bur, bone is removed at a fixed distance posterior to the articular cartilage. It is then thinned out centrally toward the intercondylar notch, and transversely and distally (E, F). (B) A knife blade is used centrally to break through where the bone is maximally thinned out. (C) A bone tamp is used to implode the medial and lateral trochlea facets to create a central sulcus. (D) The bone is fixated traditionally with a staple, but metal screws with the heads countersunk or bioabsorbable screws are now utilized. The synovium is then readvanced to the articular cartilage margin and resutured through it to maintain a soft tissue sleeve to the articular surface and the articular surface flush to the anterior femoral cortical surface. (E, F) Diagram of the subchondral bone transversely and distally. At the time of impaction of the medial and lateral trochlea facets, the entire articular surface plastically deforms to meet the anterior femoral cortex in the sagittal plane.

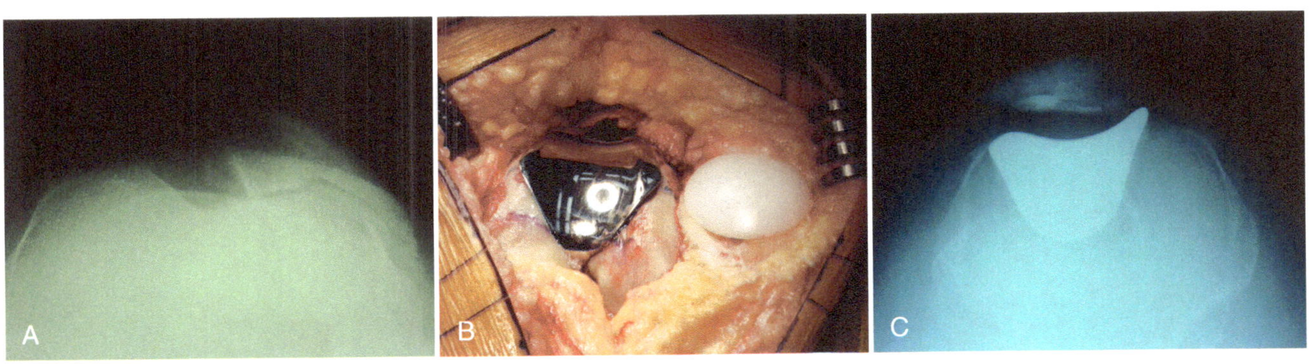

• **Fig. 12.35** (A) Merchant x-ray view demonstrating obliteration of the articular joint space. (B) Intraoperative appearance of a patella femoral prosthetic resurfacing using a standard patella from an existing knee system with a custom design inset trochlea metal implant that is 3 mm thick, which is very bone-preserving. (C) Merchant x-ray view demonstrating postoperative appearance of patellofemoral prosthesis.

tibial tubercle osteotomy with MPFL advancement and soft tissue balancing, trochleoplasty, ACI, and a unicompartmental patellofemoral prosthesis in cases of end-stage patellofemoral OA with collapse of the joint space will provide improved functionality and pain relief for young patients suffering from patellofemoral pain.

References

1. Aroen A, Loken S, Heir S, et al. Articular cartilage lesions in 993 consecutive knee arthroscopies. *Am J Sports Med.* 2004;32:211–215.
2. Curl WW, Krome J, Gordon ES, et al. Cartilage injuries: a review of 31,516 knee arthroscopies. *Arthroscopy.* 1997;13: 456–460.
3. Hjelle K, Solheim E, Strand T, et al. Articular cartilage defects in 1,000 knee arthroscopies. *Arthroscopy.* 2002;18:730–734.
4. Kaplan LD, Schurhoff MR, Selesnick H, et al. Magnetic resonance imaging of the knee in asymptomatic professional basketball players. *Arthroscopy.* 2005;21:557–561.
5. Nomura E, Inoue M, Kurimura M. Chondral and osteochondral injuries associated with acute patellar dislocation. *Arthroscopy.* 2003;19:717–721.
6. France L, Nester C. Effect of errors in the identification of anatomical landmarks on the accuracy of Q angle values. *Clin Biomech (Bristol, Avon).* 2001;16:710–713.
7. Greene C, Edwards TB, Wade MR, et al. Reliability of the quadriceps angle measurement. *Am J Knee Surg.* 2001;14:97–103.
8. Aglietti P, Insall JN, Cerulli G. Patellar pain and incongruence. I: measurements of incongruence. *Clin Orthop Relat Res.* 1983;176:217–224.
9. Dejour H, Walch G, Nove-Josserand L, et al. Factors of patellar instability: an anatomic radiographic study. *Knee Surg Sports Traumatol Arthrosc.* 1994;2:19–26.
10. Winalski C, Aliabadi P, Wright R, et al. Enhancement of joint fluid with intravenously administered gadopentetate dimeglumine: technique, rationale, and implications. *Radiology.* 1993;187:179–185.
11. Alparslan L, Winalski C, Boutin R, et al. Postoperative magnetic resonance imaging of articular cartilage repair. *Semin Musculoskelet Radiol.* 2001;5:345–363.
12. Beaconsfield T, Pintore E, Maffulli N, Petri GJ. Radiological measurements in patellofemoral disorders. A review. *Clin Orthop Relat Res.* 1994;308:18–28.
13. Schoettle PB, Zanetti M, Seifert B, Pfirrmann CWA, Fucentese SF, Romero J The tibial tuberosity–trochlear groove distance; a comparative study between CT and MRI scanning. Knee. 2006;13:26–31.
14. Caton J, Deschamps G, Chambat P, et al. Patella infera. Apropos of 128 cases [French]. *Rev Chir Orthop Reparatrice Appar Mot.* 1982;68:317–325.
15. Fulkerson JP. Anteromedialization of the tibial tuberosity for patellofemoral malalignment. *Clin Orthop Relat Res.* 1983, 177:176–181.
16. Trillat A, Dejour H, Couette A. Diagnosis and treatment of recurrent dislocations of the patella [French]. *Rev Chir Orthop Reparatrice Appar Mot.* 1964;50(Nov-Dec):813–824.
17. Pidoriano AJ, Weinstein RN, Buuck DA, et al. Correlation of patellar articular lesions with results from anteromedial tibial tubercle transfer. *Am J Sports Med.* 1997;25:533–537.
18. Minas T, Bryant T. The role of autologous chondrocyte implantation in the patellofemoral joint. *Clin Orthop Relat Res.* 2005: 436:30–39.
19. Fulkerson JP. Patellofemoral pain disorders: evaluation and management. *J Am Acad Orthop Surg.* 1994;2:124–132.
20. Gomoll AH, Minas T, Farr J, et al. Treatment of chondral defects in the patellofemoral joint. *J Knee Surg.* 2006;19:285–295.
21. Cox J. An evaluation of the Elmslie-Trillat procedure for management of patellar dislocations and subluxations: a preliminary report. *Am J Sports Med.* 1976;4(2):72–77. Mar-Apr.
22. Barber F, McGarry J. Elmslie-Trillat procedure for the treatment of recurrent patellar instability. *Arthroscopy.* 2008;24(1):77–81.
23. Bellemans J, Cauwenberghs F, Brys P, et al. Fracture of the proximal tibia after Fulkerson anteromedial tibial tubercle transfer. A report of four cases. *Am J Sports Med.* 1998;26(2):300–302. Mar-Apr.
24. Stetson W, Friedman M, Fulkerson J, et al. Fracture of the proximal tibia with immediate weightbearing after a Fulkerson osteotomy. *Am J Sports Med.* 1997;25(4):570–574. Jul-Aug.
25. Masri B, Kim W, Pagnano M. Mini-subvastus approach for minimally invasive total knee replacement. *Tech Knee Surg.* 2007;6(2):124–130.
26. Minas T, Peterson L. Advanced techniques in autologous chondrocyte transplantation. *Clin Sports Med.* 1999;18:13–44, v-vi.
27. Dejour H, Walch G, Neyret P, Adeleine P. Dysplasia of the femoral trochlea [French]. *Rev Chir Orthop Reparatrice Appar Mot.* 1990;76(1):45–54.
28. Peterson L, Karrlson J, Brittberg M. Patellar instability with recurrent dislocation due to patellofemoral dysplasia. Results after surgical treatment. *Bull Hosp Jt Dis Orthop Inst.* 1988;48:130–139.
29. Albee F. The bone graft wedge in the treatment for habitual dislocation of the patella. *Med Rec.* 1915;88:257–259.
30. Dejour H, Walch G, Nayret P, Adeleine P, Dysplasia of the femoral trochlea [French]. *Rev Chir Orthop Reparatrice Appar Mot.* 1990;76(1):45–54.
31. von Knoch F, Böhm T, Bürgi M, et al. Trochleaplasty for recurrent patellar dislocation in association with trochlear dysplasia: a 4- to 14-year follow-up study. *J Bone Joint Surg Br.* 2006;88-B:1331–1335.
32. Verdonk R, Jansegers E, Stuyts B. Trochleoplasty in dysplastic knee trochlea. *Knee Surg Sports Traumatol Arthrosc.* 2005;13:529–533.
33. Schottle P, Fucentese S, Pfirrmann C, et al. Trochleaplasty for patellar instability due to trochlear dysplasia. *Acta Orthop Scand.* 2005;76:693–698.
34. Donell ST. Deepening trochleoplasty for distal femoral dysplasia in patellar instability: thick osteochondral flap technique. *Tech Knee Surg.* 2008;7:19–26.

13

Treatment of Deep Osteochondritis Dissecans Lesions, Avascular Necrosis, and Osteochondral Defects of the Knee Using Autologous Bone Grafting

TOM MINAS, MD, MS

CHAPTER OUTLINE

Introduction

The management of an osteochondral defect in the knee is one of the most difficult conditions for the orthopedist. Although a fresh osteochondral allograft seems to be the treatment of choice for this condition, allografts are not without their own problems. A size match may be difficult to obtain and only available in certain parts of the world and resorption and collapse of the allograft are a possibility in the first 2 years after transplantation in approximately 25%–30% of cases. For these reasons, if an osteochondral defect is well contained, my preferred treatment is for the use of autologous bone graft (ABG) or ABG plus cells, i.e., matrix-induced autologous chondrocyte implantation (MACI) sandwich technique. In parts of the world where MACI is not available, ABG alone may be highly effective but not as durable. Certainly, for small focal deep osteochondral areas of damage, a cancellous ABG is a very reasonable first-choice treatment. I reserve the use of a fresh osteochondral allograft for a defect that is peripherally uncontained and not suitable for autologous bone grafting or a failed cartilage surgery such as a failed ACI procedure.

Osteochondritis Dissecans

Osteochondritis dissecans (OCD) has undergone many treatment strategies from surgical excision as advocated more than 150 years ago[1] to osteochondral autogenous transplants (OATS).[2–4]

The disease is rare under the age of 10 years and over the age of 50 years.[5] The male-to-female ratio has been reported as 2:1[6] or 3:1[7] with bilateral involvement in up to 33%.[8] The medial femoral condyle is affected approximately ¾ of the time[5] with ¾ of the lesions affecting the lateral (intercondylar) portion of the medial femoral condyle. Kindreds with clear hereditary patterns have been documented[9] as well as evidence to suggest no clear pattern of familial tendency.[10]

Many etiologies have been proposed; repetitive microtrauma and impingement of the tibial spine,[11] stress fractures with no identifying trauma,[12] as well as a vascular insult.[13] However, vascular studies of the end of the femur have demonstrated a rich vascular plexus to intramedullary cancellous bone, making this etiology unlikely,[14] and histological evaluation of specimens removed at surgery have demonstrated viable bone and cartilage and not empty lacunae.[15]

Classification and Management

The categorization of the disease process into juvenile and adult forms is important at the time of diagnosis because the treatment and prognosis may be managed by different treatment algorithms dependent on the stage of disease.[16,17]

However, there is consistent agreement that the fate of knees treated by removal of OCD fragments that are detached from the weight-bearing femoral condyles do poorly.[18–21] Linden reported that on average at 33-year follow-up of patients clinically and radiographically, 38 of 48 patients who had had the first manifestation after closure of the physes (i.e., adult form) had symptomatic and radiographic gonarthrosis. Linden noted "Symptoms and roentgenographic gonarthrosis become more frequent and approach 100 per cent with time" (see Fig. 13.1).[22]

Cystic degeneration deep to the lesion in situ may also occur and this makes bone healing especially difficult even in the juvenile form (Fig. 13.2).

Treatment by removal of the fragment and drilling to promote fibrocartilage repair is also not recommended because the repair tissue is not durable and will break down.[23–25]

Treatment aimed at assessing the stability of the OCD fragment and obtaining union, by casting immobilization in a stable juvenile fragment, or in-situ flap, to fixation with or without autogenous bone grafting by open or arthroscopic techniques is optimal treatment. This is really the treatment of choice in the adult form (Fig. 13.3). An unstable OCD lesion, assessed for the underlying bony attachment by CT scan and then fixated to the underlying bony bed by standard AO principles of a delayed union with curettage, autologous bone grafting, vascularization of the defect by drilling, and rigid internal fixation give the best results.

In the failed treatment of OCD with an empty defect or fragmented lesion, autologous chondrocyte implantation, autologous osteochondral grafting or osteochondral allograft treatments are treatment options. ACI has the advantage of being autologous tissue in a young patient, with the potential to resurface large areas without donor site morbidity, as in osteochondral autograft transfers. Most defects may be managed by ACI alone when bone deficiency centrally is less than 6–8 mm deep (see Chapter 9).[26]

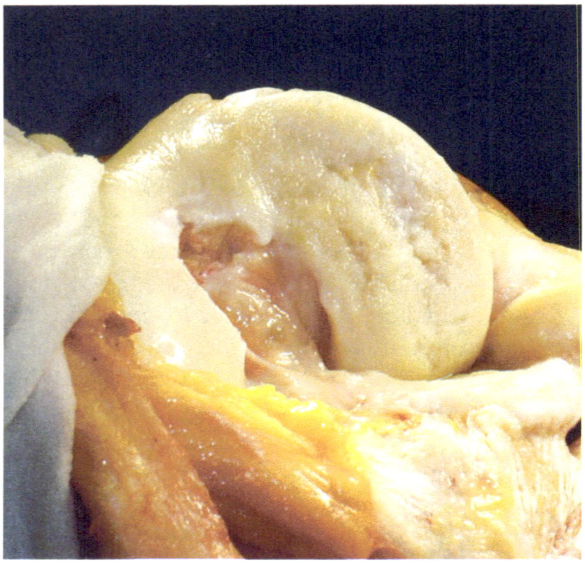

• **Fig. 13.1** A 44-year-old man with typical appearance of an osteochondritis dissecans lesion after the fragment had been removed.

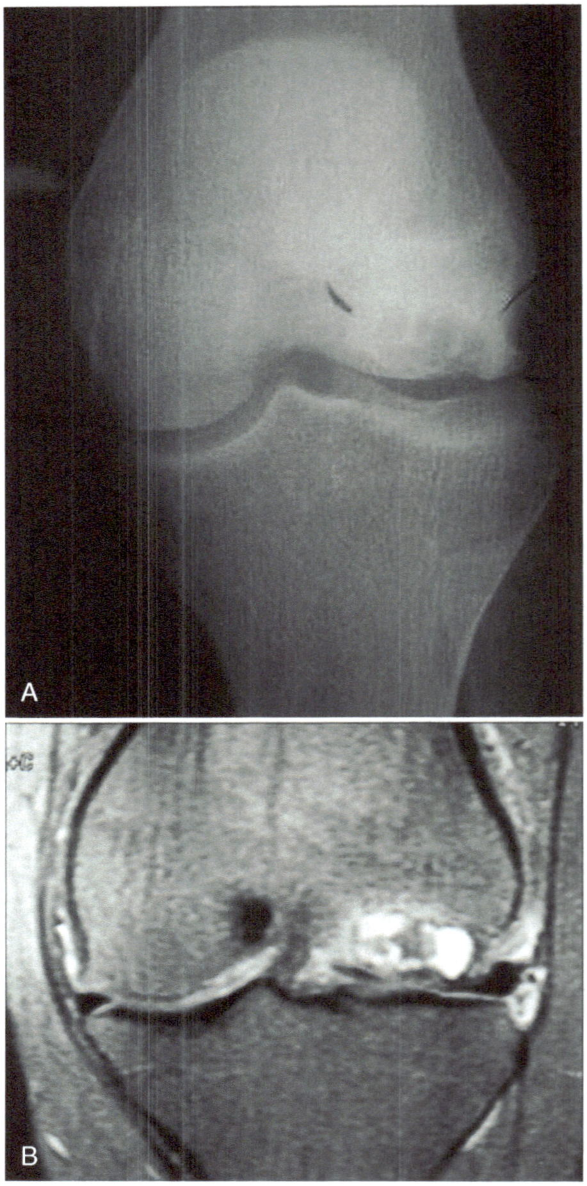

• **Fig. 13.2** (A) Anteroposterior x-ray film in an 18-year-old woman with lateral femoral condyle osteochondritis dissecans that has not been surgically treated. A degenerative cystic form of the condition is apparent by x-ray film and by magnetic resonance imaging (B).

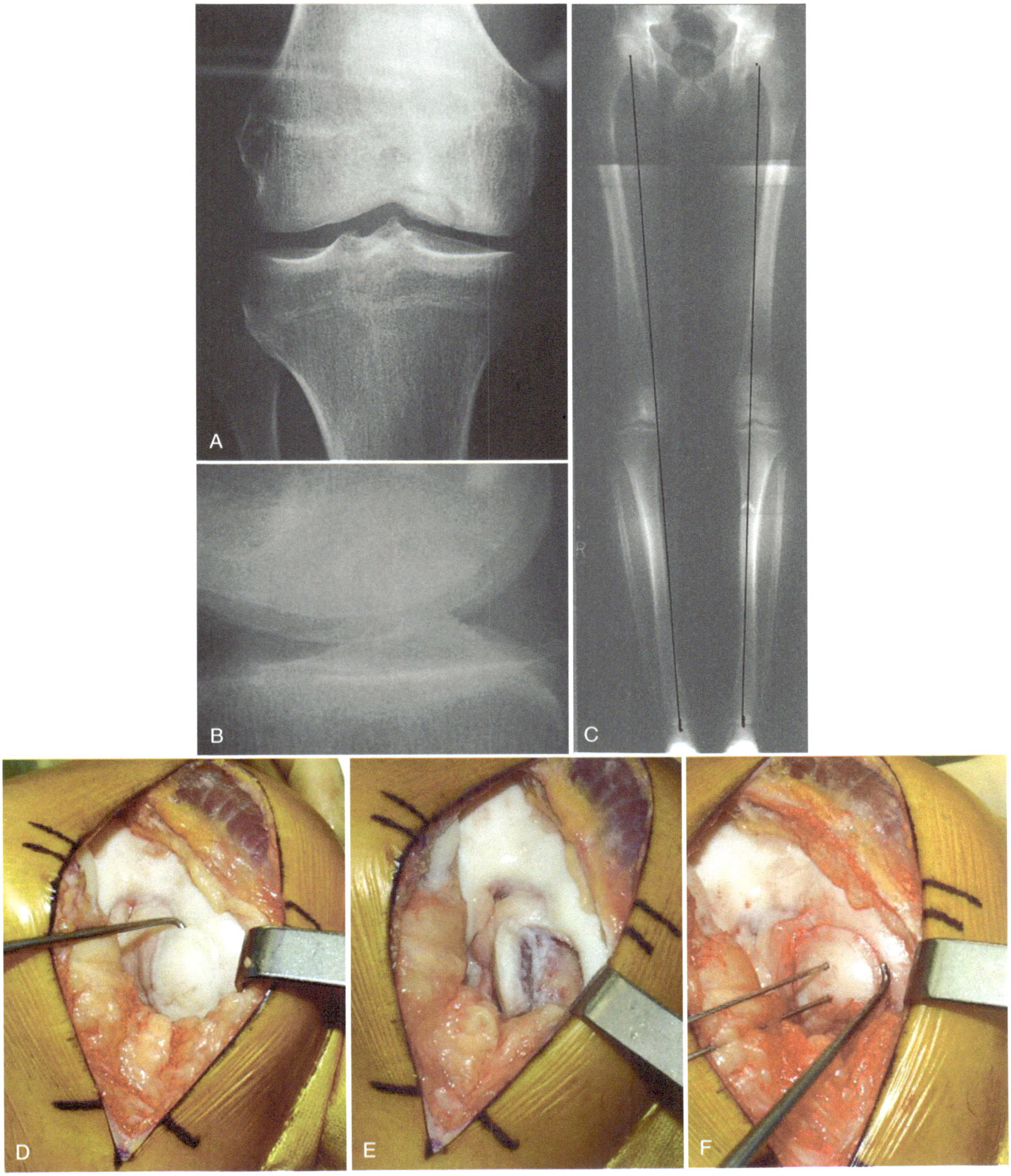

• **Fig. 13.3** A 21-year-old male college hockey player with an unstable painful medial femoral condyle osteochondritis dissecans (OCD) lesion that has failed arthroscopic stabilization with absorbable tack fixation. Persistent catching, swelling, pain, and limp are presenting symptoms. The treatment plan includes open surgical reduction internal fixation, removal of fibrous tissue at the base of the defect and undersurface of the fragment, drilling the subchondral bone to promote vascularization of the fragment, and autologous bone grafting with stable internal fixation per classic principles of treatment of a nonunion. Later removal of the internal fixation is performed. (A) Anteroposterior x-ray film demonstrates classic medial OCD lesion with a large bony fragment. (B) Lateral x-ray film. (C) Long alignment x-ray films demonstrate a varus knee with mechanical axis in the medial compartment. (D) Open appearance of un-united fragment in situ with cracked articular cartilage surface. (E) The fragment is hinged on its vascular attachment to the posterior cruciate ligament synovium toward the intercondylar notch. This maintains stability of the fragment so that it does not fall out of the wound. Note the chronic appearance of the defect base. The fragment is covered with fibrous tissue and has underlying sclerotic bone. (F) The underlying fibrous tissue and sclerotic bone are removed, autogenous bone graft from the upper tibia is placed to restore the proper anatomic location of the fragments because they tend to subside, and cannulated screw guidewires are used to check the reduction before screw fixation is performed.

Continued

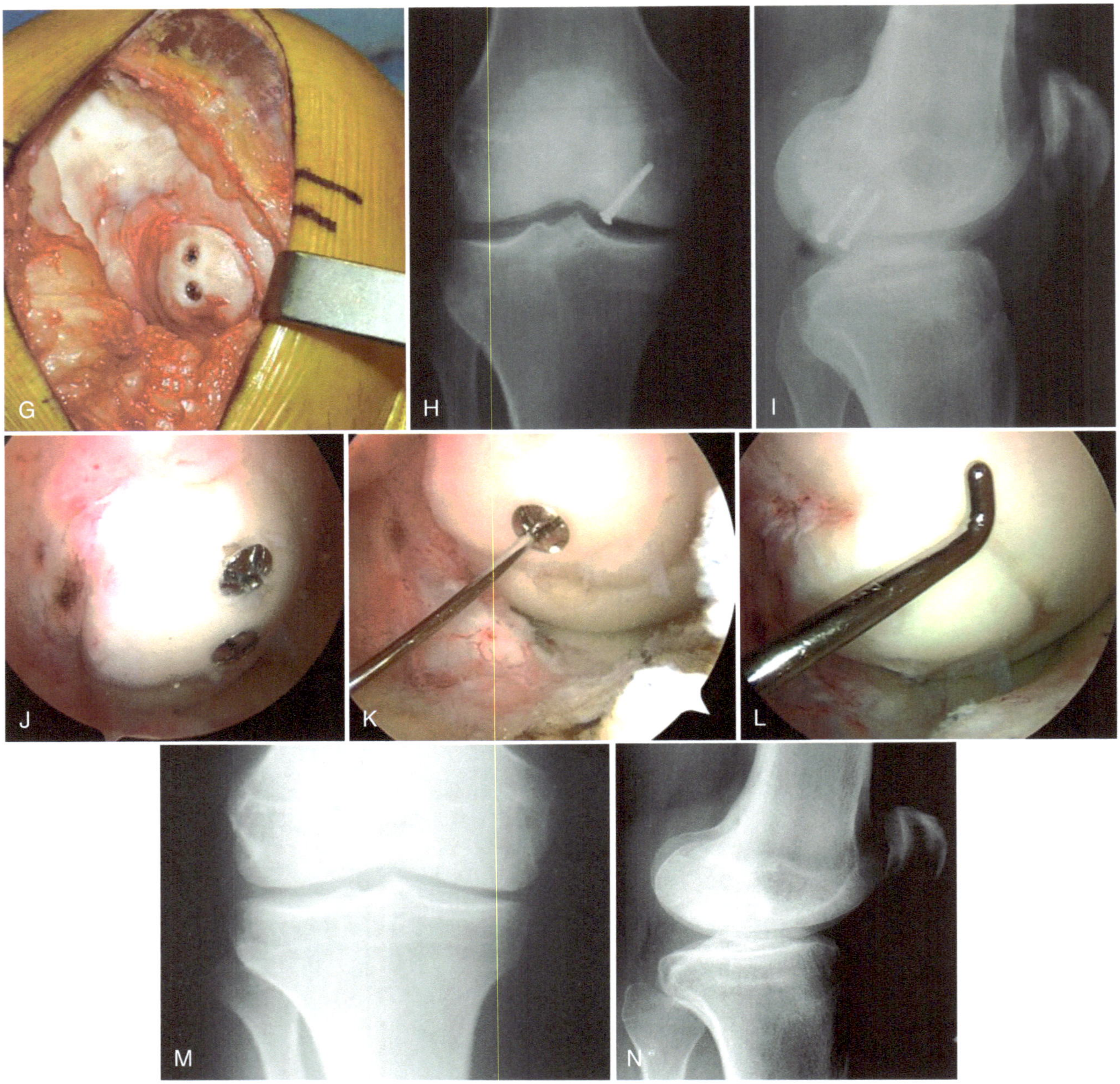

• **Fig. 13.3 Cont'd** (G) Cannulated screw fixation with anatomic reduction after curettage and bone grafting. The screw heads are buried below the articular surface to avoid damaging the tibial surface. (H) Postoperative anteroposterior x-ray film showing anatomic reduction. (I) Postoperative lateral x-ray film. (J) Eight weeks postoperatively, the hardware is removed arthroscopically before weight bearing is permitted. (K) The cannulated screw guidewires simplify screw removal. (L) The fragment is probed carefully to assess congruency and stability. Full weight bearing is allowed postoperatively, but sports are restricted for another 4 months to allow solid healing and bone remodeling. Anteroposterior (M) and lateral (N) x-ray films 1 year after treatment show solid healing of the OCD fragment. The patient returned the following season to varsity-level hockey. He remains asymptomatic after 7 years of follow-up.

When there are cystic changes under the defect as in Fig. 13.2 or the defect has near vertical walls and is greater than 8–10 mm deep or is very sclerotic due to a chronic lesion that may have undergone drilling, abrasion, or microfracture, it is safer to remove the unhealthy bed and bone graft the defect. The bone grafting technique is much like the preparation of a dental amalgam and is described in detail in Fig. 13.4.

In situations with defects requiring bone grafts, a staged bone grafting and later ACI (6–9 months) is an option. It is more likely that Stage 2 ACI will be necessary if the defects are large (>8–10 cm^2) (Fig. 13.5).

When the defects are smaller, 2–3 cm^2, it is more likely that ABG will be successful; however, attention to axial alignment is crucial (Fig. 13.6).[26] This had been our preferred treatment some 20 years ago before the development of the ACI sandwich technique. However, with the excellent and superior clinical outcomes and survivorship of ACI sandwich technique over ABG, this is no longer the case.

I feel that for large defects (average surface area 7 cm² with >1 cm deep), ACI sandwich technique is the best first-line treatment. Our clinical results with ACI sandwich technique compared with ABG alone demonstrate a 10-year survivorship of 87% versus 45%.[27]

For those few ACI sandwich cases that fail, the last biologic preservation prior to a unicompartmental knee arthroplasty remains a fresh osteochondral allograft. I prefer osteochondral allograft treatment as a salvage option for the management of OCD and not the preferred treatment. A failed allograft is a difficult problem to salvage biologically.

Avascular Necrosis

Osteonecrosis of the knee classically includes two distinct entities: spontaneous or secondary osteonecrosis.[28–31] Spontaneous osteonecrosis occurs most often in patients over 55 years of age, unilaterally and in one compartment of the knee. Secondary osteonecrosis could be secondary to corticosteroid therapy, renal and systemic disease, or barotrauma, and occurs most often in younger patients with bilateral multicompartmental disease. For both types of osteonecrosis, the natural evolution without treatment is arthritis.[28,31]

Four stages of the radiographic evolution of the lesion have been described according to Mont et al.[30] In the first stage, the knee maintains a normal aspect. In the second stage, cystic or osteosclerotic lesions are observed with normal contour, whereas subchondral collapse is observed in Stage 3. In Stage 4, a narrowing of the joint is observed.[30] For Stages 1, 2, and 3, core decompression,[30] arthroscopic debridement, or high tibial osteotomy[32] have been used with success. Stage 4 is associated with severe clinical symptoms and unicompartmental or total knee arthroplasty is recommended in the literature.

I have found that the idiopathic form of osteonecrosis is frequently isolated to the medial femoral condyle in a middle-aged male with a varus knee. My treatment for Ficat Stage III and IV disease would include a valgus-producing

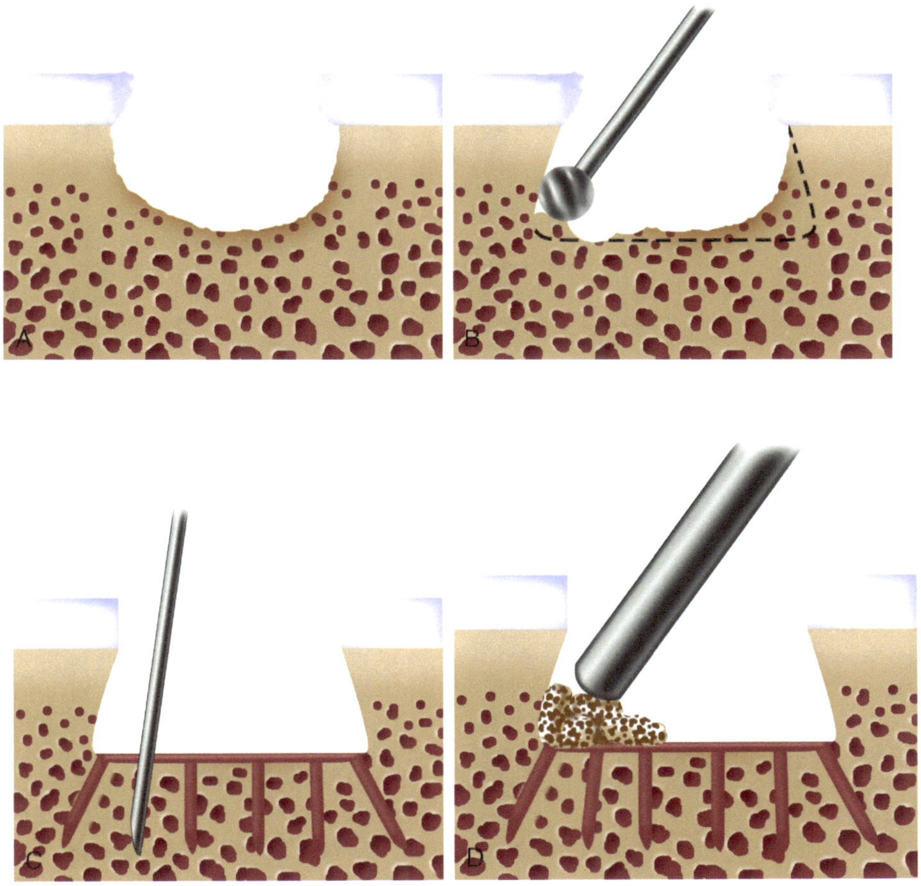

• **Fig. 13.4** Technique for autologous bone grafting of an osteochondral defect. (A) Defect that is suitable for bone grafting has steep side walls, subchondral cysts, or sclerotic subchondral bone after failed prior marrow stimulation techniques. (B) The defect is prepared as if it were a dental amalgam preparation. A high-speed bur, usually 5-mm diameter, removes all the subchondral sclerotic bone back to healthy-appearing spongy bone. The cartilage margins are undermined so that the deeper area of the defect is larger than the opening to assist in containing the morselized spongy bone after the defect is adequately prepared. (C) The base of the defect is drilled to assist in vascularizing the bone graft. (D) Autologous cancellous morselized bone chips are impacted peripherally and then centrally up to the level of the native subchondral bone plate. The autograft is usually harvested from the proximal tibial metaphysic using a 10-mm osteochondral autograft transfer system harvester (OATS, Arthrex, Naples, FL), with allograft bone substitute backfill (cadaver cancellous chips preferred).

Continued

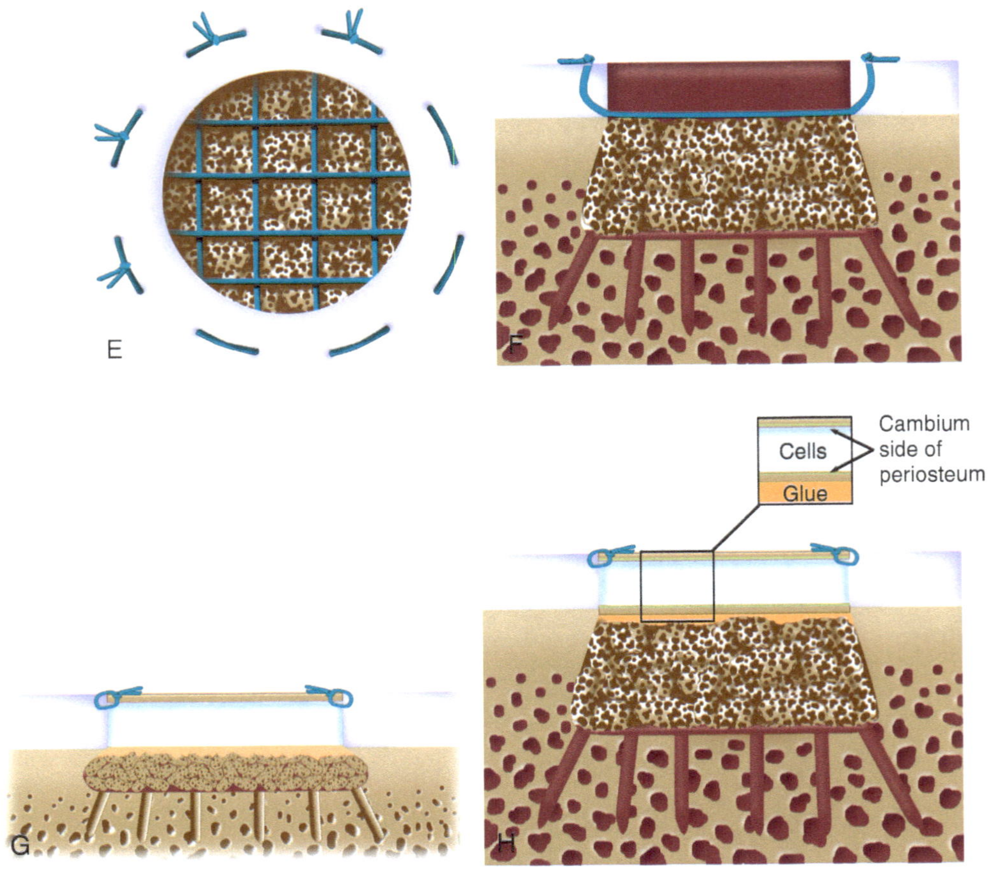

• **Fig. 13.4 Cont'd** (E) To ensure that the chips remain in place, an absorbable 5.0 or 6.0 Vicryl suture is woven across the articular surface. This is done only if there is concern about bone graft stability and is required only occasionally. (F) With the knee joint in full extension to allow the bone grafted area to be further contained by the opposing tibial surface, the tourniquet is let down. The knee is left alone for 3 to 5 minutes to allow the marrow elements to permeate the bone graft to the articular surface and form a "super clot" as in the technique of microfracture. The joint is not irrigated to avoid disturbing the "super clot." A drain, if used, is placed away from the treated defect. This marrow-derived clot allows fibrocartilage resurfacing of the bone graft (see panel H). (G) Alternatively, the bone graft and clot can be protected with a membrane of periosteum or synthetic type I to III collagen. (H) Sandwich technique autologous chondrocyte implantation in addition to autologous bone grafting. When periosteum is used, the two cambium layers face each other, and the cells are injected and "sandwiched" between them (see Chapter 9).

osteotomy with autologous bone grafting to the necrotic segment. The osteotomy is usually a closing wedge valgus-producing osteotomy to provide a source of bone for the autograft after excision of the diseased medial osteochondral segment (Fig. 13.7). The osteonecrotic bone segment secondary to steroid usage usually involves a more generalized segment of the entire distal femur. In these cases, I have found that fresh osteochondral allografts are more useful as the area of resorption and collapse is more diffuse and not amenable to a localized autologous bone graft.

Clinical Results—Case Series—Technique for the Treatment of Deep Contained Osteochondral Defects

This study was a prospective, non-randomized trial of 14 patients, 10 (Group 1) with large OCD defects and 4 (Group 2) with avascular necrosis (AVN) of the knee. Patients were treated with autologous bone grafting after excision of necrotic bone or sclerotic defects (first presented at the ICRS Congress Meeting 2002, Toronto, Canada). Concomitant realignment procedures of the patellofemoral joint and femorotibial joint were performed if indicated to correct patellar maltracking or varus deformity with medial joint space narrowing. The autologous bone graft was held in place with a suturing technique or periosteum if autologous bone graft (ABG) was unstable. Symptoms at 6 to 12 months after autologous bone grafting warranted subsequent treatment with ACI in four of the ten Group 1 OCD patients and one of the four Group 2 AVN patients.

The average surface area of the Group 1 defects was 6.6 cm^2 (range 2–12 cm^2). These lesions had an average depth of 1.5 cm (range 0.8–3.0 cm). Average preoperative and postoperative femorotibial angles for Group 1 were 3.5 degrees and 6.5 degrees, and 8 degrees valg respectively; 5/10 had high tibial valgus osteotomy (HTO). The average surface area of the Group 2 defects was 6.7 cm^2 (range

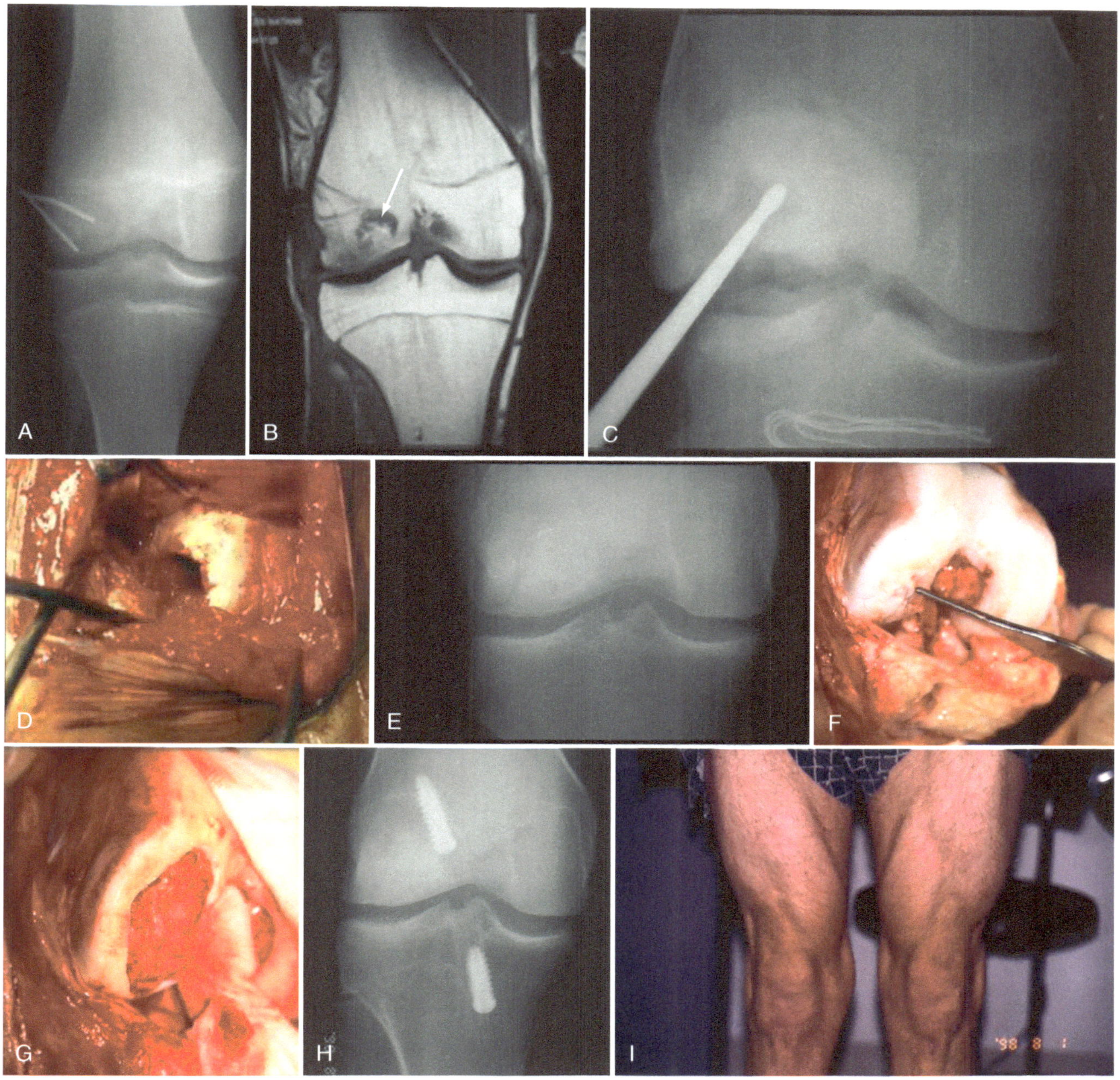

• **Fig. 13.5** Case presentation of a 17-year-old boy with chronic lateral femoral condyle osteochondritis dissecans lesion that has failed open reduction internal fixation and debridement and now has cystic degeneration in addition to anterior cruciate ligament (ACL) insufficiency. He presents with severe leg atrophy, effusions, and laterally based pain and requires double crutch ambulation. (A) Anteroposterior x-ray film showing failed open reduction internal fixation. (B) Magnetic resonance imaging demonstrates a large subchondral lateral femoral condyle cyst. (C) Anteroposterior x-ray images of the intraoperative appearance to demonstrate complete removal of the cystic cavity. (D) Open lateral arthrotomy photo after curettage. Autologous bone grafting (ABG) followed from the ipsilateral iliac crest (performed in 1995). Today ABG would be harvested with osteochondral autograft transfer system harvesters from the proximal tibia with a single-entry corticotomy and the tibia would be backfilled with allograft freeze-dried cadaver cancellous bone chips. (E) Anteroposterior radiograph 9 months later demonstrating well-healed lateral femoral condyle. (F) Intraoperative appearance with fibrous repair over lateral femoral condyles. Some of the condyles have not repaired with fibrous tissue and remain bare bone. (G) After radical debridement of fibrous repair tissue and autologous chondrocyte implantation (ACI). (H) Anteroposterior radiograph after ACI to lateral femoral condyles with ACL autogenous bone tendon bone autograft patellar tendon reconstruction and interference screw fixation. (I) Final clinical appearance 2 years postoperatively shows marked improvement of muscle tone and lessened atrophy of the right thigh after reconstruction. The patient remains asymptomatic and functioning at a high level 14 years later.

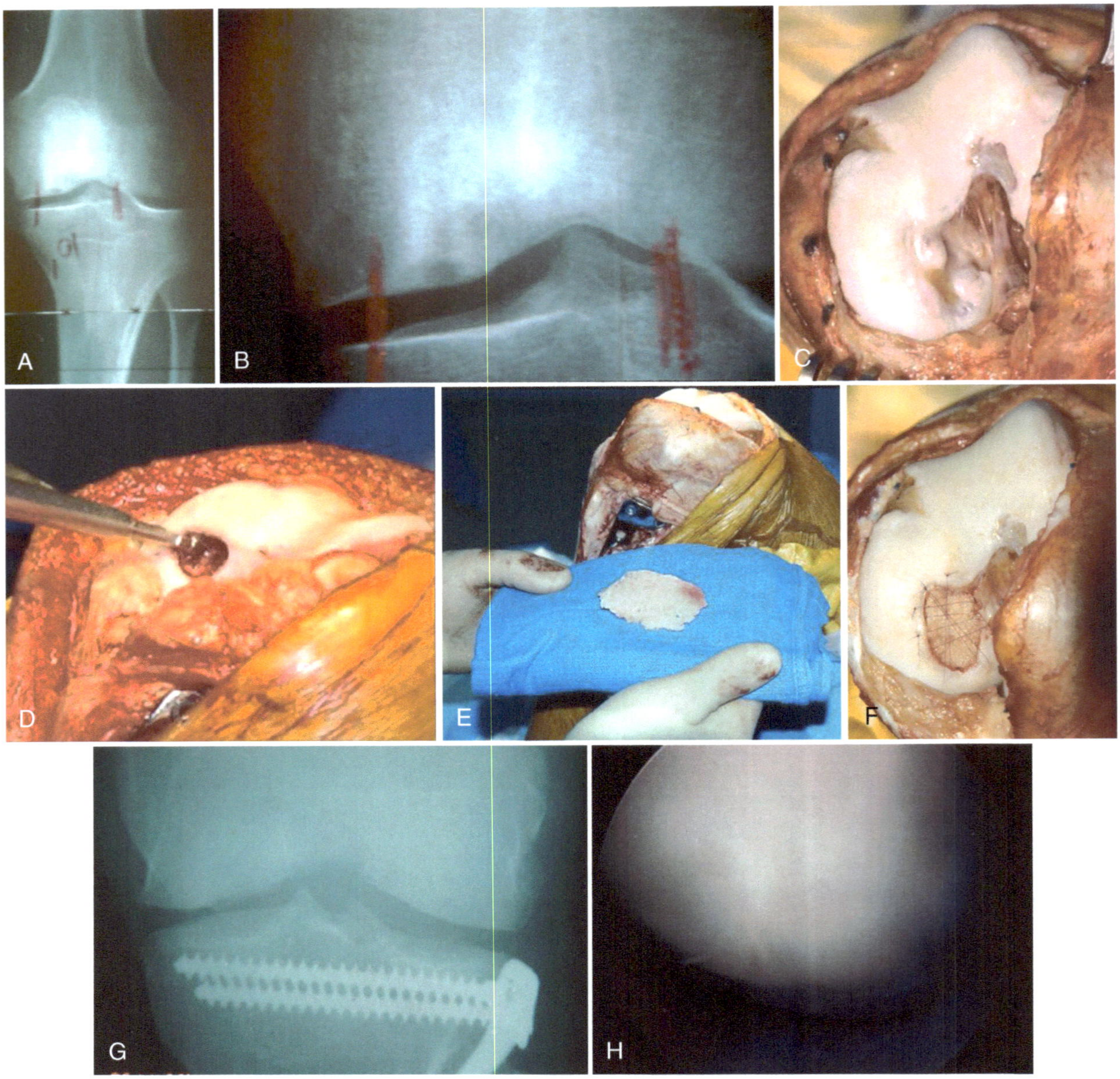

• **Fig. 13.6** Case presentation of a 23-year-old man who has chronic left medial joint pain after arthroscopic removal of loose fragments to the medial femoral condyle osteochondritis dissecans. The patient has varus malalignment with medial compartment pain. He is treated with a closing wedge valgus-producing osteotomy and autologous bone grafting to the medial femoral condyles with an excellent long-term clinical result. (A) Anteroposterior radiograph demonstrates medial femoral condyle osteochondritis dissecans empty defect. A 10-degree correction is required to place the mechanical axis to the lateral tibial spine. (B) Close-up radiograph demonstrates the cystic nature of the medial femoral condyle. (C) Open appearance of the empty defect on the medial femoral condyle adjacent to the intercondylar notch posterior cruciate ligament. (D) Radical debridement of the sclerotic and cystic changes on the medial femoral condyles requires a high-speed bur to develop an amalgam type of defect for autologous bone grafting and repair of the medial femoral condyle defect. (E) A 10-degree corrective closing wedge tibial valgus-producing osteotomy is performed. The cancellous bone from the closing wedge osteotomy and the lateral L-plate for the closing wedge osteotomy are shown. This bone is morselized and used to fill the defect, which has been prepared with a high-speed bur to the medial femoral condyle. (F) The morselized cancellous bone is compacted into the medial femoral condyle until it is flush with the subchondral bone. It is reinforced with absorbable 5.0 Vicryl sutures as a fishnet type of reinforcement to the surface to prevent loss of bone graft. The knee is brought into full extension, the tourniquet is let down, and a marrow clot fills the surface of the bone graft. A rehabilitation program per a marrow stimulation technique with continuous passive motion and protected weight bearing for 6 weeks is followed to allow fibrocartilage repair to the surface of the medial femoral condyle. (G) Postoperative anteroposterior x-ray film after complete healing of the tibial valgus-producing osteotomy with maintenance of joint space on weight-bearing film. (H) Second-look arthroscopy 1 year later demonstrates excellent repair tissue fill over the medial femoral condyle. The patient has become completely asymptomatic and requests no further treatment. Twelve years later, this fibrocartilaginous repair tissue remains stable and has not broken down. Careful surveillance postoperatively to ensure a good clinical result with physical examination for crepitus and effusions as well as maintenance of joint space on standing x-ray films is performed. If any symptoms appear, a high-resolution magnetic resonance imaging scan would be performed to assess the status of the repair tissue on the surface of the medial femoral condyle and the possibility of second-stage autologous chondrocyte implantation repair.

6–8.8 cm^2). These lesions had an average depth of 1.1 cm (range 1–1.5 cm). Average preoperative and postoperative angles for Group 2 were 2.3 degrees varus and 8 degrees valgus, respectively (4/4 had HTO). The AVN group were all in varus prior to surgery and the correction was felt to be critical to the success.

Results

The results of the autologous bone grafting for OCD (Group 1) were effective for 6 of the 10 patients treated at 4-year follow-up. Four of the patients developed recurrent symptoms of weight-bearing pain, catching and swelling

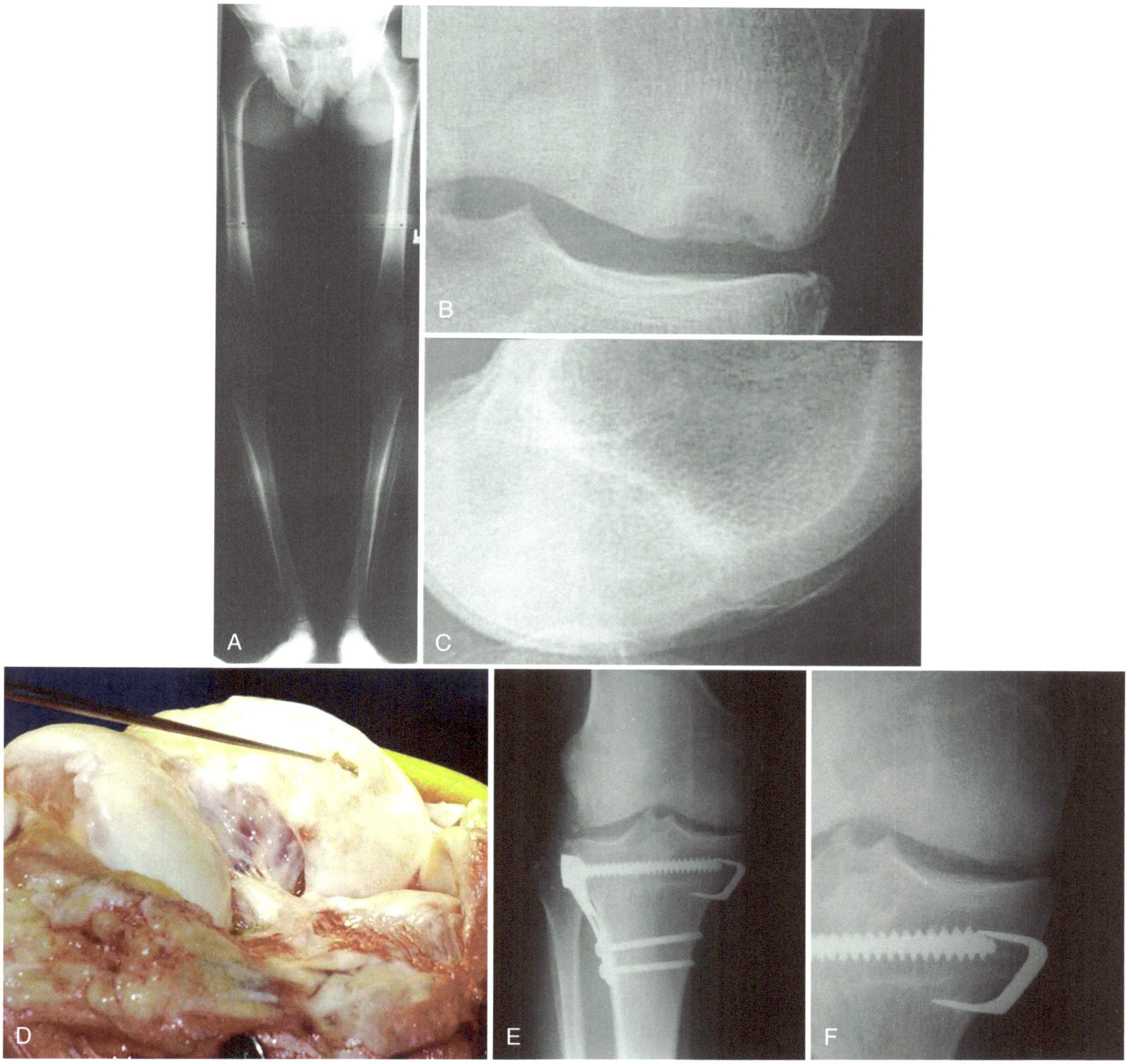

• **Fig. 13.7** Active 54-year-old man presents with medial pain in the right knee. The clinical and radiographic workup is compatible with osteonecrosis of the medial femoral condyle that is idiopathic. A closing wedge tibial valgus-producing osteotomy with curettage and autologous bone grafting of the medial femoral condyle (as in the case shown in Fig. 11.6) is performed. At latest follow-up more than 10 years later, he remains asymptomatic and without a prosthesis. (A) Long alignment x-ray films demonstrate varus alignment of both lower extremities, right greater than left. (B) Close-up anteroposterior x-ray film demonstrates resorptive cyst formation and flattening of the medial femoral condyle. (C) Lateral x-ray film demonstrates cyst formation and flattening of the medial femoral condyle. (D) Intraoperative appearance of the knee with a nerve hook falling into a resorptive cavity to the medial femoral condyle prior to radical debridement and curettage with autologous bone grafting of the medial femoral condyle. (E) Postoperative anteroposterior x-ray film demonstrating correction of axial malalignment and restoration of bone stock to the medial femoral condyle. (F) Close-up anteroposterior x-ray film demonstrating restoration of the medial femoral condyle with preservation of the joint space on standing anteroposterior x-ray film 1 year postoperatively.

Continued

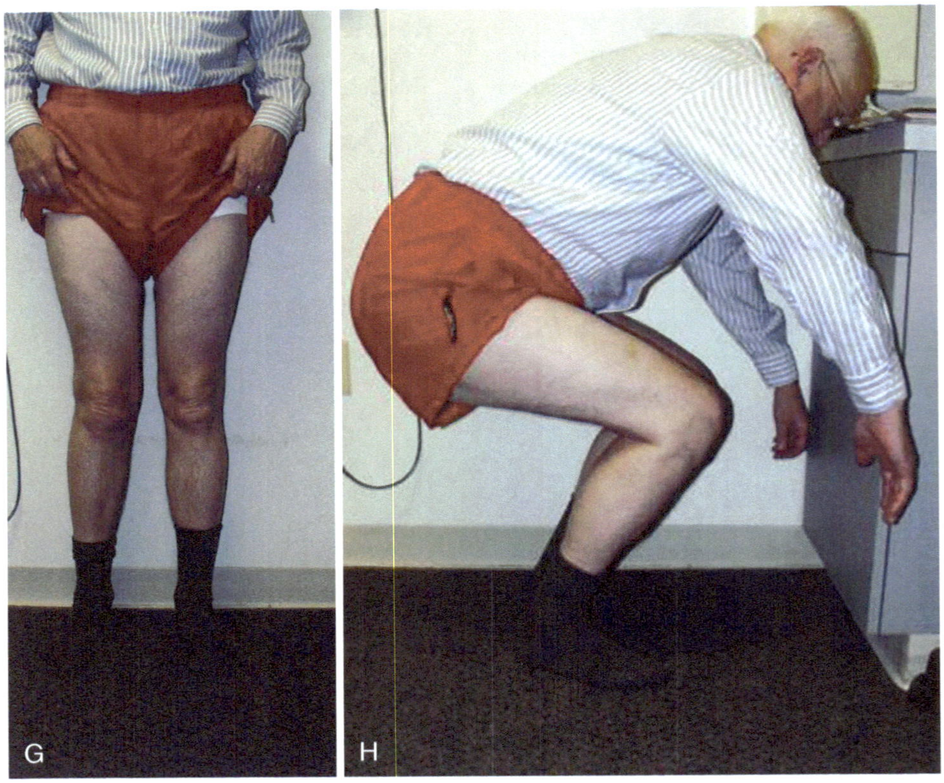

• **Fig. 13.7 Cont'd** (G) Clinical appearance 10 years postoperatively. Frontal alignment of the right leg demonstrates mild mechanical valgus, which is cosmetically acceptable to the patient. (H) Lateral clinical appearance demonstrating good active range of motion with squatting and kneeling. The patient remains asymptomatic.

over time requiring second stage ACI. At the time of ACI the repair tissue over the autologous bone graft was fibrous in nature, gelatinous, and soft. ACI provided excellent pain relief once the subchondral bone had been restored with the autologous bone graft.

The other six patients have been followed every 2 years with x-ray examinations and MRI scans to assess the repair tissue noninvasively. These patients remain asymptomatic today and demonstrate a stable repair tissue on MRI.

Three of the four patients in Group 2, AVN, did well with autologous bone graft and HTO, not requiring ACI. Although the fourth patient was relatively asymptomatic 9 months postoperative, because of his desire to maintain a high level of physical activity at the age of 47 years he requested a second stage ACI, which was performed. At the time of open ACI, the repair tissue over the autologous bone graft was of very good quality. There was a complete coverage of the bone graft with a white fibrocartilaginous tissue. ACI was performed after removal of the repair tissue. The patient remains asymptomatic 20 years after ACI. Surprisingly, the other three patients who underwent osteotomy with autologous bone graft also remained without symptoms.

Based on our early results with bone grafting for large osteochondral defects (approximately 7 cm^2 in both groups) it is recommended that, for younger patients with OCD, bone grafting with ACI as a single-staged sandwich technique be performed if the surgeon is skilled in such a technique. Alternatively, a more conservative approach of an isolated bone grafting with careful follow-up via clinical examination, MRI, and x-ray examination to evaluate the repair tissue over the bone graft prior to the possibility of ACI is a very reasonable approach. The defects are large with an average of approximately 7 cm^2 and therefore the possibility of fibrocartilage breakdown is more likely in this young active population.

In this small case series of males with idiopathic avascular necrosis with varus knees, it appears that a closing wedge osteotomy to correct alignment with autologous bone grafting to an osteonecrotic Ficat Stage III or IV lesion results in an excellent clinical result and is our recommended treatment of choice.

Our long-term follow-up of this group of patients was later published.[27] A synopsis of these results follows.

We compared the clinical outcomes and graft survivorship of patients undergoing the ACI sandwich technique with autologous bone grafting (ABG) ($n = 24$) to a historical, matched patient cohort who underwent ABG treatment alone ($n = 13$). The average defect size measured 6.9 $\pm$ 3.5 cm^2 and 7.1 $\pm$ 3. 5 cm^2 for the respective groups. The mean depth measured 1.2 $\pm$ 0.4 cm for the ABG group and 1.1 $\pm$ 0.3 cm for the ACI full sandwich group. Over the course of the study, the ACI full sandwich cohort consistently experienced greater improvement in clinical outcome and satisfaction scores. Radiographic studies and

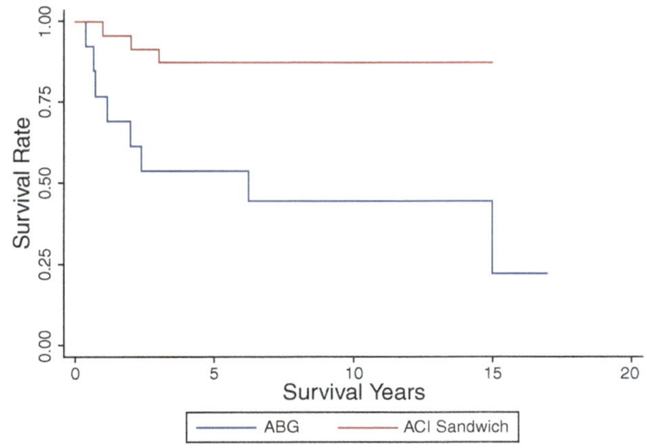

• **Fig. 13.8** The 10–15 years survivorship of autologous chondrocyte implantation (ACI) sandwich technique versus autologous bone graft (ABG) alone is greater than twice at 15 years postoperative. From Minas T, Ogura T, Headrick J, Bryant T. Autologous chondrocyte implantation "sandwich" technique compared with autologous bone grafting for deep osteochondral lesions in the knee. *Am J Sports Med*. 2018;46(2):322–332.

survivorship analysis results correlated with the reported clinical outcomes. As demonstrated in Fig. 13.8, the ACI full sandwich group had a significantly higher survival rate of 87% at 5 and 10 years postoperatively compared with the ABG group (54% at 5 years and 45% at 10 years postoperative). In total, 11 patients were considered clinical failures: eight patients in the ABG group and three patients in the ACI full sandwich group. The three ACI full sandwich failures underwent subsequent arthroscopic chondroplasty, which resolved their symptoms. Of the eight ABG failures, five proceeded with ACI revision surgery; one patient had a re-revision ACI treatment, eventually followed by a unicompartmental knee arthroplasty at 6.2 years postoperative; the other patient was converted to a total knee arthroplasty 15 years after ACI index surgery. One patient was revised with bone allograft followed by ABG and then ACI revision treatment at 8.3 post index surgery. Clinical results and survival analysis demonstrated superior outcomes in the ACI full sandwich technique group than the ABG group.

Conclusion

Osteochondral defects include OCD, osteochondral cysts, and avascular necrosis. In the adult form of OCD with an unstable fragment, the optimal treatment is open reduction internal fixation with autologous bone grafting to allow revascularization and healing of the fragment.

When there is an empty defect after failed fixation techniques or spontaneous fragmentation of an OCD fragment, assessment of the defect by a CT arthrogram is recommended. If there are no subchondral bone cysts and the defect is relatively shallow, 6 to 8 mm centrally at its deepest, which is typical, then ACI in isolation is recommended. However, if the margins of the defect are steep, the subchondral bone is thickened and sclerotic after repeated surgeries, or there are deep subchondral bone cysts, then restoration of the osteochondral unit by cartilage and bone grafting with an ACI sandwich technique is optimal. Alternatively, isolated autologous bone grafting, rehabilitation as per marrow stimulation techniques with clinical follow-up provides a safe and effective method of restoration of the osteochondral unit. The surgical technique with autologous bone grafting uses local bone graft when available and a dental amalgam type of preparation of the osseous defect. However, the repair tissue at the surface is less predictable and requires surveillance and the possibility of second stage ACI.

When an osseous defect is secondary to idiopathic avascular necrosis, this is generally in combination with varus alignment in a middle-aged male. Closing wedge valgus producing osteotomy with autologous bone grafting of the osteonecrotic fragment via the same surgical technique of autologous bone grafting of an osseous defect usually provides good and excellent results in Ficat Stage III and IV disease.

Secondary forms of avascular necrosis often have multiple necrotic segments and are more amenable to osteochondral allograft treatment or total knee replacement.

References

1. Pare A. *Ouevres Completes*. Vol.3. Paris: J.B. Balliere; 1840-1841:32.
2. Yamashita F, Sakakida K, Suzu F, Takai S. The transplantation of an autogeneic osteochondral fragment for osteochondritis dissecans of the knee. *Clin Orthop*. 1985;201:43–50.
3. Muller W. Osteochondrosis dissecans. In: Hastings DE, editor. *Progress in Orthopedic Surgery*. Vol. 3. Berlin: Springer Verlag; 1978:135.
4. Outerbridge HK, Outerbridge AR, Outerbridge RE. The use of a lateral patellar autologous graft for the repair of a large osteochondral defect in the knee. *J Bone Joint Surg Am*. 1995;77-A (1):65–72.
5. Linden B. The incidence of osteochondritis dissecans of the femur. *Acta Orthop Scand*. 1976;47:664–667.
6. Pappas AM. Osteochondritis dissecans. *Clin Orthop*. 1981;158:59–69.
7. Nagura S. The so-called osteochondritis dissecans of König. *Clin Orthop*. 1960;18:100–122.
8. Green WT, Banks HH. Osteochondritis dissecans in children. *J Bone Joint Surg Am*. Jan. 1953;35-A:26–47.
9. Mubarick SJ, Carrol NC. Familial osteochondritis dissecans of the knee. *Clin Orthop*. 1979;140:131–136.
10. Petrie PWR. Aetiology of osteochondritis dissecans. Failure to establish a familial background. *J Bone Joint Surg Br*. 1977;59-B(3): 366–367.
11. Fairbank HA. Osteo-chondritis dissecans. *Br J Surg*. 1933;21:67–82.
12. Cahill BR, Berg BC. 99m-Technetium phosphate compound joint scintigraphy in the management of juvenile osteochondritis dissecans of the femoral condyles. *Am J Sports Med*. 1983;11(5):329–335.
13. Enneking WF, ed. *Clinical Musculo-Skeletal Pathology*. 3rd ed. Gainesville, FL: University of Florida Press; 1990:166.
14. Rogers WM, Gladstone H. Vascular foramina and arterial supply of the distal end of the femur. *J Bone Joint Surg Am*. Oct. 1950;32-A:867–874.

15. Chiroff RT, Cooke III CP. Osteochondritis dissecans: a histologic and microradiographic analyses of surgically excised lesions. *J Trauma*. 1975;15:689–696.
16. Cahill BR. Osteochondritis dissecans of the knee: treatment of juvenile and adult forms. *J Am Acad Orthop Surg*. 1995;3:237–247.
17. Cahill BR, Phillips MR, Navarro R. The results of conservative management of osteochondritis dissecans using joint scintigraphy: a prospective study. *Am J Sports Med*. 1989; 17:601–606.
18. Almgard LE, Wikstad I. Late results of surgery for osteochondritis dissecans of the knee joint. *Acta Chir Scand*. 1964;127:588–596.
19. Cahill B. Treatment of juvenile osteochondritis dissecans and osteochondritis dissecans of the knee. *Clin Sports Med*. 1985;4:367–384.
20. Green JP. Osteochondritis dissecans of the knee. *J Bone Joint Surg Br*. 1966;48-B(1):82–91.
21. Hughston JC, Hergenroeder PT, Courtenay BG. Osteochondritis dissecans of the femoral condyles. *J Bone Joint Surg Am*. 1984;66-A: 1340–1348.
22. Linden B. Osteochondritis dissecans of the femoral condyles. A long-term follow-up study. *J Bone Joint Surg Am*. 1977;59-A: 769–776.
23. Landells JW. The reactions of injured human articular cartilage. *J Bone Joint Surg Br*. 1957;39-B(3):548–562.
24. Mitchell N, Shepard N. The resurfacing of adult rabbit articular cartilage by multiple perforations through the subchondral bone. *J Bone Joint Surg Am*. 1976;58-A:230–233.
25. DePalma AF, McKeever CD, Subin DK. Process of repair of articular cartilage demonstrated by histology and autoradiography with tritiated thymidine. *Clin Orthop*. 1966;48:229–242.
26. Peterson L, Minas T, Britterg M, et al. Two- to nine-year outcome after autologous chondrocyte transplantation of the knee. *Clin Orthop*. 2000;374:212–234.
27. Minas T, Ogura T, Headrick J, Bryant T. Autologous chondrocyte implantation "sandwich" technique compared with autologous bone grafting for deep osteochondral lesions in the knee. *Am J Sports Med*. 2018;46(2):322–332.
28. Aglietti P, Insall JN, Buzzi R, Deschamps D. Idiopathic osteonecrosis of the knee: aetiology, prognosis and treatment. *J Bone Joint Surg Br*. 1983;65:588–597.
29. Ahlbäck S, Bauer GCH, Bohne WH. Spontaneous osteonecrosis of the knee. *Arthritis Rheum*. 1968;11:705–733.
30. Mont MA, Baumgarten KM, Rifai A, Bluemke DA, Jones LC, Hungerford DS. Atraumatic osteonecrosis of the knee. *J Bone Joint Surg Am*. 2000;82:1279–1290.
31. Muheim G, Bohne WH. Prognosis in spontaneous osteonecrosis of the knee. *J Bone Joint Surg Br*. 1970;52:605–612.
32. Koshino T. The treatment of spontaneous osteonecrosis of the knee by high tibial osteotomy with and without bone-grafting or drilling of the lesion. *J Bone Joint Surg Am*. 1982;64:47–58.

14

Meniscal Allograft Transplantation

ANDREAS H. GOMOLL, MD AND TOM MINAS, MD, MS

CHAPTER OUTLINE

Introduction

Loss of meniscal tissue drastically alters the biomechanical environment of the knee joint, especially in the lateral compartment, where contact stress can increase by 200% to 300% after total meniscectomy. Compartment overload syndrome can ensue, presenting with weight-bearing pain and recurrent effusions. Secondary osteoarthritis is a predictable endpoint,[1,2] which has led to increased awareness among orthopedic surgeons of meniscal transplantation in cases where subtotal or total meniscectomy was unavoidable. In carefully selected patients, meniscal allograft transplantation can provide improved biomechanics and function while providing good pain relief.[3–5]

Several techniques exist for allograft meniscus transplantation, including bone-plug and bone-bridge techniques, with additional variations within these groups based on different proprietary instrumentation sets. Regardless of the specific technique used, the majority of current transplantations are performed with bony fixation rather than relying on soft tissue healing of the meniscal roots to a prepared bed on the recipient tibial plateau.

This chapter discusses the techniques for open and arthroscopic meniscal allograft transplantation.

Indications

The ideal patient for meniscal allograft transplantation has a history of prior total or subtotal meniscectomy, usually followed by a symptom-free interval of varying duration. This is followed by the onset of weight-bearing pain localized to the involved compartment, frequently with recurrent effusions. The articular surfaces should be without full-thickness chondral defects, ligaments should be stable, and the knee should be normally aligned; otherwise, these comorbidities must be addressed in concurrent or staged fashion. Several reports that investigated the outcomes of concurrent meniscal transplantation and cartilage repair demonstrated results comparable to isolated meniscal transplantation.[6,7] Therefore, repairable, focal chondral defects should not be viewed as a contraindication.

Contraindications include diffuse arthritic changes and significant joint space narrowing, especially when associated with advanced femoral condyle and tibial flattening, history of inflammatory arthritis, or marked obesity.

Planning

The preoperative radiographic evaluation includes weight-bearing anteroposterior (AP) and posteroanterior 45-degree flexion radiographs, non–weight-bearing 45-degree flexion lateral view, axial view of the patellofemoral joint, and a long-leg mechanical axis view to evaluate malalignment. Furthermore, we routinely perform magnetic resonance imaging to evaluate the joint for articular comorbidities, such as ligamentous or chondral injury.

Meniscal allografts are size-, side-, and compartment-specific; therefore, they must be individually measured and ordered for each patient. Preoperative measurements are obtained from AP and lateral radiographs with magnification markers placed on the skin at the level of the joint line. After accounting for radiographic magnification, meniscal width is measured on the AP radiograph from the edge of the ipsilateral tibial spine to the edge of the tibial plateau. Meniscal length is calculated by multiplying the depth of the tibial plateau (as measured on lateral radiographs) by 0.8 for medial and 0.7 for lateral meniscal grafts (Fig. 14.1).

Technique

Special Instrumentation

Based on the surgeon's preferred technique, a meniscal allograft workstation is used to shape the bone block or plugs containing the meniscal root attachment sites and prepare a corresponding recipient site on the tibia. Various proprietary systems are available and are usually provided by the company through which the transplant was ordered. Furthermore, meniscal repair equipment, such as zone-specific cannulas and double-armed needles, are needed for the meniscocapsular repair.

Graft Preparation

The graft should be prepared before the start of the procedure (e.g., while the patient is being induced) to reduce surgical and tourniquet time.

Depending on the specific system used, the bone bridge or plugs are prepared and sutures are placed. For our preferred technique, pull sutures are placed in the posterior horn (Fig. 14.2) to assist in reducing the meniscus under the femoral condyle. Additional sutures can be placed through the bone bridge/plugs and around the meniscal roots to assist in graft fixation. After the graft has been prepared, any residual marrow elements should be removed from the bone using pulse lavage.

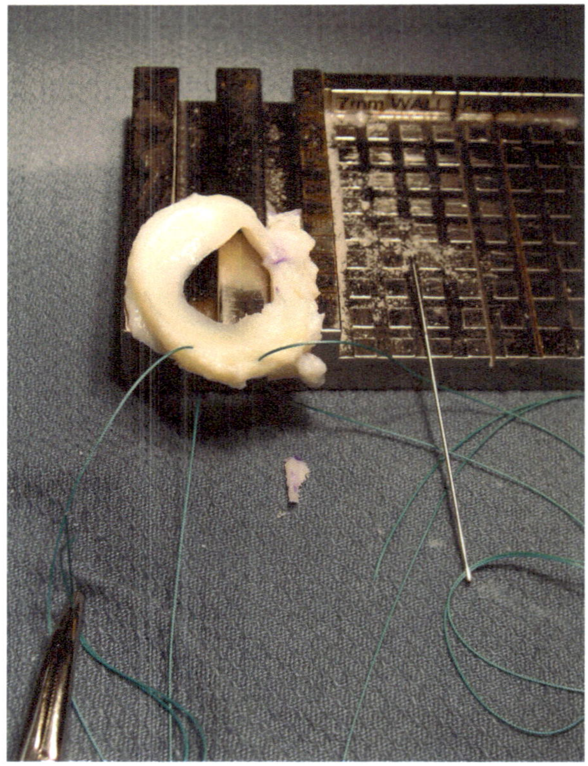

• **Fig. 14.2** Prepared meniscal allograft. A bone bridge has been fashioned from the donor tibial plateau and two pull sutures have been placed through the posterior horn to assist in reduction and fixation.

Positioning

The patient is positioned supine on a standard operating room table, with a thigh tourniquet. The posteromedial or posterolateral aspect of the knee must be easily accessible to perform inside-out meniscus suturing. For arthroscopic

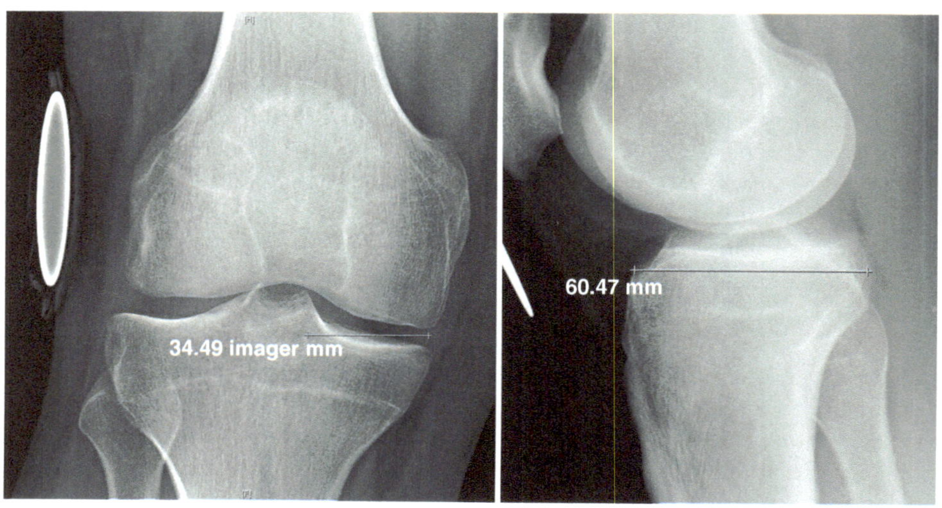

• **Fig. 14.1** Anteroposterior *(left)* and lateral *(right)* radiographs of the knee with sizing disks. The width and length of the medial tibial plateau have been measured.

techniques, it is often helpful to use a thigh holder and drop the foot of the bed. A side post and foot rest can be used for open techniques.

Surgical Anatomy

Useful surgical landmarks include the patella, patellar tendon, tibial plateau, and fibular head. Structures at risk during the procedure include the peroneal nerve, popliteal tendon, and lateral collateral ligament during the posterolateral approach. The posteromedial approach risks injury to the saphenous vein and nerve, potentially resulting in a painful neuroma. Creation of the tibial slot and needle passage during the meniscocapsular repair can injure the popliteal neurovascular bundle.

Surgical Approach

Arthroscopic techniques use standard medial and lateral portals as well as two accessory incisions: an anterior transpatellar tendon approach to introduce the meniscus into the joint and a posteromedial or posterolateral approach to the knee for inside-out meniscocapsular repair. The transpatellar tendon approach is made with spinal needle localization in line with the anterior and posterior meniscal root attachments and extends from the inferior pole of the patella to the tibial tubercle. Care should be taken to cut in line with the fibers of the patellar tendon to avoid detaching a portion of the tendon. Resection of the fat pad just anterior to the anterior root attachment is helpful to visualize the root and facilitate graft insertion, passage, and fixation. The accessory posteromedial and posterolateral incisions are standard meniscal repair techniques.

For open meniscal transplantation, a longitudinal incision is made shifted slightly from the midline toward the respective compartment. Medially, a full-thickness fasciocutaneous flap is raised around the side of the knee to allow posteromedial access to the capsule through a triangle between the semimembranosus inferiorly, the medial head of the gastrocnemius posteriorly and superiorly, and the joint capsule anteriorly. Laterally, first a full-thickness fasciocutaneous flap is raised around the lateral side of the knee (Fig. 14.3A). The iliotibial band (ITB) overlies the capsule and either it is split in line with its fibers or the patellar contribution of the ITB is divided, allowing the ITB to slide posteriorly with knee flexion. The plane between the ITB and capsule is developed to allow suturing (Fig. 14.3B). This plane is followed posteriorly past the lateral collateral ligament, which is embedded in capsular tissue. The interval between the biceps femoris inferiorly and the lateral head of the gastrocnemius posteriorly is developed to provide access to the posterior capsule. For both approaches, the surgeon should be able to palpate the area of the tibial posterior cruciate ligament insertion as well as the popliteus tendon during a lateral approach. A spoon is placed in this interval to protect the posterior neurovascular bundle (Fig. 14.3C).

An anterior arthrotomy is performed by incising the capsule just medial or lateral to the border of the patellar tendon and the fat pad is transected. A retractor is placed into the notch to displace the patellar tendon toward the other compartment. The anterior meniscal root is divided and a full-thickness capsular flap with the anterior meniscal horn attached is raised around the side of the knee toward the medial or lateral midline by subperiosteal dissection of the tissues from the proximal tibia. Medially, this flap includes the superficial and deep medial collateral ligament; laterally it includes the ITB insertion on Gerdy's tubercle. Another retractor is placed around the medial or lateral femoral condyle, providing full exposure (Fig. 14.3D).

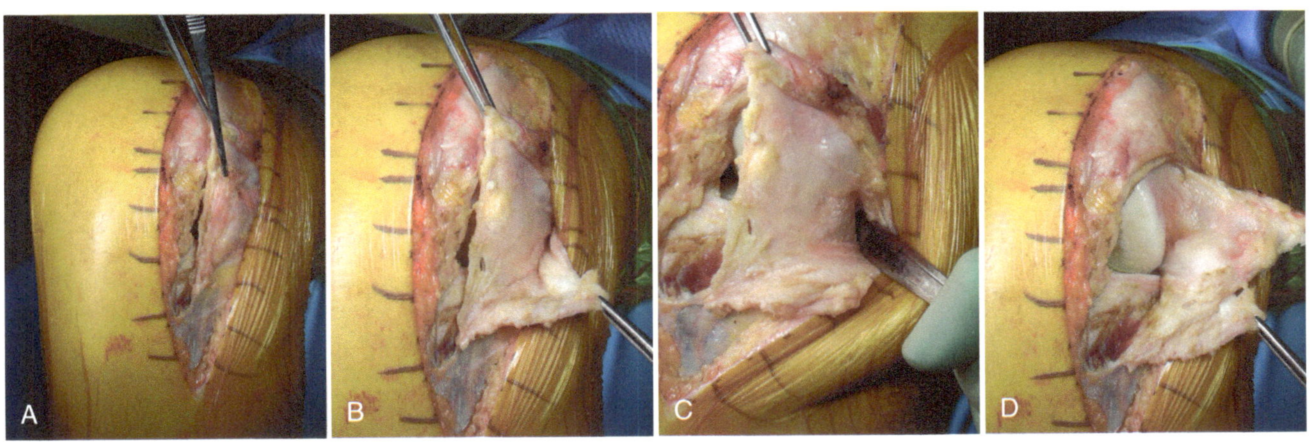

• **Fig. 14.3** Exposure for open lateral meniscal transplantation. (A) Full-thickness fasciocutaneous flap has been raised. The two forceps hold the capsule and iliotibial band. (B) The plane between the iliotibial band (reflected) and capsule has been developed. (C) The interval between the lateral head of the gastrocnemius muscle and the capsule has been developed and a spoon has been placed to protect the posterior neurovascular bundle. (D) The capsule and iliotibial band insertion on Gerdy's tubercle have been reflected by subperiosteal dissection from the lateral proximal tibia, exposing the lateral femoral condyle.

Completion Meniscectomy

The meniscal remnant must be removed in order to prepare a vascularized bed for the transplant. However, leaving a thin shell of meniscal tissue at the meniscocapsular junction (Fig. 14.4) is thought to help reduce the risk of meniscal extrusion by providing more mechanical support than the thin capsular tissue alone. The meniscal roots should be left in place at this point because they represent an important landmark for later placement of anatomically correct attachment sites.

Tibial Preparation

Depending on the specific instrumentation used, a recipient slot for bony fixation of the meniscal roots is prepared on the tibia. An inferior notchplasty as well as limited soft tissue debridement of the most inferior aspects of the anterior cruciate ligament or posterior cruciate ligament fibers can assist in visualization of the posterior root attachment site. In a line connecting the two root attachment sites (Fig. 14.5A), the tibial plateau is cleared of cartilage (Fig. 14.5B), and a slot is created with the technique-specific instrumentation (Fig. 14.5C). Two bone tunnels for later fixation of the graft can be created in the posterior and anterior aspects of the slot with a standard tibial aiming guide from the anterior cruciate ligament set (Fig. 14.6).

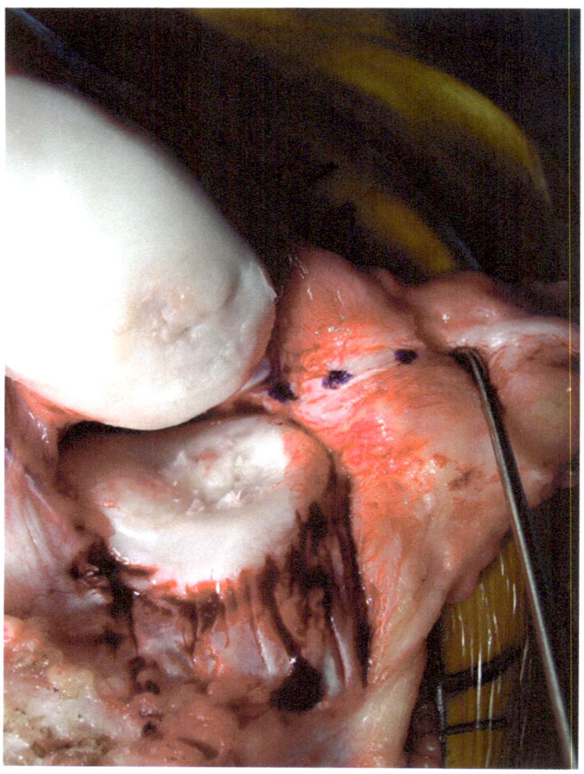

• **Fig. 14.4** Completion meniscectomy has been performed, leaving the sturdier tissue of the meniscocapsular junction *(dots)* intact.

Graft Placement and Fixation

The previously placed pull suture at the junction of the posterior horn and body of the meniscal graft is shuttled through a corresponding location of the joint capsule. This can easily be performed using zone-specific cannulas and a needle-tip suture passing wire (Fig. 14.7). If fixation sutures were placed around the meniscal roots of the graft, they are shuttled through the tibial bone tunnels at this point. Reduction of the meniscus requires a combination of pulling on the sutures and pushing the bone bridge into the slot while flexing and extending the knee with varus or valgus stress. Once the meniscus is seated under the femoral condyle (Fig. 14.8), the knee should be ranged to assess stability.

Fixation of the graft is divided into bony fixation of the meniscal root attachments and soft tissue fixation at the meniscocapsular junction. Some systems create a trapezoidal or keyhole-shaped tibial slot that provides a secure fit for the bone bridge. Others require additional fixation with sutures or a screw. The sutures that were placed around the meniscal roots and pulled through the tibial bone tunnel are tied over a bone bridge on the medial aspect of the tibia for fixation. Alternatively, the bone bridge of the graft can be fixed in the slot with an interference screw or, in open meniscal allograft transplantation, secured to the tibial plateau under direct visualization with heavy, nonresorbable suture.

For arthroscopic techniques, the meniscus is circumferentially repaired to the capsule using standard meniscal repair techniques with inside-out and all-inside techniques for the posterior horn and body and outside-in techniques for the anterior horn. For open techniques, the posterior horn is secured with inside-out techniques. The body and anterior horn are repaired with heavy nonresorbable sutures, which are placed through the capsule, meniscus, and tibial plateau sequentially back to front before all sutures are tied at the end (Fig. 14.9). This not only repairs the meniscocapsular junction but also secures the previously released capsular flap back to the proximal tibia. If necessary, the medial collateral ligament and ITB can be additionally secured with suture anchors.

Postoperatively, patients are kept on partial weight-bearing restrictions for 2 weeks and then advanced to weight bearing as tolerated. A knee immobilizer is used for 6 weeks during ambulation. Flexion exercises are limited to 90 degrees for 2 weeks, then advanced as tolerated. If meniscal allograft transplantation is performed in conjunction with other procedures such as autologous chondrocyte implantation or osteotomy, the most conservative of the various rehabilitation protocols should be used, usually extending the weight-bearing restrictions for 6 to 8 weeks. Continuous passive motion can be used for 3 weeks for isolated meniscal allograft transplantation and 6 weeks for associated cartilage repair procedures.

Summary

Meniscal allograft transplantation is successful in redistributing joint reactive forces, even though complete normalization does not occur. Patients experience good pain relief

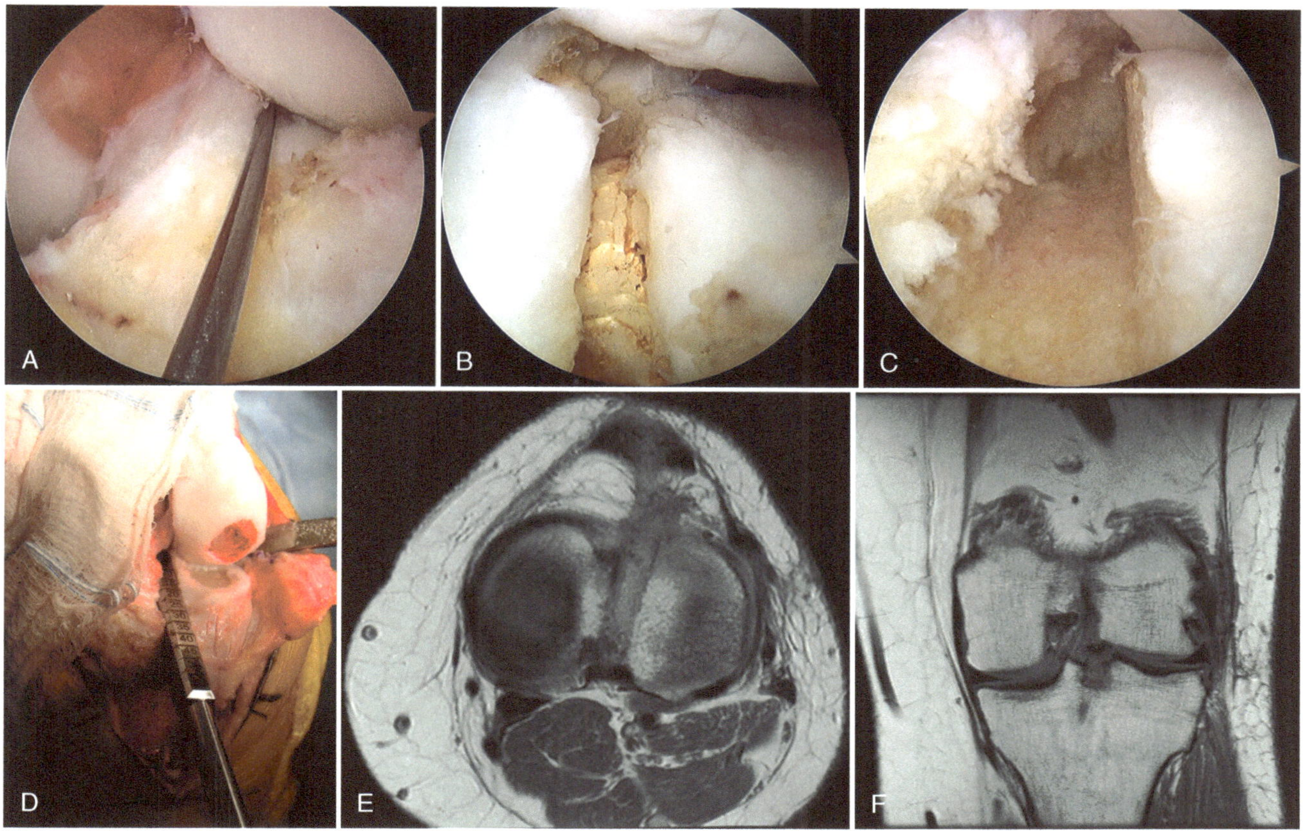

• **Fig. 14.5** Creation of the tibial slot. (A) A spinal needle is placed connecting the anterior and posterior root attachment sites. (B) Overlying cartilage is removed with the electrothermal device. (C) A recipient slot has been created on the tibial plateau. (D) Using a rasp to finish the tibial slot in an example of open meniscal allograft transplantation. (E) Postoperative axial magnetic resonance imaging after arthroscopic lateral meniscal allograft transplantation showing the orientation of the tibial slot and surgical changes in the fat pad. (F) Postoperative coronal magnetic resonance imaging showing the position of the tibial slot.

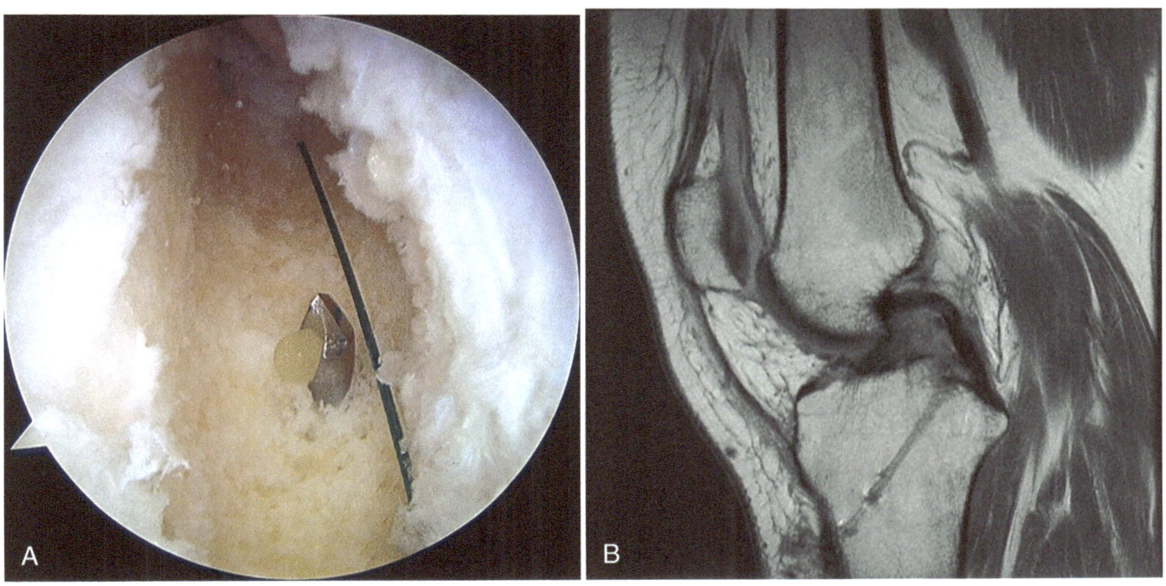

• **Fig. 14.6** Suture fixation of the bone bridge by transosseous tunnels. (A) Arthroscopic anterior view of the tibial slot. A tunnel has already been drilled into the posterior aspect of the slot and a pull suture has been placed. A standard tibial pin (tip visible) as used for anterior cruciate ligament reconstruction has been drilled into the anterior aspect of the slot using the standard tibial anterior cruciate ligament guide (removed). (B) Postoperative sagittal magnetic resonance imaging view showing the oblique bone tunnel used for suture fixation of the posterior aspect of the bone bridge. The second, anterior bone tunnel is not visible on this cut.

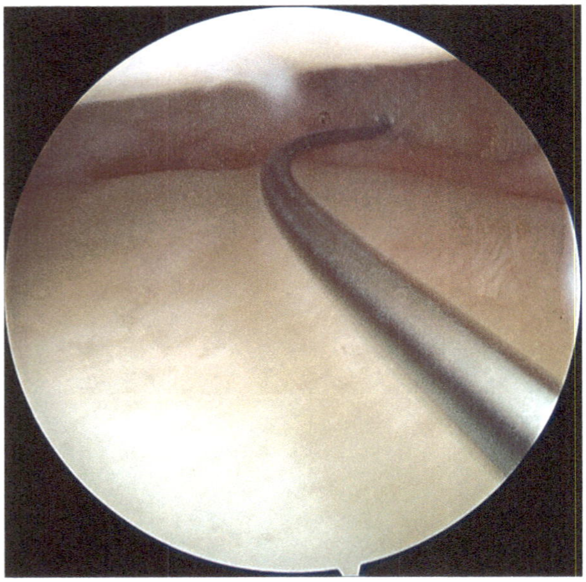

• **Fig. 14.7** Arthroscopic view of a nitinol suture passing wire that has been placed through the capsule.

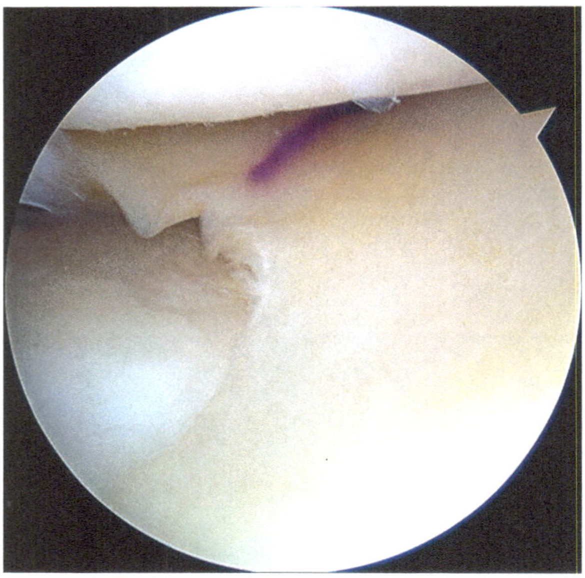

• **Fig. 14.8** The meniscus has been reduced under the femoral condyle. The junction of the body and posterior horn has been marked to assist in orienting the graft.

and are frequently able to return to higher activity levels, although pivoting and cutting sports are discouraged to reduce the risk of reinjury. Long-term outcomes still demonstrate the development of degenerative changes, possibly due to imperfect size matching with current techniques, which can result in meniscal extrusion.

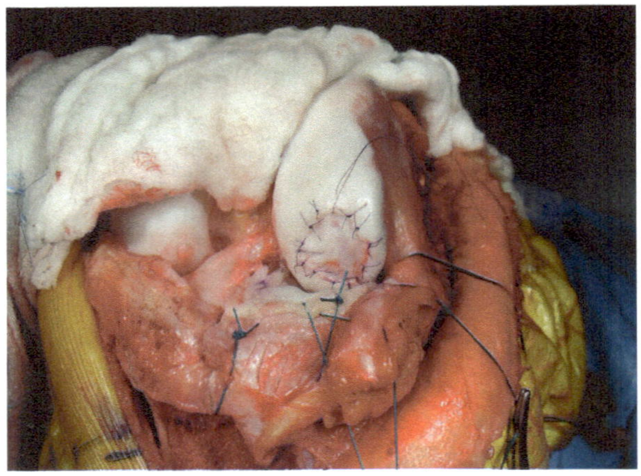

• **Fig. 14.9** Open meniscal allograft transplantation in conjunction with autologous chondrocyte implantation to the lateral femoral condyle and plateau with concurrent tibial tubercle osteotomy. The meniscus has been secured to the tibial plateau with heavy nonabsorbable suture and additional sutures have been placed through the capsule and meniscus to repair the meniscocapsular junction.

References

1. Alford W, Cole BJ. The indications and technique for meniscal transplant. *Orthop Clin North Am*. 2005;36:469–484.
2. Cameron JC, Saha S. Meniscal allograft transplantation for unicompartmental arthritis of the knee. *Clin Orthop Relat Res*. 1997;337:164–171.
3. Cole BJ, Rodeo S, Carter T. Allograft meniscus transplantation: indications, techniques, results. *J Bone Joint Surg Am*. 2002;84A:1236–1250.
4. Cole BJ, Dennis MG, Lee SJ, et al. Prospective evaluation of allograft meniscus transplantation: a minimum 2-year follow-up. *Am J Sports Med*. 2006;34(6):919–927.
5. Carter TR. Meniscal allograft transplantation. *Sports Med Arthrosc Rev*. 1999;7:51–62.
6. Rue JP, Yanke AB, Busam ML, McNickle AG, Cole BJ. Prospective evaluation of concurrent meniscus transplantation and articular cartilage repair: minimum 2-year follow-up. *Am J Sports Med*. 2008;36(9):1770–1778.
7. Farr J, Rawal A, Marberry KM. Concomitant meniscal allograft transplantation and autologous chondrocyte implantation: minimum 2-year follow-up. *Am J Sports Med*. 2007;35(9):1459–1466.

15

Complex Cases in Cartilage Repair: Tricks and Tips

TOM MINAS, MD, MS

CHAPTER OUTLINE

My residents and clinical fellows have often asked me where they can find a well written technique for a medial subvastus exposure as well as the tips and tricks that I use in more complex joint-preserving reconstructions. For this reason I have included a chapter to demonstrate in detail the technique for a medial subvastus exposure and several complex clinical cases that illustrate the principles and techniques involved in joint preservation in more extreme cases. A major improvement in my clinical practice has been in perioperative pain management, which allows me to continue performing these complex cases with minimal hospitalization, reduced patient discomfort, improved satisfaction, and a better initial experience for the patient leading to a quicker recovery.

The other major improvement with autologous chondrocyte implantation (ACI) is the generational change from periosteum to collagen to matrix-induced ACI (MACI). This has made the technique much easier for the surgeon, less invasive for the patient, and I believe improved clinical outcomes will follow. I have included periosteal ACI (pACI), collagen ACI (cACI), MACI, as generation 1, 2, and 3 because they may still exist in different parts of the world. In addition, to have a more comprehensive approach I have included allografts as particulated fresh juvenile articular allograft and fresh large osteochondral allograft.

Case 1. Medial Subvastus Approach to the Knee: Surgical Technique[1]

Introduction

There has been a recent emphasis on minimally invasive and muscle-sparing approaches in orthopedic surgery. The subvastus approach to the knee joint has been described as an alternative to traditional approaches that involve a large arthrotomy with partial division of the quadriceps mechanism. I have found the technique very useful for joint-preserving surgeries and prosthesis implantations when the soft tissue mobility of the extensor mechanism is supple and a careful surgical technique is pursued as described.

The step-by-step surgical technique for the medial subvastus approach to the knee follows. As with any procedure, patient selection is paramount to success and not all patients are appropriate for this approach. However, in patients who meet our criteria, we feel that this approach offers significant benefit to patients over traditional approaches.

These include less postoperative pain and easier, quicker rehabilitation in the early postoperative period. The long-term benefits, if any, are unknown.

Surgical Technique

I perform a medial subvastus approach whenever possible; however, some patients are better served with a standard medial parapatellar approach. Suitable candidates for a subvastus approach must have relatively mobile subcutaneous tissues in order to create a "mobile window" for performing the various aspects of the planned procedure. The mobility of the soft tissues can be assessed during a preoperative clinic visit, but the ultimate decision is made on the day of surgery with the patient under anesthesia. Obesity, contractures, and deformity are relative contraindications; however, with experience, the indications can be expanded. Revision surgery is usually contraindicated because of scar tissue formation and obliteration of tissue planes.

The patient is positioned supine in the standard fashion. We generally use a lateral post at the level of the thigh tourniquet and a post to support the foot, such that the knee can be flexed and maintained at 90 degrees of flexion. The skin incision can be made directly midline or slightly medial to midline, depending on the nature of the pathology. The length of the incision is based on the underlying pathology. Generally, it extends from the superior pole of the patella to the inferior aspect of the tibial tubercle (Fig. 15.1A). The incision is carried sharply through the subcutaneous tissue down to the retinacular tissue. Full-thickness medial and lateral flaps are then created sharply with careful hemostasis (Fig. 15.1B). The creation of large, full-thickness flaps is important because this allows the extensor mechanism to be mobilized deep to the subcutaneous tissues.

The distal insertion of the vastus medialis obliquus (VMO) on the patella is exposed (Fig. 15.1C). The fascia overlying the VMO is released sharply, taking care not to injure any underlying muscle fibers (Fig. 15.1D). The fascia is released posteriorly toward the attachment of the VMO on the medial intermuscular septum, which exposes the entire distal extent of the VMO (Fig. 15.1E). Using blunt dissection, a finger can be placed underneath the VMO at its inferior border. The VMO is then retracted proximally and laterally while maintaining its attachment to the patella. A Z-retractor is inserted anterior to the distal femur and deep to the muscle to maintain retraction (Fig. 15.1F).

Two no. 1 Vicryl marking sutures are placed at the level of the VMO attachment to the patella (Fig. 15.1G). An oblique capsular incision is then made just distal to the VMO, beginning posteriorly at the level of the intermuscular septum and extending laterally, parallel to the inferior border of the muscle, toward the medial border of the patella. The incision is made between the marking sutures, which then serve as a guide for later repair. At the medial border of the patella, the arthrotomy is extended distally, taking care to leave a cuff of tissue attached to the patella for closure (Fig. 15.1H).

The arthrotomy incision is carried distally across the joint line and parallel to the medial border of the patellar tendon. Care is taken to avoid damaging the anterior horn of the medial meniscus if a biologic procedure is being performed. If necessary, the retropatellar bursa and fat pad can be incised to gain additional exposure.

Next, attention is turned to the suprapatellar pouch where the synovial capsular attachments to the undersurface of the quadriceps tendon are released completely from medial to lateral (Fig. 15.1I). This is the key maneuver for being able to mobilize the extensor mechanism fully as it detaches the quadriceps muscle from the anterior femoral synovial supracondylar attachments. After completing this, the patella can then be subluxed into the lateral gutter. Creating a large, full-thickness, lateral subcutaneous flap during the initial exposure is necessary to create a pocket into which the patella can be subluxed. A 90-degree bent Hohman or Z-retractor is placed in the lateral gutter at the level of the quadriceps tendon insertion above the patella to maintain retraction of the patella. Flexing the knee to approximately 90 degrees provides excellent exposure of the entire joint and the appropriate procedure can be performed (Fig. 15.1J). A standard closure is performed at the end of the case (Fig. 15.1K). The closure is quite simple because no muscle needs to be repaired.

Discussion

The medial subvastus approach was originally described in the German literature by Erkes in 1929.[2] A modified version was re-introduced by Hoffman in 1991.[3] A so-called "mini" subvastus approach has since been described.[2,4,5] There are currently multiple reports in the literature describing the results with respect to total knee arthroplasty. Although concerns have been raised regarding appropriate component positioning, many studies demonstrate more rapid recovery, better pain scores, less blood loss, and better short-term knee range of motion when comparing the subvastus approach with more traditional appproaches.[6–12] Recently, Schroer et al. published their results of 600 primary total knee arthroplasties performed through a subvastus approach.[13] Follow-up was short-term, averaging 28 months. A historical group of 150 total knee arthroplasties performed through a standard medial parapatellar arthrotomy was used as a control. Overall, there were 11 major complications (1.8%) requiring reoperation in the subvastus group and 6 (4.0%) in the traditional group. The rate of both major and minor complications was found to be independent of surgical technique. The rate of major complications in the subvastus group was found to be associated with surgical experience; the rate was reduced by 16% for each additional 50 procedures performed. Mean knee flexion after 1 year averaged 125 degrees in the subvastus group and 114 degrees in the traditional group. Average operative time was initially higher in the subvastus group, but decreased with experience so that it was less than the traditional group in the last 400 subvastus procedures

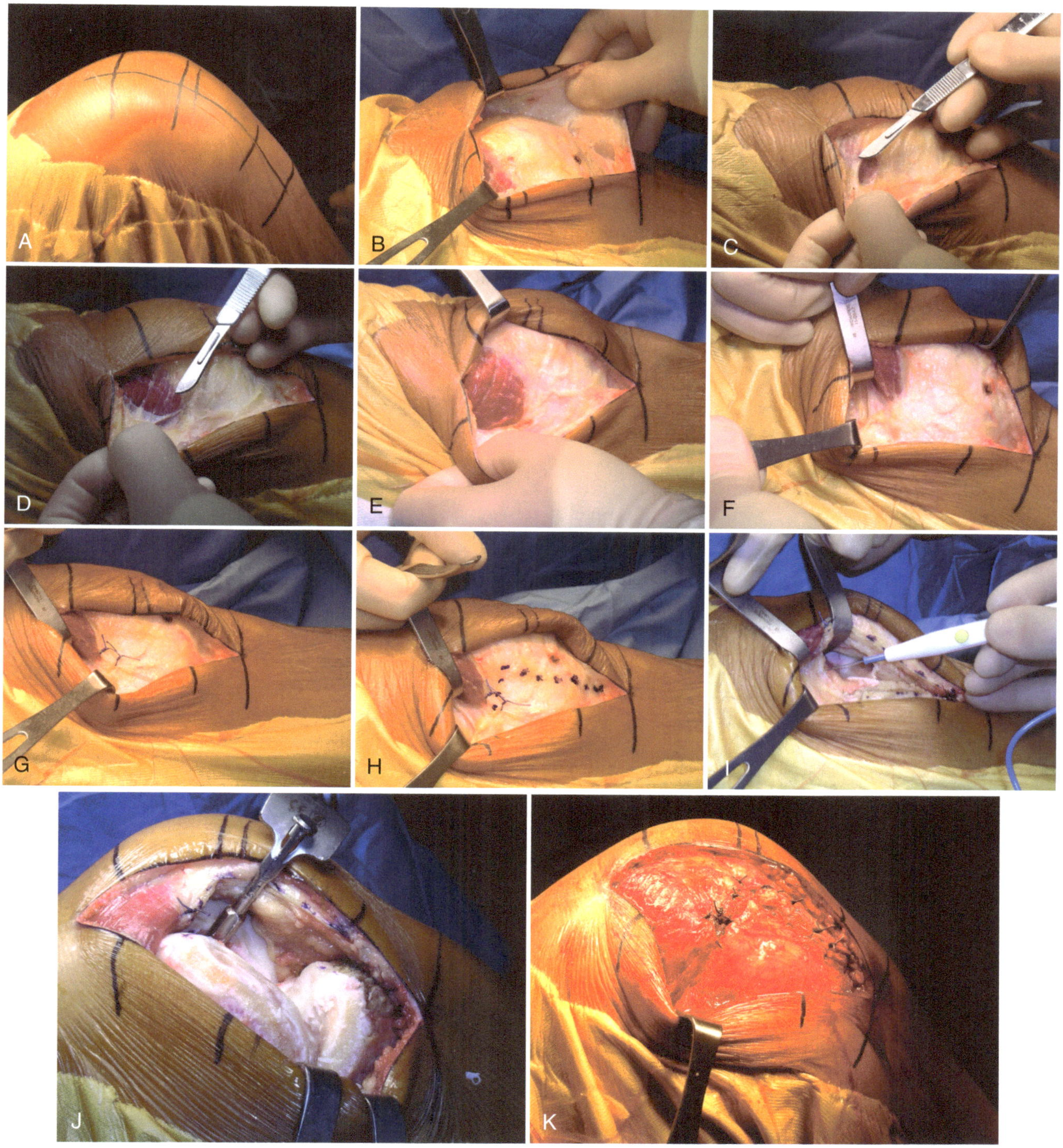

• **Fig. 15.1** (A) Typical skin incision extending from superior pole of patella to tibial tubercle. (B) Development of medial and lateral full-thickness subcutaneous flaps. (C) Exposure of vastus medialis obliquus (VMO) insertion. (D) Subfascial dissection of VMO. (E) Complete exposure of distal VMO insertion. (F) Placement of Z-retractor underneath distal VMO. Note insertion on patella is left completely intact. (G) Tagging sutures marking distal extent of insertion of VMO on patella. (H) Proposed line of incision for performing medial arthrotomy. (I) Release of synovial attachments from femur to undersurface of quadriceps from medial to lateral. The superior retractor is placed above the synovial attachments and the inferior retractor is intraarticular. This clearly delineates the synovial tissue that must be released to mobilize the extensor mechanism and expose the joint. (J) Exposure of articular surfaces. In this example, a medial unicompartmental arthroplasty is being performed. During total knee arthroplasty, we routinely place a knurled pin in the patellar tendon insertion to protect it from detachment during the case. (K) Standard closure of the arthrotomy. The VMO is left completely intact.

performed. Of note, the authors stated that 99% of total knee arthroplasties performed during the study period were done through a subvastus approach with 91% of patients classified as overweight and 11% as morbidly obese.

We have found the subvastus approach to provide excellent exposure and allow quicker advancement of rehabilitation after knee surgery. As with any procedure, there is a definite learning curve associated with the subvastus approach. My technique and indications have evolved with time and experience. Less emphasis is placed on the length of the skin incision and more emphasis placed on careful dissection of large medial and lateral skin flaps and atraumatic mobilization of the muscle. In addition to total knee arthroplasty and medial unicompartmental knee arthroplasty, we have applied the subvastus approach to the treatment of other intraarticular pathologies, primarily chondral defects. Procedures such as autologous chondrocyte implantation and osteoarticular allografts can easily be performed through this approach.

Case 2. Perioperative Pain Management

Perioperative pain management is essential for the initial perception of the patient's comfort and well-being as well as postoperative range of motion and avoiding stiffness. As mentioned in earlier chapters, choosing a patient who does not have addictive behavior is important. Weaning patients off narcotics, alcohol, or tobacco is essential prior to surgery.

At the time of surgery, preoperative preemptive analgesia can be helpful with the use of preoperative oral Tylenol 650 mg and Celebrex 200 mg as well as intravenous Decadron and intravenous TXA-Transemic Acid to manage bleeding. I use intravenous Decadron 6 mg, TXA 1 g, and intravenous antibiotics at the onset of surgery. The anesthesiologist then administers 1 g of TXA at the end of surgery. (Of course, prior DVT, pulmonary embolus, or stroke are contraindications to TXA.)

Prior to wound closure, I use a pericapsular infiltration that I have been utilizing successfully for all open knee surgeries since 2010. This eliminates the need for regional blocks and I prefer a general anesthetic with minimal gas inhalation and mostly TIVA-total intravenous anesthesia. Patients will awaken quickly, comfortably, and with minimal pain especially after the local infiltration.

The medications in the injection solution are mixed by the pharmacy and delivered to the operating room labeled with the patient's name. The total volume is 100 cc: 80 mcg clonidine, 0.5 mg epinephrine, 30 mg Ketorolac, 49.25 mL 0.5% ropivacaine, mixed with normal saline to a final volume of 100 ml.

I use an 18-gauge spinal needle or 22-gauge spinal needle in large 30 or 60 mL syringes and infiltrate everything that is pain-sensitive. This includes the periosteum and synovium circumferentially around the femur, the tibia, the quadriceps, the subcutaneous envelope, and specifically along the medial intermuscular septum at the site of the saphenous nerve exiting anteriorly over the anterior knee. When injecting, I first aspirate, especially over the saphenous nerve, to ensure that the mixture will not be injected into a blood vessel. The other point of caution is to be careful laterally and stay away from the peroneal nerve where a postoperative nerve palsy can occur as a result of the injection of ropivacaine. I have found this block to be extremely successful in alleviating pain from 24 to 72 hours postoperative before it dissipates, after which time it is easy to manage postoperative pain by transitioning to oral pain medications.

In addition, a continuous ice cryotherapy system is placed around the knee on top of a light dressing and sent home with the patient to assist in swelling and pain management.

Case 3. c-ACI-Multiple Defects Salvage Case With HTO-TTO

A 33-year-old occupational therapist has had several years of left pain, recurrent effusions, and grinding. She reports a prior medial meniscectomy and chondroplasty surgery of the left knee. Activities that she cannot perform include hiking, yoga, and Zumba.

Varus alignment is present on the limb alignment x-ray images with the mechanical axis line falling through the center of the medial tibial plateau. There is narrowing of medial cartilage joint spaces (Fig. 15.2A–E).

ACI (autologous cultured chondrocytes) using four vials of Carticel (Genzyme, Cambridge, MA, USA) with Bio-Gide membrane (Geistlich Industries, Wolhusen, Switzerland) was performed to the medial femoral condyle anterior (40 × 20 mm), posterior (25 × 15 mm), medial tibial plateau (25 × 15 mm), lateral femoral condyle (15 × 15 mm), trochlea (30 × 20 mm) combined with an opening wedge tibial valgus osteotomy and a tibial tubercle anteromedialization osteotomy (Fig. 15.2F–H).

Four years after surgery, the medial joint space is restored as seen in postoperative AP x-ray examination (Fig. 15.2I–J). Six years after surgery, the patient is doing well with a 96.4 KOOS score (preoperative 61.3) (Table 15.1), VAS score of 2 (preoperative 6) (Fig. 15.2K), and modified Cincinnati rating of 10 (preoperative 5) (Table 15.2). The patient reports full return of her knee function with minimal discomfort and has resumed recreational activities, including hiking, yoga, and even sports, and work without pain.

Case 4. MACI of Chronic Uncontained Patellofemoral Lesion With HTO-TTO

A 51-year-old former gymnast has dealt with chronic anterior knee pain and retropatellar crepitus as a result of patellofemoral lateral maltracking in the right knee.

The long alignment x-ray image demonstrates varus malalignment with the mechanical axis falling to the downslope of the medial tibial spine. In addition there is early narrowing of the lateral patellofemoral facet noted on skyline and lateral x-ray images (Fig. 15.3A–D). However, the overall cartilage spaces remain intact. Arthroscopy revealed full-thickness patellofemoral bipolar lesions with superficial fissuring of the medial tibial plateau (Fig. 15.3E–G).

As a result of the chronic lateral maltracking of the patellofemoral joint and the early fissuring noted on the medial tibial plateau in combination with slight varus malalignment, it was felt that realignment was required with both tibial valgus osteotomy and tibial tubercle osteotomy to

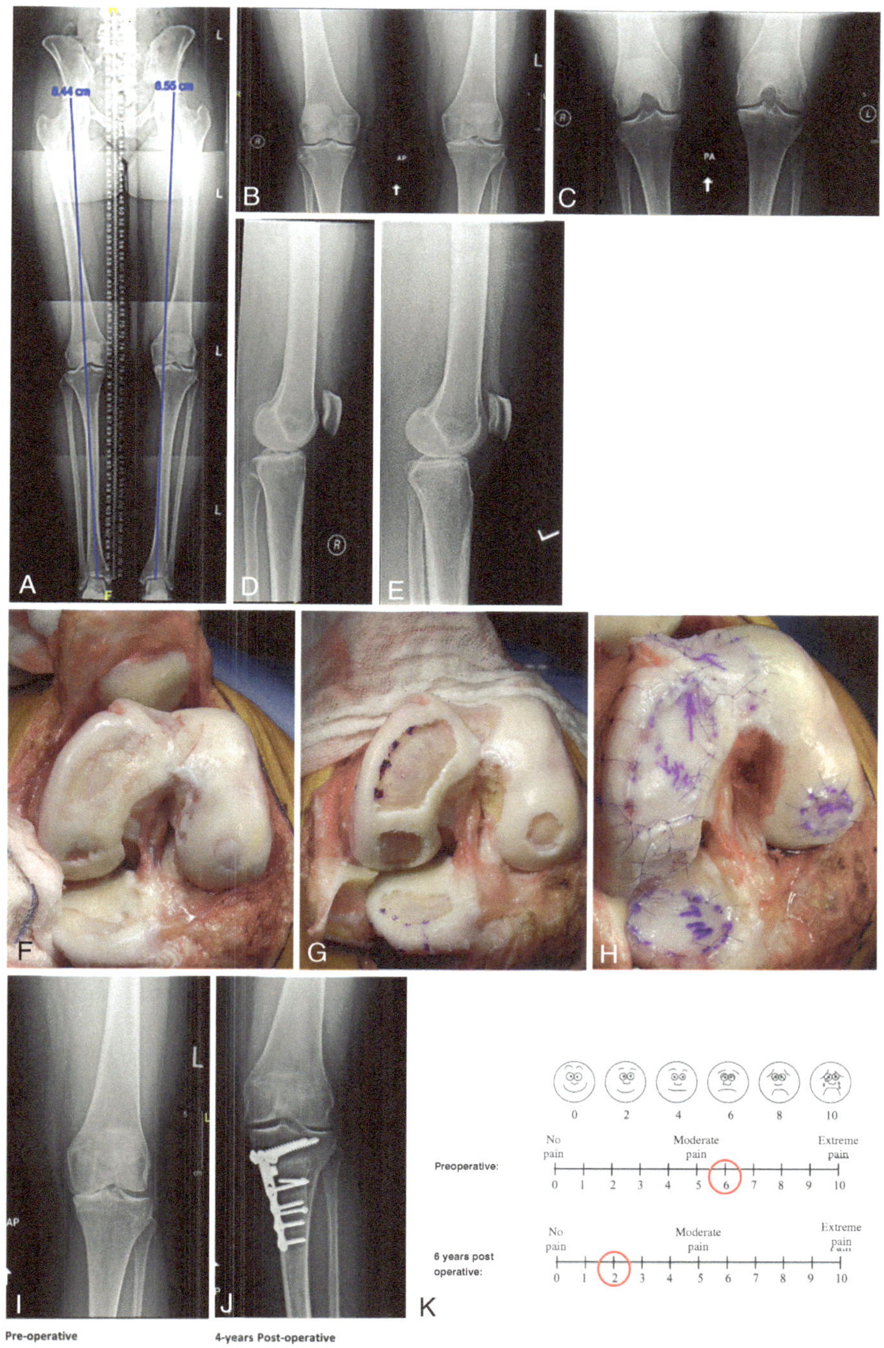

• **Fig. 15.2** (A) Long alignment x-ray image demonstrates weight-bearing axis to fall through the center of the medial joint compartment. (B) Standing AP x-ray image demonstrates loss of joint space anterior in the medial compartment. (C) Standing PA x-ray image demonstrates well-preserved posterior medial joint compartment. (D and E) Well-preserved patellofemoral joint space of both knees. (F) Large articular defects noted on the medial femoral condyle, medial tibial plateau, lateral femoral condyle, and trochlea. The exposure is facilitated by a tibial tubercle osteotomy that has been flipped up and a takedown of the medial meniscus. (G) Radical debridement of all the articular cartilage is performed back to stable intact full-thickness cartilage. The blue dots represent the location of transosseous drill holes made to secure the collagen membrane and chondrocytes using a small C-wire on a wire driver. The sutures are passed by straightening out the P3 cutting needle with a needle driver. (H) Final appearance of c-ACI after microsuturing, sealing the areas with fibrin glue, and injecting autologous cultured chondrocytes to fill the defects. The medial meniscus is then brought back to the intermeniscal ligament in near full extension and repaired with transosseous sutures through the medial meniscus anteriorly through the metaphyseal bone with a tapered needle no. 1 Vicryl suture. The tibial tubercle is then repositioned to center patellar tracking and fixated with two anterior to posterior lag screws followed by the medial patellofemoral ligament reattached to the mid-patellar pole and the lateral retinaculum being lengthened. Postoperative range of motion is instituted the morning after surgery using patellar mobilizations with manual therapy and a continuous passive motion machine. Touch weight-bearing for 6 weeks was followed by progressive weight-bearing to full body weight at 10 weeks with a medial compartment unloader braces. Because of the lateral femoral condyle defect the axial alignment is not overcorrected into the lateral compartment but just brought back to the midline. (I) Preoperative standing AP x-ray image shows loss of the anterior medial joint space with bone-on-bone changes. (J) Four-year postoperative weight-bearing x-ray image showing complete restoration of the medial joint compartment. It is a full weight-bearing AP x-ray image with mechanical axis corrected to the midline and not into the lateral compartment because of the lateral femoral condyle transplant. (K) VAS scores preoperative and postoperative.

TABLE 15.1 KOOS Scores Preoperative and 6 Years Postoperative

	Preoperative	6 years postoperative
Subtotal symptoms and stiffness:	46.43%	96.43%
Subtotal pain:	61.11%	97.22%
Subtotal function, daily living:	83.82%	100.00%
Subtotal function, sports and recreational activities:	30.00%	85.00%
Subtotal quality of life:	31.25%	93.75%
Total KOOS:	**61.3**	**96.4%**

TABLE 15.2 Modified Cincinnati Health Survey Overall Score Preoperative and 6 Years Postoperative

Poor (1–2)	I have significant limitations that affect activities of daily living.
Fair (3–4)	I have moderate limitations that affect activities of daily living. No sport possible.
Good (5–6)	I have some limitations with sports but I can participate; I compensate.
Very good (7–8)	I have only a few limitations with sports.
Excellent (9–10)	I am able to do whatever I wish (any sport) with no problem.

Modified Cincinnati Health Survey
Preoperative: 5 and **6 years postoperative**: 10

restore normal alignment in addition to MACI to the patella and trochlea of the patient's right knee. She wished to avoid a prosthesis and to preserve her own joint (Fig. 15.3H–N).

Case 5. MACI Sandwich Technique for Failed Microfracture of the Trochlea

A 39-year-old man sustained an injury playing volleyball when he jumped and landed on his left knee in a flexed position. He was diagnosed with an articular cartilage injury of the trochlea, which was then treated with microfracture. The microfracture surgery failed to resolve his symptoms. He worked as a telecommunications technician and despite surgery was unable to climb up and down cell tower ladders without persistent knee pain, rating 6/10, and recurrent effusions.

MRI revealed a full-thickness trochlear cartilage defect with associated intraarticular osteophyte formation and underlying bone marrow edema (Fig. 15.4A–B). These findings were later confirmed arthroscopically (Fig. 15.4E–F). The patellofemoral joint space remained intact on skyline and lateral x-ray images (Fig. 15.4C–D).

Following the failed microfracture, the patient's defect was treated with the MACI sandwich technique (Fig. 15.4G–I). A concomitant tibial tubercle osteotomy was performed to offload the large area of damage (Fig. 15.4J–L).

Case 6. ACI for End-Stage Patellofemoral OA in Elite Athlete Using Combined Cartilage Repair Techniques

A 42-year-old elite female athlete has a 1-year history of rapidly worsening anterior knee pain with recurrent effusions. The pain limits activities of daily living such as climbing up and down stairs, walking on uneven grounds, and stops her from participating in any sports or lower extremity resisted weight training. She sought a consultation for possible surgical solution to allow her to participate comfortably in activities of daily living and possibly return to competing in competitive swimming.

She has undergone arthroscopic debridement of the affected left knee for loose articular fragments and the patellofemoral joint with minimal improvement. She has had aspirations and steroid injections as well as plasma-rich protein injections with no improvement.

Clinical examination demonstrates a fit 42-year-old woman appearing younger than her stated age. She has atrophy to her left thigh musculature. A large intraarticular effusion and a Baker cyst are present in the left knee. Flexion of the left knee is limited secondary to the intraarticular effusion and Baker cyst. She has an increased quadriceps angle clinically. As a result of the large effusion crepitations, the knee cannot be palpated. The collateral and ligamentous examinations are normal.

AP, lateral, and skyline x-ray images (Fig. 15.5A–C) demonstrate erosive changes to the retropatellar surface of the left knee with intact tibiofemoral joint spaces. A CT scan of the knee in full extension with the quadriceps relaxed (Fig. 15.5D) and then contracted (Fig. 15.5E) demonstrates subluxation of the patellofemoral joint, subchondral bony cysts on the median ridge and lateral facet of the patella, complete loss of joint space of the lateral patellofemoral articulation, and a tibial tubercle-tibial groove distance (TT-TG) of 19 mm. Arthroscopic assessment of the left knee joint demonstrates intact tibiofemoral articulations with evidence of partial medial and lateral meniscectomies, advanced loss of articular cartilage to the patella with only a median ridge of articular cartilage remaining, and near complete loss of articular cartilage to the entire lateral trochlear facet surface. A biopsy for cultured articular chondrocytes is performed at the time of arthroscopy.

In order to reconstruct damaged patellofemoral surfaces of this patient's left knee biologically, the options include tibial tubercle osteotomy combined with kissing matched fresh osteoarticular allografts of the patella and trochlea or ACI to the patella and trochlea. However, when treating with ACI, the subchondral bone cysts, the sclerotic subchondral bone surface, and the near complete loss of articular surface

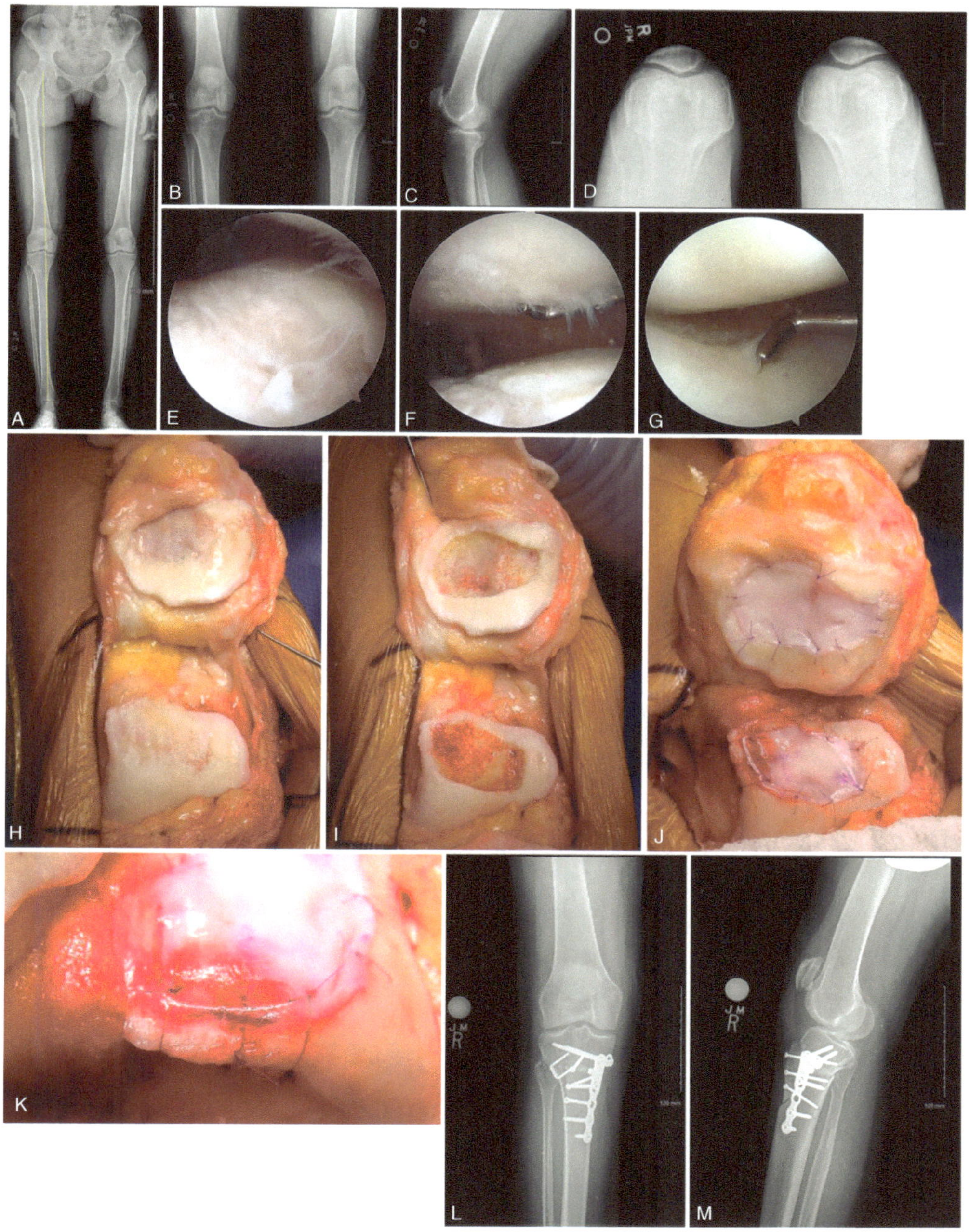

• **Fig. 15.3** (A) Long alignment x-ray images demonstrate the mechanical axis to follow through the downslope of the medial tibial spine with slight varus alignment. (B) Standing AP x-ray image demonstrates preservation of the tibiofemoral joint. (C) Lateral x-ray image of the right knee demonstrates some loss of the patellofemoral joint space with mild dysplasia of the trochlea. (D) Skyline x-ray image demonstrates bilateral early symmetrical lateral patella facet joint space narrowing. (E) Arthroscopic appearance of the trochlea with loss of articular cartilage centrally with containment noted except for peripheral and lateral. (F) The patella also shows articular cartilage loss to the lateral patella facet. (G) There is early grade 2 fissuring of the medial tibial plateau with an intact articular surface of the femoral condyle and medial meniscus. Note that long alignment x-ray images previously showed mild varus deformity and now objective evidence of medial compartment overload with fissuring on the tibial surface. The lateral tibiofemoral compartment is intact. (H) Exposure of the patellofemoral joint with tibial tubercle osteotomy flip-flop technique. Note the very chronic and sclerotic articular surfaces with bare bone exposed and peripheral osteophytes remaining. (The proximal tibial valgus osteotomy is performed next.) (I) A very careful radical debridement of the damaged articular cartilage is performed back to healthy articular cartilage, preserving the peripheral osteophytes using a ring curet to start with and a no. 15 blade. As the bone is prominent and sclerotic, it is deepened with a high-speed 6-mm diameter egg-shaped bur to produce a well-contained defect from which the matrix-induced autologous chondrocyte implantation (MACI) membrane can grow from the bottom to the surface. This is done as the soft tissues are being protected with wet sponges from any bony debris created by the bur under continuous saline irrigation. (J) The MACI membranes are glued with the cell layers facing the subchondral bone using fibrin glue and secured secondarily with 6-0 Vicryl sutures to prevent dislodgment of the membranes. The uncontained lateral trochlea utilizes the osteophyte to secure the membrane to the subchondral bone using transosseous tunnels created by a small C-wire on a mini wire driver marking the entry and exit holes with a sterile marking pen. The P3 cutting needle is straightened with a needle driver and passed through the transosseous drill hole to capture the MACI membrane securing it. On the patella surface, the synovial margin around the edge of the patella is utilized as a suturing anchor for the membrane where it is uncontained distally. In this way uncontained defects can be secured and the defects can be deepened to allow the tissue to grow to the surface. (K) A close-up of the trochlea attachment to the lateral trochlea osteophyte through transosseous drill holes. (L) Realignment postoperative AP x-ray image demonstrating realignment of the tibia to neutral mechanical axis. (M) Lateral x-ray image demonstrating repositioning of the tibial tubercle and stabilization.

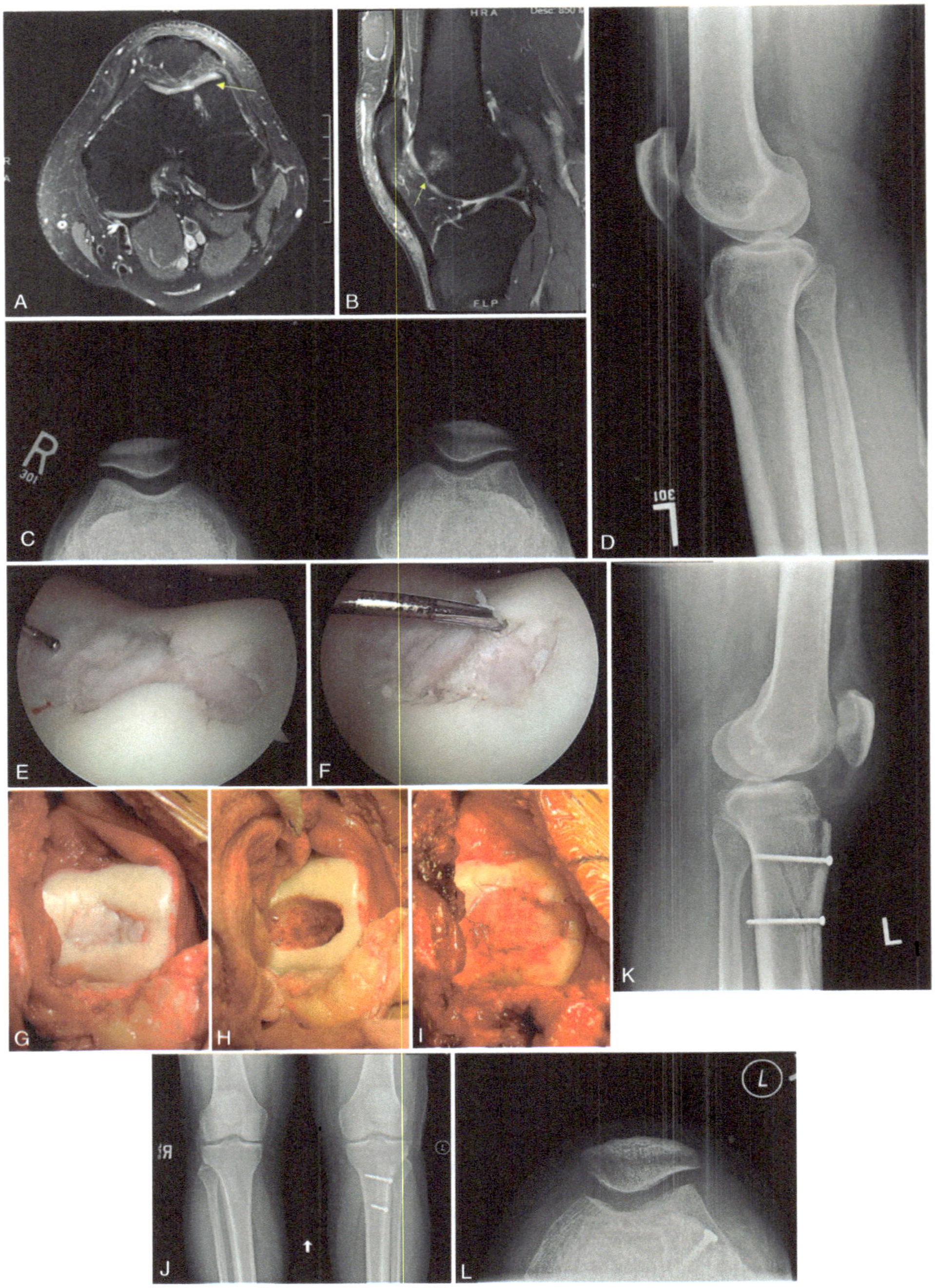

• **Fig. 15.4** (A) Axial fat-suppressed MRI scan demonstrates intralesional osteophyte thickening with adjacent bone marrow edema. (B) Sagittal fat-suppressed MRI scan demonstrates full-thickness cartilage loss, intralesional osteophyte formation, and subchondral bone marrow edema. Skyline (C) and lateral (D) x-ray images demonstrate well-preserved patellofemoral joint space suitable for cartilage repair and joint preservation. (E and F) Arthroscopic images of the area prior to microfracture demonstrate healing by intralesional osteophyte formation that is prominent to the articular surface with a thin film of fibrous tissue on its surface. (G) Intralesional osteophyte formation with a thin fibrous film is very clearly observed prior to radical debridement of the trochlear defect, which is well-contained but encompasses most of the surface. (H) Radical debridement of the defect involves first identifying native full-thickness cartilage with a no. 15 blade and a ring curet surrounding the area of damage. The ring curet is used to try to pare off all the fibrous tissue on the surface of the intralesional osteophytes. Surrounding soft tissues are protected with wet sponges. A high-speed 6-mm diameter H-shaped bur is used to remove all the intralesional osteophytes back to healthy subchondral bone, i.e., to the level of or slightly below the adjacent subchondral bone. (I) A sandwich technique is performed by using fibrin glue on the base of the subchondral bone with an MACI glued with the cell layer facing outward and the smooth layer toward the subchondral bone. The tourniquet is then let down and a small neural patty is kept on the MACI membrane that is immersed in saline to apply gentle pressure to prevent dislodgment of the membrane. The neural patty is carefully removed revealing a dry subchondral bone with layer one MACI membrane in position. A small amount of fibrin glue is applied to the surface of the first membrane and the second membrane is then applied face downward toward the first such that the cells are sandwiched between the two smooth layers of membrane. The edges are secured with interrupted 6-0 Vicryl sutures and fibrin glue on the edges. In this way the marrow-derived cells in the underlying cancellous bone are separated from the end-differentiated autologous cultured chondrocytes for the best chance to have a uniform repair tissue without admixture of bone elements or fibrous elements to the repair tissue. (J–L) AP, lateral, and skyline x-ray images demonstrate well-positioned tibial tubercle and centered patella.

to the entire patella need to be dealt with. ACI was chosen because it is a surface treatment to the articular surfaces that can be salvaged with a fresh osteoarticular allograft if it were to fail.

The surgery consists of a lateral subvastus arthrotomy with inspection of the damaged articular surfaces. The damaged patellar surfaces and the tracking can be assessed and a tibial tubercle osteotomy can be performed to medialize and normalize the tracking of the extensor mechanism. The osteotomy is performed with a transverse proximal cut, a length of 6 cm with a sloping distal cut, and anteromedialization that centralizes and minimally unloads the lateral facet of the patella. The entire extensor mechanism can then be reflected proximally and medially. This allowed excellent exposure to the patellofemoral joint without filing the quadriceps extensor mechanism. The appearance of the patella reveals only a small rim of medial facet cartilage (Fig. 15.5F–G), and proximal pole cartilage. The trochlea lateral facet demonstrates vertical ridging of the tendon remaining proximal cartilage with a central erosive full-thickness cartilage loss (Fig. 15.5H). Radical debridement of both defects requires removal of all subchondral bone cysts on the patella with a high-speed bur and trying to retain a thin margin of articular cartilage to sew peripherally and circumferentially on both the trochlea and the patella. The sclerotic subchondral bone is also deepened

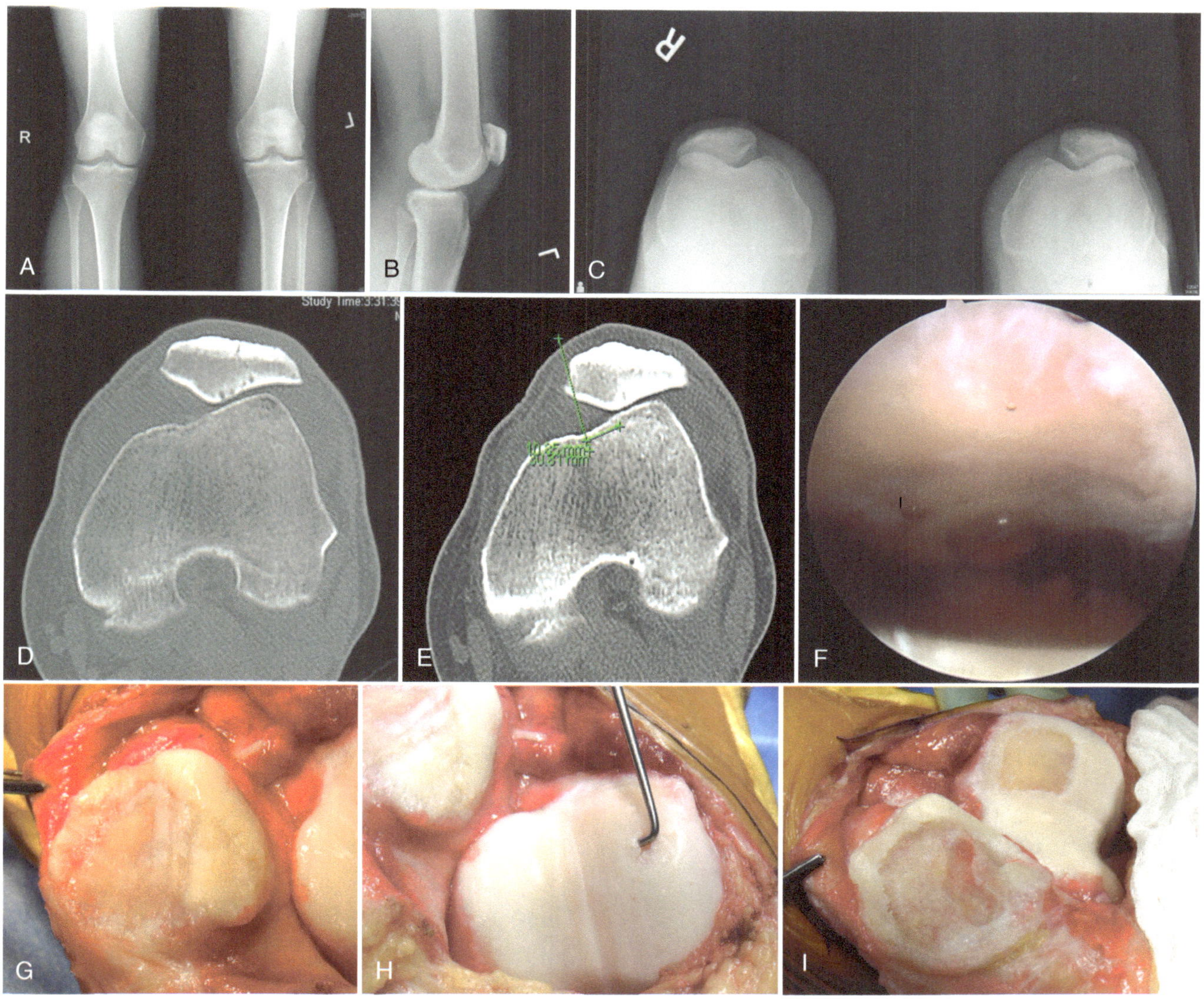

• **Fig. 15.5** (A) AP radiograph. (B) Lateral radiograph demonstrating retropatellar subchondral erosive changes. (C) Skyline radiograph demonstrating left patellar subchondral bone changes with tilt and subluxation. (D) Computed tomographic (CT) scan with the quadriceps relaxed demonstrates subchondral bone cysts on the median ridge lateral facet of the patella with loss of lateral facet articular space. (E) CT scan of the quadriceps contracted demonstrates further subluxation of the patella laterally. (F) Arthroscopic appearance of patella demonstrates near pan-patellar cartilage loss with bare bone exposed. (G) Open appearance of patella demonstrates only a small rim of median ridge cartilage remaining, with complete loss of articular surface to the lateral facet and median ridge. (H) Open appearance of trochlea shows global thinning of lateral trochlea facet and breakdown as demonstrated by a nerve hook with bare bone exposed and undermining of articular cartilage. (I) Open appearance of trochlea and patella after radical debridement of damaged articular cartilage with removal of subchondral bone cysts using high-speed bur to the patella.

Continued

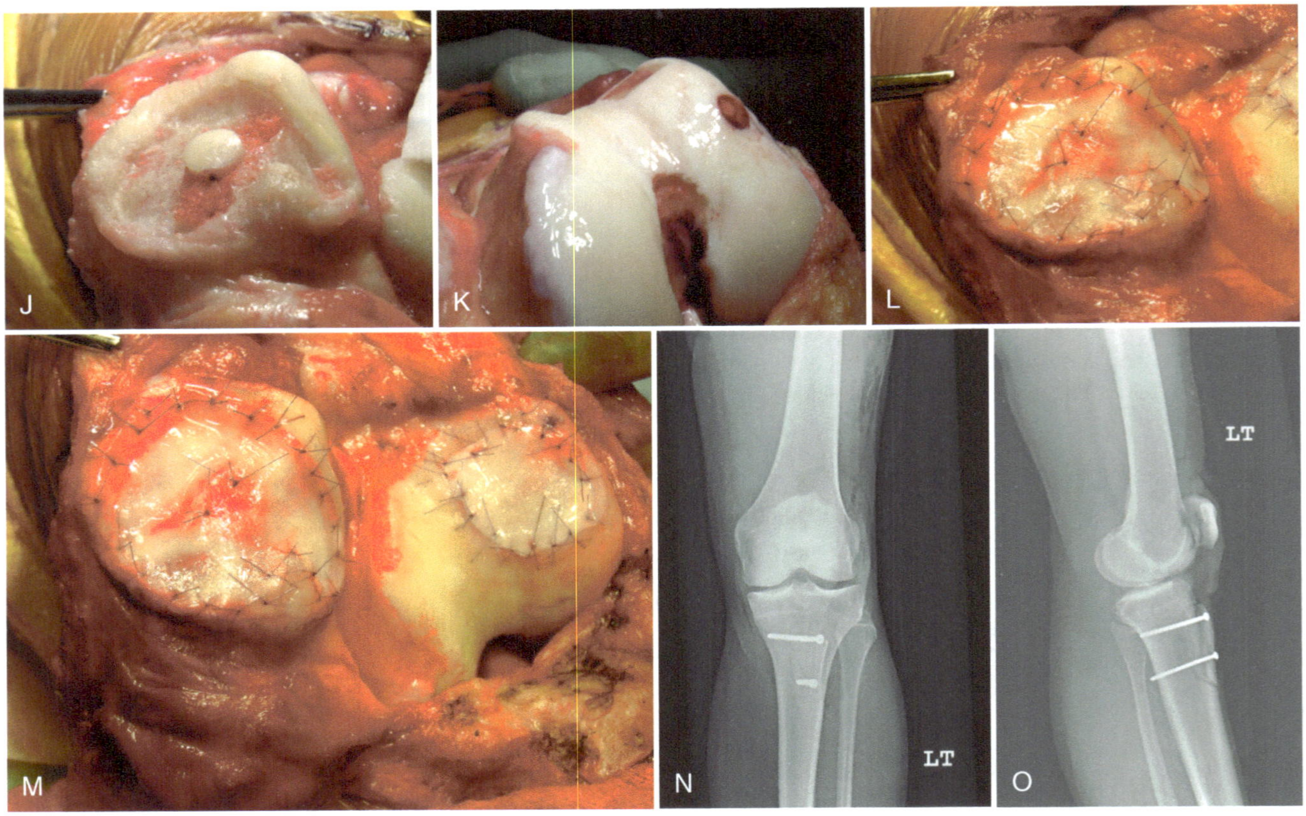

• **Fig. 15.5 —cont'd** (J) Appearance of patella with osteochondral graft placed at the area of the central median ridge in order to restore the volume of the articular surface of the patella after membrane microsuturing and bone grafting of the subchondral bone loss. (K) TruFit plug to sulcus terminalis of the distal lateral trochlea for backfill of the osteochondral dowel used to repair the patella. (L) Appearance of patella after autologous chondrocyte implantation (ACI). (M) Open appearance of patella and trochlea after ACI. (N) AP radiograph after tibial tubercle osteotomy. (O) Lateral radiograph after tibial tubercle osteotomy.

and thinned out with a high-speed bur. The peripheral synovium around the patella that is well attached to its margins is incised and reflected 5 mm circumferentially to assist in suture anchorage of the membrane that will cover the transplanted surface (Fig. 15.5I). The area of subchondral cysts that are removed with a high-speed bur was bone grafted with proximal tibial cancellous bone taken from the osteotomy site. The median ridge is maintained centrally in this area with a 10-mm osteochondral graft harvested from the distal pole sulcus terminalis and transplanted into the osseous deficient region centrally (Fig. 15.5J). The donor site for the 10-mm osteochondral graft taken from the sulcus terminalis of the distal lateral trochlea set is backfilled with a TruFit plug (Smith & Nephew, Andover, MA) (Fig. 15.5K). The patella is then resurfaced with a collagen type I-III porcine membrane (Bio-Gide). The microsuturing is performed with 60 Vicryl circumferentially in a manner that restores the V-shaped articular surface to the patella anchoring specifically at the osteochondral graft median ridge centrally (Fig. 15.5L–M). Fifty million autologous articular chondrocytes are then injected underneath the membranes and sealed. The tibial tubercle osteotomy is repositioned centrally and held with two interfragmentary compression screws (Fig. 15.5N–O).

A gentle rehabilitation program with emphasis on patellar mobility in the proximal, distal, medial, and lateral directions to prevent retropatellar adhesions, lower extremity muscle tone to the quadriceps, hamstring and gluteal muscles and a functional rehabilitation results in an excellent early functional return. The goals of a pain-free quality of life with activities of daily living are restored and further athletic endeavors pursued.

The patient returned to competitive elite-level swimming and 10 years later remains symptom-free with a well-preserved patellofemoral joint space.

Case 7. Cartilage Repair for the Lateral Meniscectomy Cascade With a Valgus Knee in a Young Athlete

A 16-year-old woman sustained a lateral meniscus tear to the left knee while playing soccer. An arthroscopy was performed and the meniscus was completely removed. Within 12 to 18 months of her subtotal lateral meniscectomy she developed recurrent effusions, laterally based joint pain, and inability to participate in sports as well as limitations of activities of daily living.

She had a second arthroscopy, which demonstrated cartilaginous loss throughout the weight-bearing surface of the lateral femoral condyle and lateral tibial plateau. A biopsy for ACI was taken. She was then referred for definitive reconstruction of her left knee.

Long alignment x-ray images demonstrate that her mechanical axis falls to the lateral compartment of her left knee (Fig. 15.6A). Standing PA radiographs (Fig. 15.6B–C) demonstrate that at 17 years old she already has 50% loss of the articular space of the lateral compartment of her left knee. Skyline x-ray images demonstrate tilt and subluxation of the patella of the left knee. A lateral x-ray image demonstrates a normal patellar height (Fig. 15.6D).

The planned reconstruction involves a tibial tubercle anteromedialization to centralize her extensor mechanism with a lateral subvastus approach to expose the distal lateral femur and lateral tibiofemoral joint surfaces (Fig. 15.6E). After radical debridement of the damaged articular cartilage to the distal femur and lateral tibial plateau (Fig. 15.6F), a trough is prepared in preparation for a lateral meniscus allograft. The lateral meniscus is prepared on the back table with type 0 Ethibond sutures through the posterior horn of the lateral meniscus (Fig. 15.6G) to allow passage of the lateral meniscus allograft through the posterior capsule, which has been carefully dissected from the posterior aspect of the knee joint. The ACI grafts are first microsutured and prepared (Fig. 15.6H) and then the lateral meniscus allograft is passed and repaired (Fig. 15.6I), prior to the opening wedge distal femoral varus osteotomy being performed, which tightens the lateral column of the knee (Fig. 15.6J–K). The tibial tubercle osteotomy is finally repositioned centrally and fixated at the end of the surgery (Fig. 15.6L).

Postoperatively, the patient undergoes continuous passive motion, touch weight-bearing, and isometric quadriceps contractions for the first 6 weeks. A custom lateral compartment unloader brace is fitted and the patient progresses with weight-bearing as comfort allows based on pain in the lateral tibiofemoral compartment. A stationary bicycle is also permitted at 6 weeks postoperatively with isometric quadriceps straight leg raises. She is off her crutches by 10 weeks postoperative.

The unloader brace is worn for 6 months at which time she is pain-free and resumes normal activities of daily living and gradually resumes non-impact sports at 9–12 months after reconstruction.

Case 8. Cartilage Repair With ACI Segmental Sandwich Technique After Failed Osteobiologic (OBI) Plugs

A 23-year-old young woman sustains an anterior cruciate ligament (ACL) tear with an articular cartilage injury to the medial femoral condyle, which is treated by an ACL reconstruction with allograft patellar bone tendon bone and TruFit OBI plug (Smith & Nephew) to the medial femoral condyle. Her medial pain persists as well as persistent effusions and anterior knee pain. She undergoes repeat arthroscopy and the treating surgeon notes large trochlea and lateral femoral condyle defects and harvests cartilage for ACI. She is then referred for definitive treatment.

A clinical examination demonstrates neutral alignment to the right lower extremity, a large effusion in the right knee, and antalgic gait pattern. She has a stable ligamentous examination, mild retropatellar crepitus, and medial joint line tenderness.

Her standing PA x-ray examination demonstrates an intralesional osteophyte to the lateral femoral condyle and well-preserved tibiofemoral joint spaces (Fig. 15.7A). Her lateral x-ray examination (Fig. 15.7B) demonstrates an increased tibial posterior slope with hardware intact from previous ACL reconstruction. Her skyline x-ray image demonstrates a well-preserved joint space (Fig. 15.7C).

At the time of the open ACI procedure it is noted that there is a large intralesional osteophyte to the lateral femoral condyle, a large trochlear defect, and evidence of a TruFit plug to the medial femoral condyle that is in situ but that has not incorporated with surrounding cartilage degradation (Fig. 15.7D). The TruFit plug is easily removed with forceps with no evidence of incorporation or healing (Fig. 15.7E). The osseous defect to the medial femoral condyle is filled with autologous bone harvested from the proximal femoral metaphysis with a core harvester. The autologous cancellous bone graft is morselized and fills in the bony deficiency to the medial femoral condyle (Fig. 15.7F). It is covered with a collagen membrane (Fig. 15.7G), the other defects are radically debrided, and the tourniquet is removed (Fig. 15.7H). The ACI grafts are microsutured into place over the defects in the usual fashion (Fig. 15.7I). The patient undergoes a standard rehabilitation for ACI to the weight-bearing condyle with trochlear defect. Six months postoperatively an MRI scan (Fig. 15.7J) demonstrates minimal bone marrow edema, excellent bone graft incorporation to the osseous defect from the previous TruFit plug, and a good cartilage repair developing. Three years postoperatively the patient remains symptom-free.

Case 9. ACI to Salvage Failed Osteochondral Autologous Transplantation Plugs for Patella Cartilage Repair

A 42-year-old man underwent bilateral staged tibial tubercle osteotomies with intractable anterior knee pain. The left knee also underwent cartilage repair with osteochondral graft transfers from the lateral trochlea to the patella with worsening of symptoms. The patient presents with severe bilateral anterior knee pain, left worse than right, and inability to work. He wishes to pursue biologic preservation of his knee joints if possible.

Physical examination demonstrates an overweight 42-year-old man appearing to be his stated age. He walks with a stiff-legged antalgic bilateral lower extremity gait pattern. He has severe palpable and audible patellofemoral crepitus on the left knee with a large effusion and mild

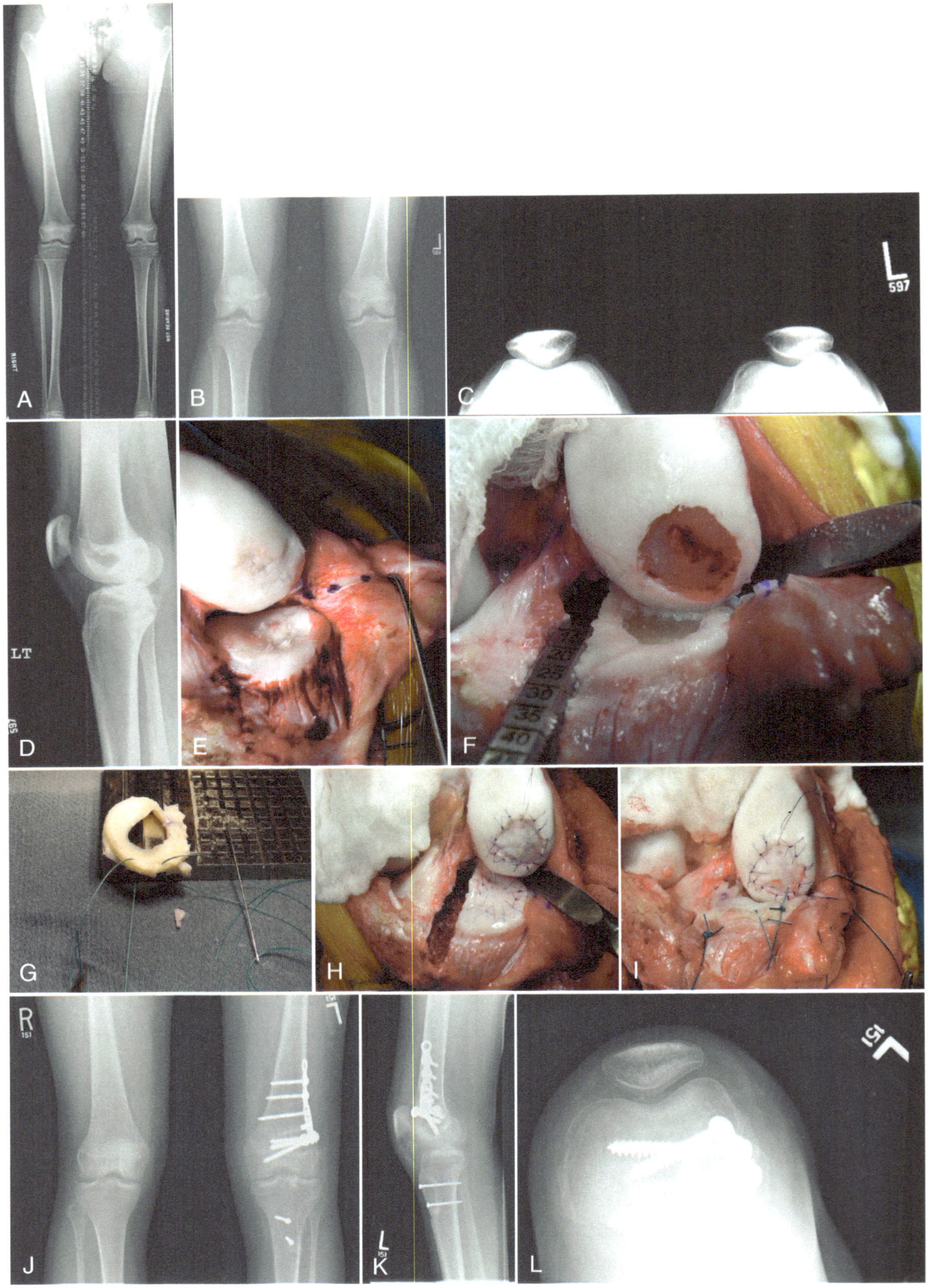

• **Fig. 15.6** (A) Long alignment x-ray films. (B) Standing posteroanterior radiographs demonstrate 50% cartilage loss to the left knee lateral tibiofemoral joint. (C) Skyline x-ray films demonstrate lateral tilt and subluxation to the left patella. (D) Lateral x-ray film. (E) Grade 3 and grade 4 central cartilage loss to lateral tibial plateau and lateral femoral condyles. (F) Lateral tibial femoral compartment after radical debridement to damaged articular cartilage surfaces and trough preparation for lateral meniscus allograft passage. (G) Lateral meniscus allograft preparation on back table with sutures through the posterior horn of the lateral meniscus. (H) Autologous chondrocyte implantation grafts sutured in position. (I) Lateral meniscus allograft passed into lateral compartment. (J) Postoperative anteroposterior radiograph of left knee following femoral osteotomy with tibial tubercle osteotomy. (K) Lateral radiograph. (L) Skyline radiograph.

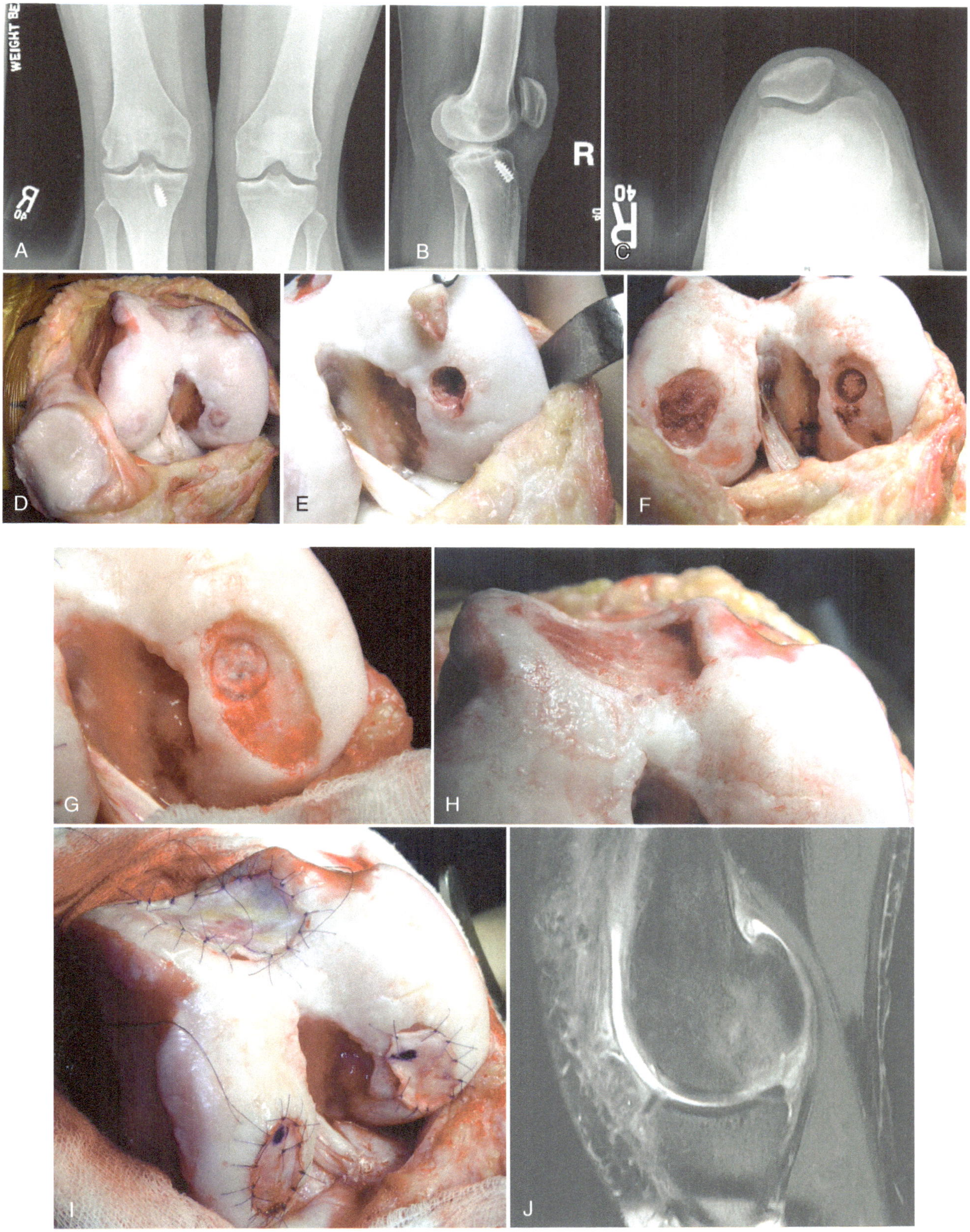

• **Fig. 15.7** (A) Posteroanterior radiograph demonstrates intralesional osteophyte to lateral femoral condyles with well-preserved tibiofemoral joint. (B) Lateral x-ray film. (C) Skyline x-ray film. (D) Medial parapatellar arthrotomy. Intralesional osteophyte to lateral femoral condyles, large trochlear defect, and TruFit plug to medial femoral condyle with surrounding cartilage thinning are evident. (E) TruFit plug to medial femoral condyles is easily removed with forceps and unincorporated. (F) Open appearance of knee after radical debridement. Intralesional osteophyte to lateral femoral condyles is removed. Autologous bone grafting to medial femoral condyle TruFit plug recipient site is performed. (G) Medial femoral condyle, after collagen cover, to autologous bone graft to recipient site for failed TruFit plug. (H) Trochlear defect. (I) Autologous chondrocyte implantation defects prepared. (J) Sagittal fat-suppressed magnetic resonance imaging scan 6 months postoperative demonstrating incorporated autologous bone graft and cartilage repair to surface of the medial femoral condyle.

to moderate palpable crepitus on the right. He has anterior midline incisions bilaterally. The soft tissue envelope is healthy bilaterally.

Standing AP x-ray images (Fig. 15.8A) demonstrate well-preserved tibiofemoral joints with mild varus alignment of both knees. There is evidence of bilateral tibial tubercle elevation with a synthetic bone substitute used for the elevation on the left (Fig. 15.8B). The skyline x-ray images (Fig. 15.8C) demonstrate well-preserved patellofemoral joint spaces. Further evaluation with CT arthrogram demonstrates loss of patellar articular surface (Fig. 15.8D), lateral trochlea articular surface (Fig. 15.8E), and thinning of the medial femoral condyle cartilage surface (Fig. 15.8F).

At the time of open reconstruction with ACI, it is evident that the cartilage cap for two of the three osteochondral graft transfers to the patella have delaminated (Fig. 15.8G) and only one remains intact for further reconstructive advantage after radical debridement (Fig. 15.8H). The patella ACI graft is then performed incorporating the osteochondral graft transfer that has remained intact (Fig. 15.8I). There is poor repair tissue fill to the donor sites of the lateral trochlea (Fig. 15.8J). After radical debridement (Fig. 15.8K) the donor sites in the trochlea and medial femoral condyle can be transplanted with ACI in the usual fashion (Fig. 15.8L).

The postoperative rehabilitation is as per ACI to the patella, focus on patellar mobility quadriceps tone, and a functional recovery resulted in an excellent clinical outcome to the patient.

This case illustrates donor site complications when osteochondral grafts are harvested from the proximal lateral

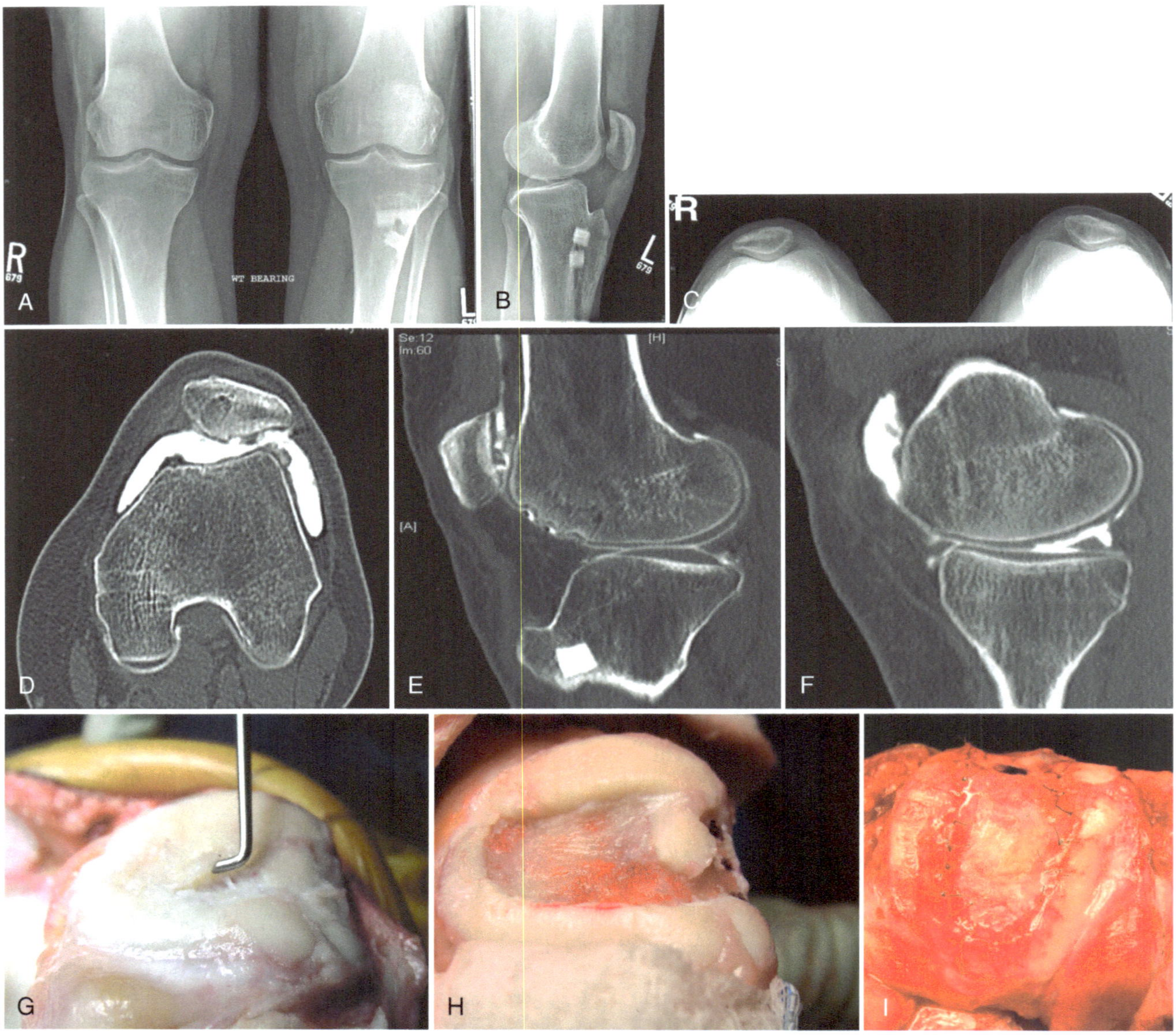

• **Fig. 15.8** (A) Anteroposterior radiograph. (B) Lateral radiograph of left knee with tibial tubercle elevation using synthetic bone substitute. (C) Skyline x-ray films demonstrate intact patellofemoral joint spaces. (D) Computed tomographic (CT) arthrogram axial view. (E) CT arthrogram sagittal view over donor sites. (F) CT arthrogram sagittal view over medial femoral condyle. (G) Failed osteochondral graft to lateral patella facet. (H) Radical debridement of patella with only one of three osteochondral grafts remaining intact to the patella. (I) Patella autologous chondrocyte implantation (ACI).

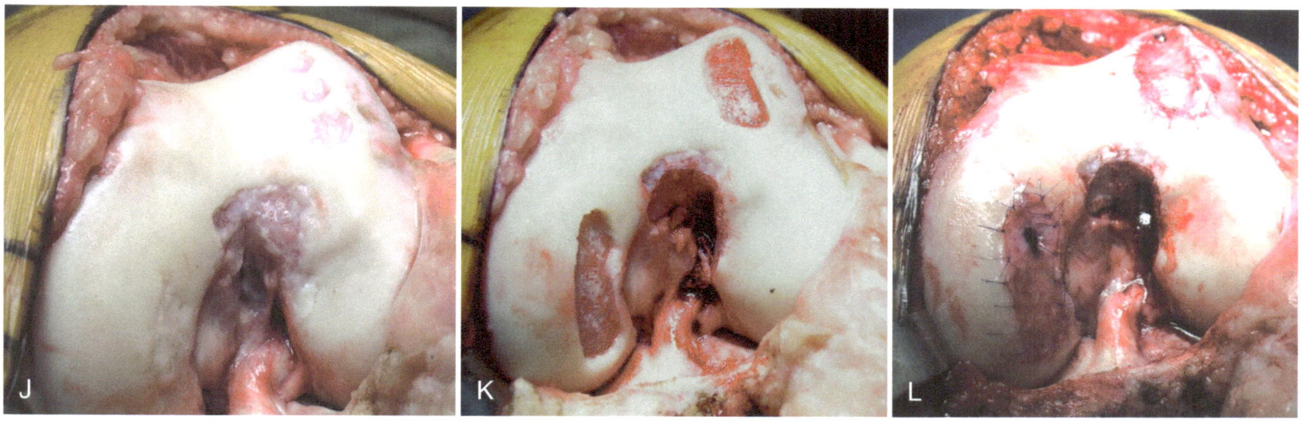

• **Fig. 15.8 —cont'd** (J) Donor sites to lateral trochlea incompletely filled with repair tissue and medial femoral condyles grade 3 defect. (K) Radical debridement of lateral trochlea donor sites and medial femoral condyles in preparation for ACI. (L) ACI to medial femoral condyle and lateral trochlea facet.

trochlea facet. Crepitation and pain are common when this high contact area is utilized. Second, osteochondral autografting to the patella is a relative contraindication. Resorption and collapse of grafts is common in the patella because the cartilage surface thickness of the donors is only 2 to 3 mm compared with 5 to 7 mm normally found in the patella cartilage surface. This mismatch leads to poor vascularity to the prominent bone of the donor osteochondral dowel, which undergoes creeping substitution resorption and collapse.

Case 10. Tibial Tubercle Osteotomy, Trochleoplasty, and Patella Cartilage Repair With Adolescent Fresh Preserved Morselized Allograft

A 27-year-old woman presents with severe bilateral anterior knee pain greater in the right knee than in the left. She has undergone bilateral tibial tubercle realignment osteotomies with proximal soft tissue realignment. She continues to have a sense of bilateral knee patellar instability and severe anterior pain.

Clinical examination demonstrates a healthy 27-year-old woman who walks with a stiff-legged, circumduction gait. She is very apprehensive about the clinical examination. She is able to flex and extend her knees on her own with a positive J-sign bilaterally, audible patellofemoral crepitus on the right worse than on the left, and a tremendous sense of instability with a fear of dislocation especially on the right side. She comments that her surgeries have not helped her sense of instability or reduced her pain.

Preoperative CT arthrography (not shown) demonstrates patellar subluxation, near pan-patellar cartilage loss, and dysplasia of the trochlea. Based on the severe degree of dysplasia that is noted at the time of CT arthrography, trochleoplasty with the possibility of revision tibial tubercle osteotomy, soft tissue realignment, and cartilage repair with adolescent minced allograft tissue is discussed. The patient is in agreement.

At the time of open medial arthrotomy, severe erosive change to the concave patella (Fig. 15.9A) and reciprocal convex dysplasia to the trochlea are noted (Fig. 15.9B). A radical debridement to the patella is performed as per ACI, the minced allograft adolescent cartilage (DeNovo NT, Zimmer, ISTO Technologies) is applied to the base of the defect and sealed with fibrin glue with a collagen membrane then circumferentially microsutured as per ACI technique to the surrounding rim and synovial tissue is present (Fig. 15.9C). After the tibial tubercle osteotomy has been revised to centralize the tubercle underneath the tibial spines, instability persists and it is felt that a trochleoplasty is necessary to allow the patella to centralize without subluxation medially or laterally. The center of the trochlea is marked with dotted sterile marking pen (Fig. 15.9D–E) and the most proximal portion of the trochlea cartilage and bone is removed and contoured toward the anterior femoral cortex as noted in Chapter 12, synovial advancement trochleoplasty. The synovium is then advanced and sutured through the articular surface. The final appearance of the reconstruction with tibial tubercle osteotomy, cartilage repair to the patella, and synovial interposition trochleoplasty is noted in Fig. 15.9F. The wound is then closed and the medial and lateral retinaculum are balanced through a range of motion.

Rehabilitation consists of continuous passive motion, patellar mobilizations, isometric quadriceps contractions, and progression to full weight-bearing with functional activities as previously described in Chapter 9 for ACI to the patella. The postoperative radiographs are noted in Fig. 15.9G–H.

This case demonstrates the difficulty encountered when standard techniques are used for stabilizing patellofemoral maltracking in the presence of trochlear dysplasia. The history is classic: recurrent instability episodes unresponsive to conservative measures and then proximal and distal realignment procedures that have failed. Trochlear dysplasia should be considered the major cause of recurrent instability in this situation, which is the case presented in Fig. 15.10.

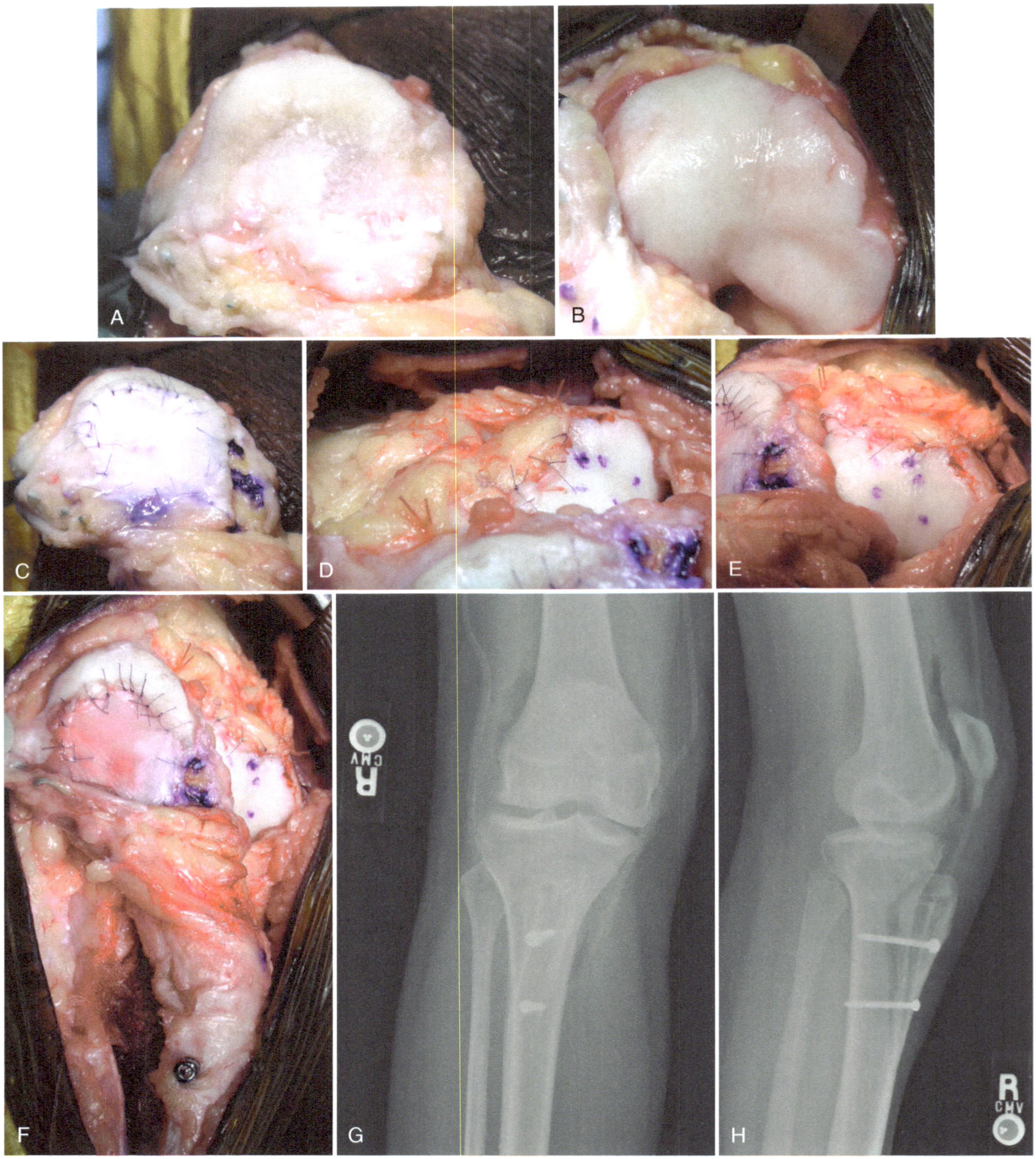

• **Fig. 15.9** (A) Open appearance of patella with articular damage. (B) Open appearance of dysplastic trochlea. (C) Cartilage repair to patella with morselized adolescent allograft cartilage (DeNovo NT, Zimmer-ISTO Technologies) with collagen cover membrane. (D) Lateral view of synovial interposition advancement trochleoplasty. (E) Frontal view of synovial interposition advancement trochleoplasty. (F) Frontal view of final reconstruction, which includes revision tibial tubercle osteotomy, lateral patellar release, cartilage repair to patella, synovial advancement trochleoplasty, and vastus medialis obliquus quadricepsplasty. (G) Anteroposterior x-ray film. (H) Lateral x-ray film.

Case 11. ACI Segmental Sandwich Technique for Failed Large Osteochondral Allograft in Division 1 Football Player

A 22-year-old intercollegiate athlete playing football at Michigan State University has had several episodes of the right knee locking and catching with significant pain to the medial aspect of his joint. He has suffered articular injury to his medial joint compartment and undergone surgical repair including an OATS procedure followed by a failed microfracture and then an osteochondral allograft to the medial femoral condyle. Because of persistent medially-based pain he underwent repeat arthroscopy demonstrating progression of disease around his allograft as well as the trochlea and lateral femoral condyle. A cartilage biopsy for ACI was taken. His long mechanical alignment x-ray examinations demonstrated a neutral mechanical axis. Because of the large trochlear defect it was felt that a tubercle osteotomy was necessary to unload the trochlea and transplant the other sites.

At the time of open ACI surgery, it was found that the cartilage cap of the osteochondral dowel allograft had completely delaminated and was unstable. There was also progression of articular damage around the medial femoral

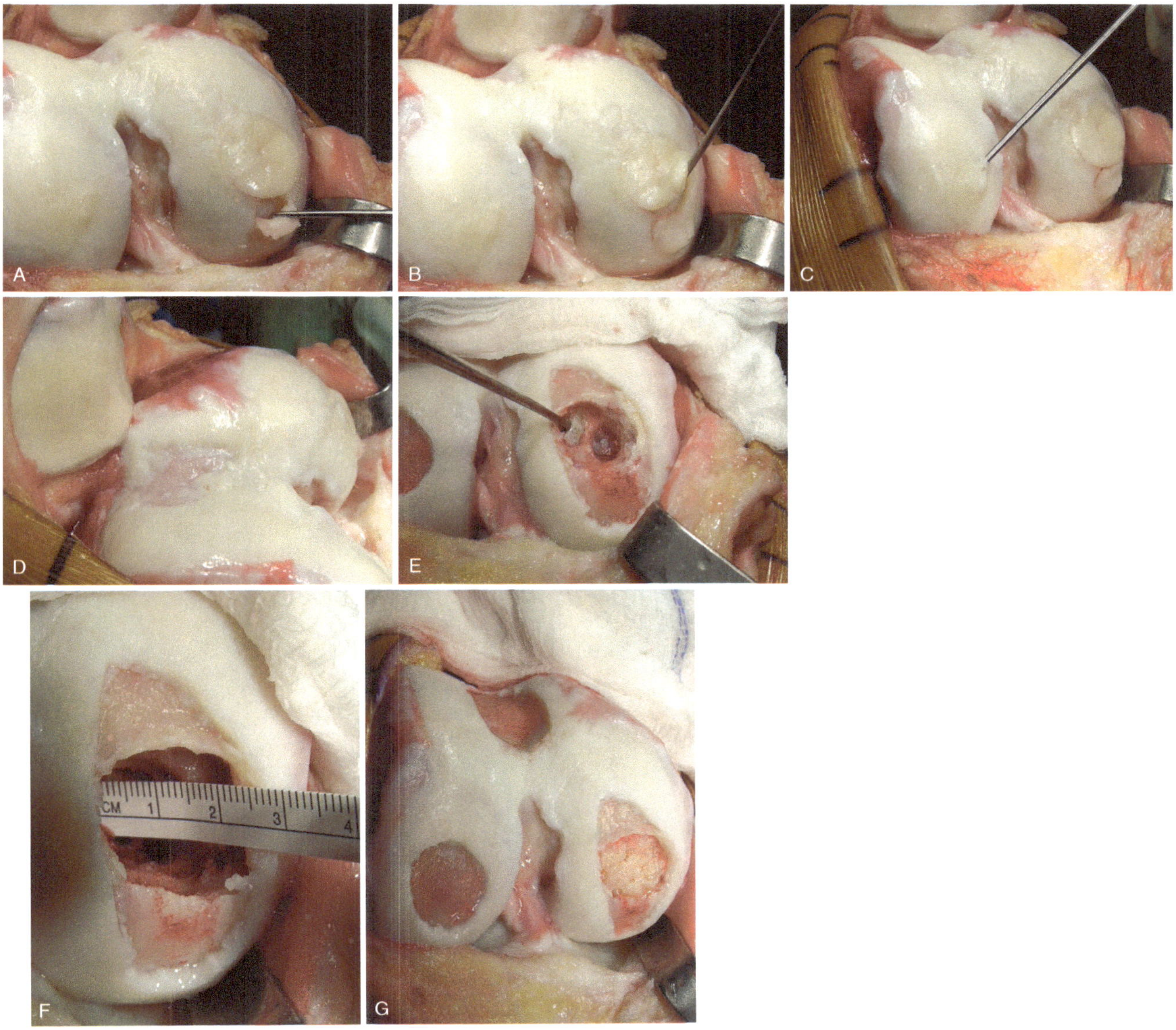

• **Fig. 15.10** (A) Intraoperative probing of the posterior smaller osteochondral allograft reveals detachment of the cartilage. (B) Failure of the larger anterior allograft results in the same way. (C) The probe demonstrates delamination of cartilage on the lateral femoral condyle. (D) There is a large grade 4 defect exposing subchondral bone on the trochlea. (E) Appearance of the femur after radical debridement of all the damaged and delaminating articular cartilage. Note there is no blood coming from the center of the two osteochondral allograft regions on the medial femoral condyle. (F–I) Sequential bony debridement with a high-speed bur under continuous saline irrigation back to healthy subchondral bone demonstrates a very large defect measuring approximately 2 x 2 cm and 2 cm deep.

Continued

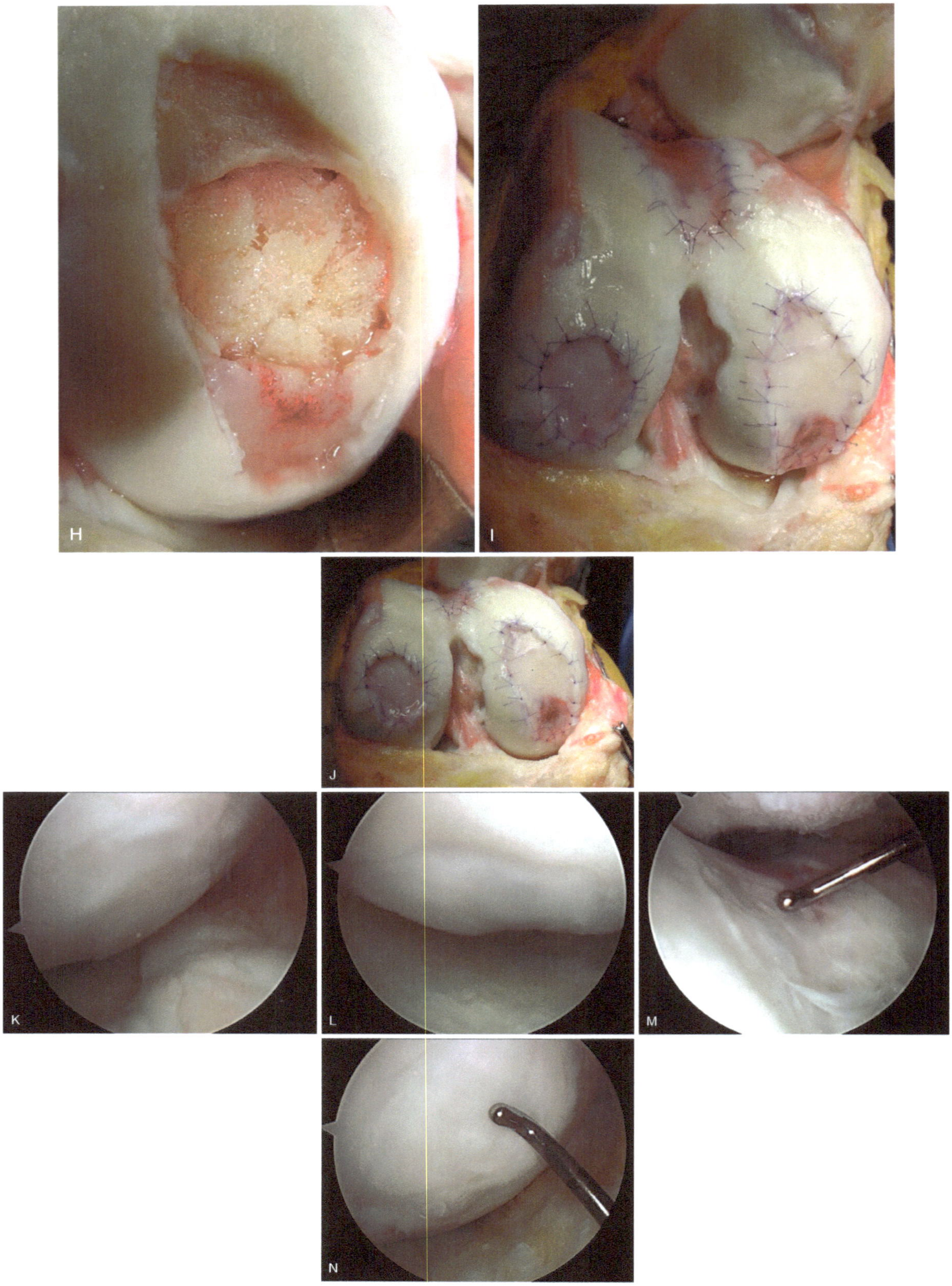

• **Fig. 15.10—cont'd** (J) Appearance of the knee after radical debridement and bone grafting of the osseous defect with autologous cancellous bone taken from the upper tibia. (K) Close-up of the autologous bone graft with surrounding native subchondral bone. A collagen membrane will be glued to the autologous bone graft with fibrin glue and pressure placed on this while the tourniquet is let down. A second membrane is then microsutured to the surrounding full-thickness chondral defect, sealed with fibrin glue, and the cavity filled with autologous cultured chondrocytes producing a sandwich technique where only a portion undergoes bone grafting, hence the term segmental sandwich technique with bone graft. (L and M) Final appearance of the transplanted knee from different views. The tibial tubercle is repositioned to unload the trochlear defect, the MPFL is secured medially, and a lateral lengthening performed. The knee is rehabilitated with a standard protocol for a weight-bearing condyle and trochlea. (N) Medial femoral condyle sandwich technique.

condyle osteochondral allograft. There was blistering centrally on the lateral femoral condyle with intact subchondral bone. The trochlea had grade IV changes. Patellar tracking was slightly lateral (Fig. 15.10A–J).

A Fulkerson osteotomy was performed to anteriorize the patella. The segmental sandwich technique using autologous bone graft from the proximal tibia was taken at the time of the tibial tubercle osteotomy. The donor site was then backfilled with cancellous allograft bone chips.

The failed osteochondral allograft was completely removed back to healthy subchondral bone with a high-speed bur and then grafted with autologous bone taken from the upper tibia. A segmental sandwich c-ACI technique was then performed over the medial femoral condyle and a standard collagen ACI to the trochlea and lateral femoral condyles.

An arthroscopy was performed 1 year later (Fig. 15.10K–N) to remove some mild adhesions in Hoffa's fat pad but more importantly to assess his transplants to determine a return to play. It was noted that he had excellent graft fill and quality throughout. He remains asymptomatic 10 years later.

Case 12. Bilateral Multiple Osteochondral Allografts for Avascular Necrosis

A 31-year-old woman presented with debilitating bilateral knee pain caused by advanced avascular necrosis of both knees from chronic prednisone use for ulcerative colitis. Bilateral knee MRI scans demonstrated multicompartmental chondral disease with large high-grade chondral lesions accompanied by adjacent subchondral bone marrow edema and osseous cystic changes. Figs. 15.11A and 15.11B highlight these findings in the patient's right knee.

Upon open surgery of the right knee, the trochlear articular surfaces had collapsed and crumbled, notably the lateral median ridge. The medial trochlear facet remained intact. The articular surfaces of the lateral femoral condyle were stable and healthy. However, the medial femoral condyle had completely collapsed with unstable cartilage surfaces. The surgical technique is thoroughly detailed and illustrated in the case of the patient's left knee. In this instance, the press-fit (dowel) technique was used to achieve dowel stability in both locations

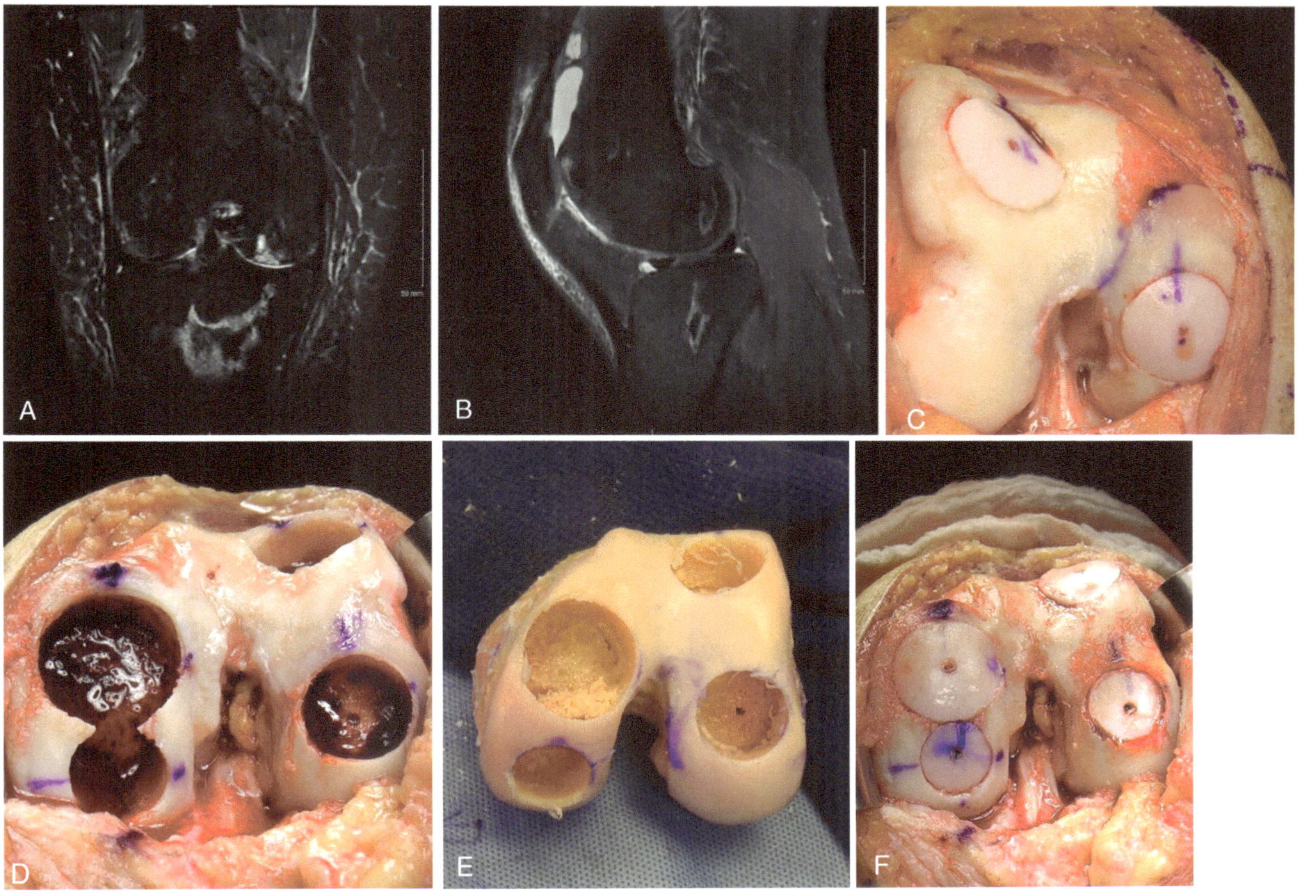

• **Fig. 15.11** (A) Coronal view of the right knee demonstrating collapse of medial femoral condyle. (B) Sagittal view of the right knee showing underlying signals of avascular necrosis in the lateral trochlear facet. (C) Final outcome of the right knee with osteochondral allografts of the medial femoral condyle and lateral trochlear facet. (D) Following inspection and palpation with a probe, the chondral defects were measured and removed as osteochondral dowels, each with a depth of approximately 10 mm. (E) Fresh matched osteochondral distal femur allograft. (F) Final outcome following press fit and screw fixation of osteochondral allografts.

(Fig. 15.11C). Fixation was not required. Following surgery, the patient experienced excellent pain relief within the first 6 weeks. We proceeded with her left knee reconstruction 6 months later.

The area of osteochondral damage in the patient's left knee was vast (Fig. 15.11D). At the time of arthrotomy, the medial femoral condyle was found to be flattened with Ficat stage 3 collapse. There was fissuring and softening of the lateral trochlear facet and the weight-bearing surface of the lateral femoral condyle. All three areas had underlying evidence of AVN confirmed on MRI scan. The three locations were then radically debrided and reamed down until there was healthy bleeding bone.

All four dowels were accurately measured to within 1 mm so that on the back table the donor distal femur could be accurately reproduced to the recipient socket (Fig. 15.11E). Multiplug osteochondral allografting using the inverted snowman technique was performed on the medial femoral condyle. The position of the dowels to the recipient site were measured precisely in reference to the intercondylar notch and the sulcus terminalis was utilized to ensure that the contour of the surface was accurate. All four dowels were then harvested, measured to the depths, and then press fit to the recipient sockets such that they were flush to the articular surface (Fig. 15.11F). Given the large defects, cannulated Acutrak headless screws were used to secure them in addition to the press fit because all four were large dowels (Fig. 15.11F). Immediate range of motion was possible with stable ridged fixation.

Osteochondral allograft transplantation has shown to be an excellent clinical resolution of pain and mobility for this young, active patient. She reports significant pain relief and continues to increase her levels of activity.

Summary

These case presentations are meant to assist surgeons in dealing with the more complex situations that are encountered occasionally in practice. Total knee replacement, although an excellent operation for the low-demand patient, is fraught with problems in young active patients and has a satisfaction rating of less than 50% in contrast to biologic reconstruction with satisfaction amongst patients >90%. Attention to the principles of assessing background factors and meticulous technique and follow-up aftercare for patients will result in excellent clinical outcomes in the majority of patients. I hope that the previous cases have helped to alert the surgeon to the breadth of possibility for joint preservation.

References

1. Endres NK, Minas T. Medial subvastus approach: surgical technique. *Harvard Orthopedic Journal*. 2010;10:62–65.
2. Masri BA, Kim WY, Pagnano M. Mini-subvastus approach for minimally invasive total knee replacement. *Tech Knee Surg*. 2007;6(2):124–130.
3. Hofmann AA, Plaster RL, Murdock LE. Subvastus (Southern) approach for primary total knee arthroplasty. *Clinical Orthopaedics & Related Research*. 1991(269):70–77.
4. Pagnano MW, Meneghini RM. Minimally invasive total knee arthroplasty with an optimized subvastus approach. *Journal of Arthroplasty*. 2006;21(4 Suppl 1):22–26.
5. Sporer SM. The minimally invasive subvastus approach for primary total knee arthroplasty. *The Journal of Knee Surgery*. 2006;19(1):58–62.
6. Aglietti P, Baldini A, Sensi L. Quadriceps-sparing versus mini-subvastus approach in total knee arthroplasty. *Clinical Orthopaedics & Related Research*. 2006;452:106–111.
7. Berth A, Urbach D, Neumann W, Awiszus F. Strength and voluntary activation of quadriceps femoris muscle in total knee arthroplasty with midvastus and subvastus approaches. *Journal of Arthroplasty*. 2007;22(1):83–88.
8. Boerger TO, Aglietti P, Mondanelli N, Sensi L. Mini-subvastus versus medial parapatellar approach in total knee arthroplasty. *Clinical Orthopaedics & Related Research*. 2005;440:82–87.
9. Chang CH, Chen KH, Yang RS, Liu TK. Muscle torques in total knee arthroplasty with subvastus and parapatellar approaches. *Clinical Orthopaedics & Related Research*. 2002;398:189–195.
10. Dalury DF, Dennis DA. Mini-incision total knee arthroplasty can increase risk of component malalignment. *Clinical Orthopaedics & Related Research*. 2005;440:77–81.
11. Roysam GS, Oakley MJ. Subvastus approach for total knee arthroplasty: a prospective, randomized, and observer-blinded trial. *Journal of Arthroplasty*. 2001;16(4):454–457.
12. Weinhardt C, Barisic M, Bergmann EG, Heller KD. Early results of subvastus versus medial parapatellar approach in primary total knee arthroplasty. *Archives of Orthopaedic & Trauma Surgery*. 2004;124(6):401–403.
13. Schroer WC, Diesfeld PJ, Reedy ME, LeMarr AR. Evaluation of complications associated with six hundred mini-subvastus total knee arthroplasties. *Journal of Bone & Joint Surgery - American*. 2007;Volume. 89(Suppl 3):76–81.

16

Emerging Technologies

TOM MINAS, MD, MS

CHAPTER OUTLINE

Introduction

New biologic options are being developed throughout the world to enhance existing techniques, offer new off-the-shelf options, and provide reproducible structural repair.

I contacted several companies worldwide and asked them to share their core technologies, preclinical development, clinical trial outcomes, and postmarketing surveillance outcomes, as available. The following list is by no means complete but offers a sampling of what potentially may be available to our patients in the United States after regulatory approval.

The categories of technology roughly translate to marrow stimulation improvement using gels or scaffolds to enhance marrow stimulation techniques; use of minced autograft and allograft cartilage; second-generation autologous chondrocyte implantation (ACI) techniques, which use scaffolds of different biomaterials precultured with cells to deliver the cells to the injury site; and third-generation tissue-engineered cartilage, which is preformed histologically and physically.

Marrow Stimulation Technique Augmentation

BST-CarGel

Background

BST-CarGel (BioSyntech Canada, Laval, Quebec, Canada), a new medical device for cartilage repair, was developed to improve outcomes of bone marrow stimulation procedures while preserving the intrinsic low cost and simple arthroscopic approach. With traditional marrow stimulating techniques, clot shrinkage and detachment from lesion surfaces occur. BST-CarGel was designed to stabilize the blood clot in the cartilage lesion by dispersing a soluble and adhesive chitosan scaffold throughout autologous, fresh whole blood. Chitosan, a cationic linear polysaccharide composed predominately of polyglucosamine, is derived from the deacetylation of chitin, the structural component of crustacean shells.[1,2] By dissolving chitosan in an aqueous glycerol phosphate buffer, BST-CarGel is uniquely obtained as a liquid chitosan solution having physiologic pH and osmolarity, intrinsic cytocompatibility, and biodegradability.[2,3] When mixed with blood (BST-CarGel-to-blood ratio of 1:3), the viscous mixture can easily be applied to cartilage lesions that have been prepared by bone marrow stimulation (microfracture, drilling), where it permits normal clot formation while simultaneously reinforcing the clot and impeding clot retraction. Furthermore, the cationic nature of the chitosan increases the adhesivity of the mixture to cartilage lesions, ensuring longer clot residency. This maintenance of critical blood components above the marrow access holes allows activation of the tissue repair process, while chitosan itself brings an intrinsic ability to stimulate wound repair.[4] Box 16.1 summarizes the primary mode of action for BST-CarGel, an approach that has been termed *scaffold-guided regenerative medicine*, where BST-CarGel provides in situ chondroinduction for cartilage repair.[5]

Nonclinical Studies

The efficacy and underlying mechanisms of action of BST-CarGel were examined in several animal studies. A skeletally mature (8–15 months) rabbit model that used drilling of surgically prepared bilateral trochlear defects elucidated BST-CarGel early reparative events and compared them with drilled controls.[6,7] Box 16.2 summarizes the key findings of BST-CarGel–mediated cartilage repair.

• Box 16.1 BST-CarGel Primary Mode of Action

Physical biomaterial scaffold for natural cartilage repair
Stabilizes blood clot
Impedes clot retraction, providing a space-filling provisional matrix
Generates an adhesive bond between clot and cartilage lesion
Provides structural framework for subsequent repair processes

• Box 16.2 BST-CarGel Stabilized Blood Clots

Mechanisms of Action for Cartilage Repair

Chitosan clearance via neutrophil phagocytosis after approximately 1 month
Chemotaxis of marrow stromal cells toward the lesion
Transient increase in vascularization in subchondral bone
Greater porosity, remodeling, and vascularization of subchondral bone
Induction of chondrogenic foci from repair tissue near 1 month
Increased quality of hyaline cartilage repair arising from subchondral bone
Improved integration of repair cartilage within the lesion
All comparisons were made to drilled-only contralateral controls ($n = 49$).[11,12]

• Box 16.3 BST-CarGel Stabilized Blood Clots

Six-Month Efficacy in Sheep

Greater adhesion of CarGel blood clot to bone and cartilage
Increased volume of repair tissue
Improved hyaline character of repair tissue
Increased GAG and collagen content of repair tissue
Reduced incidence of subchondral cyst formation
No treatment-specific safety issues
All comparisons were made to microfracture-only control group. BST-CarGel ($n = 8$), microfracture only ($n = 6$).

In another large study in adult (3–6 years) sheep, repair of surgically prepared 1-cm^2 condylar and trochlear defects was investigated by measuring the quantity and quality of BST-CarGel repair tissue after 6 months compared with microfracture-only defects.[8] Box 16.3 summarizes the efficacy of BST-CarGel treatment for cartilage repair. Fig. 16.1 shows a best case repair from a sheep condylar lesion treated with BST-CarGel. After 6 months of repair, a relatively mature articular cartilage containing superficial, transitional, and radial zones with a reestablished tidemark was observed.

Overall, the BST-CarGel device has been shown statistically to increase the volume and hyaline character of repair tissue compared with microfractured or microdrilled controls. The chondrogenic foci observed resemble endochondral processes and are believed to be responsible for the synthesis of cartilaginous repair tissue. Notably, the specific mechanisms underlying BST-CarGel–mediated repair (see Boxes 16.2 and 16.3) were independent of species or bone marrow stimulation technique.[7]

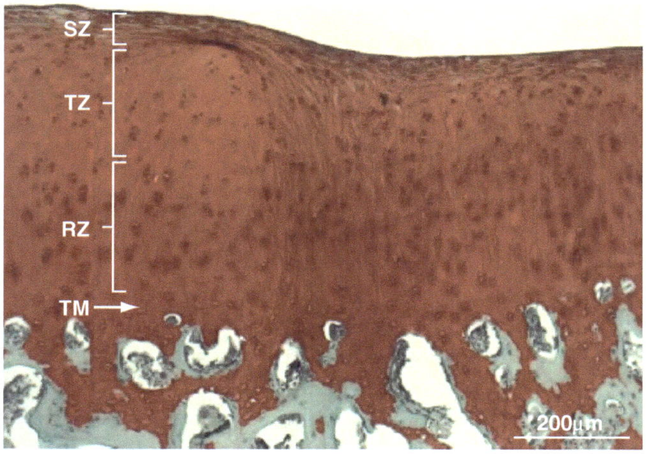

• **Fig. 16.1** Best case cartilage repair of 1-cm² defects in adult sheep treated with BST-CarGel. At 6 months, uniform cartilage resurfacing was observed. Safranin O/fast green-stained section from this block reveals relatively mature articular cartilage containing superficial (SZ), transitional (TZ), and radial (RZ) zones with a reestablished tidemark (TM) above an actively remodeling bone bed.

Clinical Experience

In 2003 and 2004, 33 human subjects were treated with BST-CarGel under Health Canada's Special Access Program for medical devices (compassionate use on a case-by-case basis; not considered a clinical trial). Treated patients encompassed the spectrum of both traumatic and degenerative lesions, along with other pathologies. Lesions ranged in size from 0.5 to 12 cm² (mean 4.3 cm²). In 16 cases, opposing tibial lesions (kissing lesions) were debrided and treated with microfracture only. One case of osteochondritis dissecans and one exposed subchondral cyst were treated; two concomitant anterior cruciate ligament replacements were performed. BST-CarGel delivery by arthroscopic (22 patients) as well as mini-open approaches (11 patients) was confirmed (Fig. 16.2). Physiotherapy follow-up was standardized and required 6 weeks of non–weight-bearing exercise and early passive range of motion by physiotherapists (i.e., no continuous passive motion). Western Ontario McMaster (WOMAC)[9] osteoarthritis index questionnaires were administered preoperatively and again postoperatively after 3, 6, and 12 months. WOMAC scores for pain, stiffness, and function improved substantially over preoperative baseline scores, although the absence of a control group and the wide-ranging patient demographics and lesion types prevent overinterpretation of outcomes.[5]

In 2005, BioSyntech initiated a multicenter randomized level 1 clinical trial in Canada and Europe comparing BST-CarGel treatment with microfracture in the repair of grade 3 or 4 articular cartilage lesions on the femoral condyles in the knee. The study was designed to measure repair tissue structure at 12 months as the primary endpoint through quantitative magnetic resonance imaging (MRI) of repair tissue volume and quality (T2, delayed gadolinium-enhanced magnetic resonance imaging of cartilage [dGEMRIC]) and microscopic analysis of biopsies (when available).

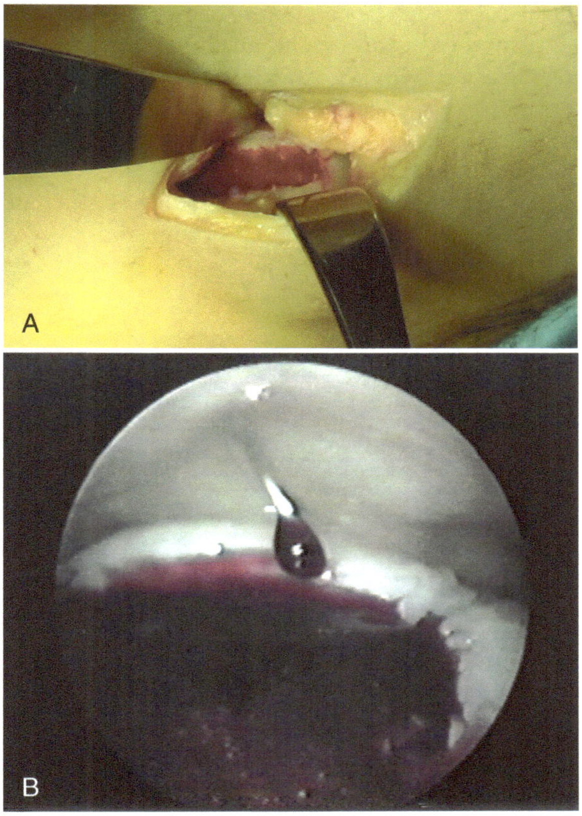

• **Fig. 16.2** (A) BST-CarGel open surgical technique includes a mini-arthrotomy to facilitate visualization of the horizontal lesion and delivery of BST-CarGel. Using a syringe, the BST-CarGel/blood mixture is applied in a controlled dropwise manner over all of the bone marrow access holes and then into the entire lesion, taking care not to overfill. (B) Arthroscopic delivery of BST-CarGel is performed when the entire lesion can be observed within the arthroscopic field of view. Prior to BST-CarGel application, the joint and lesion are fully suctioned of perfusion liquid and blood to create a "dry field" in the horizontal lesion. The delivery needle is positioned directly perpendicular and central to the lesion, and the BST-CarGel/blood mixture is delivered in dropwise fashion, being sure not to overfill. Both approaches (A and B) require a 15-minute solidification period, followed by incision closure.

The secondary endpoint assessed clinical benefit (Visual Analog Scale [VAS], WOMAC, Medical Outcomes Study 36-Item Short-Form Health Survey [SF-36]) and safety. The trial enrolled 80 patients and an interim histologic analysis of 22 available biopsies (13 BST-CarGel and 9 microfracture patients) using International Cartilage Repair Society (ICRS) Histological Scoring systems I and II[10] provided statistically significant evidence that BST-CarGel improved the quality and quantity of repair tissue compared with microfracture. The ICRS II overall score, which assimilates all the parameters listed in the grading system and generates an overall assessment of tissue repair, was significant ($P < .05$), as were individual parameters of cell morphology, cell viability, and superficial zone morphology on the biopsies. Macroscopic grading of the cartilage repair by the surgeon at the time of biopsy, which included the extent of lesion filling, tissue surface characteristics, and integration with surrounding tissue, was also statistically significant. Full study analysis on all 80 patients after 12-month follow-up revealed statistically improved quantity and quality of repair tissue in the microfracture with BST-CarGel compared with microfracture treatment alone.[11] Similar findings were observed 5 years postoperative with fewer overall failures in the BST-CarGel + microfracture group.[12] BST-CarGel received regulatory approval in numerous countries, including Australia, Canada, and most European countries.

Scaffolds

MaioRegen

Because the intrinsic ability of articular cartilage to self-repair is poor due to the lack of blood support and lymph and nervous systems, the development of effective therapies for articular cartilage and subchondral bone regeneration is an important goal in orthopedic surgery. After achondral damage, the repair tissue shows histologic and mechanical properties lower than the native tissue, which may lead to impaired functionality of the joint itself. Many treatment options have been proposed, but no optimal long-lasting solutions have been achieved, particularly for deep cartilaginous and osteochondral defects.

MaioRegen (Fin-Ceramica Faenza S.p.A., Faenza, Italy) is a novel composite osteochondral monolithic scaffold. It is a multilayered structure that reproduces the chemical gradient naturally found inside the osteocartilaginous compartment.[13,14] MaioRegen is composed of equine tendon-derived type I collagen on the upper side, which mimics the cartilaginous layer, and a blending of type I collagen and magnesium-enriched nonstoichiometric hydroxyapatite (Mg-HA) on the bottom side, which mimics the subchondral bone (Fig. 16.3). Due to its high similarity with the anatomic osteocartilaginous portion to be replaced, in terms of chemical, biologic, and structural composition, the scaffold is defined as a biomimetic device, able to be recognized as self by the recipient connective tissues. Toxicologic profile, performed in compliance to EN ISO 10993–1 European regulation on class III medical devices, showed high biocompatibility and tolerability.

An in vivo, randomized controlled study has been performed to assess the safety and efficacy of MaioRegen in an osteochondral reconstruction sheep model.[15] An osteochondral lesion was induced in the right knee, either on the medial or lateral condyle, of each animal (n = 8). Animals were then randomly assigned to three treatment groups. The objective of the study was to demonstrate a substantial equivalence (in terms of effectiveness) between the acellular approach using MaioRegen alone (group A) and chondrocytes cultured on the scaffold (cell-engineered scaffold, group B). Comparisons were made with an untreated control group (group C). No adverse events were observed in all groups, and the device was completely tolerable and fully biocompatible. At 6 months postoperative, animals were euthanized, and macroscopic and histologic investigations showed complete absorption of MaioRegen. The newly

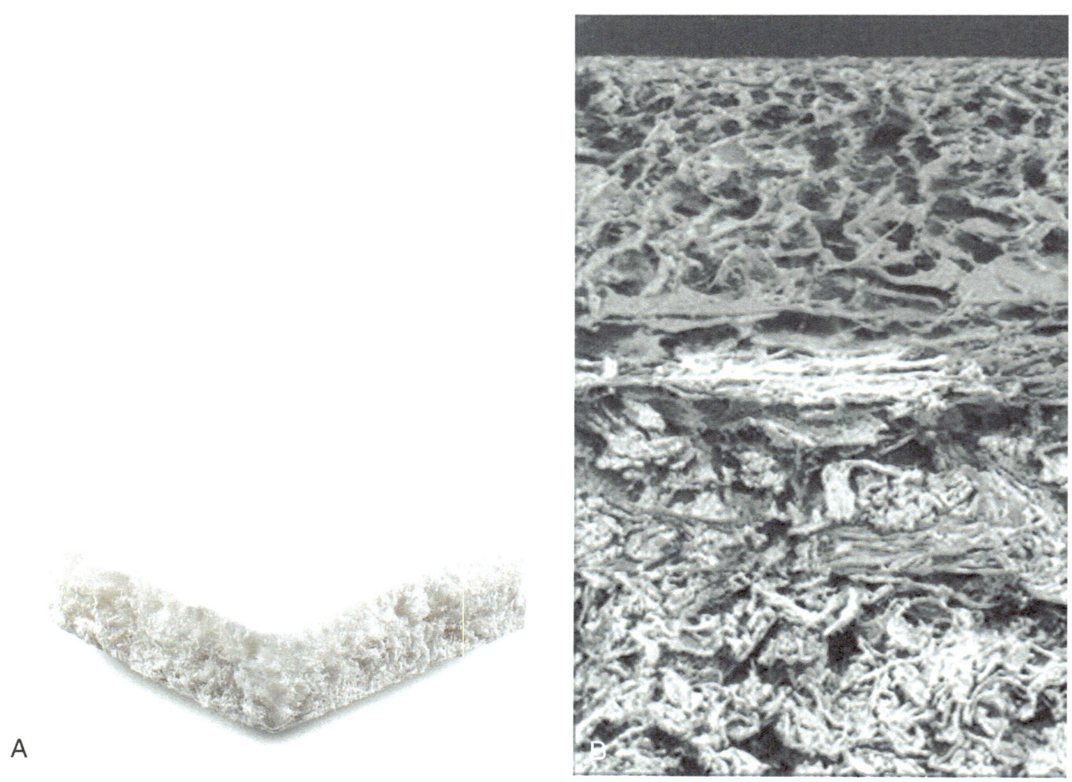

• **Fig. 16.3** (A) MaioRegen osteochondral scaffold. Scanning electron micrograph of inner structure of MaioRegen. (B) Cartilaginous layer (100% type I collagen); tidemark (60% type I collagen, 40% Mg-HA); bone layer (30% type I collagen, 70% Mg-HA).

formed tissues in the treated groups were well integrated, whereas a gap on the defect was still noticeable in the control group. Applying a Fortier score (0–15),[16] no statistical differences in average score values were seen between scaffold alone (2.63 ± 0.71) and cell-engineered scaffold (4.00 ± 0.53), whereas both groups exhibited statistical difference ($P < .05$) versus the control group (12.88 ± 0.95). Histologic evaluation showed newly formed tissue that was well organized and characterized by chondrocytes with tangential orientation in the upper part. In the two treated groups, tissues were differentiated at either the chondral or subchondral bone level, whereas fibrous tissue was evident in the control group (Fig. 16.4).

The hypothesis of a scaffold-guided tissue regeneration process is that mesenchymal and progenitor cells from subchondral bone marrow blood after surgical curettage are able to migrate inside and wholly colonize the scaffold, then differentiate along either a chondrogenic or osteogenic lineage based on the peculiar physical–chemical gradient composition found. Therefore, MaioRegen itself promoted osteoblast differentiation and bone regeneration in the deepest portions while restoring the tidemark in the intermediate portion and hyaline cartilage formation in the upper surface (chondrogenic differentiation). After the preclinical and toxicologic studies, a pilot, uncontrolled, prospective clinical trial of 30 patients has been designed and approved by an institutional review board to investigate the performance and safety of MaioRegen. Inclusion criteria for study admission were patients ranging in age from 15 to 60 years who were affected by traumatic, posttraumatic, or degenerative osteochondral defects of the knee (grade III and IV Outerbridge classification) sizing 1–9 cm^2. After arthrotomy, a curettage of the defect was made and scaffold was implanted dry by simple press fit, without fixation with suture or surgical glue (Fig. 16.5). Early stability of MaioRegen assessed 30 days postoperative by MRI revealed neither migration from the implant site nor delamination. With regard to the safety outcome, patients were monitored for the onset of any adverse events. Most of the episodes reported were considered related to surgery and not to the device itself and most occurred within the immediate postoperative period. In addition, clinical assessment by MRI performed 6 and 12 months postoperative evaluated the quality of regenerated osteochondral tissue and integration with recipient tissues applying the MRI MOCART Scoring System. Functional joint recovery, improvement of the patient's quality of life, and return to normal sport

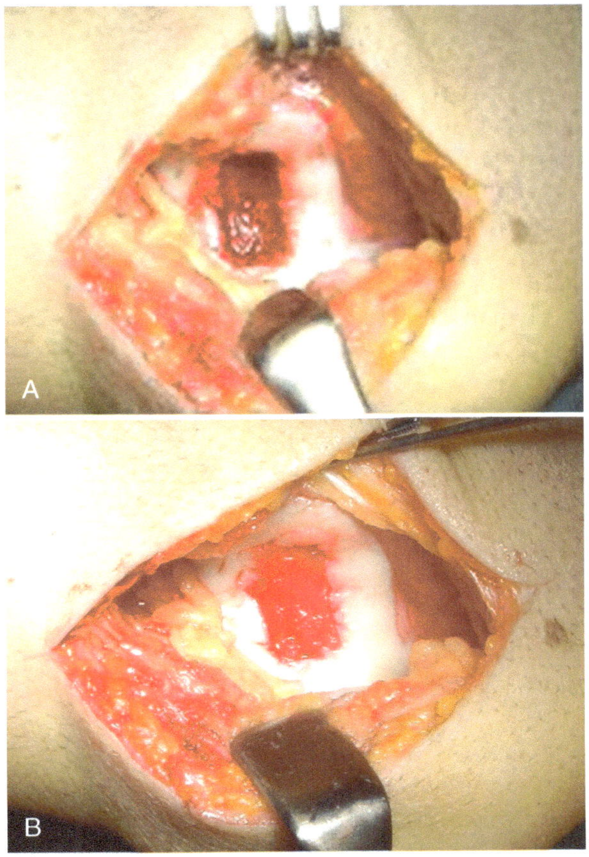

• **Fig. 16.5** (A) Osteochondral (OC) defect curettage. (B) OC defect filled with MaioRegen.

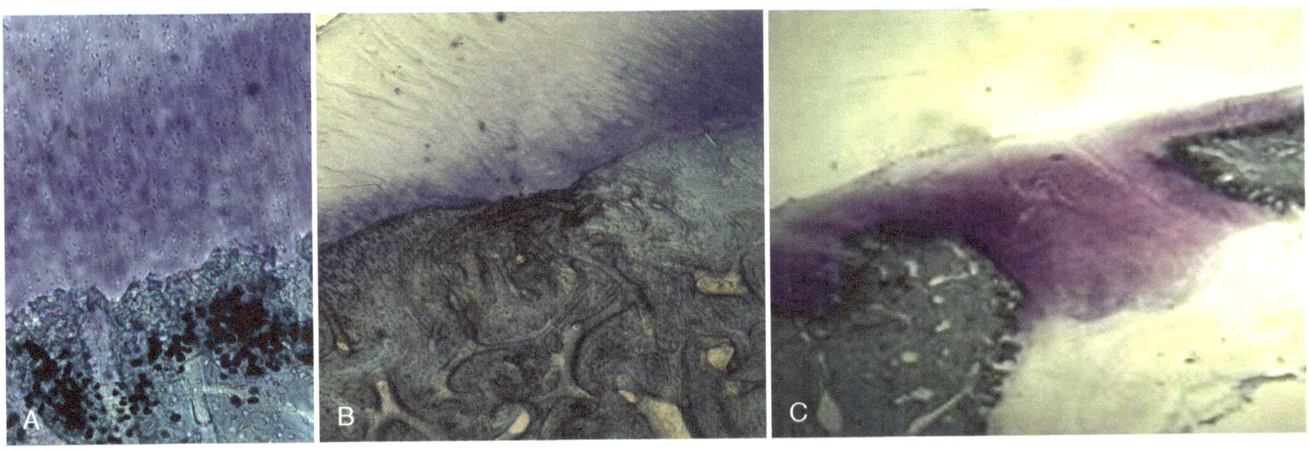

• **Fig. 16.4** (A) MaioRegen alone group (hematoxylin–eosin/fast green stain). (B) Autologous chondrocyte-engineered MaioRegen group. (C) Control group.

activity were further evaluated by applying ICRS evaluation package questionnaires and Kujala and Tegner scores. Results of statistical data analysis highlighted positive results for each observed variable with respect to both surgeon and patient evaluations at each follow-up visit. Modifications of the result for each examined variable, comparing 6- and 12-month postsurgery scores to the preoperative score, were statistically significant ($P <.05$). Upon study planning, the modification of study variables between preoperation and postoperation was identified as a success index. Because modifications in the study were reported as positive (i.e., sustained by statistical relevance), they were considered indexes of study success. Moreover, all of the parameters evaluated improved significantly after 12 months compared with 6 months, confirming good progression and enhancement of quality of life.

The preliminary results of the clinical trial at intermediate follow-up appear promising.[17,18] MaioRegen may be considered a potential innovative surgical treatment of severe osteochondral lesions; however, longer follow-up would be essential to validate fully this one-step acellular approach.

Chondro-Gide

Chondro-Gide (Geistlich Pharma AG, Wolhusen, Switzerland) is a CE-marked product for covering articular cartilage defects that are treated with either ACI or bone marrow stimulation techniques (autologous matrix-induced chondrogenesis [AMIC]).

The proprietary manufacturing process of Chondro-Gide involves several steps before the unique bilayer design consisting of a compact side and a porous side is achieved (Fig. 16.6). Standardized processes under clean room conditions and rigorous in-process and end controls guarantee a high-quality natural product. Chondro-Gide consists of porcine type I and III collagen, which is naturally resorbed. Collagenases, gelatinases, and proteinases are responsible for the breakdown of Chondro-Gide into oligopeptides and finally single amino acids.

The compact layer consists of a smooth, cell-occlusive surface that prevents cells, chondrocytes, and mesenchymal stem cells from diffusing into the joint space and protects them from mechanical stress. The porous layer of the matrix consists of loose collagen fibers that support cell invasion and attachment. The arrangement of the fibers provides high tensile strength and resistance to tearing.

Thorough biocompatibility safety testing according to international standards proves that all elements that could cause an undesirable local or systemic response are removed during the manufacturing process and that the immunogenic potential of the matrix is reduced to a minimum.

The Chondro-Gide matrix is available in sizes of 20 × 30 mm, 30 × 40 mm and now up to 60% thicker than the largest size 40 × 50 mm.

Autologous Chondrocyte Implantation

Preclinical Results for Chondro-Gide in ACI

Ovine animal models and preclinical culture condition studies have validated the proof of concept that a porcine collagen membrane may be successfully used in cartilage repair with good tissue repair and no rejection response.[19–24]

Clinical Results for Chondro-Gide in ACI

Chondro-Gide used in several human ACI studies has demonstrated clinical results equal to periosteum without hypertrophy.[21,25–32] Ease of handling, lessened operative time, and arthroscopic delivery are possible.

Autologous Matrix-Induced Chondrogenesis

AMIC as an enhanced microfracture technique combining microfracturing with the collagen I/III matrix Chondro-Gide has become a recognized cartilage repair technique. Studies evaluating the performance of this new treatment option are ongoing.

An initial study by Behrens et al.[33] showed that costs were significantly reduced by AMIC compared to ACI and

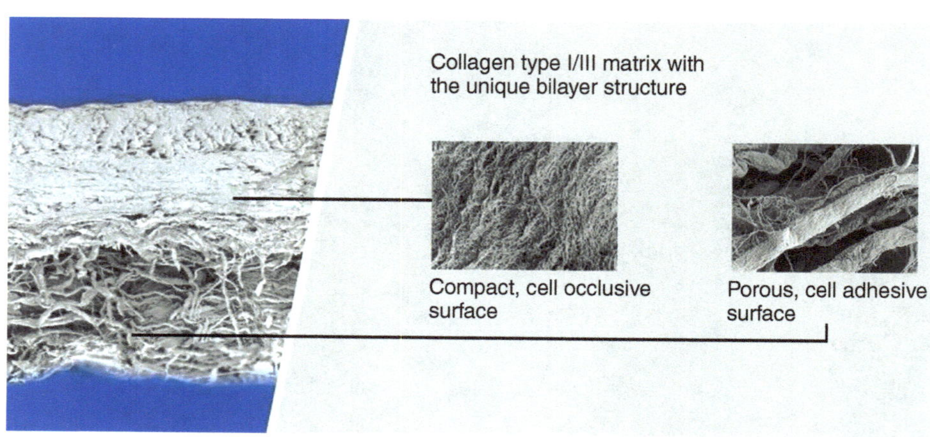

• **Fig. 16.6** Bilayer structure of Chondro-Gide porcine type I–III membrane.

immediate cartilage repair was possible in a single procedure. Improved tissue repair to ACI has not yet been studied.

Preclinical Results for AMIC

Preclinical animal work confirms that marrow clot is contained and repair tissue develops.[34,35]

Clinical Results for AMIC

Numerous early reports on the femoral condyles support positive short-term clinical results.[36–41]

AMIC Registry

At the beginning of 2007, Geistlich Surgery successfully launched the AMIC Registry online database "to offer surgeons worldwide an easy platform to collect and share their AMIC data." Data entry is standardized, simple, and rapid. Patient evaluation is based on the Lysholm knee score, VAS pain scale, and magnetic resonance testing (MRT) analysis. All data can be easily exported and graphically illustrated. By October 2008, 179 patients (67 female and 112 male, age 14–64 years, mean 36.8 years) with focal cartilage defects (Outerbridge grade II–IV) of the knee in the medial or lateral condyle (62%), patella (29%), and/or trochlea (9%) underwent AMIC and were included in the AMIC Registry.

Excellent 2-year results ($n = 57$) showed improvement of knee function as assessed by the Lysholm score from an average of 50 to 85 points and pain reduction from 6.7 to 2.0 (VAS). After 3 years ($n = 28$), the mean Lysholm score improved from 56.6 to 87.0 points. Pain on a VAS diminished from 6.2 to 2.3. During the 3-year observation period, the AMIC technique resulted in a considerable increase in knee function, with 75% reporting good to excellent results and 10% satisfactory results and exceptional pain reduction.

Kensey Nash Corporation Cartilage Repair Device

The Kensey Nash Corporation (Exton, PA) cartilage repair device (CRD) has been designed to address many of the concerns regarding current cartilage repair procedures. Significant preclinical research and development has yielded a bioresorbable, acellular, biphasic scaffold for cartilage repair. This technology uses an implant design that contains two phases, each specifically engineered to favor the growth of the histologically distinct tissues of articular cartilage and subchondral bone.

Implant Description

The Kensey Nash CRD is a porous biphasic scaffold consisting of type I collagen, β-tricalcium phosphate (β-TCP), and polylactic acid (PLA), three well-known biomaterials with a long history of use in orthopedics. The implant (Fig. 16.7) has 100% interconnected porosity that enables movement of cells and biologic fluids throughout the entire implant. The chondral phase of the implant consists of a type I collagen formulation. The collagen provides a malleable, biocompatible scaffold for repair of cartilage tissue that can be contoured to the surrounding joint surfaces. The implant's subchondral bone phase contains 80% β-TCP and 20% PLA by mass. The ceramic provides an osteoconductive

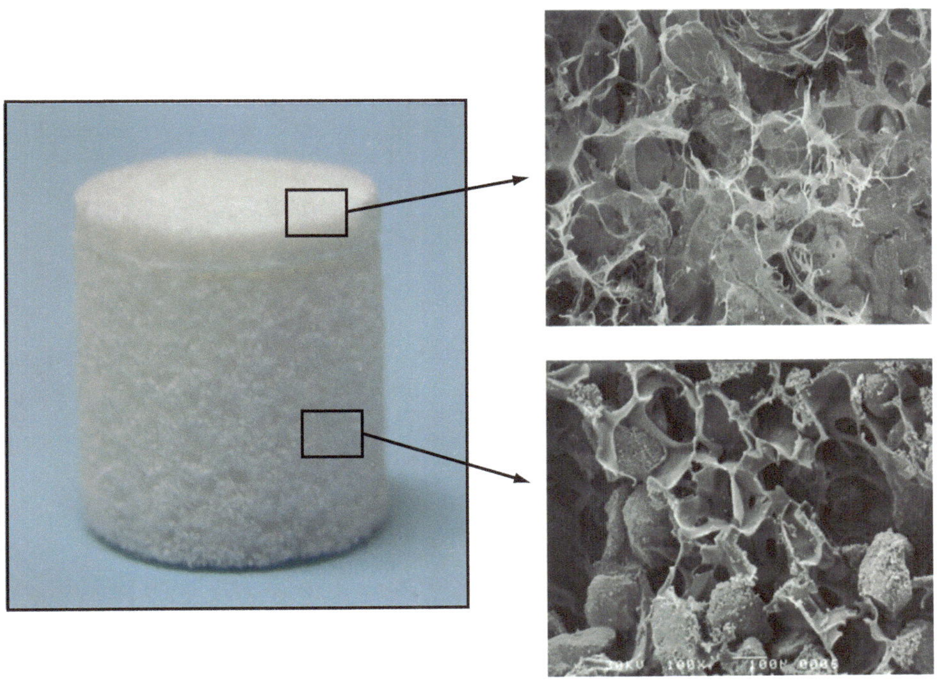

• **Fig. 16.7** The Kensey Nash cartilage repair device implant is a biphasic plug, designed as a resorbable scaffold for the repair of articular cartilage and subchondral bone. The chondral region is composed of type I collagen *(top)*, with a subchondral bone region of β-tricalcium phosphate suspended within a polylactic acid lattice *(bottom)*. Scanning electron micrograph (magnification ×100).

element to the subchondral phase of the CRD implant while supplying a source of calcium and phosphorous ions necessary for natural bone mineralization.[42,43] The PLA scaffold provides biomechanical support and three-dimensional structure for this region and ultimately breaks down into natural body metabolites via the Krebs cycle.[44,45] As a result of Kensey Nash's proprietary process, the ceramic granules are suspended within, not coated by, the polymer scaffold so that the ceramic is immediately available to the host upon implantation. The implant is available in a range of diameters and is loaded in an insertion tool that facilitates implant hydration and arthroscopic placement.

Preclinical Studies

Kensey Nash conducted a caprine study that evaluated the performance of the CRD in a 6-mm × 6-mm defect on the medial femoral condyle of 38 Nubian Cross goats at 6-, 12-, and 18-month time points (Fig. 16.8). Histology, biomechanical testing, immunohistochemistry, MRI, gross evaluations, and radiographs were the evaluation methods used. The study concluded that, by 6 months, CRD-treated defects displayed a rapid repair that was sustained through the 12-month[46] and 18-month time points. Repair tissue at each time point appeared hyaline, stained positively for type II collagen, and was biomechanically similar to healthy articular cartilage. The repair tissue also displayed excellent integration not only with the host cartilage but with the host bone as well.

Kensey Nash is also studying the performance of the CRD in healing a 10-mm × 10-mm osteochondral defect on the lateral trochlear ridge of 12 horses (Fig. 16.9). The repair of CRD-treated defects will be evaluated over a 2-year study, with interim arthroscopies at 4- and 12-month time points. Interim arthroscopies are scored using a modified ICRS system for safety and efficacy. At time of sacrifice, histology, biomechanical testing, immunohistochemistry, MRI, gross evaluations, and radiographs will be used to evaluate the repair compared to a microfracture control. Four-month interim arthroscopy showed equivalency to microfracture in terms of safety scores and a significant improvement over microfracture in efficacy scoring.[47]

Together, these studies are being used to support an Investigational Device Exemption application to commence clinical investigation of the CRD in the United States. Kensey Nash is pursuing regulatory approvals for the CRD in both the United States and Europe.

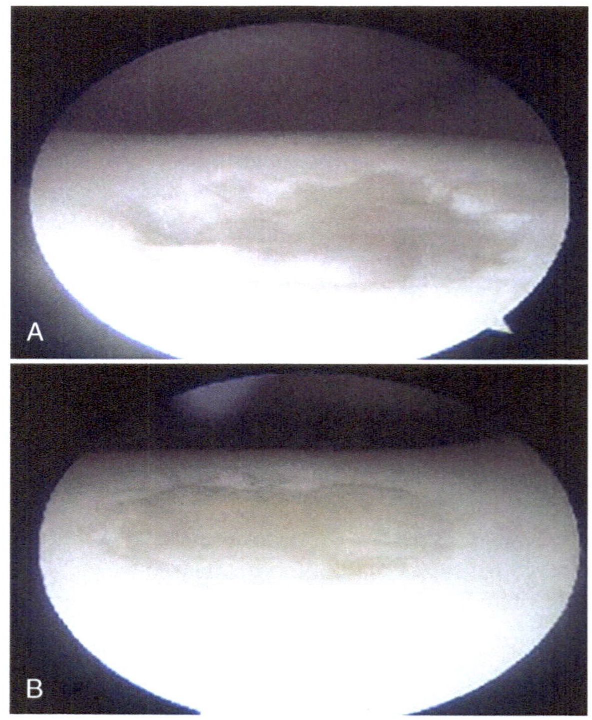

• **Fig. 16.9** Four-month interim arthroscopy images for microfracture control (A) and defect treated with Kensey Nash cartilage repair device (CRD) (B) in equine lateral trochlear ridge. CRD treatment group scored significantly higher than microfracture in terms of efficacy and equivalent to microfracture in terms of safety using a modified International Cartilage Repair Society scoring system.

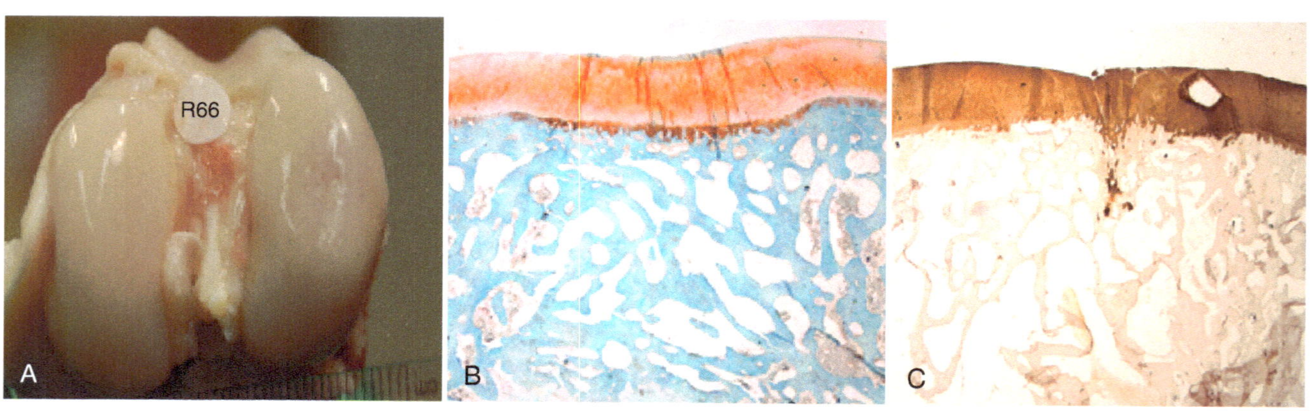

• **Fig. 16.8** Caprine stifles treated with cartilage repair device at 12 months. (A) Grossly, the defects were well filled with smooth resurfacing. (B) Histologically, safranin O staining showed the presence of proteoglycan within the repair tissue. (C) Repair tissue also stained strongly positive for type II collagen.

TRUFIT CB for Cartilage Repair

Properties of TRUFIT CB

The TRUFIT CB scaffold (Smith & Nephew, Andover, MA) is a cartilage repair option for small chondral or osteochondral lesions. It comes in preformed cylindrical plugs with diameters ranging from 5 to 11 mm. This synthetic resorbable scaffold has two phases to mimic the critical portions of osteochondral healing. Each phase is designed to initially approximate the physical and mechanical properties of the adjacent cartilage and bone (Fig. 16.10). TRUFIT CB is made of Polygraft, a porous material composed of 85:15 poly(d l-lactide-co-glycolide) copolymer, polyglycolide (PGA) fibers, calcium sulfate, and a trace amount of surfactant. Slivka et al.[48] showed that PGA reinforcement fibers improved the early structural integrity of the scaffold and provided a mechanically stable environment for cell migration and tissue repair. Calcium sulfate in the bone phase releases calcium ions, which are known to enhance osteoconductivity,[49,50] whereas the top phase is malleable to allow contouring with the adjacent articular surface after implantation. During the surgery, the original chondral/osteochondral defect is cored out with TRUKOR instrumentation to create a uniform circular defect. The implant is press-fit into the defect site using the preloaded delivery device. Because the TRUFIT CB scaffold is hydrophilic, fluids such as blood and marrow containing nutrients, proteins, and cells can be easily wicked up into the pores. TRUFIT CB then acts as a scaffold for microfracture to hold the blood and marrow cells from subchondral bleeding. Its 70% porosity and interconnected pores promote cell infiltration across the scaffold and provide a mechanically stable environment for tissue repair. TRUFIT CB is currently sold in Europe, Canada, and Australia but is not available in the United States and its territories.

Preclinical Study Using an Ovine Osteochondral Model

In an ovine study assessing cartilage repair by TRUFIT CB implants in osteochondral defects at 18 months, a unilateral circular (5.1 mm diameter × 5 mm) osteochondral defect was created in the medial femoral condyle of skeletally mature sheep.[51] The defects were repaired by TRUFIT CB (5.3 mm diameter × 5 mm; $n = 6$) and press-fit into the site or left empty in the empty defect control group ($n = 3$). Outcome of cartilage repair was assessed 18 months after surgery. None of the sheep showed any lameness and had regained a full range of motion. The medial condyle of all animals in the TRUFIT CB group had no abnormalities. By 18 months, the material of TRUFIT CB had predominantly resorbed, and the defect sites were filled with repair tissue. Cartilage restoration was evident in all TRUFIT CB specimens. The repaired cartilage was well integrated with the adjacent tissue and had a similar thickness and contour (Fig. 16.11). Safranin O staining revealed a highly cellular tissue in the repair by TRUFIT CB with the same intensity of proteoglycan staining as the adjacent hyaline cartilage. The organized collagen patterns of the mid and deeper levels of TRUFIT CB repair were similar to those of normal cartilage (Fig. 16.12). In contrast, repair cartilage in the empty defect control was thinner than normal cartilage tissue and the adjacent cartilage showed signs of degeneration, including proteoglycan loss (see Fig. 16.11). The subchondral bone portion of the defect repaired by TRUFIT CB was replaced by bone with a statistically similar bone volume

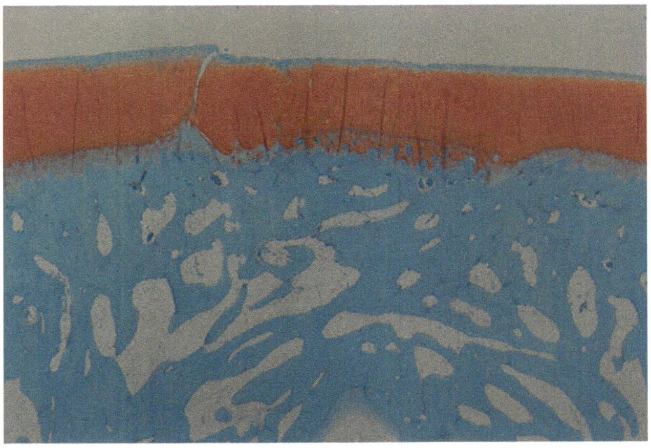

• **Fig. 16.11** Safranin O–stained sections of TRUFIT CB–treated defect and empty osteochondral defect.

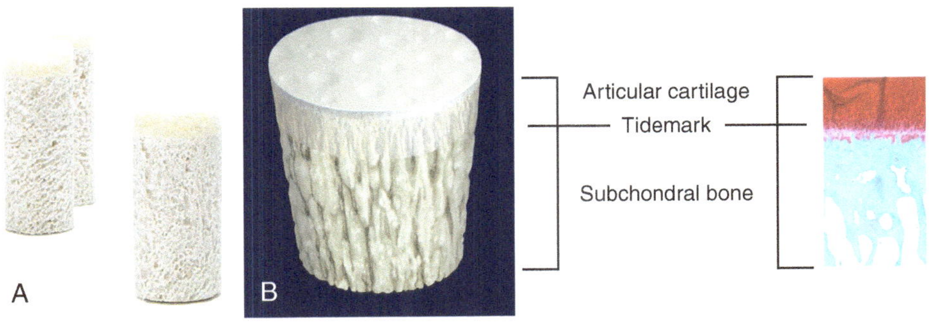

• **Fig. 16.10** (A) TRUFIT CB scaffolds. (B) TRUFIT CB mimics cartilage, tidemark, and subchondral bone in osteochondral healing.

as the untreated contralateral control (66.4% and 63.0%, respectively). Areas of new bone growth with active osteoblasts, increased cellularity, and nonlamellar structure were observed in the repair, indicating that subchondral bone remodeling was ongoing and expected to continue to completely remodel to mature bone over time.

Clinical Case Series

A prospective series by the Spalding group reported the outcome of 24 patients (mean age 34 years, range 19–50 years) with 12- to 36-month follow-up for treatment of chondral or osteochondral lesions in the knee with TRUFIT CB implants.[52] There were 13 primary procedures and 11 revision procedures (microfracture 7, osteochondral grafting 1, matrix-induced autologous chondrocyte implantation [MACI] 1, and failed fixation osteochondritis dissecans 2). Mean lesion size was 1.8 cm^2, 14 of which were on the medial femoral condyle, 4 on the lateral femoral condyle, and 6 on the lateral or central trochlea. Up to four implants were used in the repair. After surgery, patients who had undergone repair on the weight-bearing femoral condyle surface were allowed partial weight bearing at 2 weeks and full weight bearing at 4 weeks.

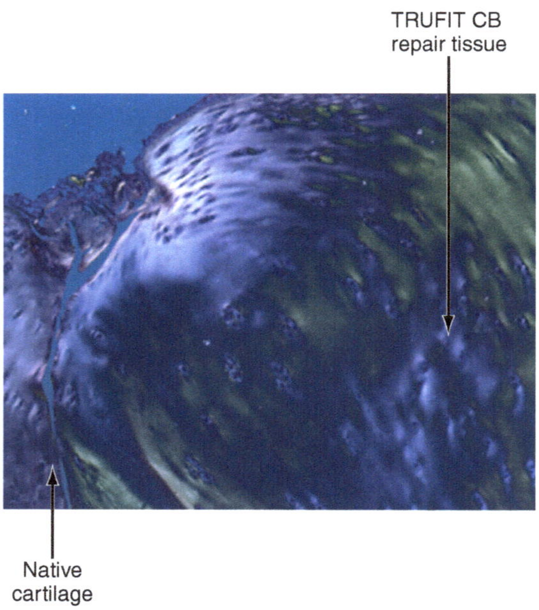

• **Fig. 16.12** Polarized light photomicrograph (hematoxylin-eosin stain, magnification ×100) of TRUFIT CB repair tissue at 18 months. The pattern of collagen is organized, similar to that of normal cartilage.

Lysholm score, International Knee Documentation Committee (IKDC) score, and Knee Injury and Osteoarthritis Outcome Score (KOOS) showed statistically significant improvement ($P < .001$) at 12 months compared with preoperatively (Fig. 16.13). Activity levels and hence the mean Tegner activity score ($P = .05$, see Fig. 16.4) improved after 12 months when return to sport was allowed. MRI showed maintenance of the thickness of the new articular surface, gradual differentiation of the implant, and remodeling of the bony component over time (Fig. 16.14). Subchondral lamina formation also was evident. Five patients underwent second-look arthroscopy, which showed that although TRUFIT CB stayed soft up to 8 months or more, excellent defect fill and integration with surrounding cartilage were seen. In one patient with slow incorporation of the plugs, patience and perseverance with rehabilitation allowed full resolution of symptoms and return to semiprofessional soccer.[53]

Following the treatment of chondral or osteochondral lesions in the knee with TRUFIT CB, the most active patients in the series returned to semiprofessional sports; the remainder returned to their previous level of activity by 12 months, with no deterioration to date. This series of patients demonstrated outcome comparable to microfracture at 12 months. The improvement of KOOS (see Fig. 16.13) was

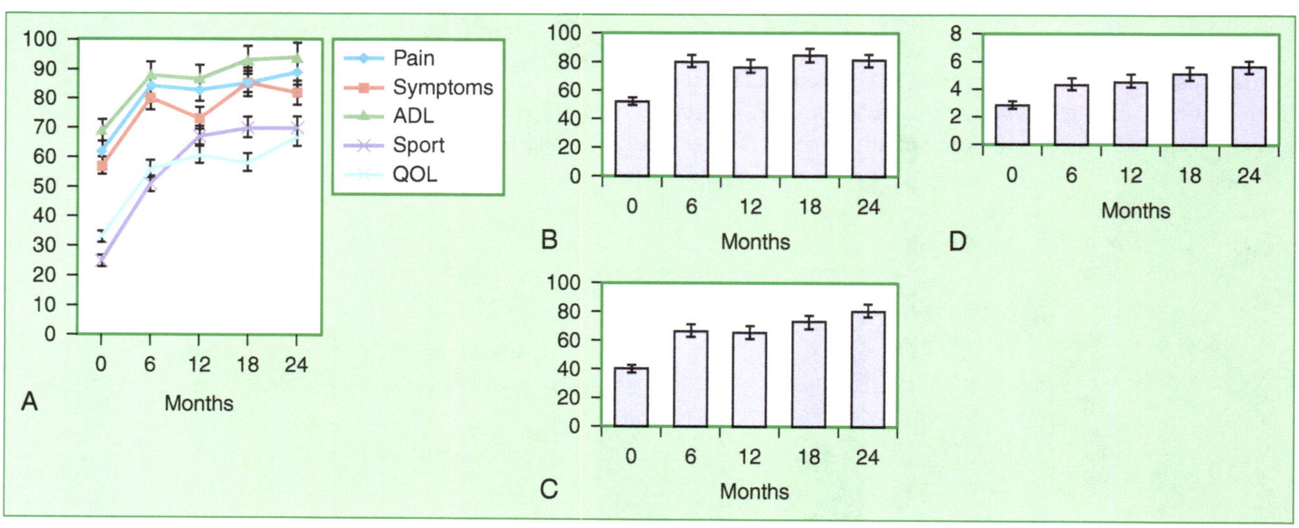

• **Fig. 16.13** (A) Knee Injury and Osteoarthritis Outcome Score (KOOS); (B) Lysholm score; (C) International Knee Documentation Committee score; and (D) Tegner activity level score. Mean KOOS pain, symptom, activities of daily living (ADL), sport, and quality-of-life (QOL) scores increased 21, 16, 18, 42, and 28 points at 12 months from baseline, respectively (all $P < .004$).

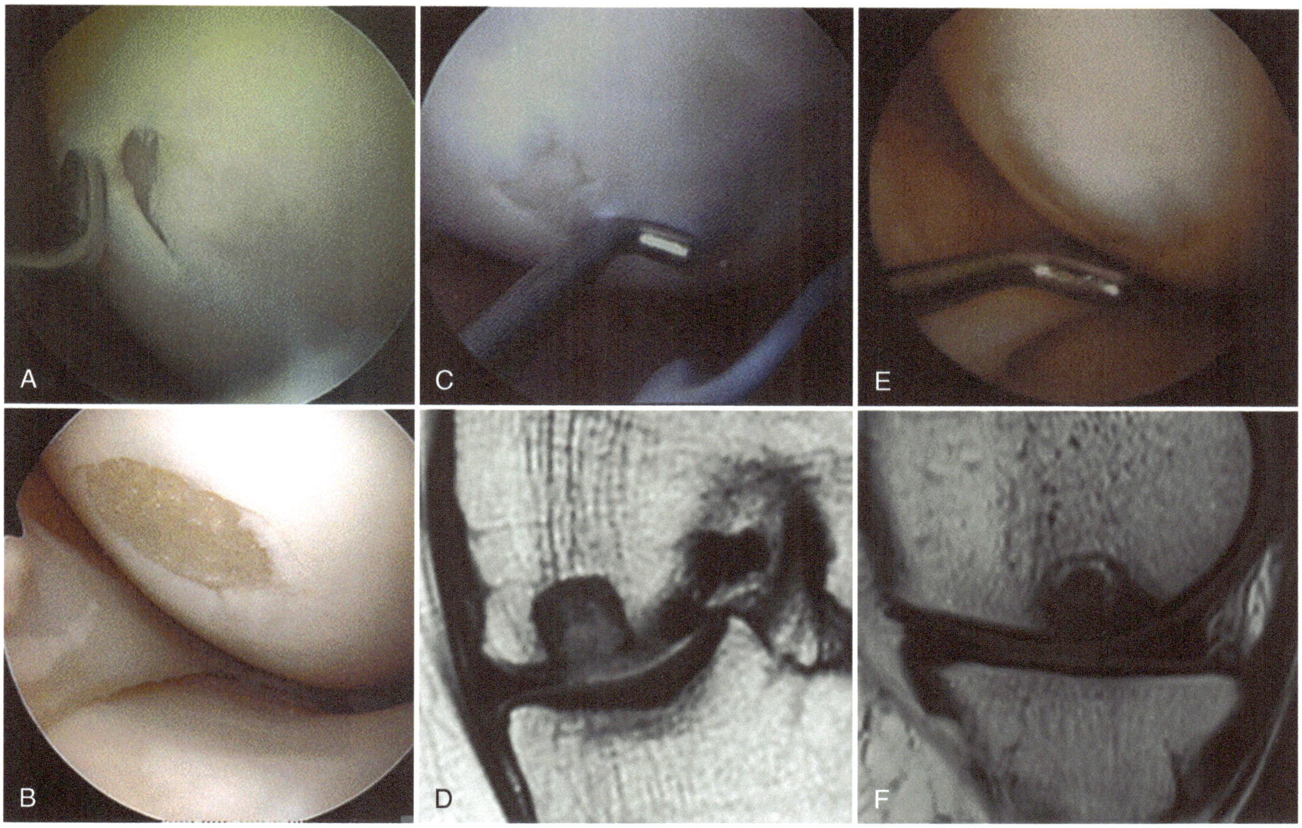

• **Fig. 16.14** A 37-year-old patient in the series undergoing repair of defect on medial femoral condyle. (A) Initial operative view showed delamination. (B) Repair with a 9-mm TRUFIT CB implant. (C) Second-look arthroscopy at 8 months showed soft area of repair. (D) Magnetic resonance imaging (MRI) at 8 months. (E) Arthroscopy at 3 years postoperative showed a smooth articular surface. (F) MRI showed reformation of the subchondral lamina and well-integrated articular cartilage.

similar to Saris' report on patients who received microfracture at 12 months (mean KOOS pain, symptom, activities of daily living [ADL], and quality-of-life [QOL] scores increased 13, 11, 12, and 16 points, respectively, from baseline).[54] TRUFIT CB provides a stable scaffold for early mobilization of the knee postoperatively, avoiding the prolonged period of limited weight bearing in microfracture. Other benefits of TRUFIT CB include its availability as an "off-the-shelf" product, the avoidance of donor site morbidity associated with osteochondral grafting, and the ease of the procedure. The results from this case series indicate that TRUFIT CB provides a one-step solution in managing small (<2-cm diameter) areas of chondral or osteochondral injury, particularly in patients who require rapid rehabilitation and a high level of activity.

Agili-C

Agili-C (CartiHeal Ltd., Israel) is another cartilage repair technology designed to treat chondral and osteochondral defects with favorable outcomes. It is a cell-free aragonite-based scaffold impregnated with hyaluronic acid at the articular surface. The aragonite-hyaluronate (Ar-HA) scaffold aims to restore the osteochondral unit through two mechanisms of action: (1) promote subchondral bone tissue repair through the recruitment of progenitor cells from the localized bone marrow edema, while simultaneously (2) stimulating the migration of MSCs and chondrocytes into the superficial cartilaginous layers with new cartilage formation at the articular surface.[55,56] Pre-clinical and histological studies have supported the potential of the Agili-C scaffold in facilitating a suitable environment for hyaline-like cartilage formation and cartilage regeneration.[55,56] CartiHeal Ltd. currently reached interim analysis of their Agili-C phase III multicenter, 2:1 randomized, clinical trial. Initial analysis revealed positive results with a predictive probability of trial success greater than 95%.[57] Enrollment is closed and we now wait for final study results to be announced. The Agili-C implant is an appealing one-step scaffold-based strategy for the treatment of osteochondral defects.

Minced Cartilage

One-Stage Autologous Procedure for Cartilage Regeneration

One-stage and two-stage surgical therapies to repair or restore articular cartilage in the treatment of focal chondral defects have been explored. Point-of-care techniques include marrow stimulation (e.g., microfracture) and osteochondral autografting and allografting; two-stage therapies include ACI and MACI. Each therapy has clinical advantages and limitations in terms of applicable defect size and location, patient age, and long-term durability of the repair tissue. Although ACI-based procedures have demonstrated promising clinical results, the requirement for multiple surgical exposures and ex vivo cell expansion can impact rehabilitation time, surgical/anesthesia risk, and health care costs. As a result, several emerging technologies are being studied either to improve existing single-stage therapies or to enable point-of-care chondrocyte-based implantation.

Cartilage Autograft Implantation System

The CAIS cartilage autograft implantation system (DePuy Mitek, Raynham, MA) has been developed as a point-of-care therapy composed of mechanically fragmented autologous cartilage implanted on a bioresorbable scaffold. (*Note:* CAIS is an investigational device limited by federal and local regulations to investigational use only.) This one-stage approach uses a customized harvester device to morselize donor tissue from an unaffected, low–weight-bearing region of the knee (intercondylar notch, trochlear ridge or other minor load-bearing site) into small fragments to promote cell outgrowth from the dense cartilaginous matrix (Fig. 16.15A). These cartilage fragments are overlaid onto a bioresorbable scaffold that provides both structural integrity and a defined three-dimensional architecture to support cell outgrowth, proliferation, and matrix deposition in the repair site. The CAIS scaffold is a synthetic composite matrix composed of polycaprolactone-co-glycolide polymeric foam reinforced with a polydioxanone mesh. Cartilage fragments are uniformly distributed over the scaffold surface using a custom dispersion device and subsequently coated with a layer of fibrin sealant to promote fragment retention during implant templating and fixation (Fig. 16.15B). Following debridement of the cartilage lesion to healthy margins, the implant is cut to size (Fig. 16.15C) and rigidly affixed in the repair site using bioresorbable polydioxanone staples (Figs. 16.15D and 16.16). Cyclic testing (10,000 cycles at 1 Hz) of this staple-based fixation in human cadaveric knees demonstrated robust scaffold retention with no detectable wear of adjacent cartilage or meniscus.[58]

In vitro studies have demonstrated chondrocyte viability as well as time-dependent cellular outgrowth into the CAIS scaffold following tissue fragmentation and seeding. In a subcutaneous implantation model, outgrowth cells from morselized cartilage exhibit more prominent neocartilaginous tissue formation than subculture-expanded chondrocytes, as revealed by safranin O staining.[59] These studies indicate that morselized cartilage fragments are a viable repository of chondrocytes capable of outgrowth and synthesis of a cartilaginous repair tissue.

Large animal cartilage repair models implementing this one-stage technique demonstrated safranin O–positive, hyaline-like tissue repair that was well integrated with adjacent cartilage and subchondral bone as early as 6 months postsurgery.[59] Empty defects or those treated with scaffold alone typically resulted in repair tissue of inferior quality and staining intensity compared to lesions treated with morselized cartilage fragments (Fig. 16.17). In addition, results from a 12-month equine study suggested that this one-step

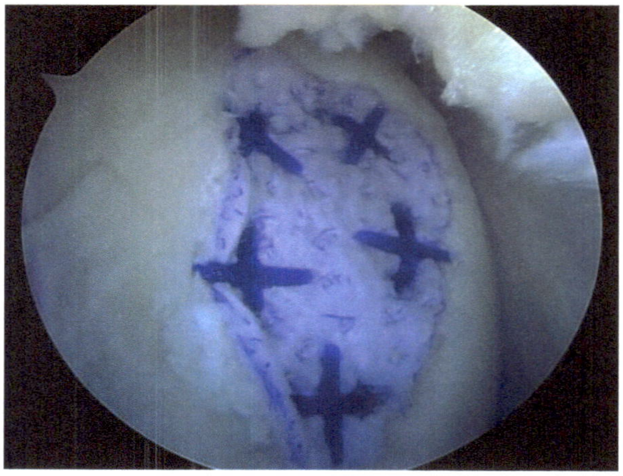

• **Fig. 16.16** Cartilage autograft implantation system implant affixed with bioresorbable staples.

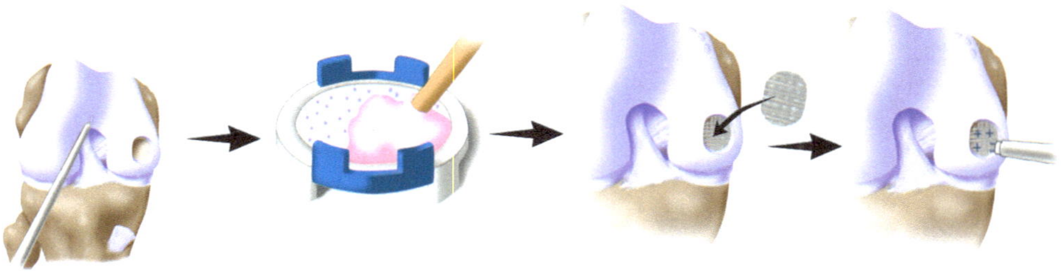

• **Fig. 16.15** Procedural steps of the cartilage autograft implantation system surgical technique, including harvest of donor cartilage (A), dispersion and fixation of cartilage fragments using fibrin sealant (B), sizing of the implant (C), and fixation with bioresorbable staples (D).

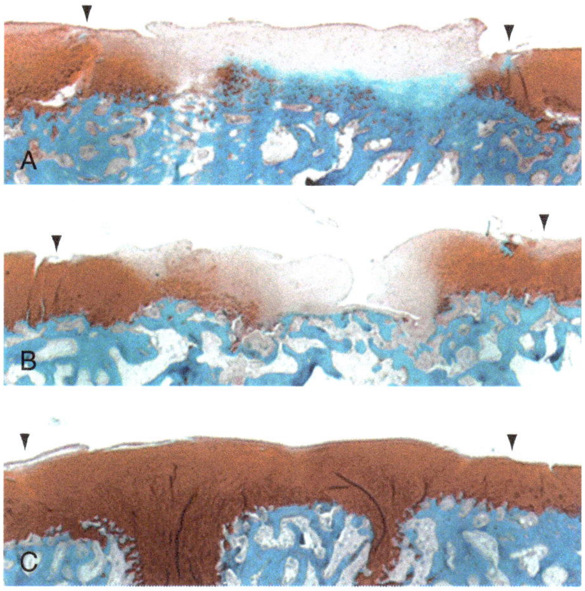

• **Fig. 16.17** Representative histology micrographs (safranin O staining) showing chondral defect repair in a goat model at 6 months: empty defects (A), scaffold only (B), and scaffold with morselized cartilage tissue fragments (C).

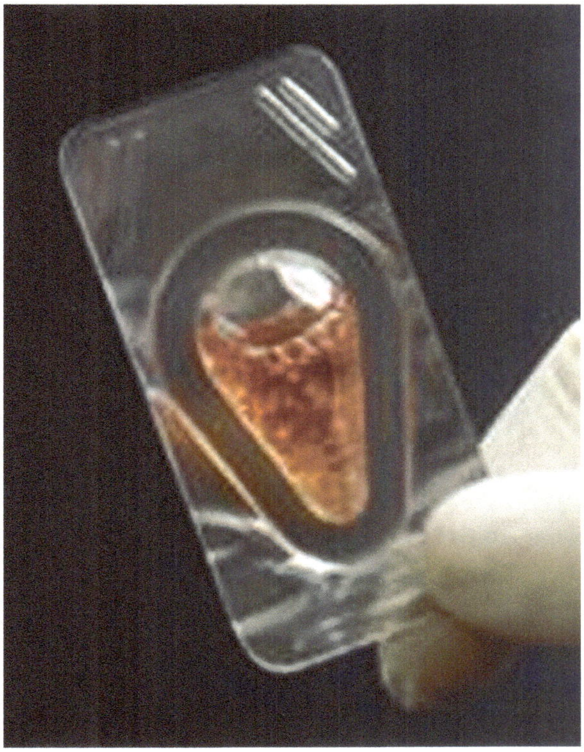

• **Fig. 16.18** DeNovo natural tissue graft.

approach may provide similar or improved healing progression and hyaline-like tissue repair compared to a modified ACI technique.[60,133] Human clinical studies evaluating the safety and efficacy of CAIS compared with microfracture are ongoing in North America and Europe.

In summary, CAIS, a one-stage cartilage regeneration therapy, potentially offers several practical advantages over other cell-based techniques. Delivery of morselized cartilage provides a direct source of primary autologous chondrocytes to the site of repair as opposed to a heterogeneous population of marrow-derived cells resulting from marrow stimulation procedures. The incarcerated chondrocytes subsequently outgrow and proliferate in vivo, thereby reducing the time, cost, and multiple procedures required for two-step ACI-based techniques. Morselized cartilage-derived chondrocytes may retain a more potent chondrogenic phenotype than culture-expanded cells because they are not exposed to the environmental trauma associated with ex vivo expansion. CAIS is a promising first-line cartilage regeneration therapy for the treatment of focal chondral defects in a single surgical procedure.

DeNovo Natural Tissue Graft

DeNovo natural tissue (NT) graft (Zimmer, Warsaw, IN/ISTO Technologies, St. Louis, MO) is composed of aseptically processed particulated cartilage tissue recovered from donated juvenile human knee joints (Fig. 16.18). No biologic manipulation or chemical processing is performed. The tissue pieces are packaged in a sterile blister package filled with a proprietary nutrient medium. The cartilage pieces are implanted into articular cartilage defects using fibrin adhesive for graft fixation. In an equine study in which human juvenile cartilage pieces were implanted to repair chondral defects of horse knee joints, no inflammation/immune rejection caused by the xenograft transplantation was observed (D. Frisbie, unpublished data). The DeNovo NT graft is considered to be human tissue per section 361 of the Public Health Service (PHS) Act and is therefore regulated solely under 21 CFR 1271 in the same way as many other allograft products, such as fresh osteochondral allografts and bone–tendon–bone allografts. Since May 2007, this product has been implanted to repair cartilage defects in more than 300 patients in various anatomic locations (knee, ankle, shoulder, hip, elbow, and great toe). Early clinical data on patients receiving DeNovo NT graft treatment have been encouraging.[61] Patients who were implanted with DeNovo NT Graft more than 2 years ago are reporting good clinical outcomes.

Second-Generation Cell-Based ACI

Matrix-Induced Autologous Chondrocyte Implantation

Background

MACI is a second-generation ACI therapy for repair of full-thickness cartilage defects. Developed by Verigen and later acquired by Genzyme Biosurgery (Cambridge, MA), MACI was designed to overcome the surgical complexity and

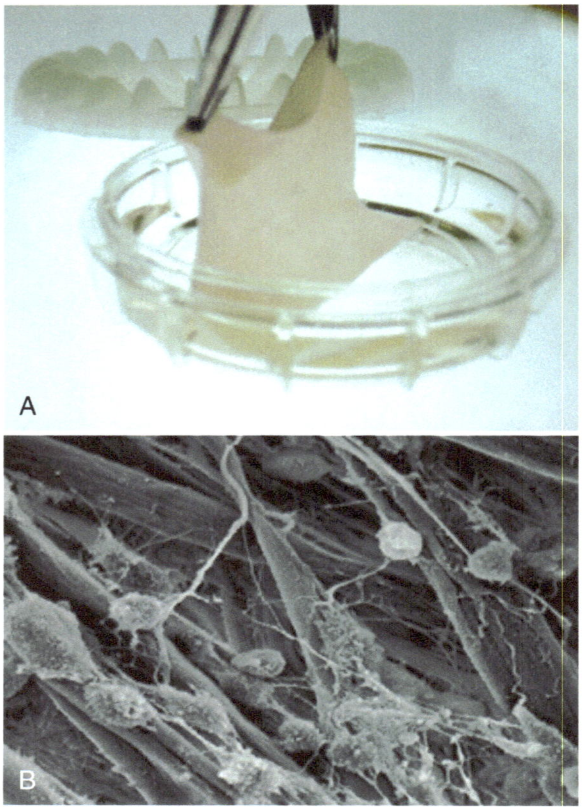

• **Fig. 16.19** (A) Matrix-induced autologous chondrocyte implantation (MACI). Collagen type I–III membrane is preseeded with autologous cultured chondrocytes and cultured, which is then ready for surgical implantation. (B) Scanning electron micrograph of autologous chondrocyte seeded MACI. (Courtesy Dr. Ming-Hao Zheng, School of Surgery and Pathology, University of Western Australia, Perth, Australia.)

invasiveness associated with first-generation ACI, Carticel (cultured ACI). For Carticel, cells are delivered in a liquid suspension, implanted in the defect, and secured with an autologous periosteal cover that is harvested from the proximal tibia. MACI is a surgically convenient delivery method in which cells are implanted attached or "seeded" onto the surface of a purified porcine biodegradable type I/III collagen membrane (Fig. 16.19). MACI is typically secured in the defect with fibrin sealant and sutures are used if supplemental fixation is deemed necessary (Fig. 16.20). Patients are not exposed to a second incision that is needed to harvest the periosteum and a large arthrotomy that is required to accommodate periosteal fixation. Arthroscopic delivery of MACI has been reported.[62]

Manufacturing Process

For MACI, chondrocytes are isolated from a cartilage biopsy using an enzymatic process, expanded in a monolayer cell culture, and seeded onto an absorbable purified type I/III collagen membrane. When cells are grown in monolayer cell culture, they dedifferentiate; that is, they change their phenotype and down-regulate expression of cartilage matrix genes. To ensure proper cell expression and phenotype within the final product, MACI implants

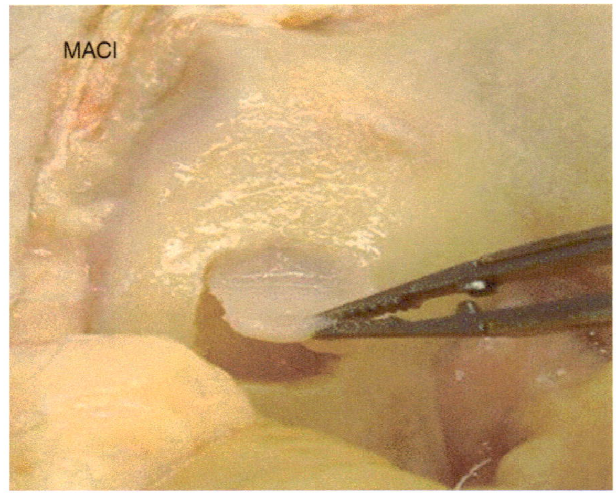

• **Fig. 16.20** Matrix-induced autologous chondrocyte implantation of a femoral condyle with fibrin glue fixation.

are characterized for cell potency, identity, and viability using proprietary assays that were designed to meet regulatory guidelines. MACI also undergoes extensive quality control release testing, including sterility, mycoplasma, and endotoxin assays.

Commercial Availability

MACI has been commercially available in several European member states and Australia since 1998. Because of the EU Advanced Therapy Medicinal Products regulation, commercial availability of MACI after December 2012 has required formal approval by the centralized European Medicines Agency (EMEA) process. In response to this regulation, Genzyme is conducting a phase III prospective, randomized, open-label, parallel-group, multicenter study, known as SUMMIT (Superiority of MACI vs. Microfracture Treatment), to demonstrate the superiority of MACI versus arthroscopic microfracture for the treatment of symptomatic articular cartilage defects of the femoral condyle, including the trochlea. The endpoints of SUMMIT include patient-reported assessments of pain and function, MR assessments, and histology assessments. MACI is not currently available in the United States.

Clinical Outcomes

Results from several studies demonstrate significant reductions in pain and functional impairment at early follow-up (2 years). Although longer-term data are limited, results from two studies demonstrate significant improvement from baseline out to 5-year follow-up.[63,64] Although no comparative ACI and MACI studies have been published, comparable rates of good/excellent results have been reported. After treatment with MACI, 70% to 89% of patients reported good/excellent results.[65–67] Overall, results of MRI, histology, and arthroscopic (macroscopic) assessments of the repair tissue demonstrate that treatment with MACI can yield repair tissue with hyaline-like cartilage (Fig. 16.21),[68–70] complete defect fill,[71] complete integration

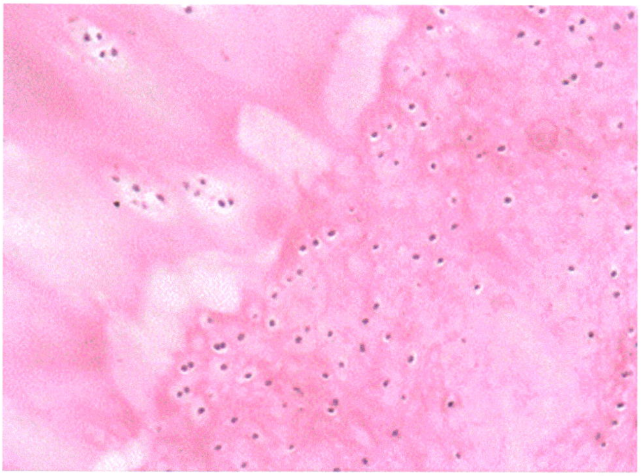

• **Fig. 16.21** Integration of native and regenerative cartilage (with appearance of hyaline-like cartilage) by matrix-induced autologous chondrocyte implantation. (Courtesy Dr. Ming-Hao Zheng, School of Surgery and Pathology, University of Western Australia, Perth, Australia.)

with surrounding cartilage,[72] and ICRS score of grade I/II.[68] Some studies have reported that MACI repair tissue was fibrocartilage and failed to integrate completely or fill the defect, findings that may be a result of the negative bias associated with limiting objective assessments to patients with only postoperative complications and not a representative sample of patients in the entire study.[66,71] The reported incidence of postoperative complications associated with the MACI procedure is low (range 0%–6.3%).[66,68,72,73] Reported postoperative complications include tissue hypertrophy, partial graft detachment, infections, and subsequent surgical procedures. The reported incidence of treatment failure, defined as graft detachment or bone to bone contact, also is low (range 0%–6.3%).[66,68,72,73]

Hyalograft C Autograft

Preclinical Findings

Hyalograft C autograft (Fidia Advanced Biopolymers, Abano Terme, Italy) is a second-generation ACI product.[74,75] It is a graft composed of autologous chondrocytes grown on a three-dimensional hyaluronan-based scaffold. The scaffold is a nonwoven pad composed of HYAFF 11, a hyaluronic acid benzyl ester polymer.[76]

Chondrocytes can be easily isolated from small biopsies and expanded in vitro; however, when cultured in two dimensions they tend to lose their characteristic phenotype, namely, collagen type II and aggrecan expression.[77] In vitro characterization studies confirmed that maintenance of a differentiated phenotype is favored by the use of a three-dimensional scaffold. Studies have clearly demonstrated that Hyalograft C scaffolds not only allow chondrocyte attachment but also provide adequate support to permit expression of the differentiated chondrocytic phenotype.[78,79] Excellent functional integration of Hyalograft C seeded with chondrocytes with the surrounding native bone and cartilage was demonstrated via the assessment of structure, biochemical composition, and mechanical behavior of the construct in an ex vivo model.[80] Moreover, an in vitro study has been conducted to analyze the growth and differentiation behavior of human articular chondrocytes on Hyalograft C scaffold compared with a porcine collagen scaffold and a gelatin gel matrix.[81] Results demonstrated that Hyalograft C scaffold was superior to the other scaffolds in terms of supporting rapid redifferentiation of chondrocytes after monolayer culture, as shown by electron microscopic evaluation of cell phenotype and the differentiation index (calculated as collagen II/I ratio), which was ~1 and stable during the observation period. The same index was only 10^{-3} for the collagen and gelatin scaffolds. Only Hyalograft C scaffold enabled the formation of a relatively large amount of cartilage-like differentiated cells, indicating that the nature of the matrix greatly influences the differentiation behavior of dedifferentiated human chondrocytes.

Expanded human chondrocytes cultivated on Hyalograft C scaffold and then subcutaneously implanted in athymic mice for up to 3 months confirmed that this scaffold is an adequate support for cartilage formation. Explant examination after implantation showed formation of hyaline-like cartilage.[82] Moreover, a study using a functional animal model verified that chondrocyte transplantation using Hyalograft C induces the regeneration of injured articular cartilage.[83] Nonclinical protocols in small and large animal models have also been performed to assess the biocompatibility and feasibility of Hyalograft C autograft for use in a clinical setting.[84–88]

Based on the nonclinical findings, Hyalograft C autograft was evaluated in clinical settings for the treatment of full-thickness articular cartilage defects.

Clinical Development

Since Hyalograft C autograft became available in clinical practice, more than 4800 patients have been treated with this technology. Of these patients, 230 have been evaluated in investigator-initiated clinical studies and the results of more than 900 patients have been reported in the published literature.

Preliminary clinical experience derived from pilot clinical studies indicated that the Hyalograft C autograft was well tolerated. The studies also showed that the surgical technique was substantially simpler than ACI (Fig. 16.22) because the product could be shaped to fit the lesion and could be applied by mini-invasive arthrotomy without the need for a periosteal flap, thus significantly reducing operation times and morbidity.

Consequently, in 2001, an Italian investigator initiated a multicenter observational study of more than 200 consecutive patients (mean age 37.4, mean lesion size 3.7 cm^2) who were treated with the Hyalograft C autograft and prospectively followed for 5 years, with 4-year follow-up data available to date.[75,89,90] The durability results suggest that clinical improvements obtained 2 years after implantation

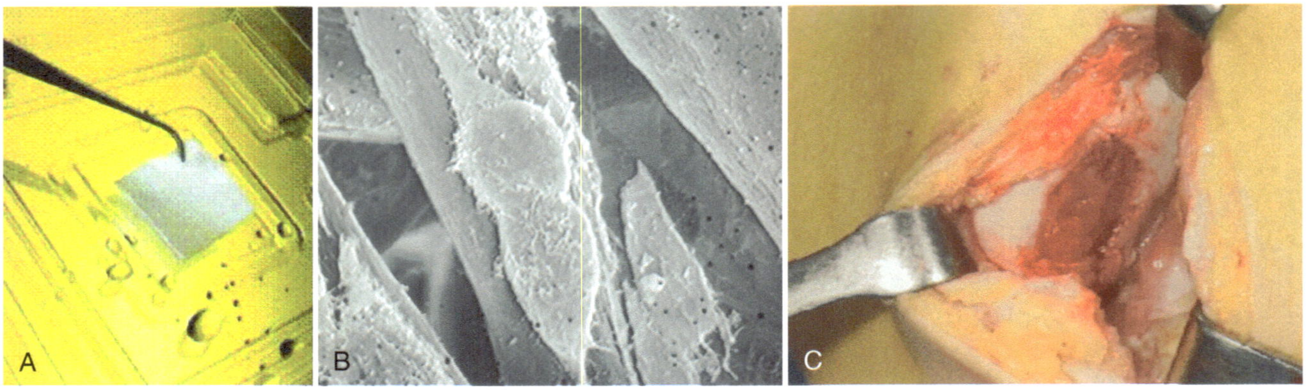

• **Fig. 16.22** (A) Hyalograft C. Membrane seeded with cultured autologous chondrocytes ready for surgical implantation. (B) Scanning electron micrograph of chondrocyte attachment to hyaluronan-based scaffold. (C) Mini-arthrotomy for delivery of Hyalograft C with fibrin glue fixation.

are maintained at 5-year follow-up. After an average of 4 years (n = 179) from implantation, 86% of patients had a significant benefit in knee symptoms and function. A mean IKDC subjective score of 78.6 points was obtained postoperatively, reflecting high levels of function and sports activities and low level of symptoms, compared with a mean IKDC preoperatively of 39.9 ($P < .0001$). After clinician-performed examination, 95.7% of the knees were rated as normal and nearly normal based on objective IKDC score. Significant improvements (86.4%, $P < .0001$) were obtained for health-related quality of life (EuroQol EQ-5D), particularly for pain and mobility aspects that overlap those obtained in an age- and gender-matched reference population.

In 2009, Kon et al.[91] reported a prospective, comparative, nonrandomized study with 5-year follow-up. In their study, the clinical outcome of patients treated with Hyalograft C autograft was compared with the microfracture technique. Eighty active symptomatic patients (mean age 29.8 years) with grade III to IV chondral lesions of femoral condyles or trochlea (mean defect size 2.4 cm^2) were enrolled and treated with arthroscopic Hyalograft C autograft (40 patients; Fig. 16.23) or microfracture (40 patients) techniques. More patients who had undergone previous surgery (47.5% vs. 25%, $P < .05$) and had fewer traumatic cartilage lesions (45% vs. 67.5%, $P < .05$) were enrolled in the Hyalograft C autograft group than in the microfracture group.

Both groups showed statistically significant improvement of all clinical scores from preoperative to 5-year follow-up ($P < .001$). In the microfracture group, the IKDC objective score increased from 2.5% normal and nearly normal knees before surgery to 75% at 5-year follow-up, and the subjective score increased from 41.1 preoperatively to 70.2 at 5-year follow-up. In the group treated with Hyalograft C autograft, the IKDC objective score increased from 15% normal and nearly normal before surgery to 90% at 5-year follow-up and the subjective score increased from 40.5 preoperatively to 80.2 at 5-year follow-up. When comparing the groups, better clinical results assessed with objective ($P < .001$) and subjective ($P = .003$) IKDC scores at 5-year follow-up were found in the group treated with arthroscopic Hyalograft C autograft transplantation. Also, no decrease in the resumption of sports activities evaluated with the Tegner score from 2- to 5-year follow-up was observed in patients treated with Hyalograft C autograft transplantation

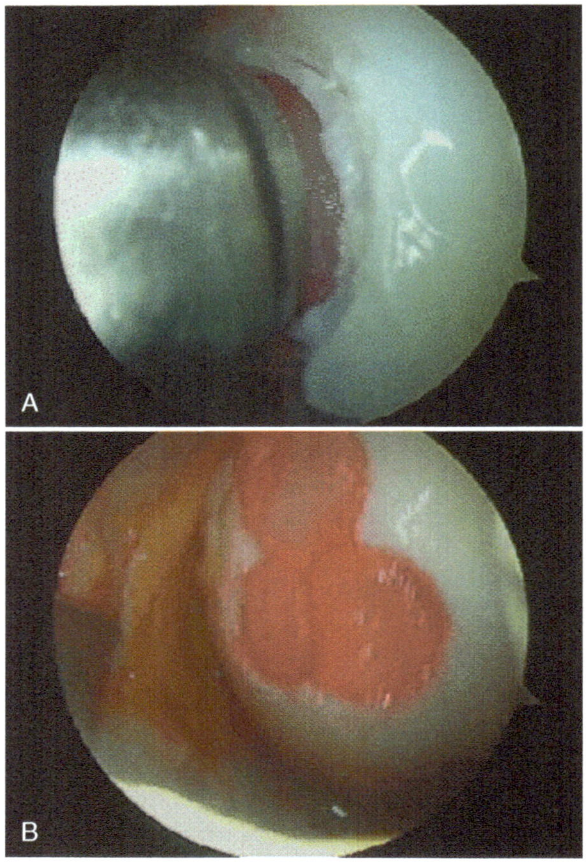

• **Fig. 16.23** (A) Arthroscopic delivery of Hyalograft C in an air environment after preparation of the defect in a mosaic pattern. Debridement of the chondral defect is performed in a saline environment using specially sized and cannulated guide instruments that facilitate the technique. (B) Final arthroscopic appearance of arthroscopically transplanted chondral defect in a mosaic pattern with Hyalograft C.

versus a decrease in sports activity in the group treated with microfracture.

These findings confirm the clinical superiority and durability of Hyalograft C autograft over microfracture in treating large articular cartilage defects.

Since Hyalograft C autograft became available in clinical practice, a total of 70 biopsies have been harvested from consenting patients from 5 to 33 months (mean 14.1 months) after Hyalograft C autograft implantation, both for purely investigative and for diagnostic purposes (i.e., in symptomatic patients).[92,93] The data were analyzed as a function of time from implantation and biopsies taken after a longer follow-up time appeared to show a significantly ($P = .0042$) higher percentage of hyaline cartilage (45.4% in hyaline specimens vs. 23.7% in biopsies taken within the first 18 months). Evidence of cartilage maturation over time was confirmed by analysis of the third-look biopsies. Hyaline tissue was present in all third-look specimens (mean time from implantation 30.6 months) but not in second-look biopsies (mean time from implantation 13.6 months) of the same patients. Taken together, these data indicate that after Hyalograft C autograft implantation, cartilage resurfacing is achieved, with consistent integration with subchondral bone, tidemark formation, and clear evidence of hyaline-like maturation over time. Evidence of cartilage maturation over time using Hyalograft C autograft has also been reported in studies using high-resolution MRI techniques, which confirmed stability of the implant postimplantation and analyzed the in vivo kinetics of defect filling.[94–96]

Other clinical reports have confirmed these observations in both the knee (Table 16.1) and ankle.[97] Table 16.1 summarizes some of the findings of clinical studies on the use of Hyalograft C autograft in the knee.[98–104]

The population treated is uniform in terms of age, lesion etiology, and lesion size and severity and is very similar to the demographics of first-generation ACI patients. Candidates for Hyalograft C autograft treatment were a relatively young, active, and clinically challenging patient population that presented, on average, with severe pain and functional impairment resulting from moderate to large chondral defects.

The 2- to 5-year follow-up data demonstrate that after Hyalograft C autograft treatment, the improvements in pain and mobility are durable and that patients have resumed their preinjury levels of activity.

These findings support algorithms that recommend cell-based therapies for treatment of large, disabling, articular cartilage lesions of traumatic origin or consequent to osteochondritis dissecans.

Taken together, the long-term clinical evidence available on Hyalograft C autograft indicates that, following treatment, the improvements in pain and mobility are durable and that patients have resumed their preinjury levels of activity, suggesting that Hyalograft C autograft is a safe and effective cartilage substitute for the indication proposed.

TABLE 16.1 Clinical Studies on Use of Hyalograft C Autograft in the Knee

--	Marcacci (2006)[99]	Marlovits and Nehrer (2004)[101]	Kon et al. (2009)[103]	Ferruzzi et al. (2008)[102]	Nehrer (2008)[105]	Marlovits et al. (2006)[100]	Gobbi et al. (2009)[104]
No. of patients treated	206	24	40	50	53	13	32
Mean age (years)	37.4	32.4	29.8	31.0	32	34	30.5
Mean defect size (cm²)	3.7	5.98	2.4	5.9	4.4	5.3	4.7
Outerbridge defect grade	III-IV	III-IV	III-IV	III-IV	III-IV	III-IV	III-IV
Previous surgeries (%)	45.6	87.5	47.5	–	77.8	–	59.4
Previous failed cartilage treatment (%)	33	29.1	20		32		21.9
Patients improved after minimum 2-year follow-up (%)	86	70.8	90	77	84.6	81.6	90.7

Clinical demographics and outcomes from studies.

ChondroCelect

Introduction

ChondroCelect (TiGenix N.V., Leuven, Belgium) is a characterized cell therapy product (according to the European regulatory framework for Advanced Therapy Medicinal Products) that consists of autologous cartilage cells expanded ex vivo via a highly controlled and consistent manufacturing process.

In order to culture cells with the best potential to generate stable cartilage, it is critical that the cell culture process not cause the cells to lose their cartilage phenotype.[77] Maintaining the ability of the cells to conserve maximally their preculture phenotype and high-quality cartilage-forming capacity was the key element for product development.

The initial research conducted by Dell'Accio et al.[105,106] was used as the basis to develop both the ChondroCelect process and the ChondroCelect score, which is used as a quality measure before the release of each cell batch.

Translational Research Background

Dell'Accio et al.[105,106] tested different mesenchymal cell populations (including precursor cells, chondrocytes, primitive cells, stem cells) in nude (immunosuppressed) mice for their basic ability to form stable cartilage. This research led to the development of an in vivo model: the ectopic cartilage formation assay (ECFA). This assay tests the potency and capacity of a cell population to form a cartilage implant in an in vivo environment. It is now used as one of the pillars in the ChondroCelect research and development process.

The ECFA potency test consists of the following steps (Fig. 16.24):

- The cells are injected into the thigh of a nude mouse.
- The cells are allowed to grow in this ectopic site (i.e., in vivo) for a period of 3 to 4 weeks.
- The tissue, which has developed at the injection site, is removed for histologic examination, including scoring using toluidine blue and safranin O staining.

In this model, the cells' intrinsic capability to form cartilage is tested in a stringent, noncartilaginous environment. Hence, it provides a direct measure of the relevant biologic properties of the cells in regenerating hyaline cartilage. This is accomplished by assessing some of the main characteristics of cartilage formation, such as extracellular matrix (ECM) deposition leading to tissue formation, absence of vascular invasion, and absence of pathologic mineralization.

The following insights were gained through these initial experiments:

- Identification of cell populations that retain their ability (their phenotype) to form cartilage implants in vivo and those that either had no potential or had lost that capability (laying the foundation for the ChondroCelect score).

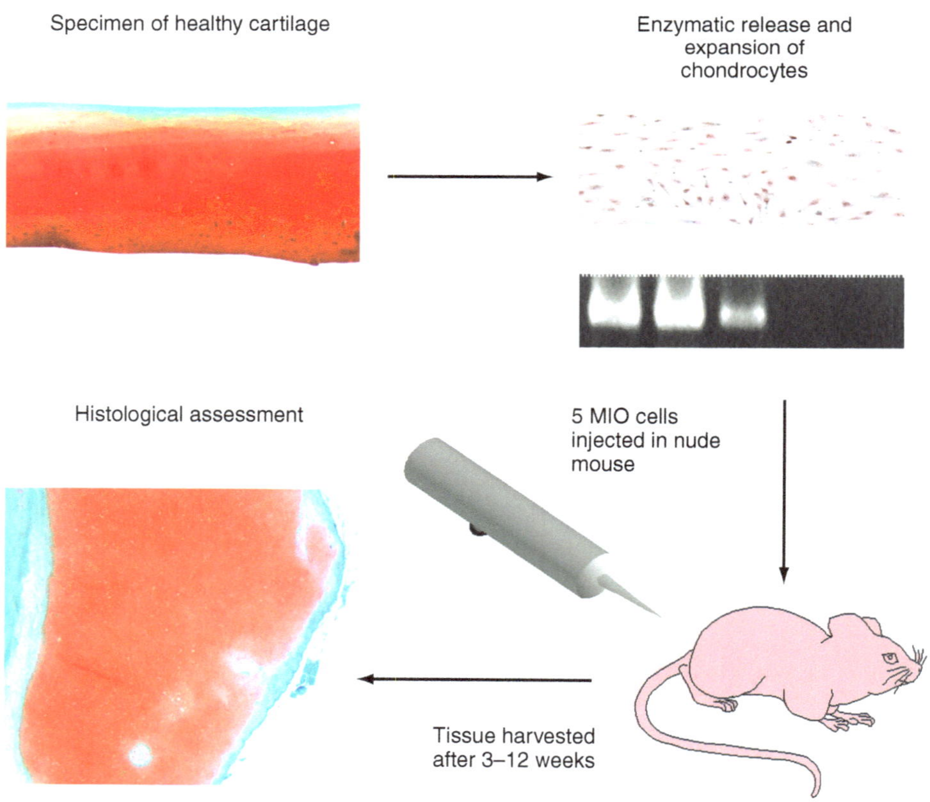

• **Fig. 16.24** Potency testing in the ectopic nude mouse assay.

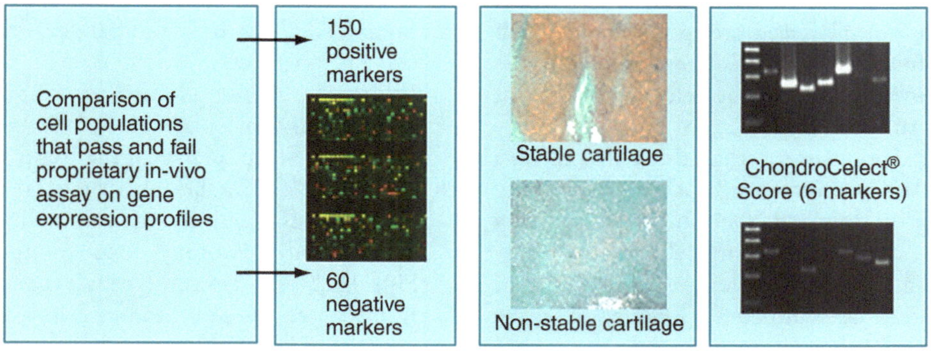

• **Fig. 16.25** Development of surrogate marker assay.

- Development of a cell culturing process with the goal of preserving the chondrocyte phenotype in cells (the precursor of the ChondroCelect process).

Refining Predictive Power: Development of the ChondroCelect Score

Although the ECFA is a powerful assay for demonstrating a cell population's ability to regenerate stable cartilage, it is not practical for use as a quality test in a routine manufacturing setting. A quicker, less cell consuming, preferably in vitro assay was needed.

In order to develop an in vitro assay, the same cell populations tested in the ECFA were analyzed in a comparative microarray analysis (Fig. 16.25). This assay looks at the expression of a large number of genes with the goal of identifying both positive and negative markers relevant for cartilage formation.

Through this assay, 150 positive markers (genes that are highly expressed in the cells that produced a cartilage implant in the ECFA and are not or are very lowly expressed in the cells that have no ability to form cartilage) and 60 negative markers (genes that are highly expressed in cells that have no ability to form cartilage in the ECFA) were identified.

Of these 210 markers, six markers were selected (four positive and two negative) based on their capacity to generate cartilage tissue in the ECFA. These markers form the basis of the ChondroCelect score.

To determine the prediction threshold of the score in cartilage formation, a correlation was drawn between the score and the outcome of the ECFA histology score. The histology score is based on the presence and brightness of staining of the ECM of cartilage cells.

When analyzing the results between the in vitro assay of cells and the in vivo capacity of cells to form cartilage in the ECFA implants, a clear correlation was noted between cells having a good score and a good histology score.

In routine manufacturing, the marker gene expression profile of these six markers can be measured using reverse transcriptase polymerase chain reaction (RT-PCR) methodology. Each of the individual markers can be scored based on its overall expression level in the assay. The combination of these individual scores gives the ChondroCelect score.

Developing the ChondroCelect Manufacturing Process

The second major development push and product differentiation was through the creation of the ChondroCelect process. As stated in the scientific rationale, the goal during cell culture is for the cells to maintain their phenotype. For proper cartilage defect filling, 1,000,000 cells/cm^2 are required and must be cultured from the original biopsy material. The problem is the well-documented issue of gradual cell dedifferentiation during routine cell culturing.

In order to develop the process, factors influencing the cell culture process were varied in a controlled manner. The expanded cells obtained from each of these batches were qualified for their ability to produce cartilage in vivo. The goal of these tests was to identify which factors during the cell culture process influenced the cells' ability to maintain their chondrocyte phenotype.

The ChondroCelect process strictly controls the different factors during the culturing process that support the multiplication of chondrocyte cells while preventing these cells from becoming too dedifferentiated.

At the end of each individualized patient batch production, the potency is measured to verify that the cultured cells have retained their ability to grow cartilage. By using this controlled and consistent culturing process, an optimal quality product is obtained.

Proof of Concept in a Large Animal Model

In order to evaluate the validity of the process, a preclinical experiment in a large animal model was initiated. The experiment compared autologous goat cells cultured according to the ChondroCelect process with dedifferentiated and fibroblast cells.

Stable chondrocyte cells (obtained through the ChondroCelect culturing method) showed good filling of the defect at 10 weeks. In contrast, the dedifferentiated cells gave only limited filling at the edges and little or no filling at the center of the defect.

Consequently, the cells cultured by the ChondroCelect process had a higher overall modified O'Driscoll Score (MODS) and much higher integration score than the dedifferentiated cells, which had scores only slightly better than the negative control fibroblast cell group at 10 weeks. In addition, the cells cultured by the ChondroCelect process gave a high-quality overall filling of the defect with superior integration into the surrounding tissue.

Further research demonstrated that the cells cultured by the ChondroCelect process were capable of resorbing and then reforming the calcified layer and were signaling to the environment, thereby recruiting cells from the surrounding tissues (Fig. 16.26). This led to better filling of the defect and superior basal and lateral integration in the ChondroCelect process cell group.

In contrast, the dedifferentiated cells did not demonstrate any reforming of the calcified layer or signaling capabilities to surrounding cells.

This experiment confirmed the original rationale that differentiated cells are needed to form cartilage. The dedifferentiated cells, in addition to the fibroblast-negative control group, did not yield good cartilage implants.

Clinical Development: The TIGACT01 Study

The objective of the TIGACT01 study was to evaluate the efficacy and safety of ChondroCelect (CC) versus microfracture (MF) in the repair of symptomatic full-thickness cartilage defects of the femoral condyles.

CC ($n = 51$) was compared to MF ($n = 61$) in patients with grade III to IV symptomatic cartilage defects of the femoral condyles in a prospective, multicenter, randomized controlled trial. Structural repair was assessed at 1 year by histopathologists blinded to the treatment using computerized histomorphometry and the Overall Histology Assessment Score (item 1 of the ICRS II score).

CC resulted in better structural repair than MF at 1 year as assessed by histomorphometry ($P = .003$) and Overall Histology Assessment Score ($P = .010$) (Fig. 16.27). Structural repair parameters relating to chondrocyte phenotype and tissue structure also were superior with CC.[54]

Mean improvement in overall KOOS at 36 months compared with baseline was higher in the CC group versus the MF group (21.65 ± 3.05 vs. 15.27 ± 3.07, respectively).

When applying a mixed linear model analysis, statistically significantly greater improvement was shown for the CC group versus the MF group with regard to change from baseline in overall KOOS as well as in four of five KOOS subdomains (ADL, pain, symptoms/stiffness, and QOL).

Two failures (defined as need for reintervention) occurred in the CC group versus seven in the MF group at 36 months (Fig. 16.28).

Patients treated within 3 years of symptom onset had a better clinical outcome (as measured by overall KOOS)

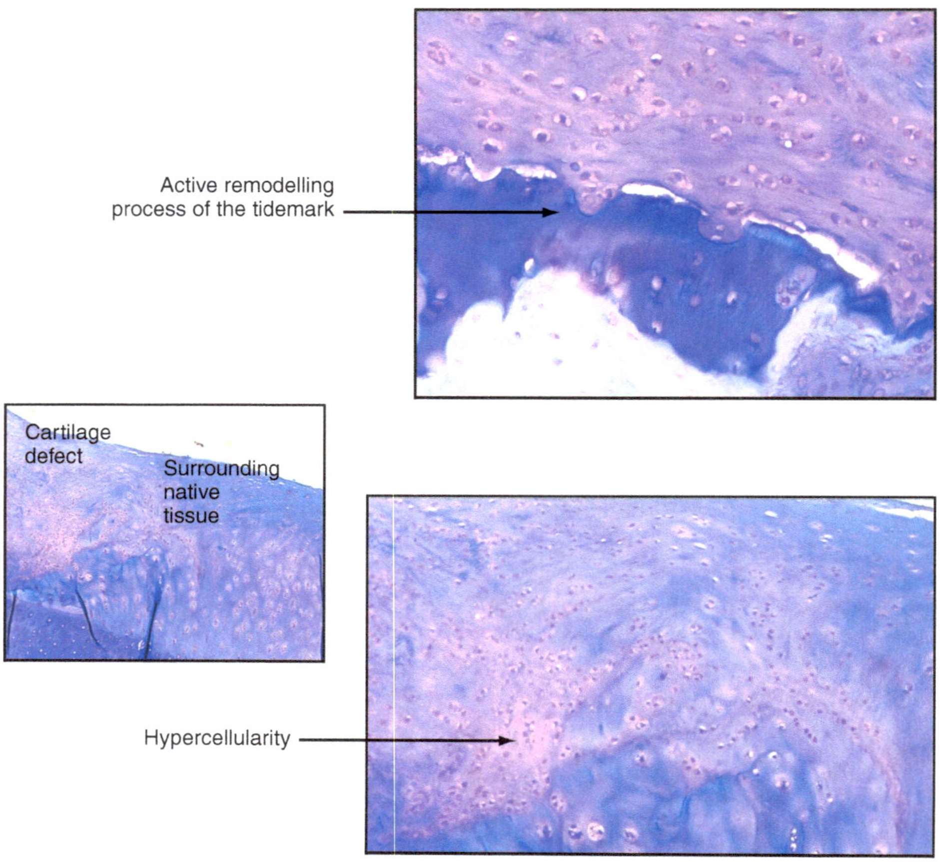

• **Fig. 16.26** Mode of action studies in goat.

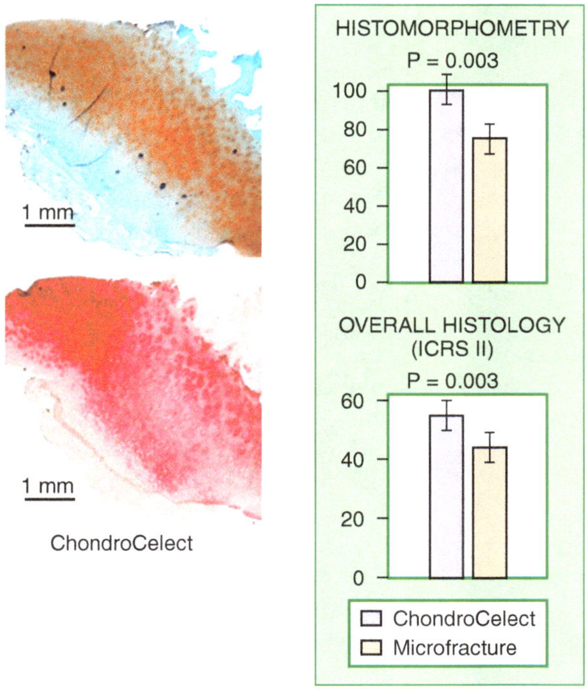

• **Fig. 16.27** Superior structural repair at 12 months.

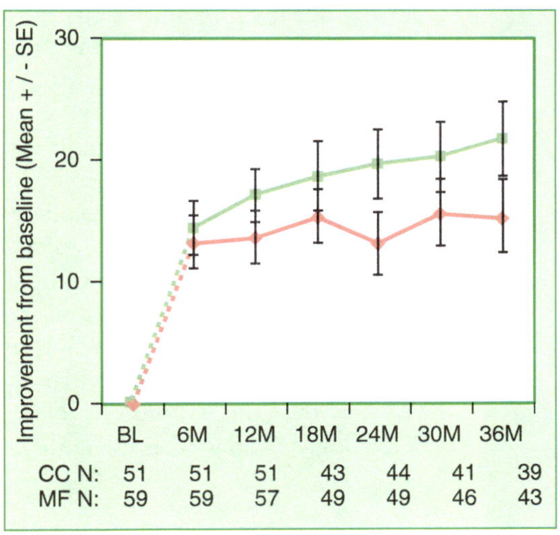

Longitudinal analysis:
treatment effect at 36 months
(mixed linear model)

KOOS	*P*-value***
Overall*	0.018
Pain	0.028
Symptoms	0.020
Activity (ADL)	0.035
Sports	0.200
Quality of life	0.041

Treatment failures
(reinterventions)
CC: 2 MF: 7

*Average of all KOOS domains, except Sports
**FAS without imputation for missing data of failures
***Between group KOOS changes from baseline

• **Fig. 16.28** Superior clinical outcome at 36 months.[54] *KOOS*, Knee Injury and Osteoarthritis Outcome Score; *FAS*, full analysis set.

than did patients treated beyond 3 years of symptom onset (and compared with MF).

MRI scans were performed at 12, 24, and 36 months and were assessed using the Magnetic resonance Observation of Cartilage Repair Tissue (MOCART) score and nine additional items.

On MRI, several parameters (e.g., filling of the defect) were comparable between the two treatment groups. However, more patients in the MF group than in the CC group reported having subchondral bone reaction and enhanced elevation of the subchondral bone plate at 36 months. This resulted in a thinner "covering" layer of cartilage, which could potentially explain failure after MF.

ChondroCelect is currently under regulatory review for EU market authorization. It is not approved for use in the United States.

CaReS Cartilage Regeneration System

The CaReS cartilage regeneration system (Arthro Kinetics, Esslingen, Germany) is a minimally invasive method for treating large cartilage defects in knees. Using the patient's own cartilage cells and a biologically purified collagen type I matrix derived from rat tail collagen, CaReS is a cartilage transplant with ease of application.

With the cartilage regeneration system, isolated autologous cultured chondrocytes (passage 0) are embedded in the purified collagen type I matrix, which solidifies within 25 minutes at room temperature. The construct is then incubated for 8 to 13 days and then implanted. The cell count is that of healthy cartilage and the cells are outside their accustomed three-dimensional matrix environment for only a few hours (Fig. 16.29). The size and thickness of the transplant are variable during manufacture of the transplant and may be sized during the operation with the cutting instruments provided (Fig. 16.30A–C). The operative time is significantly reduced because microsuture of a cover to secure the implant is not required. The transplant is fixated using standard fibrin glue.

The transplant is manufactured by Arthro Kinetics under an extensive total quality management system (QMS). The manufacturing is based on pharmaceutical law (German drug law Arzneimittelgesetz [AMG]) and Good Manufacturing Practices (GMP), internationally established.

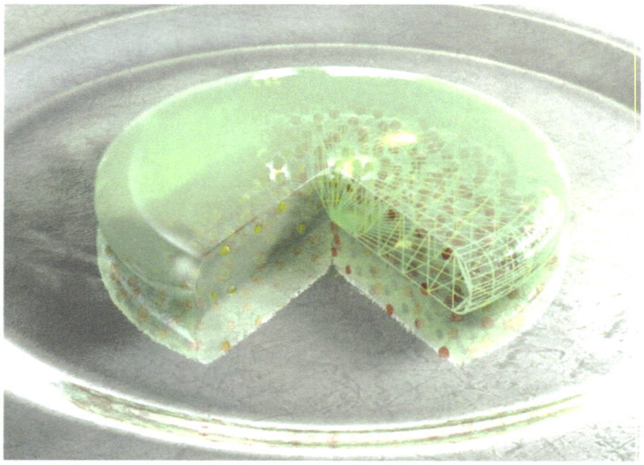

• **Fig. 16.29** Schematic representation of cellular suspension in a three-dimensional collagen–gelatin matrix ready for implantation.

Requirements for the surgery are grade III or IV Outerbridge chondral defects measuring 2.5 to 10 cm^2. Intact and healthy surrounding cartilage is necessary for the graft to remain stable within its implanted bed. A maximum of two defects are allowed. Contraindications include joint stiffness, ligamentous instability, infectious disease, and background factors that have not been addressed, such as varus or valgus malalignment.

BioCart II

Optimal repair of focal articular cartilage lesions requires physiologically active chondrocytes delivered in biocompatible, self-instructive scaffolds. Such integrated products should result in the deposition of authentic cartilage matrix, duplicating both the structure and function of the native tissue. A novel approach combining growth factor–driven chondroprogenitors that do not proliferate but rapidly produce cartilage matrix in a true three-dimensional, fibrin–hyaluronan scaffold has enabled successful repair of full-thickness cartilage defects.

Mature articular cartilage is composed primarily of postmitotic cells separated from each other by a thick and dense matrix (ECM); as a result, it has a highly restricted ability for self-repair. Chondrocyte cell functions are primarily regulated through specific cell–matrix interactions mediated by both integrin and nonintegrin receptors as well as mechanosensitive ion channels with direct implications for the expression and deposition of physiologic, hyaline-type cartilage.

In tissue culture, the cells can be expanded but their proliferation is frequently accompanied by dedifferentiation in which their "chondrocytic" phenotype is lost and their ability to produce high-quality ECM upon reimplantation is compromised. Therefore, despite pioneering successes, the regeneration of physiologic hyaline cartilage, the goal of tissue regeneration, is not reproducibly attained.

An optimal scaffold for implantation should be both highly porous and permeable, facilitating homogeneous cell seeding, cell attachment, and diffusion of nutrients and

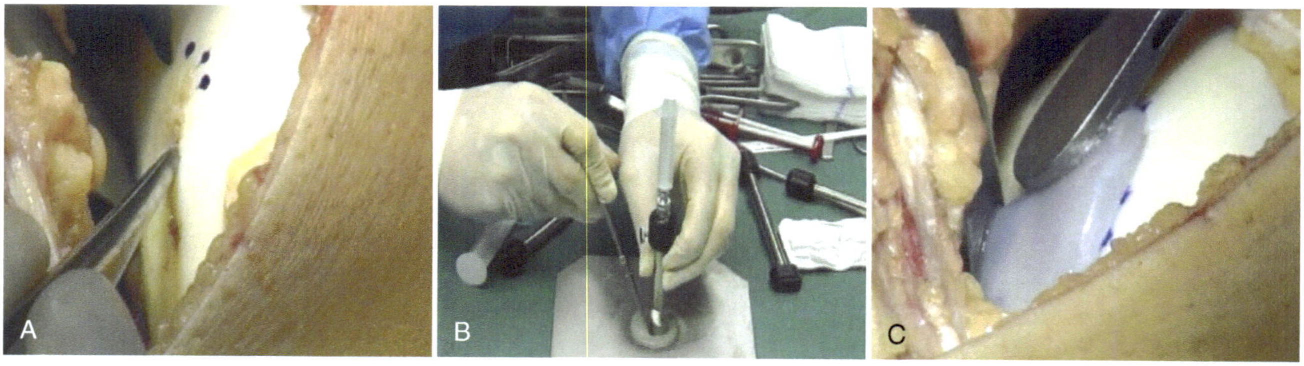

• **Fig. 16.30** (A) Chondral defect being outlined for radical debridement. (B) The cartilage regeneration system transplant being cut precisely to the defect on the back table. (C) The cartilage regeneration system transplant being glued with fibrin sealant to the chondral bed after it has been cut precisely to the defect. Pressure is maintained for up to 5 minutes to allow the collagen gel implant to mold to the defect and become secure.

instructive molecules. It should have the ability to support the deposition of authentic cartilage matrix until the cells have produced sufficient ECM and then be biodegradable, allowing for the replacement of scaffold with cartilage.

BioCart II (ProChon Biotech, Ness Ziona, Israel) uses growth factor–directed autologous chondrocytes in a fibrin–hyaluronan matrix for enhanced focal articular cartilage repair. In designing BioCart II, the conditions for ex vivo expansion of primary human chondrocytes are used, consisting of autologous serum supplemented with a recombinant variant of fibroblast growth factor 2 (rFGF2v) in cultures that promote rapid expansion of the cells while preserving their chondrogenic potential. Chondrocytes cultured for 10 days with FGF2v yield 10 times as many cells as cultures without the growth factor and, most importantly, can generate, in mass cultures, extensive, highly differentiated, cartilage-like structures (Fig. 16.31A). The cells are subsequently seeded throughout a three-dimensional scaffold composed of human plasma–derived fibrin and hyaluronic acid.

Fibrin is the naturally occurring matrix through which healing occurs in the human body. However, in marked contrast to a fibrin clot environment, this particularly designed scaffold does not support chondrocyte proliferation; rather, it provides the correct microenvironment for the embedded chondrocytes to express a mature chondrocyte phenotype and build-up of ECM.

The scaffold is a highly porous structure (Fig. 16.31B) that allows for even cell distribution (Fig. 16.31C). This semisolid construct is unique because it combines the tensile, resistant, cross-linked fibrin fibers with the viscoelastic properties of an intercalated fibrinogen hyaluronan hydrogel. Such a unique composite provides enough mechanical resilience to support cell attachment and mechanical loads combined with a highly conductive microenvironment optimized to support cell survival and matrix deposition. Indeed, static mechanical testing demonstrated a dramatic increase in tensile strength a few days after cell seeding contributed by deposition of ECM, giving the implant distinct mechanical properties that allow it to be easily handled and cut to a defined shape during the implantation procedure.

The clinical experience with BioCart II has extended to the almost 100 BioCart II implantations performed to date. The majority of the recipients of the BioCart II have significantly improved by most measurable clinical parameters,[107] in good agreement with radiologic evidence by MRI demonstrating complete filling of defects after 1 and 2 years of follow-up in most implanted cases.[108] Most interesting is the very high rate of success in highly active individuals and athletes. This may be a result of the unique combination of a differentiation supportive environment with the mechanotransduction features of the BioCart II scaffold responding to the mechanical stimuli exerted during the enhanced and highly disciplined rehabilitation program of these particular patients.

It is rather ambitious to try and recapitulate the stepwise progression that occurs during normal chondrogenesis. However, understanding and successfully implementing some of the key necessary signals may guide the direction of cells along physiologic routes of differentiation, thereby dramatically improving the quality of the derived tissue and the clinical outcome.

CARTIPATCH

Second-Generation Autologous Chondrocyte Transplantation Technique

TBF Tissue Engineering Company (Mions, France) developed and validated CARTIPATCH, an autologous chondrocyte transplantation technique that includes a biomaterial scaffold designed according to the three following criteria:

1. Ability to obtain differentiated cells as a result of a three-dimensional environment;
2. Ease of handling and implantation;
3. Potential to make the transplanted chondrocytes evolve into an osteochondral functional tissue.

The combination of agarose and alginate was selected based on their safety and performance.[109–111] They both are of nonanimal origin, show high biocompatibility properties when properly purified, and can be steam-sterilized. Once mixed with a cell suspension, the gel can be molded (at 37°C) into complex shape implants, which solidify at

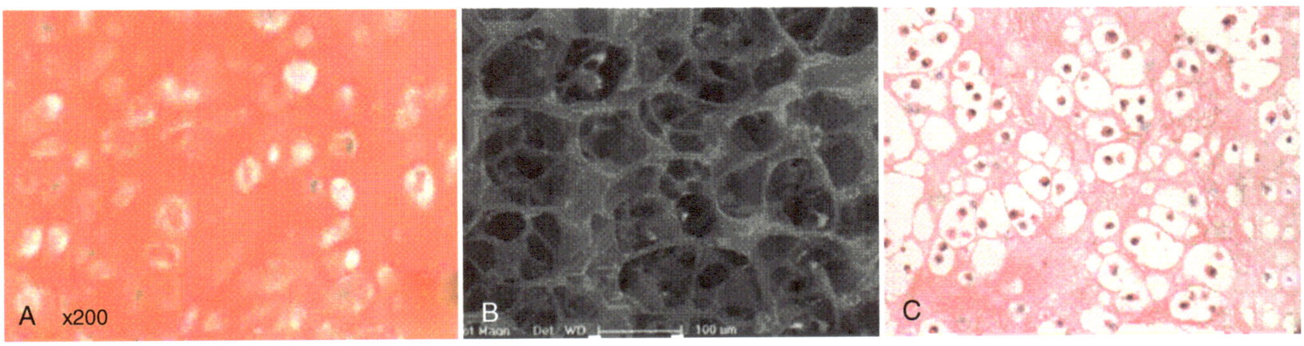

• **Fig. 16.31** (A) Standard mass pellet culture of chondrocytes cultured in vitro with FGF2v showing cartilage structure formed during the culture. (B) Scanning electron micrograph of BioCart scaffold showing the porous structure of the matrix. (C) Cross section of scaffold loaded with cells and stained with hematoxylin-eosin stain showing the cells distributed throughout the pores of the scaffold.

approximately 25°C in conditions that do not stress the cells. Even cell distribution is obtained by quick gelation. Hydrogel porosity allows culture medium diffusion, ensuring good cell viability. Alginate provides matrix elasticity,[112] improving ease of handling during production and surgery. Because the implant is not porous to cells once implanted, the biomaterial can protect the chondrocytes from immunogenic cells and allows cell maturation through protein synthesis. The hydrogel is patented in Europe (1 355 981) and a patent has been submitted in the United States (2004-0047912).

Dedicated instrumentation was developed to press-fit one or several premolded implants in the debrided lesion during an open knee surgical procedure. One or several cylindrical implants of various diameters, with a conical bottom, can be used to obtain adequate coverage of the lesion (Fig. 16.32). The CARTIPATCH surgical procedure is easy, reproducible, and precise and can be performed within 1 hour.[113]

Chondrocyte viability and distribution in CARTIPATCH were validated in vitro. Cell potency and functionality were assessed after 14 days of incubation using both real-time quantitative PCR and immunostaining techniques. Real-time quantitative PCR showed a positive evolution of the ratio between type II and type I collagen when the expansion phase was compared with the incubation phase. Immunostaining showed that more than 50% of the chondrocytes included in the matrix were marked positively for both type II collagen and aggrecan.[114]

An in vivo proof of concept on agarose gel implanted in sheep condyles allowed development of a surgical procedure and evaluation of biocompatibility. At 6 months, a hyaline-type cartilaginous repair was observed. An in vivo safety and efficacy study on the final gel formulation is in progress, including condyle and trochlear implantation in 11 sheep up to 12 months. The preliminary results obtained after 6 months showed good cartilage repair.

The CARTIPATCH phase II prospective, multicenter clinical study (sponsored by TBF, main investigator Philippe Neyret, CHU de Lyon, period January 9, 2002, to January 6, 2006) enrolled 20 patients and was completed in 2006 after 2 years of follow-up.[115] The evaluation included clinical, radiologic, arthroscopic, and histologic parameters and allowed demonstration of the following:

1. Surgical feasibility of the CARTIPATCH technique;
2. Absence of serious unexpected adverse events;
3. First clinical encouraging results: significant improvement ($P < .001$ by t-test) of mean subjective IKDC score at 1 and 2 years (+39 and +41, respectively);
4. Significant decrease of mean defect size measured by MRI, from 2.7 cm^2 preoperatively to 0.4 cm^2 at final follow-up ($P < .001$ by t-test);
5. Reconstruction of predominant hyaline-like cartilage observed in 8 of 13 biopsied patients and reconstruction of hyaline-like cartilage mixed with fibrocartilage in 3 of 13 patients;
6. Both chondral and osteochondral reconstruction of the cartilage.

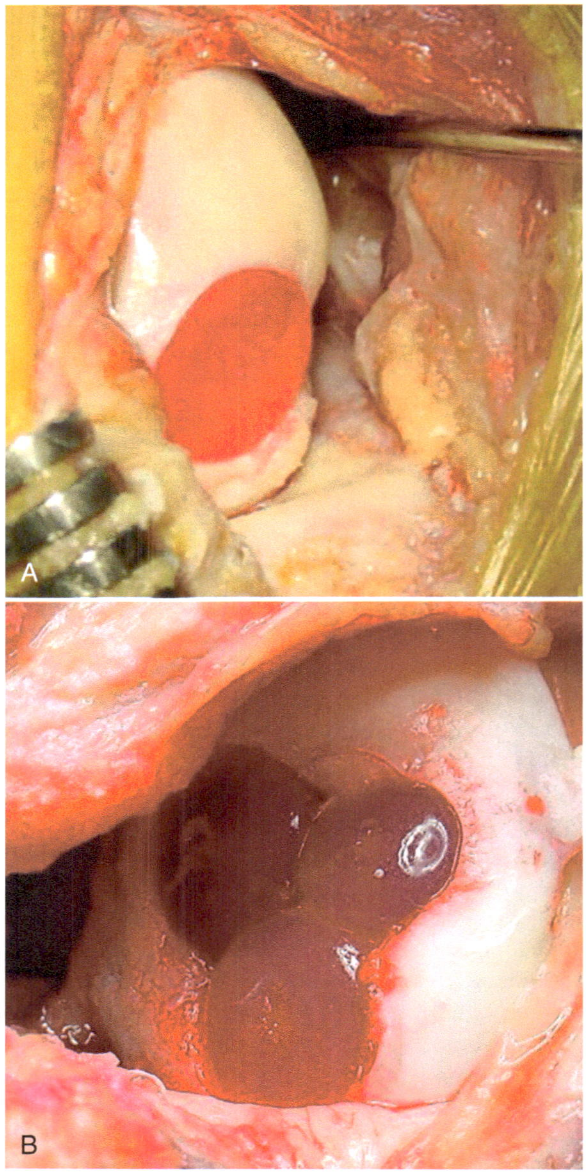

• **Fig. 16.32** (A) CARTIPATCH implantation: single implant. (B) CARTIPATCH implantation: mosaic pattern.

Two separate Phase III clinical multicentric studies comparing CARTIPATCH with mosaicplasty or microfracture are in progress.

Third-Generation Cell-Based Therapies

NeoCart System

The Concept

The NeoCart autologous cartilage implant (Histogenics Corporation, Waltham, MA) is designed to restore articular cartilage of chondral lesions. The NeoCart system applies concepts of cell biology, materials science, and tissue engineering to develop, ex vivo, a regenerated tissue with the characteristics of hyaline neocartilage, that is, the NeoCart implant, when newly placed in the lesion, actively produces ECM components. At the same time, individual cells continue to divide and are free to migrate and exchange with the surrounding tissue. By simulating the biophysical and biochemical conditions in the joint environment, the chondrocytes retain their phenotype and respond with increased ECM production.

The NeoCart implant is produced by seeding autologous chondrocytes into a type I collagen honeycomb-type scaffold with pores that permit diffusion of nutrients throughout the construct. This construct is placed in a tissue processor that regulates the hydrostatic pressure and oxygen levels to mimic the physiologic stresses experienced by chondrocytes in native articular cartilage within the joint.[116–126] This process results in a neocartilage with well-distributed chondrocytes in lacunae and ECM containing sulfated glycosaminoglycans and type II collagen. Implantation of this neocartilage will result in accelerated repair of the lesion site and continued maturity of the tissue into hyaline cartilage.

Fixation of the implant into the chondral lesion without adversely affecting adjacent tissue or underlying bone is a concern that has prompted investigation into alternatives to current techniques, such as sutures. In the NeoCart system, fixation is accomplished using a bioadhesive that is strong, biodegradable, biocompatible, and easy to use. It is composed of methylated collagen and polyethylene glycols (PEGs) that, when combined, polymerize to form a clear viscous solution that effectively seals the implant in the lesion, is an order of magnitude stronger than fibrin glue, and is more benign.

The Procedure

NeoCart uses non–weight-bearing cartilage retrieved by arthroscopic biopsy and digested with collagenase to isolate the chondrocytes. Once the cells have attained the desired expansion index in two-dimensional culture, they are transferred to the NeoCart type I collagen scaffold and placed in a tissue processor under hydrostatic pressure and low oxygen to promote ECM production (Fig. 16.33).

Six to eight weeks after biopsy, the NeoCart implant, approximately 3 cm in diameter and 2 mm thick, is returned to the surgeon for implantation, which is performed via mini-arthrotomy. The lesion is debrided of all damaged tissue and the calcified cartilage layer is removed carefully to avoid penetration of the subchondral plate and osseous bleeding into the site. The lesion site is templated and the NeoCart is cut to size using the template. NeoCart is secured by applying a thin layer of the proprietary bioadhesive CT3 onto the lesion bed prior to positioning the implant and then across the top of the NeoCart overlaying the adjacent cartilage.

Preclinical Animal Studies

In the porcine chondral defect model, NeoCart constructs, produced from autologous chondrocytes retrieved from the contralateral knee and grown in culture as described, were secured to 4-mm defect sites using the bioadhesive. At 3 and 6 months after implantation, the NeoCart system demonstrated biocompatibility, with no inflammation or other adverse effects. Histologic evaluations of the defect sites at 6 months showed that chondrocytes in the defect site were oriented in a columnar fashion throughout the newly formed matrix and that the autologous implant was integrated well with the adjacent cartilage and subchondral bone. The chondrocytes in the NeoCart construct continued to produce ECM that, by 6 months, was equivalent to the host tissue (Fig. 16.34).

Clinical Trials

A phase I clinical trial enrolled 10 patients and reported results up to 24 months for eight patients.[127] The first two of the 10 implantation procedures were unsuccessful because

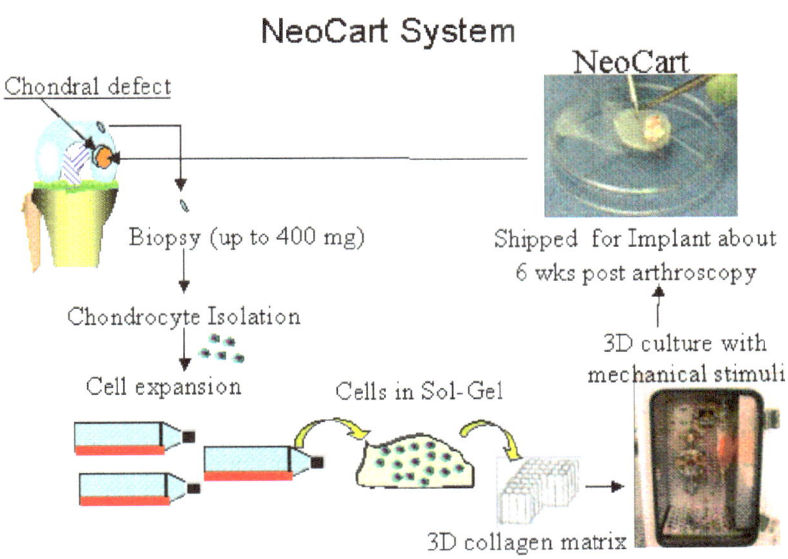

• **Fig. 16.33** Schematic drawing of the NeoCart system process.

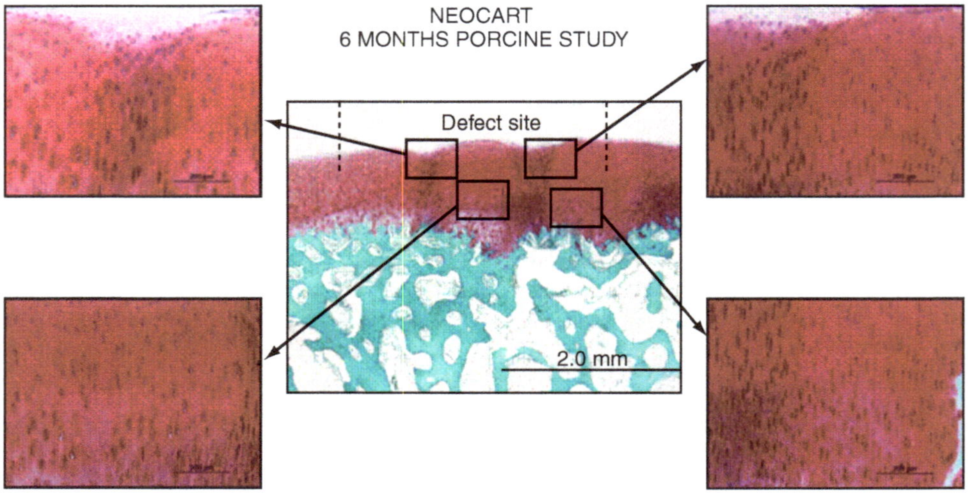

• **Fig. 16.34** Photomicrograph of histologic section (stained with safranin O) of porcine chondral defect site 6 months after implantation with NeoCart. The NeoCart implant has integrated with the host tissue and has sulfated glycosaminoglycan (S-GAG) content and chondrocyte organization similar to that of the host.

sutures that were used to augment the bioadhesive damaged the NeoCart implant when it was subjected to intraoperative range of motion. All subsequent procedures were sutureless and intraoperative motion was limited to full extension for closure of the incision and placement of the knee immobilizer.

The rehabilitation program was analogous to that used after microfracture and ACI-type procedures and included use of a continuous passive motion machine for 6 hours per day during the 6 weeks after removal of the immobilizer approximately 10 days postsurgery.[2,128–132] In accordance with the protocols mentioned, the first 6 weeks were non–weight-bearing with unrestricted weight bearing permitted thereafter.

Outcomes were assessed using the VAS pain scale and the IKDC subjective score and by measuring range of motion. Clinical evaluations were performed at 6 and 12 weeks after surgery, at 6 and 12 months after surgery, and annually thereafter. As a secondary outcome, analysis of cartilage repair quality was evaluated by MRI obtained at 12 weeks after surgery, 6 and 12 months after surgery, and annually thereafter.

No serious adverse events associated with the NeoCart implant occurred and the implant remained stable within the lesion site. A second-look arthroscopy performed on one patient 3 months after NeoCart implantation showed uniform fill with good integration to adjacent cartilage (Fig. 16.35). By 12 months, all patients had decreased pain scores (average 0.9 ± 1.5) compared with baseline (average 3.3 ± 2.8). At 24 months, pain scores remained statistically significantly lower than baseline and IKDC scores increased in seven of eight patients to 76 ± 17 from 57 ± 25 at baseline.

MRI evaluations showed that seven of eight patients had good to complete fill of the defect site and improved integration with the adjacent cartilage at 1 year, and six of eight subjects had good to complete fill of the defect at 2 years. T2 mapping was also performed to assess the collagen matrix content and organization. Normal cartilage, when perpendicular to the magnetic field, has a laminar appearance or stratification.[133] At 24 months, four of eight patients had stratification of T2 values similar to the adjacent cartilage (Fig. 16.36).

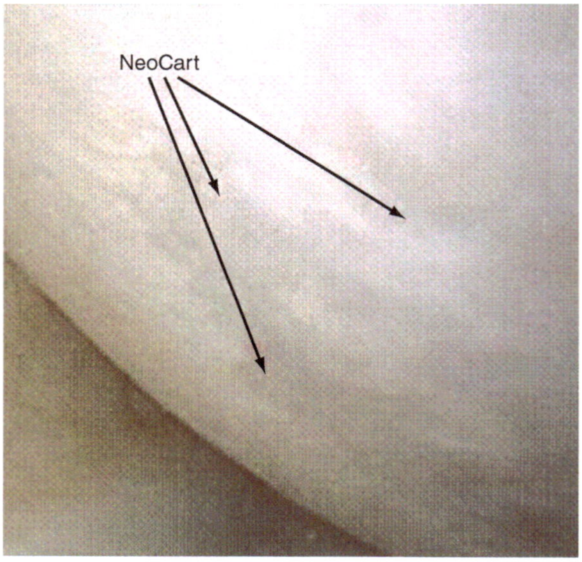

• **Fig. 16.35** Second-look arthroscopy performed on a Phase I patient 3 months after NeoCart implantation. Note excellent integration and fill throughout the lesion.

These promising results led to a 30-patient prospective, randomized Phase II trial that compared NeoCart to microfracture (2:1). Although patient enrollment and treatment have been completed, the 12-month data are still being collected and collated. Early results indicate similar trends to those seen in Phase I with the NeoCart system.

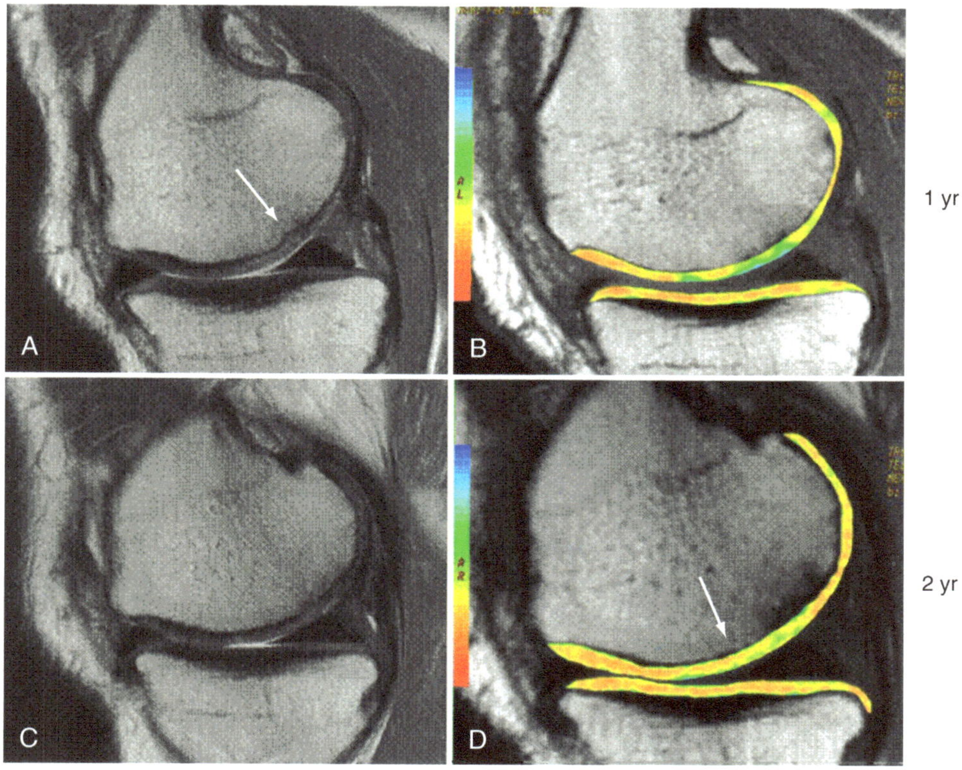

• **Fig. 16.36** Sagittal magnetic resonance images taken 1 year (A, B) and 2 years (C, D) after NeoCart implantation. Fast spin-echo images (A, C) show good fill and progressive decrease in signal intensity. Corresponding T2 mapped images (B, D) show progressive matrix organization with partial stratification or layering at 2 years.

The NeoCart System provides a biocompatible, neocartilage implant that remains stable within the site and matures in situ as the autologous chondrocytes within the construct continue to synthesize cartilage-specific ECM.

DeNovo Engineered Tissue Graft

DeNovo engineered tissue (ET) graft (ISTO Technologies, St. Louis, MO, USA) is a three-dimensional articular cartilage tissue (Fig. 16.37) grown with cultured human juvenile chondrocytes. DeNovo ET graft is currently in a Phase I/II clinical trial in the United States. After undergoing a Phase III clinical trial, a Biologics License Application (BLA) will be submitted to the FDA for approval to commercialize the product. The primary chondrocytes used to produce DeNovo ET graft are obtained by enzymatic digestion of donated juvenile cartilage. No fetal cartilage tissue is used. A proprietary cell expansion technology is then used to increase the number of cells. These expanded cells are subsequently cultured by a proprietary process to produce a large number of grafts for implantation. This process uses a defined serum-free medium *without* a scaffold and the resulting engineered tissue can be physically handled with forceps and trimmed to required sizes to fill cartilage defects. A fibrin adhesive is used to fix the graft in the defect.

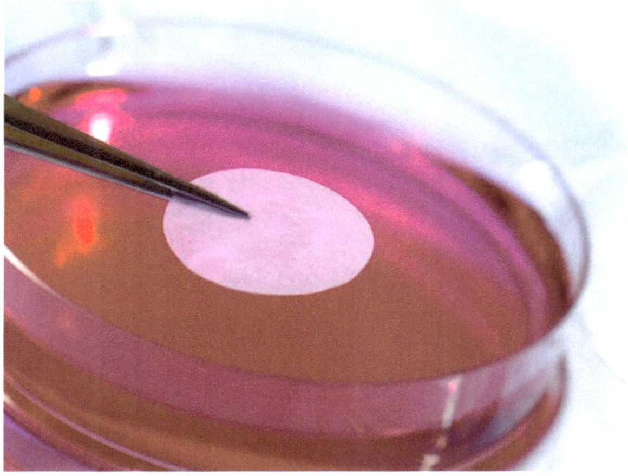

• **Fig. 16.37** DeNovo engineered tissue graft can be handled with forceps and trimmed to required sizes to fill cartilage defects. A fibrin adhesive is applied to fix the graft in the defect.

Conclusion

The field of cartilage repair is rapidly advancing. Many of the new techniques offer simplicity of application with less arduous rehabilitations and excellent clinical outcomes. They may offer improvements to existing techniques and have unique profiles that could fill in the voids in existing treatment algorithms.

Assessment of procedural cost-effectiveness will be difficult. Head-to-head comparative, randomized, blinded, multicenter clinical trials may be necessary. However, it has proved problematic in the past to obtain homogeneous populations of injuries treated, surgical skill, and numbers.

The future of cartilage repair is bright. We are now able to treat and cure a problem that for centuries has been known to "be a troublesome thing."[2]

Acknowledgments

I thank the following companies and their representatives for their contributions to this chapter: Matthew Shive, PhD (BioSyntech, Laval, Quebec, Canada); Claudio De Luca, PhD, and Daniele Presato (Fin-Ceramica Faenza S.p.A., Faenza, Italy); K. Martin, MD (Geistlich Pharma AG, Wolhusen, Switzerland); Gino Bradica, PhD (Kensey Nash Corp., Exton, PA); Ada Au, PhD (Advanced Biomaterials Group, Smith & Nephew Endoscopy, Andover, MA); Ben Byers, PhD, and Chris Kilburn-Peterson (DePuy Mitek, Raynham, MA); Jian Yao, PhD (Zimmer, Warsaw, IN); Steve Duguay, PhD, and Prudence Roaf (Genzyme Corp., Cambridge, MA); Alessandra Pavesio, PhD, Manuela Minto, PhD, and Cristina Longinotti, PhD (Fidia Advanced Biopolymers, Abano Terme, Italy); Micheline Wille (TiGenix N.V., Leuven, Belgium); Arthro Kinetics (Esslingen, Germany); ProChon (Ness Ziona, Israel); Laurence Barnouin and Gaelle Regeur (TBF Tissue Engineering Company, Mions, France); and Sonya Shortkroff, PhD (Histogenics Corp., Waltham, MA).

References

1. Kumar M, Muzzarelli R, Muzzarelli C, et al. Chitosan Chemistry and Pharmaceutical Perspectives. *Chem Rev.* 2004;104:6017–6084.
2. Hunter W. On the structure and diseases of articulating cartilage. *Phil Trans R Soc Lond B Biol Sci.* 1743;9:267.
3. Chenite A, Chaput C, Wang D, et al. Novel injectable neutral solutions of chitosan form biodegradable gels in situ. *Biomaterials.* 2000;21:2155–2161.
4. Mattioli-Belmonte M, Muzzarelli B, Muzzarelli R. Chitin and chitosan in wound healing and other biomedical applications. *Carbohydrate Eur.* 1997;14(6):30–36.
5. Shive M, Hoemann C, Restrepo A, et al. BST-CarGel: In situ chondroinduction for cartilage repair. *Oper Tech Orthop.* 2006;16(4):271–278.
6. Chevrier A, Hoemann C, Sun J, et al. Chitosan-glycerol phosphate/blood implants increase cell recruitment, transient vascularization and subchondral bone remodeling in drilled cartilage defects. *Osteoarthr Cartil.* 2007;15(3):316–327.
7. Hoemann CD, Sun J, McKee MD, et al. Chitosan-glycerol phosphate/blood implants elicit hyaline cartilage repair integrated with porous subchondral bone in microdrilled rabbit defects. *Osteoarthr Cartil.* 2007;15(1):78–89.
8. Hoemann C, Hurtig M, Rossomacha E, et al. In situ chitosan-glycerol phosphate/blood implants significantly improve hyaline cartilage repair in ovine microfracture defects. *J Bone Joint Surg Am.* 2005;87(12):2671–2686.
9. Bellamy N, Buchanan W, Goldsmith C, et al. Validation study of WOMAC: a health status instrument for measuring clinically important patient relevant outcomes to antirheumatic drug therapy in patients with osteoarthritis of the hip or knee. *J Rheumatol.* 1988;15(12):1833–1840.
10. Mainil-Varlet P, Aigner T, Brittberg M, et al. Histological assessment of cartilage repair: a report by the Histology Endpoint Committee of the International Cartilage Repair Society (ICRS). *J Bone Joint Surg Am.* 2003;85-A:45–57.
11. Stanish WD, McCormack R, Forriol F, et al. Novel scaffold-based BST-CarGel® treatment results in superior cartilage repair compared with microfracture in a randomized controlled trial. *J Bone Joint Surg Am.* 2013;95:1640–1650.
12. Shive MS, Stanish WD, McCormack R, et al. BST-CarGel® treatment maintains cartilage repair superiority over microfracture at 5 years in a multicenter randomized controlled trial. *Cartilage.* 2015;6(2):62–72.
13. Tampieri A, Sandri M, Landi E, et al. Biomimetic hybrid composites to repair osteo-chondral lesions. *Key Eng Mater.* 2008;361–363:927–930.
14. Tampieri A, Sandri M, Landi E, et al. Design of graded biomimetic osteo-chondral composite scaffolds. *Biomaterials.* 2008;29:3539–3546.
15. Kon E, Delcogliano M, Filardo G, et al. Orderly osteochondral regeneration in a sheep model using a novel nano-composite multilayered biomaterial. *J Orthop Res.* 2010;28:116–124.
16. Fortier L, Mohammed H, Lust G, et al. Insulin-like growth factor-I enhances cell based repair of articular cartilage. *J Bone Joint Surg Br.* 2002;84(2):276–288.
17. Kon E, Delcogliano M, Filardo G, et al. Novel nano-composite multi-layered biomaterial for osteo-chondral regeneration: early stability evaluation. *Injury.* 2010;41(7):693–701.
18. Kon E, Delcogliano M, Filardo G, Altadonna G, Marcacci M. Novel nano-composite multi-layered biomaterial for the treatment of multifocal degenerative cartilage lesions. *Knee Surg Sports Traumatol Arthrosc.* 2009;17(11):1312–1315.
19. Russlies M, Behrens P, Ehlers EM, et al. Periosteum stimulates subchondral bone densification in autologous chondrocyte transplantation in a sheep model. *Cell Tissue Res.* 2005;319:133–142.
20. Fuss M, Ehlers EM, Russlies M, Rohwedel J, Behrens P. Characteristics of human chondrocytes, osteoblasts and fibroblasts seeded onto a type I/III collagen sponge under different culture conditions. A light, scanning and transmission electron microscopy study. *Ann Anat.* 2000;182:303–310.
21. Gille J, Meisner U, Ehlers EM, et al. Migration pattern, morphology and viability of cells suspended in or sealed with fibrin glue: a histomorphologic study. *Tissue Cell.* 2005;37:339–348.
22. Russlies M, Behrens P, Wünsch L, Gille J, Ehlers EM. A cell-seeded biocomposite for cartilage repair. *Ann Anat.* 2002;184:317–323.
23. Russlies M, Rüther P, Köller W, Stomberg P, Behrens P. Biomechanical properties of cartilage repair tissue after different cartilage repair procedures in sheep. *Z Orthop Ihre Grenzgeb.* 2003;141:465–471.
24. Scherer K, Schünke M, Sellckau R, Hassenpflug J, Kurz B. The influence of oxygen and hydrostatic pressure on articular chondrocytes and adherent bone marrow cells in vitro. *Biorheology.* 2004;41:323–333.
25. Steinwachs M, Kreuz PC. Autologous chondrocyte implantation in chondral defects of the knee with a type I/III collagen membrane: a prospective study with a 3-year follow-up. *Arthroscopy.* 2007;23:381–387.

26. Niemeyer P, Kreuz PC, Steinwachs M, et al. Technical note: the "double eye" technique as a modification of autologous chondrocyte implantation for the treatment of retropatellar cartilage defects. *Knee Surg Sports Traumatol Arthrosc.* 2007;15:1461–1468.
27. Haddo O, Mahroof S, Higgs D, et al. The use of ChondroGide membrane in autologous chondrocyte implantation. *Knee.* 2004;11:51–55.
28. Steinwachs M, Kreuz PC. *Clinical Results of Autologous Chondrocyte Transplantation Using a Collagen Membrane, in Cartilage Surgery and Future Perspectives.* Berlin: Springer Verlag; 2003:37–47.
29. Bentley G, Biant LC, Carrington RW, et al. A prospective, randomised comparison of autologous chondrocyte implantation versus mosaicplasty for osteochondral defects in the knee. *J Bone Joint Surg Br.* 2003;85:223–230.
30. Briggs TW, Mahroof S, David LA, et al. Histological evaluation of chondral defects after autologous chondrocyte implantation of the knee. *J Bone Joint Surg Am.* 2003;85:1077–1083.
31. Steinwachs M. New technique for cell-seeded collagen matrix-supported autologous chondrocyte transplantation. *Arthroscopy.* 2009;25:208–211.
32. Niemeyer P, Pestka J, Kreuz M, et al. Characteristic complications after autologous chondrocyte implantation for cartilage defects of the knee joint. *Am J Sports Med.* 2008;36:2091–2099.
33. Behrens P. Matrixgekoppelte mikrofrakturierung. *Arthroskopie.* 2005;18:193–197.
34. Kramer J, Bohrnsen F, Lindner U, et al. In vivo matrix-guided human mesenchymal stem cells. *Cell Mol Life Sci.* 2006;63:616–626.
35. Steck E, Fischer J, Lorenz H, et al. Mesenchymal stem cell differentiation in an experimental cartilage defect: restriction of hypertrophy to bone-close neocartilage. *Stem Cells Dev.* 2009;18:969–978.
36. Kusano T, Jacobi R, Jakob P. AMIC: Treatment of chondral and osteochondral defects of the knee. *Leading Opin Orthop.* 2007;20:2109–2115.
37. Wendler NO, et al. Ein neues Therapiekonzept zur Knorpeldefektbehandlung. *Med Rev.* 2006;7:2.
38. Wendler NO, et al. *Autologous Matrix-Induced Chondrogenesis (AMIC) mid-term results* Universitätsklinikum Schleswig-Holstein: 2008.
39. Anders S, et al. Autologous matrix induced chondrogenesis (AMIC) for focal chondral defects of the knee—first results. *EFFORT 2007* Florence, Italy, 2007.
40. Steinwachs MR, Guggi T, Kreuz PC. Marrow stimulation techniques. *Injury.* 2008;39(suppl 1):S26–S31.
41. Valderrabano V, et al. The AMIC technique: new option for osteochondral defects of the Talus. *Leading Opin.* 2008;04/2008:34–36.
42. Cameron H. Tricalcium phosphate as a bone graft substitute. *Contemp Orthop.* 1992;25:506–508.
43. Vaccaro A. The role of the osteoconductive scaffold in synthetic bone graft. *Orthopedics.* 2002;25(5):571–578.
44. Bostman O. Biodegradable bone repair materials: synthetic polymers and ceramics. *J Bone Joint Surg Br.* 1991;73:148–153.
45. Hollinger J, Battistone G. Biodegradable bone repair materials: Synthetic polymers and ceramics. *Clin Orthop Relat Res.* 1986;(207):290–305.
46. Ahern BJ, Engiles J, Underwood C, et al. *Single site osteochondral resurfacing – an in vivo caprine study.* Paper presented at: International Cartilage Repair Society 2009 Meeting; Miami, FL: May 26, 2009.
47. McCarrel TM, Pownder S, Gilbert S, et al. Two-year evaluation of osteochondral repair with a novel biphasic graft saturated in bone marrow in an equine model. *Cartilage.* 2017;8(4):406–416.
48. Slivka M, Leatherbury N, Kieswetter K, et al. Porous, resorbable, fiber-reinforced scaffolds tailored for articular cartilage repair. *Tissue Eng.* 2001;7(6):767–780.
49. Gao C, Gao J, You X, et al. Fabrication of calcium sulphate/PLLA composite for bone repair. *J Biomed Mater Res A.* 2005;73(2):244–253.
50. Pecora G, De Leonardis D, Ibrahim N, et al. The use of calcium sulphate in the surgical treatment of a "through and through" periradicular lesion. *Int Endod J.* 2001;34(2):189–197.
51. Advanced Biomaterials Group., 2009. *Cartilage/bone repair using TRUFIT CB implants* Smith & Nephew Endoscopy: Andover, MA Technical white paper
52. Spalding T. TRUFIT CB plugs for articular cartilage repair in the knee: early experience and important considerations Presentation at the 28th Annual Meeting of the Arthroscopy Association of North. America, 2009.
53. Carmont M, Carey-Smith R, Saithna A, et al. Delayed incorporation of TRUFIT plug: perseverance is recommended. *Arthroscopy.* 2009;25:810–814.
54. Saris D, Vanlauwe J, Victor J, et al. Characterized chondrocyte implantation results in better structural repair when treating symptomatic cartilage defects of the knee in a randomized controlled trial versus microfracture. *Am J Sports Med.* 2008;36(2):236–246.
55. Kon E, Robinson D, Verdonk P, et al. A novel aragonite-based scaffold for osteochondral regeneration: early experience on human implants and technical developments. *Injury.* 2016 Dec;47(Suppl 6):S27–S32.
56. Kon E, Filardo G, Shani J, et al. Osteochondral regeneration with a novel aragonite-hyaluronate biphasic scaffold: up to 12-month follow-up study in a goat model. *Journal of Orthopaedic Surgery and Research.* 2015;10:81. https://doi.org/10.1186/s13018-015-0211-y.
57. CartiHeal Announces Positive Interim Analysis Results of Agili-C™ IDE Study. 2019, December 10. https://www.cartiheal.com/news/cartiheal-announces-positive-interim-analysis-results-of-agili-c-ide-study/
58. Zheng N, Lu Y, Boock R, Conrad B, Binette F. Retention of scaffold with staple fixation for cartilage repair during cyclic motion of human cadaveric knees. *J Musculoskelet Res.* 2008;11(4):151–159.
59. Lu Y, Dhanaraj S, Wang Z, et al. Minced cartilage without cell culture serves as an effective intraoperative cell source for cartilage repair. *J Orthop Res.* 2006;24:1261–1270.
60. Frisbie DD, Lu Y, Kawcak CE, et al. In vivo evaluation of autologous cartilage fragment-loaded scaffolds implanted into equine articular defects and compared with autologous chondrocyte implantation. *Am J Sports Med.* 2009;37(1):71–80.
61. J. Farr, 2009 *DeNovo NT Natural Tissue Graft* 8th World Congress of International Cartilage Repair Society. Miami, FL: May 26
62. Abelow S, Guillen P, Ramos T. Arthroscopic technique for matrix-induced autologous chondrocyte implantation for the treatment of large chondral defects in the knee and ankle. *Oper Tech Orthop.* 2006;16:257–261.
63. Ebert JR, Robertson WB, Woodhouse J, et al. Clinical and magnetic resonance imaging–based outcomes to 5 years after matrix-induced autologous chondrocyte implantation to address articular cartilage defects in the knee. *Am J Sports Med.* 2011;39(4):753–763.

64. Behrens P, Bitter T, Kurz B, et al. Matrix-associated autologous chondrocyte transplantation/implantation (MACT/MACI)-5-year follow-up. *Knee*. 2006;13:194–202.
65. Bartlett W, Gooding C, Carrington R, et al. Autologous chondrocyte implantation at the knee using a bilayer collagen membrane with bone graft. A preliminary report. *J Bone Joint Surg Br*. 2005;87:330–332.
66. Bartlett W, Flanagan A, Gooding C, et al. Autologous chondrocyte implantation versus matrix-induced autologous chondrocyte implantation for osteochondral defects of the knee: a prospective, randomised study. *J Bone Joint Surg Br*. 2005;87:640–645.
67. Amin A, Bartlett W, Gooding C, et al. The use of autologous chondrocyte implantation following and combined with anterior cruciate ligament reconstruction. *Int Orthop*. 2006;30:48–53.
68. Cherubino P, Grassi F, Bulgheroni P, Ronga M. Autologous chondrocyte implantation using a bilayer collagen membrane: a preliminary report. *J Orthop Surg (Hong Kong)*. 2003;11:10–15.
69. Ronga M, Grassi F, Bulgheroni P. Arthroscopic autologous chondrocyte implantation for the treatment of a chondral defect in the tibial plateau of the knee. *Arthroscopy*. 2004;20:79–84.
70. Ronga M, Grassi F, Montoli C, et al. Treatment of deep cartilage defects of the ankle with matrix-induced autologous chondrocyte implantation (MACI). *Foot Ankle Surg*. 2005;11:29–33.
71. Bachmann G, Basad E, Lommel D, et al. MRI in the follow-up after MACI(R) or microfracture [German]. *Radiologe*. 2004;44:773–782.
72. Marlovits S, Striessnig G, Kutscha-Lissberg F, et al. Early postoperative adherence of matrix-induced autologous chondrocyte implantation for the treatment of full-thickness cartilage defects of the femoral condyle. *Knee Surg Sports Traumatol Arthrosc*. 2005;13:451–457.
73. D'Anchise R, Manta N, Prospero E, et al. Autologous implantation of chondrocytes on a solid collagen scaffold: clinical and histological outcomes after two years of follow-up. *J Orthop Traumatol*. 2005;6:36–43.
74. Marcacci M, Kon E, Zaffagnini S, et al. New cell-based technologies in bone and cartilage tissue engineering. II. Cartilage regeneration. *Chir Organi Mov*. 2003;88:42–47.
75. Marcacci M, Zaffagnini S, Kon E, et al. Second generation ACI technique. *Am Acad Orthop Surg*. 2003;6:49–58.
76. Campoccia D, Doherty P, Radice M, et al. Semisynthetic resorbable materials from hyaluronan esterification. *Biomaterials*. 1998;19(23):2101–2127.
77. Benya P, Shaffer J. Dedifferentiated chondrocytes reexpress the differentiated collagen phenotype when cultured in agarose gels. *Cell*. 1982;30:215–224.
78. Grigolo B, Lisignoli G, Piacentini A, et al. Evidence for redifferentiation of human chondrocytes grown on a hyaluronan-based biomaterial (HYAFFs11): molecular, immunohistochemical and ultrastructural analysis. *Biomaterials*. 2002;22(4):1187–1195.
79. Grigolo B, Roseti L, Fiorini M, et al. Cathepsin B as a soluble marker to monitor the phenotypic stability of engineered cartilage. *Biomaterials*. 2003:1751–1757.
80. Tognana E, Chen F, Padera R, et al. Adjacent tissues (cartilage, bone) affect the functional integration of engineered calf cartilage in vitro. *Osteoarthr Cartil*. 2005;13(2):129–138.
81. Schlegel W, Nürnberger S, Hombauer M, et al. Scaffold-dependent differentiation of human articular chondrocytes. *Int J Mol Med*. 2008;22(5):691–699.
82. Aigner J, Tegeler J, Hutzler P, et al. Cartilage tissue engineering with novel nonwoven structured biomaterial based on hyaluronic acid benzyl ester. *J Biomed Mater Res (Part A)*. 1998;42(2):172–181.
83. Grigolo B, Roseti L, Fiorini M, et al. Transplantation of chondrocytes seeded on a hyaluronan derivative (hyaff-11) into cartilage defects in rabbits. *Biomaterials*. 2001;22:2417–2424.
84. Solchaga L, Dennis J, Goldberg V, et al. Hyaluronic acid-based polymers as cell carriers for tissue-engineered repair of bone and cartilage. *J Orthop Res*. 1999;17(2):205–213.
85. Solchaga L, Yoo J, Lundberg M, et al. Hyaluronan-based polymers in the treatment of osteochondral defects. *J Orthop Res*. 2000;18(5):773–780.
86. Solchaga L, Temenoff J, Gao J, et al. Repair of osteochondral defects with hyaluronan- and polyester-based scaffolds. *Osteoarthr Cartil*. 2005;13(4):297–309.
87. Buma report, data on file 1999, internal Fidia files
88. Busetto report, data on file 2001, internal Fidia files
89. Pavesio A, Abatangelo G, Borrione A, et al. Hyaluronan-based scaffolds (Hyalograft C) in the treatment of knee cartilage defects: preliminary clinical findings. *Novartis Found Symp*. 2003;249:203–217.
90. Marcacci M, Berruto M, Brocchetta D, et al. Articular cartilage engineering with Hyalograft C: 3-year clinical results. *Clin Orthop Relat Res*. 2005;(435):96–105.
91. Kon E, Gobbi A, Filardo G, et al. Arthroscopic second-generation autologous chondrocyte implantation compared with microfracture for chondral lesions of the knee: prospective non-randomized study at 5 years. *Am J Sports Med*. 2009;37:33–41.
92. Hollander A, Dickinson S, Sims T, et al. Maturation of tissue engineered cartilage implanted in injured and osteoarthritic human knees. *Tissue Eng*. 2006;12(7):1787–1798.
93. Brun P, Dickinson S, Zavan B, et al. Characteristics of repair tissue in second-look and third-look biopsies from patients treated with engineered cartilage: relationship to symptomatology and time after implantation. *Arthritis Res Ther*. 2008;10:R132.
94. Trattnig S, Pinker K, Krestan C, et al. Matrix-based autologous chondrocyte implantation for cartilage repair with Hyalograft C: two-year follow-up by magnetic resonance imaging. *Eur J Radiol*. 2006;57(1):9–15.
95. Marlovits S, Striessnig G, Resinger C, et al. Definition of pertinent parameters for the evaluation of articular cartilage repair tissue with high-resolution magnetic resonance imaging. *Eur J Radiol*. 2004;52(3):310–319.
96. Marlovits S, Singer P, Zeller P, et al. Magnetic resonance observation of cartilage repair tissue (MOCART) for the evaluation of autologous chondrocyte transplantation: determination of interobserver variability and correlation to clinical outcome after 2 years. *Eur J Radiol*. 2006;57(1):16–23.
97. Giannini S, Buda R, Vannini F, et al. Arthroscopic autologous chondrocyte implantation in osteochondral lesions of the talus: surgical technique and results. *Am J Sports Med*. 2008;36(5):873–880.
98. Marcacci M, Berruto M, Brocchetta D, et al. Articular cartilage engineering with Hyalograft C: 3-year clinical results. *Clin Orthop Relat Res*. 2005;435:96–105.
99. Marcacci report, data on file, 2006
100. Marlovits S, Zeller P, Singer P, et al. Cartilage repair: generations of autologous chondrocyte transplantation. *Eur J Radiol*. 2006;57:24–31.
101. Marlovits and Nehrer report, data on file, 2004

102. Ferruzzi A, Buda R, Faldini C, et al. Autologous chondrocyte implantation in the knee joint: open compared with arthroscopic technique. Comparison at a minimum follow-up of five years. *J Bone Joint Surg Am.* 2008;90(4):90–101.
103. Kon E, Gobbi A, Filardo G, et al. Arthroscopic second-generation autologous chondrocyte implantation compared with microfracture for chondral lesions of the knee: prospective nonrandomized study at 5 years. *Am J Sports Med.* 2009;39(10):33–41.
104. Gobbi A, Kon E, Berruto M, et al. Patellofemoral full-thickness chondral defects treated with second-generation autologous chondrocyte implantation: results at 5 years' follow-up. *Am J Sports Med.* 2009;37(6):1083–1092.
105. Dell'Accio F, De Bari C, Luyten F. Molecular markers predictive of the capacity of expanded human articular chondrocytes to form stable cartilage in vivo. *Arthritis Rheum.* 2001;44:1608–1619.
106. Dell'Accio F, De Bari C, Luyten F. Microenvironment and phenotypic stability specify tissue formation by human articular cartilage-derived cells in vivo. *Exp Cell Res.* 2003;287:16–27.
107. Nehrer S, Chiari C, Domayer S, et al. Results of chondrocyte implantation with a fibrin-hyaluronan matrix: a preliminary study. *Clin Orthop Relat Res.* 2008;466:1849–1855.
108. Domayer SE, Welsch GH, Nehrer S, et al. T2 mapping and dGEMRIC after autologous chondrocyte implantation with a fibrin-based scaffold in the knee: Preliminary results. *Eur J Radiol.* 2010;73:636–642.
109. Rahfoth B, Weisser J, Sternkopf F, et al. Transplantation of allograft chondrocytes embedded in agarose gel into cartilage defects of rabbits. *Osteoarthr Cartil.* 1998;6:50–65.
110. De Vos P, De Haan BJ, Wolters GH, et al. Improved biocompatibility but limited graft survival after purification of alginate for microencapsulation of pancreatic islets. *Diabetologia.* 1997;40:262–270.
111. Wong M. Alginates in tissue engineering. *Methods Mol Biol.* 2004;238:77–86.
112. Hutmacher DW, Ng KW, Kaps C, et al. Elastic cartilage engineering using novel scaffold architectures in combination with a biomimetic cell carrier. *Biomaterials.* 2003;24:4445–4458.
113. Selmi TA, Verdonk P, Barnouin L, Neyret P. Surgical technique: autologous chondrocyte transplantation in combination with an alginate-agarose based hydrogel. *Tech Knee Surg.* 2007;6:253–258.
114. Selmi TA, Barnouin L, Bussiere C, Neyret P. CARTIPATCH. In: Zanasi S, Brittberg M, Marcacci M, eds. Basic Science, Clinical Repair and Reconstruction of Articular Cartilage Defects: Current Status and Prospects. Bologna, Italy: Timeo; 2006;431–438.
115. Selmi TA, Verdonk P, Chambat P, et al. Autologous chondrocyte implantation in a novel alginate-agarose hydrogel: outcome at 2 years. *J Bone Joint Surg Br.* 2008;90:597–604.
116. Mizuno S, Tateishi T, Ushida T, et al. Hydrostatic fluid pressure enhances matrix synthesis and accumulation by bovine chondrocytes in three-dimensional culture. *J Cell Physiol.* 2002;193:319–327.
117. Mizuno S, Glowacki J. Low oxygen tension enhances chondroinduction by demineralized bone matrix in human dermal fibroblasts in vitro. *Cells Tissues Organs.* 2005;180:151–158.
118. Glowacki J, Mizuno S. Collagen scaffolds for tissue engineering. *Biopolymers.* 2008;89:338–344.
119. Smith R, Rusk S, Ellison B, et al. In vitro stimulation of articular chondrocyte mRNA and extracellular matrix synthesis by hydrostatic pressure. *J Orthop Res.* 1996;14:53–60.
120. Smith RL, Lin J, Trindade MC, et al. Time-dependent effects of intermittent hydrostatic pressure on articular chondrocyte type II collagen and aggrecan mRNA expression. *J Rehabil Res Dev.* 2000;37:53–61.
121. Ikenoue T, Trindade MC, Lee M, et al. Mechanoregulation of human articular chondrocyte aggrecan and type II collagen expression by intermittent hydrostatic pressure in vitro. *J Orthop Res.* 2003;21:110–116.
122. Smith RL, Carter D, Schurman D. Pressure and shear differentially alter human articular chondrocyte metabolism: a review. *Clin Orthop Relat Res.* 2004;427:S89S95.
123. Wernike E, Li Z, Alini M, et al. Effect of reduced oxygen tension and long-term mechanical stimulation on chondrocyte-polymer constructs. *Cell Tissue Res.* 2008;331:473–483.
124. Kawanishi M, Oura A, Furukawa K, et al. Redifferentiation of dedifferentiated bovine articular chondrocytes enhanced by cyclic hydrostatic pressure under a gas-controlled system. *Tissue Eng.* 2007;13:957–964.
125. Domm C, Schünke M, Steinhagen J, et al. Influence of various alginate brands on the redifferentiation of dedifferentiated bovine articular chondrocytes in alginate bead culture under high and low oxygen tension. *Tissue Eng.* 2004;10(11–12):1796–1805.
126. Kurz B, Domm C, Jin M, et al. Tissue engineering of articular cartilage under the influence of collagen I/III membranes and low oxygen tension. *Tissue Eng.* 2004;10(7–8):1277–1286.
127. Williams 3rd RJ, Harnly HW. Microfracture: indications, technique, and results. *Instr Course Lect.* 2007;56:419–428.
128. Mithoefer K, Williams 3rd RJ, Warren RF, et al. Chondral resurfacing of articular cartilage defects in the knee with the microfracture technique. Surgical technique. *J Bone Joint Surg Am.* 2006;88(suppl 1 Pt 2):294–304.
129. Reinold MM, Wilk KE, Macrina LC, et al. Current concepts in the rehabilitation following articular cartilage repair procedures in the knee. *J Orthop Sports Phys Ther.* 2006;36(10):774–794.
130. Mithoefer K, Williams 3rd R, Warren R, et al. The microfracture technique for the treatment of articular cartilage lesions in the knee. A prospective cohort study. *J Bone Joint Surg Am.* 2005;87:1911–1920.
131. Steadman JR, Rodkey WG, Briggs KK. Microfracture to treat full-thickness chondral defects: surgical technique, rehabilitation, and outcomes. *J Knee Surg.* 2002;15:170–176.
132. Steadman JR, Rodkey WG, Rodrigo JJ. Microfracture: surgical technique and rehabilitation to treat chondral defects. *Clin Orthop Relat Res.* 2001;391(suppl) S362S369.
133. Potter HG, Foo LF. Magnetic resonance imaging of articular cartilage: trauma, degeneration, and repair. *Am J Sports Med.* 2006;34:661–677.

Index

Note: Page numbers followed by "*b*" indicate boxes, those followed by "*f*" indicate figures, and those followed by "*t*" indicate tables.

B

C

P

Q

R

S